Leadership Roles and Management Functions in Nursing: Theory and Application

Leadership Roles and Management Functions in Nursing: Theory and Application

Fifth Edition

Bessie L. Marquis, RN, MSN
Professor Emeritus of Nursing
California State University
Chico, California

Carol J. Huston, RN, CNAA, MSN, DPA
Professor of Nursing
California State University
Chico, California

Senior Acquisitions Editor: Quincy McDonald
Developmental Editor: Deedie McMahon
Editorial Assistant: Marie Rim
Project Manager: Cynthia Rudy
Director of Nursing Production: Helen Ewan
Senior Managing Editor / Production: Erika Kors
Art Director: Carolyn O'Brien
Manufacturing Manager: William Alberti
Production Services / Compositor: Seven Worldwide Publishing Solutions
Printer: R. R. Donnelley—Crawfordsville

5th Edition

LIBRARY OF CONGRESS CATALOGING-IN-PUBLICATION DATA

Marquis, Bessie L.
  Leadership roles and management functions in nursing : theory and application / Bessie L. Marquis, Carol J. Huston.—5th ed.
    p. ; cm.
  Includes bibliographical references and index.
  ISBN 0-7817-9594-X (alk. paper)
  1. Nursing services—Administration. 2. Leadership. 3. Nurse administrators. I. Huston, Carol Jorgensen. II. Title.
  [DNLM: 1. Leadership. 2. Nursing, Supervisory. 3. Nurse Administrators. 4. Nursing—organization & administration. WY 105 M357L 2006]
  RT89.M387 2006
  362.17'3'068—dc22

                              2004026634

I dedicate this book to my grandchildren, who have brought me much joy: Elizabeth, Patrick and Michael Willey; Tyler McKenna; Zaida and Wyatt Marquis and Bennett Yocum; and to my life's partner, Don Marquis.

Bessie L. Marquis

I dedicate this book to my daughters Kristin and Shauna, who are an immense source of pride and joy in my life, and to my husband Tom, who continues to support me in so many ways. I love all of you.

Carol Jorgensen Huston

Reviewers

Sonia Acorn, RN, PhD
Professor
The University of British Columbia
Vancouver, British Columbia, Canada

Becky A. Burgoyne, RN, BSN, MSN, ONC
Nursing Instructor
Northwestern Oklahoma State University
Enid, Oklahoma

Verda Epp Deckert, MSN, RN
Associate Professor
Bethel College of Kansas
North Newton, Kansas

Marlene Huff, PhD, RNC
Assistant Professor, College of Nursing
The University of Akron
Akron, Ohio

Phyllis A. King, RN, CN, MSN
Assistant Professor
Milligan College
Milligan College, Tennessee

Diane Faucher Moy, MSN, RN, APRN-BC
Clinical Nursing Instructor
University of Texas at Austin School of Nursing
Austin, Texas

Beth Perry, RN, PhD
Associate Professor
Athabasca University
Athabasca, Alberta, Canada

Cheryl Slaughter Smith, MSRN
Associate Professor
Arkansas Tech University
Russellville, Arkansas

Susan G. Sochacki, MSN, RNC
Nursing Instructor
Medical College of Ohio
Toledo, Ohio

Golden M. Tradewell, RN, MA, MSN, PhD
Associate Professor
McNeese State University
Lake Charles, Louisiana

Tonya Trucks, BSN, RN
Nursing Instructor
Jefferson School of Nursing
Pine Bluff, Arkansas

Connie S. Wilson, EdD, RN
Associate Professor
University of Indianapolis
Indianapolis, Indiana

Preface

This book's philosophy has evolved during 23 years of teaching leadership and management. We entered academe from the community sector of the healthcare industry, where we held nursing management positions. In our first effort as authors, *Management Decision Making for Nurses: 101 Case Studies*, we used an experiential approach and emphasized management functions appropriate for first- and middle-level managers. The primary audience for that text was the nursing student.

Our second book, *Retention and Productivity Strategies for Nurse Managers*, focused on leadership skills necessary for managers to decrease attrition and increase productivity. This book was directed to the manager rather than to the student. The experience of completing research for the second book, coupled with our clinical observations, compelled us to incorporate more leadership content in our teaching and writing.

Leadership Roles and Management Functions in Nursing was also influenced by national events in business and finance—events that have led many to believe that a lack of leadership in management is widespread. It has become apparent that if managers are to function effectively in the rapidly changing healthcare industry, enhanced leadership and management skills are needed.

What we have attempted to do, then, is combine these two very necessary elements: leadership and management. We do not see leadership as merely one role of management, nor management as only one role of leadership. We view the two as forever symbiotic. We have attempted to show this interdependent relationship by defining the leadership components and management functions inherent in all phases of the management process. Undoubtedly, a few readers will find fault with our divisions of management functions and leadership roles. Because the effective leader–manager must be skilled in both leadership and management, we felt it necessary to first artificially separate the two components for the reader, and then reiterate the roles and functions. Adoption of this integrated role is critical for success in management.

The second concept that shaped this book was our belief in the teaching-to-think movement, especially our commitment to experiential learning and whole-brain thinking. Currently, the overwhelming majority of academic instruction is conducted in a teacher-lecturer–student-listener format, the least effective of all teaching strategies. A limited number of individuals learn best using this style. Most people learn best by methods that utilize concrete, experiential, self-initiated, and real-world learning experiences.

In nursing, theoretical teaching is almost always accompanied by concurrent clinical practice that allows concrete and real-world learning experience. However, the exploration of leadership and management theory often omits this application through practicum, presenting theory in a lecture–listener format. The learner generally has little opportunity to observe first- and middle-level managers in the leader–manager role in nursing practice. Because few individuals have a guided learning experience in this area, many novice managers have had little opportunity to practice their skills before assuming their first management position.

For us, there is little question that vicarious learning, or learning through mock experience, has tremendous value in the application of leadership and management theory. We propose that integrating leadership and management and using whole-brain thinking can be accomplished through the use of learning exercises. A type of experiential learning that has proved more effective than the traditional lecture format, learning exercises strengthen problem-solving and critical-thinking skills.

Having gradually moved away from the lecture–listener format in our classes, we currently lecture only 20% to 30% of class time. Our students, once resistant to the experiential approach, are now our most enthusiastic supporters. We also find this enthusiasm for experiential learning apparent in the many workshops and seminars we provide for registered nurses. Experiential learning enables management and leadership theory to be fun and exciting, but most important, it facilitates retention of didactic material. Research we have completed on this approach to teaching supports these findings.

Although many leadership and management texts are available, this book meets the need for an emphasis on both leadership and management and the use of an experiential approach. Over 225 learning exercises, taken from many different healthcare settings and a wide variety of learning modes, are included to give the reader many opportunities to apply theory, resulting in internalized learning.

In the first chapter we have provided the learner with guidelines for using the experimental learning exercises in the text. We have also provided guidelines for instructors using the text on the Instructor's CD, which is available for instructors who adopt the text. The Instructor's CD also has a large test bank, suggestions for using the learning exercises, additional learning exercises not found in the text and a very large selection of PowerPoint slides. We feel the Instructor's CD greatly assists instructors who use the text and recommend its use. We strongly urge readers of this book to use the learning exercises as they supplement the text.

FEATURES OF THIS EDITION

The first edition of *Leadership Roles and Management Functions in Nursing* created a stimulating learning experience by presenting the symbiotic elements of leadership and management with an emphasis on problem solving and critical thinking. This fifth edition maintains this precedent with a balanced presentation of a strong theory component with real-world scenarios in the form of case studies, clinical situations, and experiential learning exercises. However, with this latest edition we have changed the organization of the text. We have combined chapters, added chapters, and changed the sequence of some chapters. For example, we moved decision making to Chapter 1, as it is the foundation for using the experiential approach of the text.

However, previous users of the text will find most issues of leadership and management, covered in previous editions, to also be found in this fifth edition. As we have completed new editions we have retained the strengths of earlier editions, reflecting content and application exercises appropriate to the issues faced by nurse leader–managers as they practice in an era increasingly characterized by limited resources and emerging technologies.

Our faithful readers will find some of their favorite cases from our earlier editions and figures from our other books adapted for use in this text. Although we have retained essential content, this edition also includes contemporary research and theory to ensure accuracy of the didactic material.

The first unit of this book provides a broad background of decision making, problem solving, and critical thinking as well as management and leadership theory to assist with management–leadership problems presented in the text. The second unit covers ethics as well as legislative and advocacy issues, which we see as core components of leadership and management decision making. The next five units are organized using the management process of planning, organizing, staffing, directing, and controlling.

LEARNING TOOLS

This edition contains many pedagogical features designed to benefit both the student and instructor:

- **Tables, Displays, and Illustrations** are liberally supplied throughout the text to reinforce learning as well as to help clarify complex information.
- **Numerous Learning Exercises** integrated in color throughout the text foster the reader's critical-thinking skills and promote interactive discussions.
- **Additional Learning Exercises** are available at the end of each chapter for further study and discussion.
- **Key Concepts** summarize important information within every chapter.
- **A combined Instructor's Resource Manual and Test Bank is available on a CD-ROM with a large number of PowerPoint slides.**

NEW LEARNING FEATURES OF THIS EDITION

- Web links appropriate to each chapter have been updated.
- Much of the learner's guide has been added to the first chapter to ensure that readers have a more thorough introduction to experiential learning and problem solving.
- A CD including combined Test Bank, Instructor's Manual, and PowerPoint slides is available to faculty as a supplemental teaching resource. The number

of graphic enriched PowerPoint slides has been increased from 360 for the fourth edition to 621 for this edition.

- Forty-six new case studies have been added, further strengthening the problem-based element of this text. Case studies included in this book occur in all care settings such as acute care, ambulatory care, long-term care, and community health.
- Forty-seven new tables, figures and displays have been added to this edition.
- The unique challenges of working with a diverse (gender, age, culture, language) workforce and diverse clients have been integrated throughout the book.
- New or updated content has been added to reflect cutting-edge trends in healthcare, including:
  - nursing workforce issues such as the nursing shortage, the graying of the nursing workforce, and declining nursing school enrollments and the nursing shortage
  - the ongoing impact of managed care on healthcare reimbursement and quality of care and organizational concepts of magnet status, shared governance and stakeholders
  - revised ANA Code of Ethics, Standards for Administrators, expanded ethics committees
  - new and emerging roles for case managers such as the coordination of disease management programs
  - emotional intelligence, building cultural bridges, and the impact of followers on leadership
  - the critical nature of the interpersonal relationship between an employee and his or her supervisor on the employee's motivation level
  - chaos theory, learning organizations, and the need for organizational renewal
  - the ever-increasing impact of technology on organizational communication and client confidentiality
  - the introduction of performance management as an alternative to traditional performance appraisal
  - the use of benchmarking and best practices to further the standardization of outcomes measurement in healthcare
  - competency assessment and professional certification as part of career management
  - how to develop a personal portfolio, discovering joy at work, and interview techniques for the interviewee
  - electronic technology as a communication tool
  - new research that depicts current thinking in nursing management and leadership
  - socialization needs of international and minority nurses
  - mandatory overtime, minimum staffing rations, and an expanded discussion of PCSs
  - new overtime laws and union organizing strategies

Contents

Decision Making, Problem Solving, and Critical Thinking: Requisites for Successful Leadership and Management

The successful nurse executive has the ability to make good decisions consistently.

—Thomas R. Clancy

To cope with the realities of today's health care system, nurses must be prepared to be critical thinkers. They must also be ready to welcome change and thrive in rapidly changing environments. Chapter 1 explores the primary requisites for successful management and leadership: problem solving, critical thinking, and decision making. Decision making is often thought to be synonymous with management and is one of the criteria on which management expertise is judged. Much of any manager's time is spent critically examining issues, solving problems, and making decisions. It is the authors' belief that problem solving, decision making, and critical thinking are learned skills that improve with practice. So that the processes can be consistently replicated, these learned skills rely heavily on established tools, techniques, and strategies.

The quality of the leader–managers' decisions is the factor that weighs most heavily in their success or failure. Decision making is both the innermost leadership activity and the core of management. Therefore, effective leaders and managers must be able to answer the following questions:

- Do the circumstances warrant that a decision is required?
- How should the decision be made?
- Who should be involved in the decision-making process?

This unit describes the process of decision making in Chapter 1; explores the development of management theory and management decision-making tools in Chapter 2; and examines leadership theory from historical to contemporary perspectives in Chapter 3. Chapter 1 introduces the reader to problem solving, decision making, and critical thinking and provides several problem-solving and decision-making models that assist leaders and managers in making quality decisions. It also introduces the learning exercise as a new approach for gaining skill in management and leadership decision making.

DECISION MAKING, PROBLEM SOLVING, AND CRITICAL THINKING

Decision making is a complex, cognitive process often defined as choosing a particular course of action. Webster's definition—to "judge or settle"—is another view of decision making. Both definitions imply that there was *doubt* about several courses of action and that a choice was made that eliminated the uncertainty.

Problem solving is part of decision making. A systematic process that focuses on analyzing a difficult situation, problem solving always includes a decision-making step. Many educators use the terms *problem solving* and *decision making* synonymously, but there is a small yet important difference between the two. Although decision making is the last step in the problem-solving process, it is possible for decision making to occur without the full analysis required in problem solving. Because problem solving attempts to identify the root problem in situations, much time and energy are spent on identifying the real problem. Decision making, on the other hand, is usually triggered by a problem but is often handled in a manner that does not eliminate the problem. For example, a person who handled a conflict crisis when it occurred but did not attempt to identify the real problem causing the conflict, used only decision-making skills. The decision maker might later choose to address the real cause of the conflict or might decide to do nothing at all about the problem. The decision has been made *not* to problem solve. This alternative may be selected because of a lack of energy, time, or resources to solve the real problem adequately. In some situations, this is an appropriate decision.

Here is an example of a decision not to solve a problem. A nursing supervisor has a staff nurse who has been absent a great deal during the last 3 months. However, the supervisor has reliable information that the nurse will be resigning soon to return to school in another state. Because the problem will soon no longer exist, the supervisor *decides* that the time and energy needed to correct the problem are not warranted.

Critical thinking, sometimes referred to as reflective thinking, is related to evaluation and has a broader scope than decision making and problem solving. "Critical thinking is purposeful, outcome-directed thinking that is based on a body of knowledge derived from research and other sources of evidence" (Ignatavicius, 2001, p. 38). Components of critical thinking include reasoning and creative analysis. Ignatavicious (2001) has identified six cognitive skills used in critical thinking, including evaluation and analysis (see **Display 1.1**).

Various theorists define critical thinking differently, but most agree that it is more complex than problem solving or decision making, involves higher-order reasoning and evaluation, and has both a cognitive and affective component. The authors believe that insight, intuition, empathy, and the willingness to take action are additional components of critical thinking. These same skills are necessary to some degree in decision making and problem solving. See **Display 1.2** for some additional characteristics of a critical thinker.

> Insight, intuition, empathy, and the willingness to take action are components of critical thinking.

VICARIOUS LEARNING TO INCREASE PROBLEM-SOLVING AND DECISION-MAKING SKILLS

Decision making is one step in the problem-solving process, an important task that relies heavily on critical-thinking skills (Marquis & Huston, 1995). How do people become successful problem solvers and decision makers? Although successful decision making can be learned through life experience, not everyone learns to solve

Display 1.1	**Six Cognitive Skills Used in Critical Thinking**

Interpretation: involves clarifying meaning
Analysis: understanding data
Evaluation: determining outcome
Inference: drawing conclusions
Explanation: justifying actions based on data
Self-regulation: examining one's professional practice

Adapted from Ignatavicius, D. D. (2001). *Critical thinking skills for at-the-bedside nurse. Nursing Management, 32*[1], 37–39.

Display 1.2	**Characteristics of a Critical Thinker**	
Open to new ideas	Flexible	Creative
Intuitive	Empathic	Insightful
Energetic	Caring	Willing to take action
Analytical	Observant	Outcome-directed
Persistent	Risk-taker	Willing to change
Assertive	Resourceful	Knowledgeable
Communicator	"Out of the box" thinker	

problems and judge wisely by this trial-and-error method because much is left to chance.

Some educators feel that people are not successful in problem solving and decision making because individuals are not taught how to reason insightfully from multiple perspectives. Belcher (2000) maintains that managers' critical thinking skills can be improved by having students write management case studies for analysis. She thinks that improved critical thinking skills have a positive effect on the quality of a manager's decision making and problem solving skills. Ignatavicious (2001) feels that anyone can learn critical thinking, but it is a long-term process that must be practiced, nurtured, and reinforced.

The Marquis-Huston Critical-Thinking Teaching Model

The desired outcome for teaching and learning decision making and critical thinking in management is an interaction between learners and others that results in the ability to critically examine management and leadership issues. This is a learning of appropriate social and professional behaviors rather than a mere acquisition of knowledge. This type of learning occurs best in groups; therefore, when teaching management and leadership the group process should be used in some way.

Additionally, learners retain didactic material more readily when it is personalized or when they can relate to the material being presented. The use of case studies that learners can identify with assists in retention of didactic material presented.

While formal instruction in critical thinking is important, Clancy (2003) maintains that using a formal decision-making process is mandatory for successful decision making. So often new leaders and managers struggle to make quality decisions because their opportunity to practice making management and leadership decisions is very limited until they are appointed to a management position. These limitations can be overcome by creating opportunities for vicariously experiencing the problems that individuals would encounter in the real world of leadership and management.

The Marquis-Huston Critical-Thinking Teaching Model assists in achieving desired learner outcomes (**Figure 1.1**). Basically, the model depicts four overlapping spheres, each being an essential component for teaching leadership and management. There needs to be a didactic theory component, such as the material that is presented in each chapter; secondly, a formalized approach to problem solving and decision making must be used. Thirdly, there must be some use of the group

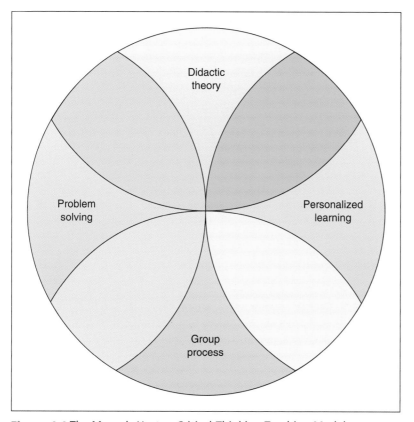

Figure 1.1 The Marquis-Huston Critical-Thinking Teaching Model.

process, which can be accomplished by the use of large and small groups and class-room discussion. Lastly the material must be made real for the learner so that the learning is internalized. This can be accomplished through writing exercises, personal exploration, values clarification, and risk-taking that is involved as case studies are examined.

This book was developed with the perspective that experiential learning provides mock experiences that have tremendous value in applying leadership and management theory. Throughout this text the authors have included numerous opportunities for readers to experience the real world of leadership and management. Some of these learning situations, which are called learning exercises, include case studies, writing exercises, specific management or leadership problems, staffing and budgeting calculations, group discussion or problem solving, and assessment of personal attitudes and values. Some exercises include opinions, speculation, and value judgments. Since almost all the learning exercises require critical thinking, problem solving, or decision making to some degree, the remainder of this chapter will focus on providing a theoretical foundation for leadership and management problem solving.

THEORETICAL APPROACHES TO PROBLEM SOLVING AND DECISION MAKING

Clancy (2003) states that there is a great tendency in decision making to bypass a thorough analysis and jump too quickly into solutions. Process and structure are beneficial to the process of decision making and force people to be specific about options and to separate probabilities from values. A structured approach to problem solving and decision making increases critical reasoning and is the best way to learn how to make quality decisions because it eliminates trial and error and focuses the learning on a proven process. A structured or professional approach involves applying a theoretical model in problem solving and decision making.

A structured approach to problem solving and decision making increases critical reasoning.

To improve decision-making ability, it is important to use an adequate process model as the theoretical base for understanding and applying critical-thinking skills. Many acceptable problem-solving models exist, and most include a decision-making step; only four are reviewed here.

Traditional Problem-Solving Process

The *traditional problem-solving model* is widely used and is perhaps the most well known of the various models. The seven steps follow. (Decision-making occurs at step 5.)

1. Identify the problem.
2. Gather data to analyze the causes and consequences of the problem.
3. Explore alternative solutions.
4. Evaluate the alternatives.
5. Select the appropriate solution.
6. Implement the solution.
7. Evaluate the results.

Although the traditional problem-solving process is an effective model, its weakness lies in the amount of time needed for proper implementation. This process, therefore, is less effective when time constraints are a consideration. Another weakness is lack of an initial objective-setting step. Setting a decision goal helps to prevent the decision maker from becoming sidetracked.

The Managerial Decision-Making Process

The *managerial decision-making model,* a modified traditional model, eliminates the weakness of the traditional model by adding a goal-setting step. Harrison (1981) has delineated the following steps in the managerial decision-making process:

1. Set objectives.
2. Search for alternatives.
3. Evaluate alternatives.
4. Choose.
5. Implement.
6. Follow up and control.

The managerial decision-making process flows in much the same manner as the nursing process. A comparison of the simplified nursing process and a model of decision-making are shown in **Table 1.1.**

Table 1.1 Comparing the Decision-Making Process with the Nursing Process

Decision-Making Process	Simplified Nursing Process
Identify the decision	Assess
Collect data	
Identify criteria for decision	Plan
Identify alternatives	
Choose alternative	Implement
Implement alternative	
Evaluate steps in decision	Evaluate

The Nursing Process

The *nursing process* provides another theoretical system for solving problems and making decisions. Educators have identified the nursing process as an effective decision-making model, although there is current debate about its effectiveness as a clinical reasoning model (Pesut & Herman, 1998).

As a decision-making model, the nursing process has a strength that the previous two models lack, namely its feedback mechanism. The arrows in **Figure 1.2** show constant input into the process. When the decision point has been identified, initial decision-making occurs and continues throughout the process by using a feedback mechanism. Although the process was designed for nursing practice with regard to patient care and nursing accountability, it can easily be adapted as a theoretical

Figure 1.2 Feedback mechanism of the nursing process.

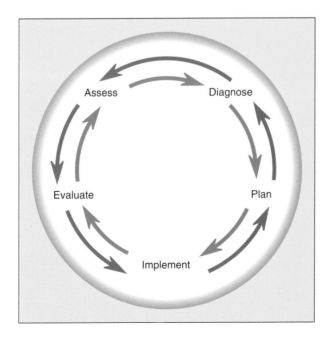

model for solving leadership and management problems. Table 1.1 shows how closely the nursing process parallels the decision-making process.

The weakness of the nursing process, like the traditional problem-solving model, is in not requiring clearly stated objectives. Goals should be clearly stated in the planning phase of the process, but this step is frequently omitted or obscured.

However, because nurses are familiar with this process and its proven effectiveness, it continues to be recommended as an adapted theoretical process for leadership and managerial decision making.

Many other excellent problem analysis and decision models exist. The model selected should be one with which the decision maker is familiar and one appropriate for the problem to be solved. Using models or processes consistently will increase the likelihood that critical analysis will occur. By cultivating a scientific approach, the quality of one's management and leadership problem solving and decision making will improve tremendously.

Intuitive Decision-Making Model

According to Hansten and Wahburn (2000), many nursing scientists in the past did not value intuition in decision making as they felt intuitive reasoning did not align itself well with the status and power of a true science. Recently, however, there has been a renewed interest in intuitive thinking and Ignatavicious (2001) identifies it as one of the characteristics of an expert critical thinker. It must be remembered, however, that intuition can be overpowered by emotions. Therefore, using an intuitive decision-making model is helpful in order to prevent emotions from clouding the decision-making process.

Romiszowski (1981) built on the nursing process in creating the intuitive decision-making model shown in **Figure 1.3**. In this model, the decision maker consciously

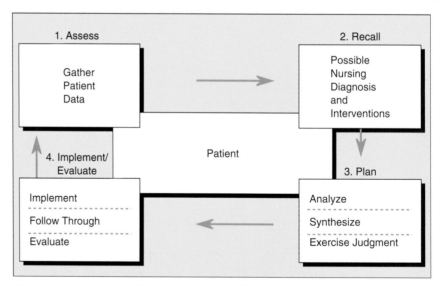

Figure 1.3 Intuitive decision-making model (Romiszowski, 1981). Reprinted with permission of *Journal of Nursing Staff Development*.

incorporates recall or cumulative knowledge that comes from education, both formal and informal, as well as experience, in planning the decision. Inexperienced or novice decision makers spend more time in the assessment, recall, and planning phases, whereas experienced decision makers gather information, recall, and often leap directly to implementation, because planning has become automatic. That novice nurses and experienced nurses process information differently has been supported by Benner (1994).

Ironically, this "leap" from information gathering to implementation may be the greatest weakness of this model. In discussing intuitive decision making, Lamond and Thompson (2000) warn that since the process is largely invisible, there is little information to evaluate if the outcome of the decision is less than positive.

 Learning Exercise 1.1

Applying Scientific Models to Decision Making
You are an RN who graduated three years ago. During the last three years, your responsibilities in your first position have increased. Although you enjoy your family (husband and one preschool-age child), you realize that you love your job, and your career is very important to you. Recently, you and your husband decided to have another baby. At that time, you discussed your career and both of you reached a joint decision that, if you had another baby, you wanted to reduce your work time and spend more time at home with the children. Last week, you were thrilled and excited when your supervisor told you the charge nurse is leaving and that she wants to appoint you to the position. Yesterday, you found out that you are pregnant.

Last night, you and your husband talked about your career future. He is an attorney whose practice has suddenly gained momentum. Although he has shared child rearing equally with you until this point, he is not sure how much longer he will be able to do so if his practice continues to expand. If you take the position, which you would like to do, it would mean full-time work. You want the decision you and your husband reach to be well thought-out as it has far-reaching consequences and concerns many people. **Assignment:** Using a scientific approach (one of the four models just discussed), determine what you should do. After you have made your decision, get together in a group (four to six people) and share your resolution. Were your decisions the same? How did you approach the problem solving differently from others in your group? Did some of the group members identify alternatives you had not considered? How did your personal values influence your decision?

CRITICAL ELEMENTS IN PROBLEM SOLVING AND DECISION MAKING

Because decisions may have far-reaching consequences, problem solving and decision making must be of high quality. Using a scientific approach to problem solving and decision making does not, however, ensure a quality decision. Special attention must be paid to other critical elements. The following elements, considered crucial in the problem-solving process, frequently result in poor-quality decisions.

Define Objectives Clearly

Decision makers often forge ahead in their problem-solving process without first determining their goal. Even when decisions must be made quickly, there is time to pause and reflect on the purpose of the decision. If a decision lacks a clear objective or if an objective is not consistent with the individual's or organization's stated philosophy, a poor-quality decision is likely. Sometimes the problem has been identified but the wrong objectives are set. Problems can be extremely complex and may need multiple objectives (Clancy, 2003).

Gather Data Carefully

Because decisions are based on knowledge and information available to the problem solver at the time the decision must be made, one must learn how to process and obtain accurate information. The acquisition of information begins with identifying the problem or the occasion for the decision and continues throughout the problem-solving process. Often the information is unsolicited, but most information is sought actively.

Acquiring information always involves people, and no tool or mechanism is infallible to human error. Human values tremendously influence our perceptions. Therefore, as problem solvers gather information, they must be vigilant that their own preferences and those of others are not mistaken for facts. Remember that facts can be misleading if they are presented in a seductive manner or taken out of context or if they are past-oriented. Numerous parents have been misled by the factual statement, "Johnny hit me." In this case, the information seeker needs to do more fact finding. What was the accuser doing before Johnny hit him? What was he hit with? Where was he hit? When was he hit? Like the parent, the manager who becomes expert at acquiring adequate, appropriate, and accurate information will have a head start in becoming an expert decision maker and problem solver.

To gain knowledge and insight into managerial and leadership decision making, individuals must reach outside their current sphere of knowledge in solving the problems presented in this text. Some data-gathering sources include textbooks, periodicals, experts in the field, colleagues, and current research.

Questions that should be examined in data gathering are:

1. What is the setting?
2. What is the problem?
3. Where is it a problem?
4. When is it a problem?
5. Who is affected by the problem?
6. Is this your problem or someone else's problem?
7. What is happening?
8. Why is it happening? What are the causes of the problem? Can the causes be prioritized?
9. What are the basic underlying issues? What are the areas of conflict?
10. What are the consequences of the problem? Which is the most serious?

Learning Exercise 1.2

Gathering Necessary Information
Identify a poor decision you recently made because of faulty data gathering. Have you ever made a poor decision because necessary information was intentionally or unintentionally withheld from you?

Generate Many Alternatives

The definition of decision-making implies there are at least two choices in every decision. Unfortunately, many problem solvers limit their choices to two when many more options usually are available. The greater the number of alternatives that can be generated during this phase, the greater the chance that the final decision will be sound. When seeking alternatives, individuals need to expand their horizons; the most common trap managers fall into is limiting the borders of their decision frames (Clancy, 2003).

Remember that one alternative in each decision should be the choice not to do anything. When examining decisions to be made using a formal process, it is often found that the status quo is the right alternative. Several techniques can help generate more alternatives. Involving others in the process confirms the adage that two heads are better than one. Because everyone thinks uniquely, increasing the number of people working on a problem increases the number of alternatives that can be generated.

Learning Exercise 1.3

Possible Alternatives in Problem Solving
In the personal choice scenario presented in Learning Exercise 1.1, some of the following alternatives could have been generated:
  Do not take the new position.
  Hire a full-time housekeeper, and take the position.
  Ask your husband to quit his job.
  Have an abortion.
  Ask one of the parents to help.
  Take the position, and do not hire child care.
  Take the position and hire child care.
  Have your husband reduce his law practice and continue helping with child care.
  Ask the supervisor if you can work four days a week and still have the position.
  Take the position and wait and see what happens after the baby is born.
Assignment: How many of these alternatives did you or your group generate? What alternatives did you identify that are not included in this list?

Brainstorming is another frequently used technique. The goal in brainstorming is to think of all possible alternatives, even those that may seem "off target." By not limiting the possible alternatives to only apparently appropriate ones, people are able to break through habitual or repressive thinking patterns and allow new ideas to surface. Although most often used by groups, people making decisions alone also may use brainstorming. Clancy (2003) suggests that once a large number of alternatives are generated that the list be revised so that the decision maker is left with three or four, as any more may create too many variables and factors to evaluate effectively.

Think Logically

During the problem-solving process, one must draw inferences from information. An inference is part of deductive reasoning. People must carefully think through the information and the alternatives. Clancy (2003) states that among other things, deep-seated biases often cloud effective decision making. Faulty logic at this point may lead to poor-quality decisions. People think illogically primarily in three ways.

1. *Overgeneralizing.* This type of "crooked" thinking occurs when one believes that because *A* has a particular characteristic, every other *A* also has the same characteristic. An example of this thinking is when stereotypical statements are used to justify arguments and decisions.
2. *Affirming the consequences.* In this type of illogical thinking, one decides that if *B* is good but he or she is doing *A*, then *A* must not be good. For example, if a new method is heralded as the best way to perform a nursing procedure and the nurses on your unit are not using that technique, it is illogical to assume that the technique currently used in your unit is wrong or bad.
3. *Arguing from analogy.* This thinking applies a component that is present in two separate concepts and then states that because *A* is present in *B*, then *A* and *B* are alike in all respects. An example of this would be to argue that because intuition plays a part in clinical and managerial nursing, then any characteristic present in a good clinical nurse also should be present in a good nurse–manager. However, this is not necessarily true; a good nurse–manager does not necessarily possess all the same skills as a good nurse–clinician.

Various tools have been designed to assist managers with the important task of analysis. Several of these tools are discussed later in Chapter 2. In analyzing possible solutions, individuals may want to look at the following questions:

1. What factors can you influence? How can you make the positive factors more important and minimize the negative factors?
2. What are the financial implications in each alternative? The political implications? Who else will be affected by the decision and what support is available?
3. What are the weighting factors?
4. What is the best solution?
5. What are the means of evaluation?
6. What are the consequences of each alternative?

Choose and Act Decisively

It is not enough to gather adequate information, think logically, select from among many alternatives, and be aware of the influence of one's values. In the final analysis, one must act. Individuals may become vulnerable at this last point in the problem-solving process and choose to delay acting because they lack the courage to face the consequences of their choices. For example, if managers granted all employees' requests for days off, they would have to accept the consequences of their decision by dealing with short staffing.

It may help the reluctant decision maker to remember that decisions, although often having long-term consequences and far-reaching effects, are not cast in stone. In many cases, judgments found to be ineffective or inappropriate can be changed. By evaluating decisions at a later time, managers can learn more about their abilities and where the problem solving was faulty. However, decisions must continue to be made, although some are of poor quality, because through continued decision making, people develop increased decision-making skills (**Display 1.3**).

INDIVIDUAL VARIATIONS IN DECISION MAKING

If each person receives the same information and uses the same scientific approach to solve problems, an assumption could be made that identical decisions would result. However, in practice, this is not true. Because decision making involves perceiving and evaluating, and people perceive by sensation and intuition and evaluate their perception by thinking and feeling, it is inevitable that individuality plays a part in decision making. Because everyone has different values and life experiences, and each person perceives and thinks differently, different decisions may be made given the same set of circumstances. No discussion of decision making would, therefore, be complete without a careful examination of the role of the individual in decision making (see **Display 1.4**).

Values

Individual decisions are based on each person's value system. No matter how objective the criteria, value judgments will always play a part in a person's decision making, either consciously or subconsciously. The alternatives generated and the final choice selected are limited by each person's value system. For some, certain choices

Display 1.3	**Critical Elements in Decision Making**

- Define objectives clearly
- Gather data carefully
- Generate many alternatives
- Think logically
- Choose and act decisively

Display 1.4	Individual Variations in Decision Making

- Values
- Life experience
- Individual preference
- Individual ways of thinking and decision making

are not possible because of a person's beliefs. Because values also influence perceptions, they invariably influence information gathering, information processing, and final outcome (Marquis & Huston, 1995). Values also determine which problems in one's personal or professional life will be addressed or ignored.

Life Experience

Each person brings to the decision-making task past experiences that include education and decision-making experience. The more mature the person and the broader his or her background, the more alternatives he or she can identify. Each time a new behavior or decision is observed, that possibility is added to the person's repertoire of choices. People vary in their desire for autonomy, so some nurses may want more autonomy than others. It is likely that people seeking autonomy may have much more experience at making decisions than those who fear autonomy. Likewise, having made good or poor decisions in the past will influence a person's decision making.

Individual Preference

With all the alternatives a person considers in decision making, one alternative may be preferred over another. The decision maker, for example, may see certain choices as involving greater personal risk than others and therefore may choose the safer alternative. Physical, economic, and emotional risks, and time and energy expenditures, are types of personal risk and costs involved in decision making. For example, those with limited finances or a reduced energy level may decide to select an alternative solution to a problem that would not have been their first choice had they been able to overcome limited resources.

Individual Ways of Thinking and Decision Making

Our way of evaluating information and alternatives on which we base our final decision constitutes a thinking skill. Individuals think differently. Some think systematically—and are often called analytical thinkers—whereas others think intuitively. It is believed that most people have either right- or left-brain hemisphere dominance (Good, 2002). Although the authors encourage whole-brain thinking, and studies have shown that people can strengthen the use of the less dominant side of the brain, most people continue to have a dominant side. Analytical, linear, left-brain thinkers process information differently than creative, intuitive, right-brain thinkers. Intuition is the ability to understand the possibilities inherent in a situation.

Some feel that there is a gender difference in how we think and behave. Rudan's research (2003) looked at how male and female leaders behaved differently and noted that males and females socialized and communicated differently; males paid much less attention to relationships and resisted being influenced. These differences have the potential to effect decision making.

The way one thinks has much to do with individual problem solving and decision making. There is no evidence that either right- or left-brain thinking is preferable. In the past, organizations openly recognized the value of logical, analytical thinkers but more recently have acknowledged that intuitive thinking is a valuable managerial resource. It is felt that right-brain thinkers are more creative, but the current emphasis in teaching and learning is to encourage whole-brain thinking (Good, 2002).

 Learning Exercise 1.4

Thinking Styles
In a group discussion, examine how each individual in the group thinks. Do you have a majority of individuals with right- or left-brain dominance in your group? Do more women than men belong to one group? Discuss what type of thinkers are represented in your family. Did most individuals in your group have a variety of thinkers in their family?

OVERCOMING INDIVIDUAL VULNERABILITY IN DECISION MAKING

How do people overcome subjectivity in making decisions? This can never be completely overcome, nor should it. After all, life would be boring if everyone thought alike. However, managers and leaders must become aware of their own vulnerability and recognize how it influences and limits the quality of their decision making. Using the following suggestions will help decrease individual subjectivity and increase objectivity in decision making.

Values

Being confused and unclear about one's values may affect decision-making ability (Huston & Marquis, 1995). Overcoming a lack of self-awareness through values clarification decreases confusion. People who understand their personal beliefs and feelings will have a conscious awareness of the values on which their decisions are based. This awareness is an essential component of decision making and critical thinking. Therefore, to be successful problem solvers, managers must periodically examine their values. Values clarification exercises are included in Chapter 7.

Life Experience

It is difficult to overcome inexperience when making decisions. Benner (1994) refers to this lack of experience as "reason in transition." However, a person can do some things to decrease this area of vulnerability. First, use available resources, including current research and literature, to gain a fuller understanding of the issues involved. Second, involve other people, such as experienced colleagues, trusted friends, or superiors, to act as sounding boards and advisors. Third, analyze decisions later to assess their success. By evaluating decisions, people learn from mistakes and are able to overcome inexperience.

Individual Preference

Overcoming this area of vulnerability involves self-awareness, honesty, and risk taking. The need for self-awareness was discussed previously, but it is not enough to be self-aware; people also must be honest with themselves about their choices and their preferences for those choices. Additionally, the successful decision maker must take some risks. Nearly every decision has some element of risk, and most involve consequences and accountability. Those who are able to do the right but unpopular thing and who dare to stand alone will emerge as leaders.

Individual Ways of Thinking

People who make decisions alone are frequently handicapped because they are not able to understand problems fully or make decisions from both an analytical and intuitive perspective. However, in most organizations, both types of thinkers may be found. Using group process, talking management problems over with others, and developing whole-brain thinking also are methods for ensuring that both intuitive and analytical approaches will be used in solving problems and making decisions. Use of heterogeneous rather than homogeneous groups will usually result in better-quality decision making. See **Display 1.5** for more information.

Indeed, learning to think "outside the box" is often accomplished by including a diverse group of thinkers to solve problems and make decisions. It is good organizational theory for leaders to surround themselves with a variety of talented people,

Display 1.5	Qualities of Successful Decision Makers

Although not all experts agree, Huston (1990) suggests that the following are qualities of successful decision makers:
- Courage. Courage is of particular importance and involves the willingness to take risks.
- Sensitivity. Good decision makers seem to have some sort of antenna that makes them particularly sensitive to situations and others.
- Energy. People must have the energy and desire to make things happen.
- Creativity. Successful decision makers tend to be creative thinkers. They develop new ways to solve problems.

including individuals who sometimes have strange ideas and are "out of the box" thinkers (Ignatavicius, 2001).

DECISION MAKING IN ORGANIZATIONS

In the beginning of this chapter the need for managers and leaders to make quality decisions was emphasized. The effect of the individual's values and preferences on the decision making process was discussed. But it is important for leaders and managers to also understand how the organization influences the decision-making process. Since organizations are made up of people with differing values and preferences, there is often conflict in organizational decision dynamics.

Effect of Organizational Power on Decision Making

Powerful people in organizations are more apt to have decisions made (by themselves or their subordinates) that are congruent with their own preferences and values. On the other hand, people wielding little power in organizations must always consider the preference of the powerful when they make management decisions. Power is frequently part of the decision factor (Good, 2003). In organizations choice is constructed and constrained by many factors, and therefore choice is not equally available to all people.

Additionally, not only does the preference of the powerful influence decisions of the less powerful, but the powerful also are able to inhibit the preferences of the less powerful. This occurs because individuals who remain and advance in organizations are those who feel and express values and beliefs congruent with the organization. Therefore, a balance must be found between the limitations of choice posed by the power structure within the organization and totally independent decision making that could lead to organizational chaos.

The ability of the powerful to influence individual decision making in an organization often requires adopting a private personality and an organizational personality. For example, some might believe they would have made a different decision had they been acting on their own, but they went along with the organizational decision. This "going along" in itself constitutes a decision; people choose to accept an organizational decision that differs from their own preferences and values. The concept of power in organizations is discussed more fully in Chapter 13.

> The ability of the powerful to influence individual decision making in an organization often requires adopting a private personality and an organizational personality.

Rational and Administrative Decision Making

For many years, it was widely believed that most managerial decisions were based on a careful, scientific, and objective thought process and managers made decisions in a rational manner. In the late 1940s, Herbert A. Simon's classic work revealed that most managers made many decisions that did not fit the objective rationality theory. Simon (1965) delineated two types of management decision makers: the *economic man* and the *administrative man*.

Managers who are successful decision makers attempt to make rational decisions, much like the economic person described in **Table 1.2.** Because they realize

Table 1.2 Comparing the Economic Man with the Administrative Man	
Economic	**Administrative**
Makes decisions in a very rational manner.	Makes decisions that are good enough.
Has complete knowledge of the problem or decision situation.	Because complete knowledge is not possible, knowledge is always fragmented.
Has a complete list of possible alternatives.	Because consequences of alternatives occur in the future, they are impossible to predict accurately.
Has a rational system of ordering preference of alternatives.	Usually chooses from among a few alternatives, not all possible ones.
Selects the decision that will maximize utility function.	The final choice is "satisficing" rather than maximizing.

Adapted from Simon, 1965.

that restricted knowledge and limited alternatives directly affect a decision's quality, these managers gather as much information as possible and generate many alternatives. Simon believed that the economic model was an unrealistic description of organizational decision making. The complexity of acquiring information makes it impossible for the human brain to store and retain the amount of information that is available for each decision. Because of time constraints and the difficulty of assimilating large amounts of information, most management decisions are made using the administrative model of decision making. The administrative person never has complete knowledge and generates fewer alternatives. Simon argued that the administrative person carries out decisions that are only "*satisficing,*" a term used to describe decisions that may not be ideal but result in solutions that have adequate outcomes. These managers want decisions to be "good enough" so that they "work," but they are less concerned that the alternative selected is the optimal choice. The "best" choice for many decisions is often found to be too costly in terms of time or resources, so another less costly but workable solution is found.

SUMMARY

This chapter has discussed effective decision making, problem solving, and critical thinking as requisites for being a successful leader and manager. The effective leader–manager is aware of the need for sensitivity in decision making. The successful decision maker possesses courage, energy, and creativity. It is a leadership skill to recognize the appropriate people to include in decision making and to use a suitable theoretical model for the decision situation.

The manager should develop a systematic, scientific approach to problem solving that begins with a fixed goal and ends with an evaluation step. Managers who make quality decisions are effective administrators.

The integrated leader–manager understands the significance that personal values, life experience, preferences, and ways of thinking have upon selected alternatives in making the decision. The critical thinker pondering a decision is aware of the areas of vulnerability that hinder successful decision making and will expend his or her efforts to avoid the pitfalls of faulty logic and data gathering.

Both managers and leaders understand the impact the organization has on decision making and that some decisions that will be made in the organization will be only satisficing. However, leaders will strive to problem solve adequately in order to reach optimal decisions as often as possible.

❋ Key Concepts

- The professional decision maker is self-aware, courageous, sensitive, energetic, and creative.
- The professional approach to problem solving begins with a fixed goal and ends with an evaluation process.
- The successful decision maker understands the significance that each person's values, life experience, preferences, and way of thinking have on selected alternatives.
- The critical thinker is aware of areas of vulnerability that hinder successful decision making and makes efforts to avoid the pitfalls of faulty logic in his or her data gathering.
- The act of making and evaluating decisions increases the expertise of the decision maker.
- There are many models for improving decision making. Using a model reduces trial and error and increases the probability that decisions made will be sound.
- Left- and right-brain dominance influences to some degree how individuals think.
- Two major considerations in organizational decision making are how power affects decision making and whether management decision making needs to only be "*satisficing.*"

More Learning Exercises and Applications

These exercises may be discussed individually, in groups, or used as written assignments.

Learning Exercise 1.5

Evaluating Decision Making
Describe the two best decisions you have made in your life and the two worst. What factors assisted you in making the wise decisions? What elements of critical thinking went awry in your poor decision making? How would you evaluate your decision making ability?

Learning Exercise 1.6

Profile Examining
Examine the process you used to decide to become a nurse. Would you describe it as fitting a profile of the economic or the administrative model?

Learning Exercise 1.7

Considering Critical Elements in Decision Making
You are a college senior and president of your nursing organization. You are on the committee to select a slate of officers for the next academic year. Several of the current officers will be graduating and you want the new slate of officers to be committed to the organization. Some of the brightest members of the junior class that are involved in the organization are not well liked by some of your friends in the organization.
Assignment: Looking at the critical elements in decision making compile a list of the most important points to consider in making the decision for selection of a slate of officers. What must you guard against and how should you approach the data gathering to solve this problem?

Learning Exercise 1.8

Examining the Decision-Making Process
You have been a staff nurse for three years, since your graduation from nursing school. There is a nursing shortage in your area and many openings at other facilities. Additionally, you have been offered a charge nurse position at your present employment. Lastly, you have always wanted to do community health nursing and know that this is also a possibility. You are self-aware enough to know that it is time for a change, but which change should you make, and how should you make the decision?
Assignment: Examine both the individual aspects of decision making and the critical elements in making decisions. Make a plan including a goal, a list of information and data that you need to gather and areas where you may be vulnerable to successful decision making. Examine the consequences of each alternative available to you. After you have done this, as an individual, form a small group and share your decision making planning with members of your group. How was your decision making like others in the group and how was it different?

Learning Exercise 1.9

Using Models in Decision Making
Do you use a problem-solving or decision-making model to solve problems? Have you ever used an intuitive model? Think of a critical decision you have made in the last year. What model, if any, did you use?
Assignment: Write a one-page essay about a problem you solved or a decision that you made this year. Describe what theoretical model you use to assist you in the process. Determine if you consciously used the model or if it was purely by accident. Did you enlist the help of other experts in solving the problem?

 Learning Exercise 1.10

Step-by-Step Problem Solving
You are a home-health nurse who makes in-home visits to a moribund elderly man with advanced cancer. He is now confined to bed, and his major care needs are comfort-based. In addition to directly providing pain medication to this man, you, as a case manager, are responsible for overseeing other personnel who assist in caring for him. These personnel include rotating health aides who are responsible for bathing the patient, preparing his meals, and providing other basic care not requiring a professional license. The patient's family generally stays with him at night.

At times, during your in-home visits, you have noticed that there are food crumbs in the bed, that the patient's hair is uncombed, and that his teeth have not been brushed, and you suspect that he has not been recently bathed.

Assignment: Use one of the problem-solving or decision-making models in this chapter and do the following:
1. Identify a brief (no longer than one or two sentences) problem statement for this case.
2. Determine who owns the problem.
3. List at least three goals or objectives to guide your problem solving.
4. Detail at least three key pieces of information you must consider in data gathering.
5. List at least six alternatives for solving this case, including the pros and cons of each.
6. Identify at least four specific criteria you will use to evaluate your final decision and/or choice of action. Be sure these criteria reflect the decision-making process you used as well as the desired outcome.
If time allows, divide into small groups and share the results of your problem solving.

⊛ Web Links

Judgment and Decision Making
http://www.sjdm.org
Promotes the study of normative, descriptive theories of decision processes.
http://www.hooah4health.com/spirit/decisions.htm
Free tools you can use to solve problems and make decisions in your life.

Mission Critical
http://www.sjsu.edu/depts/itl
The goal of this site is to teach visitors the basic concepts of critical thinking, deductive reasoning, and finding faults in dubious arguments. The site provides tutorials, exercises, and links to related Web sites.

References

Belcher, J. V. R. (2000). Improving managers' critical thinking skills. *Journal of Nursing Administration, 30*(7/8), 351–353.

Benner, P. (1994, July 17). *Engaged reasoning: Critical evaluation of critical thinking.* Paper presented at Improving the Quality of Thinking in a Changing World, The Sixth International Conference on Thinking, Cambridge, Massachusetts.

Clancy, T. R. (2003). The art of decision-making. *Journal of Nursing Administration, 33*(6), 343–349.

Good, B. (2002). A call for creative teaching and learning. *Creative Nursing, 8*(4), 4–9.

Hansten, R., & Washburn, M. (2000). Intuition in professional practice. *Journal of Nursing Administration, 30*(4), 185–189.

Harrison, E. F. (1981). *The managerial decision-making process* (2nd ed.). Boston: Houghton Mifflin.

Huston, C. J. (1990). What makes the difference? Attributes of the exceptional nurse. *Nursing 20*(5), 170–171.

Huston, C. J., & Marquis, B. L. (1995). Seven steps to successful decision-making. *American Journal of Nursing, 95*(5), 65–68.

Ignatavicius, D. D. (2001). Critical thinking skills for at-the-bedside nurse. *Nursing Management, 32*(1), 37–39.

Lamond, D., & Thompson, C. (2000). Intuition and analysis in decision making and choice. *Journal of Nursing Scholarship, 32*(4) 411–414.

Marquis, B. L., & Huston, C. J. (1994, March). Decisions, decisions. *Advanced Practice Nurse, 1,* 46–49.

Munhall, P. K. (1999). From "out of the box" to "fitting in." *Journal of Nursing Scholarship, 31*(2), 102.

Pesut, D. J., & Herman, J. (1998). OPT: Transformation of nursing process for contemporary practice. *Nursing Outlook, 46*(1), 29–36.

Romiszowski, A. J. (1981). *Designing instructional systems.* New York: HarperCollins College Publishers.

Rudan, V. T. (2003). The best of both worlds: A consideration of gender in team building. *Journal of Nursing Administration, 33*(3), 179–186.

Simon, H. A. (1965). *The shape of automation for man and management.* New York: Harper Textbooks.

Bibliography

Bohinc, M., & Gradisar, M. (2003). Decision-making model for nursing. *Journal of Nursing Administration, 33*(12), 627–638.

Chau, J. P. C., Chang, A. M., Lee, I. F. K., Ip, W. Y., Lee, D. T. F., & Wootton, Y. (2001). Effects of videotaped vignettes on enhancing students' critical thinking ability in a baccalaureate nursing programme. *Journal of Advanced Nursing, 36*(1), 112–120.

Contino, D. S. (2003). Notes from the field. What's your perspective-past, present, or future? *Nursing Management, 34*(6), 49–51.

Daly, W. M. (2001). The development of an alternative method in the assessment of critical thinking as an outcome of nursing education. *Journal of Advanced Nursing, 36*(1), 120–131.

Graf, C. M. (2003). Patients' needs for nursing care: Beyond staffing ratios. *Journal of Nursing Administration 33*(2), 76–81.

Florida, R. (2002). *The Rise of the Creative Class.* New York: Basic Books.

Havens, D. S. & Vasey, J. (2003). Measuring staff nurse decisional involvement: The decisional involvement scale. *Journal of Nursing Administration, 33*(6), 331–337.

Krairiksh, M & Anthony, M. K. (2001). Benefits and outcomes of staff nurses' participation in decision making. *Journal of Nursing Administration, 31*(1), 16–23.

Omery, A. J. (2003). Advice nursing practice: On the quality of evidence. *Journal of Nursing Administration, 33*(6), 353–360.

Ritter-Teitel, J. (2003). Nursing administrative research: The underpinning of decisive leadership. *Journal of Nursing Administration, 33*(5), 257–259.

Introduction to Management and Management Decision Making

The roles of the nurse manager and nurse executive have evolved significantly in response to changes in the healthcare industry in the last 20 years.

—Carol S. Kleinman

Throughout history, nursing has been required to respond to changing technological and social forces. The new managerial responsibilities placed on organized nursing services require nurse administrators who are knowledgeable, skilled, and competent in all aspects of management. Now more than ever there is a greater emphasis on the business of health care, with managers being involved in the financial and marketing aspects of their respective departments. To confront expanding responsibilities and demands, the manager's role must take on new dimensions to facilitate quality outcomes in patient care and meet other strategic institutional goals and objectives.

Although, management functions are similar in every discipline and across societies, changes in the healthcare industry in the last 20 years have been so dramatic that nurse managers have had to bring a new cadre of skills into a dynamic and rapidly changing managerial role (Kleinman, 2003).

The relationship between leadership and management continues to prompt some debate, although the literature demonstrates the need for both (Trent, 2003; Zaleznik, 2004). Whereas management emphasizes control–control of hours, costs, salaries, overtime, use of sick leave, inventory, and supplies–leadership increases productivity by maximizing work force effectiveness.

Leadership is viewed by some as one of management's many functions; others maintain that leadership requires more complex skills than management and that management is only one role of leadership; still others delineate between the two. But if a manager guides, directs, and motivates others and a leader empowers others, then it could be said that every manager is a leader.

Management and leadership are, however, first artificially separated in this chapter so that there is a full understanding of the functions of management. The following are some of the characteristics of managers:

- Have an assigned position within the formal organization
- Have a legitimate source of power due to the delegated authority that accompanies their position
- Are expected to carry out specific functions, duties, and responsibilities
- Emphasize control, decision making, decision analysis, and results
- Manipulate people, the environment, money, time, and other resources to achieve organizational goals
- Have a greater formal responsibility and accountability for rationality and control than leaders
- Direct willing and unwilling subordinates

Historically, strong management skills were valued more than strong leadership skills in the healthcare industry. This was true not only in nursing and health care but throughout businesses in Western society. Only in the last 50 years has the world shifted much of its research and interest onto leadership. Effective managers need to be well grounded in management theory and to understand management decision making. Leadership without management results in chaos and failure for both the organization and the individual executive. The ultimate goal for all executives is to integrate management functions and leadership roles. This chapter will focus on providing an historical overview of management theory development and provide some tools for management decision making.

HISTORICAL DEVELOPMENT OF MANAGEMENT THEORY

Management science, like nursing, develops a theory base from many disciplines, such as business, psychology, sociology, and anthropology. Because organizations are complex and varied, theorists' views of what successful management is and what it should be have changed repeatedly in the last 100 years.

Scientific Management (1900–1930)

Frederick W. Taylor, the "father of scientific management," was a mechanical engineer in the Midvale and Bethlehem Steel plants in Pennsylvania in the late 1800s. Frustrated with what he called "systematic soldiering," where workers achieved minimum standards doing the least amount of work possible, Taylor postulated that if workers could be taught the "one best way to accomplish a task," productivity would increase. Borrowing a term coined by Louis Brandeis, a colleague of Taylor's, Taylor called these principles "scientific management." The four overriding principles of scientific management as identified by Taylor (1911) are:

1. Traditional "rule-of-thumb" means of organizing work must be replaced with scientific methods. In other words, by using time and motion studies and the expertise of experienced workers, work could be scientifically designed to promote greatest efficiency of time and energy.
2. A scientific personnel system must be established so workers can be hired, trained, and promoted based on their technical competence and abilities. Taylor thought each employee's abilities and limitations could be identified so the worker could be best matched to the most appropriate job.
3. Workers should be able to view how they "fit" into the organization and how they contribute to overall organizational productivity. This provides common goals and a sharing of the organizational mission. One way in which Taylor thought this could be accomplished was by the use of financial incentives as a reward for work accomplished. Because Taylor viewed humans as "economic animals" motivated solely by money, workers were reimbursed according to their level of production, rather than by an hourly wage.
4. The relationship between managers and workers should be cooperative and interdependent, and the work should be shared equally. Their roles, however, were not the same. The role of managers, or "functional foremen" as they were called, was to plan, prepare, and supervise. The worker was to do the work.

What was the result of scientific management? Productivity and profits rose dramatically. Organizations were provided with a rational means of harnessing the energy of the industrial revolution. Some experts have argued that Taylor was not a humanist and that his scientific principles were not in the best interest of unions or workers. However, it is important to remember the era in which Taylor did his work. During the industrial revolution, laissez-faire economics prevailed, optimism was high, and a Puritan work ethic was prevalent. Taylor maintained that he truly believed managers and workers would be satisfied if increased productivity resulted in adequate financial rewards.

As the cost of labor rose in the United States, many organizations took a new look at scientific management. Healthcare organizations are using new technology, such as video cameras and computers for time and motion studies, to enable individuals to find ways to "work smarter" (Russell, 2000). The implication is that managers need to think of new ways to do traditional tasks so that work is more efficient. Meltzer (1999) maintains that time and motion studies can be used to improve performance, cut costs significantly, and improve the quality of care.

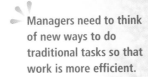 Managers need to think of new ways to do traditional tasks so that work is more efficient.

 Learning Exercise 2.1

Strategies for Efficiency
In small groups, discuss some work routines carried out in healthcare organizations that seem to be inefficient. Could such routines or the time and motion involved to carry out a task be altered to improve efficiency without jeopardizing quality of care? Make a list of ways that nurses could work more efficiently. Don't limit your examination only to nursing procedures and routines, but examine the impact other departments or the arrangement of the nurse's work area may have on preventing nurses from working more efficiently. Share your ideas with your peers.

Bureaucracy

About the same time that Taylor was examining worker tasks, Max Weber, a well-known German sociologist, began to study large-scale organizations to determine what made some more efficient than others. Weber saw the need for legalized, formal authority and consistent rules and regulations for personnel in different positions; he thus proposed bureaucracy as an organizational design. His essay, "Bureaucracy," was written in 1922 in response to what he perceived as a need to provide more rules, regulations, and structure within organizations to increase efficiency. Much of Weber's work and bureaucratic organizational design are still evident today in many healthcare institutions. His work is discussed further in Chapter 12.

Management Functions Identified (1925)

Henri Fayol (1925) first identified the management functions of planning, organization, command, coordination, and control. Luther Gulick (1937) expanded on Fayol's management functions in his introduction of the seven activities of management—*planning, organizing, staffing, directing, coordinating, reporting, and budgeting*—as denoted by the mnemonic POSDCORB. Although often modified (either by including staffing as a management function or renaming elements), these functions or activities have changed little over time. Eventually, theorists began to refer to these functions as the management process.

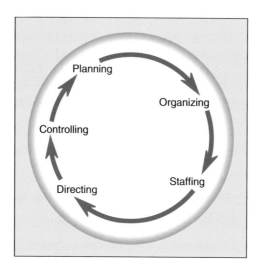

Figure 2.1 The management process.

The management process, shown in **Figure 2.1,** is this book's organizing framework. Brief descriptions of the five functions for each phase of the management process follow:

1. *Planning* encompasses determining philosophy, goals, objectives, policies, procedures, and rules; carrying out long- and short-range projections; determining a fiscal course of action; and managing planned change.
2. *Organizing* includes establishing the structure to carry out plans, determining the most appropriate type of patient care delivery, and grouping activities to meet unit goals. Other functions involve working within the structure of the organization and understanding and using power and authority appropriately.
3. *Staffing* functions consist of recruiting, interviewing, hiring, and orienting staff. Scheduling, staff development, employee socialization, and team building are also often included as staffing functions.
4. *Directing* sometimes includes several staffing functions. However, this phase's functions usually entail human resource management responsibilities, such as motivating, managing conflict, delegating, communicating, and facilitating collaboration.
5. *Controlling* functions include performance appraisals, fiscal accountability, quality control, legal and ethical control, and professional and collegial control.

In many ways, the management process is similar to the nursing process, as shown in **Figure 2.2.** Both processes are cyclic, and many different functions may occur simultaneously. Suppose that a nurse-manager spent part of the day working on the budget (planning), met with the staff about changing the patient care management delivery system from primary care to team nursing (organizing), altered the staffing policy to include 12-hour shifts (staffing), held a meeting to resolve a conflict between nurses and physicians (directing), and gave an employee a job performance evaluation (controlling). Not only would the nurse-manager be performing all phases of the management process, but each function has a planning, implementing, and controlling phase.

Just as nursing practice requires that all nursing care has a plan and an evaluation, so too does each function of management.

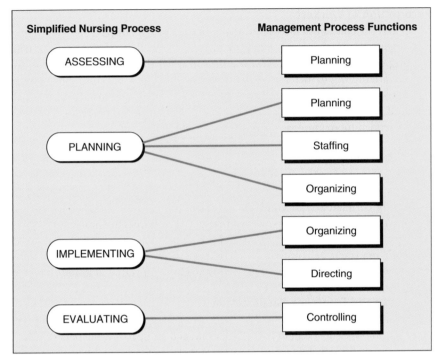

Figure 2.2 Integrating nursing and management processes.

Human Relations Management (1930–1970)

During the 1920s, worker unrest developed. The industrial revolution had resulted in great numbers of relatively unskilled laborers working in large factories on specialized tasks. Thus, management scientists and organizational theorists began to look at the role of worker satisfaction in production. This human relations era developed the concepts of participatory and humanistic management, emphasizing people rather than machines.

Participative Management

Mary Parker Follett was one of the first theorists to suggest basic principles of what today would be called *participative decision making* or *participative management*. In her essay "The Giving of Orders" (1926), Follett espoused her belief that managers should have authority with, rather than over, employees. Follett stated that to do so, a need existed for collective decision making.

The human relations era also attempted to correct what was perceived as the major shortcoming of the bureaucratic system—a failure to include the "human element." Studies done at the Hawthorne Works of the Western Electric Company near Chicago between 1927 and 1932 played a major role in this shifting focus. The studies, conducted by Elton Mayo and his Harvard associates, began as an attempt to look at the relationship between light illumination in the factory and productivity.

Recognition of Workers

Mayo and his colleagues discovered that when management paid special attention to workers, productivity was likely to increase, regardless of the environmental working conditions. This *Hawthorne effect* indicated that people respond to being studied, attempting to increase whatever behavior they feel will continue to warrant the attention. Mayo (1953) also found that informal work groups and a socially informal work environment were factors in determining productivity, and Mayo recommended more employee participation in decision making.

Employee Satisfaction

Douglas McGregor (1960) reinforced these ideas by theorizing that managerial attitudes about employees (and, hence, how managers treat those employees) can be directly correlated with employee satisfaction. He labeled this Theory X and Theory Y. Theory X managers believe that their employees are basically lazy, need constant supervision and direction, and are indifferent to organizational needs. Theory Y managers believe that their workers enjoy their work, are self-motivated, and are willing to work hard to meet personal and organizational goals.

Flexibility and Employee Participation

Chris Argyris (1964) supported McGregor and Mayo by saying that managerial domination causes workers to become discouraged and passive. He believed that if self-esteem and independence needs are not met, employees will become discouraged and troublesome or may leave the organization. Argyris stressed the need for flexibility within the organization and employee participation in decision making.

The human relations era of management science brought about a great interest in the study of workers. Many sociologists and psychologists took up this challenge, and their work in management theory contributed to our understanding about worker motivation, which will be discussed in Chapter 18. **Table 2.1** summarizes the development of management theory up to 1970.

By the late 1960s, there was growing concern that the human relations approach to management was not without its problems. Most people continued to work in a bureaucratic environment, making it difficult to always apply a participatory

Table 2.1 Developers of Management Theory

Theorist	Theory
Taylor	Scientific management
Weber	Bureaucratic organizations
Fayol	Management functions
Gulick	Activities of management
Follett	Participative management
Mayo	Hawthorne effect
McGregor	Theory X and Theory Y
Argyris	Employee participation

approach to management. The human relations approach was time-consuming and often resulted in unmet organizational goals. In addition, not every employee liked working in a less-structured environment.

The evolution of management theory has affected how managers address workers' concerns and needs. The early management theorists discounted workers' needs and focused on productivity and efficiency. Later the needs and motivation of workers became the focal point of the work of the human relation theorist's research into management science. It was not until the 1960s that it became apparent that management was a complex issue that was intertwined with leadership. The following chapter will focus on leadership and the relationship between leadership and management.

MANAGEMENT DECISION-MAKING TECHNOLOGY

As was discussed in Chapter 1, decision making is one of a manager's primary functions. Clancy (2003) maintains that even the most experienced manager cannot eliminate all uncertainty when making decisions. However, to assist the manager in making decisions, management analysts have developed tools that provide order and direction in obtaining and using information or that are helpful in selecting who should be involved in making the decision. Because there are so many of these decision aids, this chapter presents selected technology that would be most helpful to a beginning manager. Some of these aids encourage analytical thinking, others are designed to increase intuitive reasoning, and a few encourage use of both hemispheres of the brain.

Quantitative Decision-Making Tools

Some management authors label management decision-making aids as models; others use the term "tools." It is only important to remember that any decision-making aid always results in the need for the person to make a final decision and that all aids are subject to human error.

Decision Grids

A decision grid allows one to visually examine the alternatives and compare each against the same criteria. Although any criteria may be selected, the same criteria are used to analyze each alternative. An example of a decision grid is depicted in **Figure 2.3.** When many alternatives have been generated or a group or committee is collaborating on the decision, these grids are particularly helpful to the process. This tool, for instance, would be useful when changing the method of managing care on a unit or when selecting a candidate to hire from a large interview pool. The unit manager or the committee of nursing staff would evaluate all the alternatives available using a decision grid. In this manner, every alternative is evaluated using the same criteria. It is possible to weight some of the criteria more heavily than others if some are more important. To do this, it is usually necessary to assign a number value to each criterion. The result would be a numeric value for each alternative considered.

Alternative	Financial effect	Political effect	Departmental effect	Time	Decision
#1					
#2					
#3					
#4					

Figure 2.3 A decision grid.

Payoff Tables

The decision aids that fall in this category have a cost-profit-volume relationship and are very helpful when some quantitative information is available, such as the item's cost or predicted use. To use payoff tables, one must determine probabilities and use historical data, such as a hospital census or a report on the number of operating procedures performed. To illustrate, a payoff table might be appropriately used in determining how many participants it would take to make an in-service program break even.

If the instructor for the class costs $400, the in-service director would need to charge each of the 20 participants $20 for the class, but for 40 participants, the class would cost only $10 each. The in-service director would use attendance data from past classes and the number of nurses potentially available to attend to determine probable class size and thus how much to charge for the class. Payoff tables do not guarantee that a correct decision will be made, but they assist in visualizing data.

Decision Trees

Because decisions are often tied to the outcome of other events, management analysts have developed decision trees. Used to plot a decision over time, decision trees allow visualization of various outcomes. The decision tree in **Figure 2.4** compares the cost of hiring regular staff to the cost of hiring temporary employees. Here the decision is whether to hire extra nurses at regular salary to perform outpatient procedures on an oncology floor or to have nurses available to the unit on an on-call basis and pay them on-call and overtime wages. The possible consequences of a decreased and an increased volume of procedures must both be considered. Initially, costs would increase in hiring a regular staff, but over a longer period of time, this move would mean greater savings if the volume of procedures does not dramatically decrease.

Consequence Tables

Clancy (2003) used a consequence table to demonstrate how various alternatives create different consequences. A consequence table lists the objectives for solving a

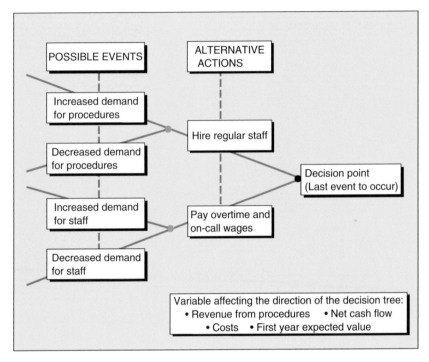

POSSIBLE EVENTS

ALTERNATIVE ACTIONS

Increased demand for procedures

Hire regular staff

Decreased demand for procedures

Decision point (Last event to occur)

Increased demand for staff

Pay overtime and on-call wages

Decreased demand for staff

Variable affecting the direction of the decision tree:
• Revenue from procedures   • Net cash flow
• Costs   • First year expected value

Figure 2.4 A decision tree.

problem down one side of a grid and rates how each alternative would meet the desired objective. For example, consider this problem: *The number of patient falls has exceeded the benchmark rate for two consecutive quarters.* After a period of analysis the following alternatives were selected as solutions:

- Provide a new educational program to instruct staff on how to prevent falls.
- Implement a night check to ensure that patients have side rails up and beds are in a low position.
- Implement a policy requiring soft restraints orders on all confused patients.

The decision maker then lists each alternative opposite the objectives for solving the problem, which for this problem might be:

- Reduces the number of falls
- Meets regulatory standards
- Is cost effective
- Fits present policy guidelines.

The decision maker(s) then ranks each desired objective and examines each of the alternatives through a standardized key, which allows a fair comparison between alternatives and assists in eliminating undesirable choices. It is important

Table 2.2 Consequence Table: An Example

Objectives for Problem Solving	Alternative 1	Alternative 2	Alternative 3
1. Reduces the number of falls	X	X	X
2. Meets regulatory standards	X	X	X
3. Is cost effective		X	X
4. Fits present policy guidelines			X
Decision Score			

to examine long-term effects of each alternative as well as how the decision will affect others. See **Table 2.2** for an example of a consequence table.

Program Evaluation and Review Technique

Program evaluation and review technique (PERT) is a popular tool to determine the timing of decisions. Developed by the Booz-Allen-Hamilton organization and the United States Navy in connection with the Polaris missile program, PERT is essentially a flowchart that predicts when events and activities must take place if a final event is to occur. **Figure 2.5** shows a PERT chart for developing a new outpatient treatment room for oncology procedures. The number of weeks to complete tasks is listed in optimistic time, most likely time, and pessimistic time. The critical path shows something that must occur in the sequence before one may proceed. PERT is especially helpful when a group of people are working on a project. The flowchart keeps everyone up-to-date, and problems are easily identified when they first occur. Flowcharts are popular, and many people use them in their personal lives.

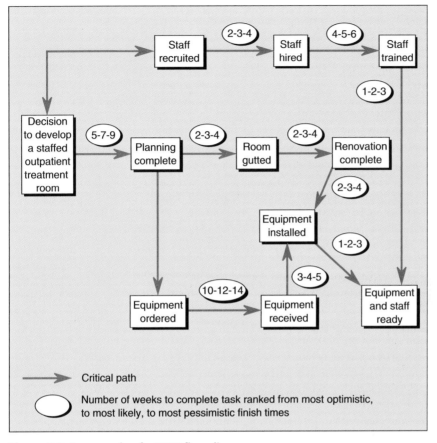

Figure 2.5 An example of a PERT flow diagram.

Learning Exercise 2.2

Charting Workflow

Think of some project you're working on; it could be a dance, a picnic, remodeling your bathroom, or a semester schedule of activities in a class.

Assignment: Draw a flowchart, inserting at the bottom the date activities for the event are to be completed. Working backward, insert critical tasks and their completion dates. Refer to your flowchart throughout the project to see if you stay on target.

PITFALLS IN USING DECISION-MAKING TOOLS

Clancy (2003) maintains that there is a strong tendency for managers to favor first impressions when making a decision and a second tendency called confirmation biases often follows. A *confirmation bias* has a tendency to affirm one's initial impression and preferences as other alternatives are evaluated. So even using consequence tables, decision trees and other quantitative decision tools will not guarantee a successful decision.

It is also human nature to focus on an event that leaves a strong impression so individuals may have preconceived notions or biases that influence decisions. Too often managers allow the past to influence current decisions. Lastly, managers often become too confident about their decision making ability and remember their good decisions and forget the negative outcomes that resulted from some of their other decisions (Clancy, 2003).

Minimizing Pitfalls

Many of these pitfalls can be reduced by choosing the correct decision making style and involving others when appropriate. It is not always necessary to involve others in decision making and frequently a manager does not have time to involve a large group, but it is important to separate out decisions needing others from those a manager can make alone.

In addition to quantitative decision technology, management analysts have developed models that assist managers in choosing the correct decision-making style. A manager can be autocratic in making decisions and have little or no input from others or can be democratic and involve others in the process. Some managers develop patterns and use the same methods, rather than looking at the particular situation and then concluding which type of decision making is needed. Vroom and Yetton (1973) developed a useful approach in selecting an appropriate decision-making style. They have identified five decision-making methods (**Table 2.3**).

Variables to Determine Decision-Making Style

Seven situation variables were identified by Vroom (1973). These situation variables determine which of the five decision-making styles is appropriate in a situation (**Table 2.4**).

1. *The information rule.* If the quality of the decision is important and the leader does not possess enough information or expertise to solve the problem by himself or herself, AI is eliminated from the feasible set. (Its use risks a low-quality decision.)
2. *The goal congruence rule.* If the quality of the decision is important and the subordinates do not share the organizational goals to be obtained in solving the problem, GII is eliminated from the feasible set. (Alternatives that eliminate the leader's final control over the decision reached may jeopardize the quality of the decision.)

Table 2.3 Types of Management Decision Styles

A1	You solve the problem or make the decision yourself, using information available to you at that time.
A11	You obtain the necessary information from your subordinate(s), then decide on the solution to the problem yourself. You may or may not tell your subordinates what the problem is when getting the information from them. The role played by your subordinates in making the decision is clearly one of providing the necessary information to you, rather than generating or evaluating alternative solutions.
C1	You share the problem with relevant subordinates individually, getting their ideas and suggestions without bringing them together as a group. Then you make the decision that may or may not reflect your subordinates' influence.
C11	You share the problem with your subordinates as a group, collectively obtaining their ideas and suggestions. Then you make the decision that may or may not reflect your subordinates' influence.
G11	You share a problem with your subordinates as a group. Together you generate and evaluate alternatives and attempt to reach agreement (consensus) on a solution. Your role is much like that of chairman. You do not try to influence the group to adopt "your" solution, and you are willing to accept and implement any solution that has the support of the entire group.

Reprinted by permission of publisher from Organizational Dynamics. Spring 1973. p. 74. New York: American Management Association. All rights reserved.

3. *The unstructured problem rule.* When the quality of the decision is important, if the leader lacks the necessary information or expertise to solve the problem alone, and if the problem is unstructured (i.e., he or she does not know exactly what information is needed and where it is located), the method used must provide a means not only to collect the information, but also to do so in an efficient and effective manner. Methods that involve interaction among all subordinates with full knowledge of the problem are likely to be both more efficient and more likely to generate a high-quality solution to the problem. Under these conditions, AI, AII, and CI are eliminated from the feasible set. (AI does not provide for collection of the necessary information; AII and CI represent more cumbersome, less-effective, and less-efficient means of bringing the necessary information to bear on the solution of the problem than methods that do permit those with the necessary information to interact.)

4. *The acceptance rule.* If the acceptance of the decision by subordinates is critical to effective implementation and it is not certain that an autocratic decision made by the leader would receive that acceptance, AI and AII are eliminated from the feasible set. (Neither provides an opportunity for subordinates to participate in the decision, and both risk the necessary acceptance.)

5. *The conflict rule.* If the acceptance of the decision is critical, an autocratic decision is not certain to be accepted, and/or subordinates are likely to be in

Table 2.4 Problem Attributes Used in the Vroom Decision-Making Model

Problem Attributes	Diagnostic Questions
A. The importance of the quality of the decision	Is there a quality requirement such that one solution is likely to be more rational than another?
B. The extent to which the leader possesses sufficient information/expertise to make a high-quality decision by himself or herself	Do you have sufficient information to make a high-quality decision?
C. The extent to which the problem is structured	Is the problem structured?
D. The extent to which acceptance or commitment on the part of subordinates is critical to the effective implementation of the decision	Is acceptance of the decision by subordinates critical to effective implementation?
E. The prior probability that the leader's autocratic decision will receive acceptance by subordinates	If you were to make the decision by yourself, is it reasonably certain that your subordinates would accept it?
F. The extent to which subordinates are motivated to attain the organizational goals as represented in the objectives explicit in the statement of the problem	Do subordinates share the organizational goals to be obtained in solving this problem?
G. The extent to which subordinates are likely to be in conflict over preferred solution	Is conflict among subordinates likely in preferred solutions?

conflict or disagreement over the appropriate solution, AI, AII, and CI are eliminated from the feasible set. (The method used in solving the problem should enable those who disagree to resolve their differences with full knowledge of the problem. AI, AII, and CI involve no interaction or only "one-on-one" relationships and therefore provide no opportunity for those in conflict to resolve their differences. Their use runs the risk of leaving some of the subordinates with less than the necessary commitment to the final decision.)

6. *The fairness rule.* If the quality of the decision is unimportant and acceptance is critical and not certain to result from an autocratic decision, AI, AII, CI, and CII are eliminated from the feasible set. (The method used should maximize the probability of acceptance because this is the only relevant consideration in determining the effectiveness of the decision. In these circumstances, AI, AII, CI, and CII create less acceptance or commitment than GII. To use them is to run the risk of getting less than the needed acceptance of the decision.)

A. DOES THE PROBLEM POSSESS A QUALITY REQUIREMENT?
B. DO YOU HAVE SUFFICIENT INFORMATION TO MAKE A HIGH-QUALITY DECISION?
C. IS THE PROBLEM STRUCTURED?
D. IS ACCEPTANCE OF DECISION BY SUBORDINATES IMPORTANT FOR EFFECTIVE IMPLEMENTATION?
E. IF YOU WERE TO MAKE THE DECISION BY YOURSELF, IS IT REASONABLY CERTAIN
   THAT IT WOULD BE ACCEPTED BY YOUR SUBORDINATES?
F. DO SUBORDINATES SHARE THE ORGANIZATIONAL GOALS TO BE ATTAINED IN SOLVING THIS PROBLEM?
G. IS CONFLICT AMONG SUBORDINATES OVER PREFERRED SOLUTIONS LIKELY?

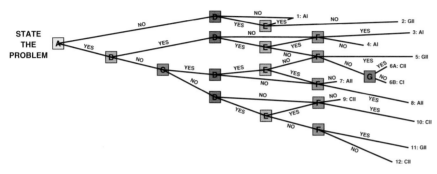

Figure 2.6 Decision tree governing group problems—Model A: Time efficient
(Vroom, Yetton, & Jago, 1976. Reprinted by permission of publisher from Organizational Dynamics.
Spring 1973. p. 74. New York: American Management Association. All rights reserved.)

7. *The acceptance priority rule.* If acceptance is critical and not ensured by an
   autocratic decision, and subordinates can be trusted, AI, AII, CI, and CII
   are eliminated from the feasible set. (Methods that provide equal partnership in the decision-making process can provide greater acceptance without
   risking decision quality. Use of any method other than GII results in an
   unnecessary risk that the decision will not be fully accepted or receive the
   necessary commitment on the part of subordinates.

In later work, Vroom and associates (1976) demonstrated how a decision tree
could assist managers in deciding which decision-making style to use (**Figure 2.6**).
Vroom and Jago (1988) maintain that this model is able to deal with complexities
in situational demands more effectively than either McGregor's Theory Y or Blake
and Mouton's managerial grid, and they demonstrated its mathematical attributes
when the model was revised in the 1980s. Later work also demonstrated the effective use of a modified model for solving individual rather than group decisions.
However, the earlier model is less complex to use and for novice managers provides
a good basis for determining decision-making style appropriate for a manager
working with a group.

MANAGEMENT FUNCTIONS

No clear-cut lists of management functions are found in the current literature.
Kleinman (2003) lists the basic components of management functions to include
planning, organizing, delegating, problem solving, evaluating, and enforcing policies

Display 2.1	**Functions of Management**		
Planning		Empower staff	Satisfy customers
Directing		Maintain quality	Organizing
Problem-solving		Staffing	Delegating
Enforcing policies		Controlling	
and procedures		Evaluating	
Manage day-to-day		Build productive	
operations		work teams	

and procedures. Nurse managers are expected to also manage day-to-day operations, empower staff, build productive work teams, maintain quality, and satisfy customers. However, others describe empowerment as a role for nurse leaders (Tourangeau, 2003; Trent, 2003) See **Display 2.1** for a list of some of the functions of management.

What soon becomes evident in reviewing the literature is that there is some overlap in management functions with leadership roles. It does seem to become increasing clear, however, that management functions are more concerned with the day-to-day activity of the organization and with maintaining the status quo, and therefore stability, for the organization while the role of leadership is more focused on moving the organization forward toward the future and thereby changing the status quo (Trent, 2003).

Throughout this text, leadership and management—the two very necessary elements—are combined. Leadership is not merely one function of management, nor management only one role of leadership. The two are forever symbiotic. However, by artificially separating the two components, leadership roles and management functions, readers can see the differences in the two but also see the need for an integrated leader manager. Zakeznik (2004) maintains that businesses must find ways to train good managers and develop leaders at the same time. Adoption of the integrated leader manager is critical for the healthcare industry.

 Learning Exercise 2.3

Questions on Management
Examine Display 2.1 and then recall your own experiences as a manager or the experiences you have had working for a manager.
Assignment: Write a one-page essay, or discuss in a group, the following questions.
 What functions of management do you feel are the most critical?
 What additional functions of management should be added to this list?
 Do you feel empowering staff is a function of management or a leadership role?

SUMMARY

Management has a unique purpose and outcome that is needed to maintain a healthy organization. The history of management science provides managers with a background into what came before so they are well grounded in the past. Managers continue to use some past theories in coping with management problems today. Since the earliest management studies, theorists have learned much about human behavior; additionally society has changed remarkably, providing current management theorists with new insights and challenges.

However, even today one of the most important functions for the manager remains that of being a successful decision maker. Decision making takes place throughout the management process and is one of the most critical functions of management

The use of management tools and models to guide decision making will assist the manager in making more effective decisions. Although there are many such tools available, the successful manger knows that they are not foolproof and often do not allow for the human element in management. Lastly, the manager is cognizant that selecting the appropriate decision making style will influence the success of the decision making.

☀ Key Concepts

- Management functions include *planning, organizing, staffing, directing, and controlling.* These are incorporated into what is known as the management process.
- Each management function has a planning and controlling phase.
- *Classical*, or *traditional, management science* focused on production in the workplace and on delineating organizational barriers to productivity. Workers were assumed to be motivated solely by economic rewards, and little attention was given to worker job satisfaction.
- The *human relations era of management science* grew out of the Hawthorne studies, which emphasized the needs of the worker for recognition. Concepts of participatory and humanistic management emerged during this era.
- Management science has produced many tools to assist in management decision making but all are subject to human error.
- Selecting an appropriate decision making style is critical in decision making.
- Management functions are not clear cut and are sometimes merged with leadership roles.

More Learning Exercises and Applications

These exercises may be discussed individually or in groups, or used as written assignments.

Learning Exercise 2.4

What's Your Management Style?
Recall times when you have been a manager. This does not only mean a nursing manager. Perhaps you were a head lifeguard or an evening shift manager at a fast-food restaurant. During those times, do you think you were a good manager? Did you involve others in your management decision making appropriately? How would you evaluate your decision-making ability? What style of decision-making (from the Vroom and Yetton model) did you use?
Assignment: Make a list of your management strengths and make a list of management skills that you felt you were lacking.

Using the decision-making guidelines developed by Vroom and Yetton, decide what type of decision-making style should be selected for Learning Exercises 2.5, 2.6, and 2.7.

Learning Exercise 2.5

What's Your Decision Making Style?
You are the manager of a 30-bed medical unit. After consultation, you recently implemented a system for incorporating nursing diagnoses on the patient care plans. Although the system was expected to reduce report time between shifts and improve the quality of patient care, to everyone's surprise, including your own, you find that the system is not working. You do not think there is anything wrong with your idea. Many other hospitals in the areas are using nursing diagnoses with success. You had a consultant come from another hospital and give an update to your nurses on use of the system. The consultant reported that your staff seemed knowledgeable and appeared to understand their responsibilities in implementing the system. You suspect that a few nurses might be sabotaging your efforts for planned change, but your charge nurses do not agree; they believe the failure may be lack of proper incentives or poor staff morale.

Your nursing administrator is anxious to implement the system in other patient care units but wants it to be working well in your unit first. You have just come from a manager's meeting where your administrator told you to solve the problem and report back to her within one week regarding the steps you had taken to solve your problem. You share your administrator's concern, but how should you solve this problem? Select the most appropriate decision style.

Learning Exercise 2.6

Who Should Go?
You are the evening shift charge nurse of the intensive care unit. Your supervisor is sending two nurses from each shift to an upcoming critical care conference in a nearby city. The supervisor wants each charge nurse to submit names of the selected nurses in two weeks. All 12 of the full-time evening shift nurses would like to go. From a staffing standpoint, any of them could go. All are active in the local critical care organization. Financial resources, however, limit your choice to two. How do you resolve this situation? Select the most appropriate decision style.

Learning Exercise 2.7

Gathering the Facts—Stat!
You are the day shift charge nurse on a surgical unit. Because of your related expertise, your supervisor has asked you to select a new type of blood-warming unit. You want to be sure that you select the right one. Several companies have provided your staff with trial units. You have not received much feedback from the staff regarding their preferences. Today, your supervisor tells you that your selection and its price must be ready to accompany her budget, which is due in two days. What do you do? Select the most appropriate decision style.

Learning Exercise 2.8

Teamwork in Hiring
Six nurses have just applied for a position in the open heart unit. Working with a group, develop an appropriate decision grid for selecting which nurse to hire. Identify six criteria for hiring. You may give each criterion weighted points so that the decision is a quantitative solution. For example, level of education could be weighted 5 to 10 points and experience, 10 to 30 points.

Web Links

Guide to project management research sites:
http://www.amanet.org/index.htm
A Web site of the American Management Associates. They offer many free learning resources.

Management Skills and Development: Interview with Warren Bennis.
http://www.managementskills.co.uk/articles.htm (under Leadership)
An interview with Leadership theorist Warren Bennis.

References

Argyris, C. (1964). *Integrating the individual and the organization*. New York: John Wiley and Sons.
Clancy, T. R. (2003). The art of decision-making. *Journal of Nursing Administration, 33*(6), 343–349.
Fayol, H. (1925). *General and industrial management*. London: Pittman and Sons.
Follett, M. P. (1926). The giving of orders. In H. C. Metcalf (Ed.), *Scientific foundations of business administration*. Baltimore: Williams & Wilkins.
Gulick, L. (1937). Notes on the theory of the organization. In L. Gulick & L. Urwick (Eds.), *Papers on the science of administration (pp. 3–13)*. New York: Institute of Public Administration.
Kleinman, C. S. (2003). Leadership roles, competencies, and education. *Journal of Nursing Administration, 33*(9), 451–455.
Mayo, E. (1953). *The human problems of an industrialized civilization*. New York: Macmillan.
McGregor, D. (1960). *The human side of enterprise*. New York: McGraw-Hill.
Meltzer, W. (1999). Time and motion study of total hip replacement: A tool to improve surgical team performance. Presented at the Annual Meeting of American Academy of Orthopaedic Surgeons in Anaheim, CA, February. Report found at *http://www.aaos.org/wordhtml/anmeet99/sciexh/se054.htm* on 07/25/2001.
Russell, V. C. (2000). Working smart. *Journal of Management in Engineering, 16*(6), 5.
Taylor, F. W. (1911). *The principles of scientific management*. New York: Harper & Row.
Trent, B. A. (2003). Leadership myths. *Reflections on Nursing Leadership, 29*(3), 8–9.
Tourangeau, A. E. (2003). Building nurse leader capacity. *Journal of Nursing Administration, 33*(12), 624–626.
Vroom, V. H. (1973). A new look at managerial decision-making: Organizational decision-making. *Organizational Dynamics*, 1(4), 66–80.
Vroom, V., & Jago, A. G. (1988). *The new leadership*. Englewood Cliffs, NJ: Prentice Hall.
Vroom, V., & Yetton, P. W. (1973). *Leadership and decision-making*. Pittsburgh: University of Pittsburgh Press.
Vroom, V., Yetton, P. W., & Jago, A. G. (1976). *Leadership and decision making: Cases and manuals for use in leadership training* (3rd ed.). New Haven, CT: Authors.
Zakeznik, A. (2004). Managers and leaders: Are they different? *Harvard Business Review, 82*(1), 74–81, 113.

Bibliography

Boswell, J. (2001). The missing link. *Nursing Management, 32*(5), 34.
Connelly, L. M. (2003). A qualitative study of charge nurse competencies. *Medical Surgical Nursing, 12*(5), 298–306.
Curran, C. R. (2000). Musings on managerial excellence. *Nursing Economic$, 15*(6), 277.

Grindel, C. G. (2003). Mentoring managers. *Nephrology Nursing Journal, 30*(5), 517–522.

Lord, R. G. (2000). Thinking outside the box by looking inside the box. *Leadership Quarterly, 11*(4), 551–580.

Middaugh, D. J. (2001). The physics of management. *Medical Surgical Nursing, 13*(4), 268–269.

Ohman, K. A. (2000). Critical care managers, change views, change lives. *Nursing Management, 31*(9), 32–35.

Seden, J. (2003). Managing mistakes and challenges. *Journal of Nursing Management (London), 10*(5), 26–29.

Thomas, D. O. (2003). Management decisions help line. *RN, 66*(10), 26.

Thompson, J. (2003). What perioperative and emerging work force nurses want in a manager. *Journal of American Operating Room Nurses, 78*(2), 246–249, 252–256.

Zimmermann, P. G. (2003). Advice for the new manager. *Journal of Clinical Systems Management, 1*(8/9), 10.

3

Developing Leadership

Leadership is leading.

—*Geraldine Bednash*

The need to develop nursing leadership skills has never been greater as reform of health care is being addressed at national, state, and community levels. Leadership skills also are necessary for team building at the organizational level. Ensuring successful recruitment, retaining a cohesive nursing staff, and maintaining a high-quality practice depend on successful team building.

The last 15 years have seen several national trends that have impacted health care. First, the increase in managed care, aimed at slowing escalation of national healthcare costs, has resulted in redesign of most healthcare organizations. Second, a shift in the locus of care has occurred, from acute hospitals to community and outpatient sites. Third, there has also been a shift from episodic care to preventive or restorative care. Lastly, the workplace is increasingly driven by innovation and technological transformation. In this fast-paced demanding environment, nurse leaders must cultivate the financial and political skills to be innovative. All of these changes have brought about a need for leaders to learn new roles and develop new skills (Porter-O'Grady, 2003).

To examine the word *leader* is to note that leaders lead. They are in the front, moving forward, taking risks, and challenging the status quo. Although leadership is clearly different from management, leadership and management are of equal importance. Trent (2003) maintains that leadership requires collaborators, but it is not a mystical process and can be performed by anyone with the appropriate resources.

DIFFERENCES BETWEEN LEADERSHIP AND MANAGEMENT

A job title alone does not make a person a leader. Only a person's behavior determines if he or she occupies a leadership position. The manager is the person who brings things about; the one who accomplishes, has the responsibility, and conducts. A leader is the person who influences and guides direction, opinion, and course of action.

What, then are some of the characteristics of leaders? **Leaders**:

- Often do not have delegated authority but obtain their power through other means, such as influence
- Have a wider variety of roles than do managers
- May or may not be part of the formal organization
- Focus on group process, information gathering, feedback, and empowering others
- Emphasize interpersonal relationships
- Direct willing followers
- Have goals that may or may not reflect those of the organization

Much greater emphasis has been placed on leadership skills in the last decade. Indeed, Bednash (2003) maintains that presently leadership is the issue of the day, not only in nursing but also in society as a whole. Leadership means getting very clear about your values, taking risks, and having a willingness to seek partners and collaborators who will commit to the common good.

Learning Exercise 3.1

Management Functions and Leadership Skills
In small or large groups, discuss your views of management and leadership. Do you believe they are the same or different? If you believe they are different, do you think they have the same importance for the future of nursing? How can novice nurse managers learn important management functions and develop leadership skills? How do they become integrated leader–managers?

HISTORICAL DEVELOPMENT OF LEADERSHIP THEORY

Thousands of books and articles, representing widely varying schools of thought, have been published on the topic of leadership. To summarize what is known about this topic in one chapter is impossible. Instead, an effort is made to introduce the idea that leadership theory is dynamic; that is, what is "known" and believed about leadership has changed considerably during the last hundred years and will continue to change in the future. Instead, conceptual definitions of leadership, the evolution of leadership theory, and contemporary theories of leadership are presented.

Defining Leadership

Although the term *leader* has been in use since the 1300s, the word *leadership* was not known in the English language until the first half of the 19th century. Despite its relatively new addition to the English language, leadership has many meanings. From Chapin's (1924) technical definition of leadership as a point of polarization for group cooperation to Bednash's (2003) assertion that "leadership is a vital component of change," (p. 258) it becomes clear that there is no single definition broad enough to encompass the total leadership process.

Leadership can occur outside of an organizational context and has been defined as the process of moving a group or groups in some direction through mostly non-coercive means. Gardner (1990) defined leadership as "the process of persuasion and example by which an individual (or leadership team) induces a group to pursue objectives held by the leader or shared by the leader and his or her followers" (p. 1). Bennis (2001) says that the leader makes a vision so palpable and seductive that others eagerly sign on. Tourangeau (2003) used a broader definition stating that "leaders are those who challenge the process, inspire a shared vision, enable others to act, model the way, and encourage the heart" (p. 625).

Because leadership researchers and theorists do not agree on exactly what leadership is, it is perhaps wiser to focus on what roles are inherent in leadership. **Display 3.1** lists some of a leader's roles.

Display 3.1	Leadership Roles	
Decision maker	Coach	Forecaster
Communicator	Counselor	Influencer
Evaluator	Teacher	Creative problem solver
Facilitator	Critical thinker	Change agent
Risk taker	Buffer	Diplomat
Mentor	Advocate	Role model
Energizer	Visionary	

Learning Exercise 3.2

Roles of a Leader
In groups or individually, add roles to the list in Display 3.1 that you believe are examples of what a leader does. Of the previously listed leadership roles, or others you have formulated, how many are also recognized as nursing roles?

EVOLUTION OF LEADERSHIP THEORY

The scientific study of leadership began in the 20th century. Early works focused on broad conceptualizations of leadership, such as the traits or behaviors of the leader. Contemporary research focuses more on leadership as a process of influencing others within an organizational culture and the interactive relationship of the leader and follower. To understand better today's beliefs about leadership, it is necessary to look at how leadership theory has evolved during the last century.

> Early leadership definitions focused on the traits or behaviors of leaders; contemporary definitions focus more on leadership as a process of influencing and interacting with others within an organizational culture.

Great Man Theory and Trait Theories

The great man theory and trait theories were the basis for most leadership research until the mid-1940s. The great man theory, from Aristotelian philosophy, asserts that some people are born to lead, whereas others are born to be led. Trait theories assume that some people have certain characteristics or personality traits that make them better leaders than others. To determine the traits that distinguish great leaders, researchers studied the lives of prominent people throughout history. The effect of followers and the impact of the situation were ignored. Contemporary opponents of these theories argue that leadership skills can be developed, and are not necessarily inborn. Trent (2003) states that scientific inquiry has proved these theories not valid and maintains that leadership requires collaborators more than charisma.

Although trait theories have obvious shortcomings (e.g., they neglect the impact of others or the situation on the leadership role), they are worth examining. Many of the characteristics identified in trait theories (**Display 3.2**) are still used to describe successful leaders today.

Learning Exercise 3.3

Leaders' Skills and Characteristics
In groups or individually, list additional characteristics you believe an effective leader possesses. Which leadership characteristics do you have? Do you believe you were born with leadership skills, or have you consciously developed them during your lifetime? If so, how did you develop them?

Behavioral Theories

During the human relations era, many behavioral and social scientists studying management also studied leadership. For example, McGregor's (1960) theories had as much influence on leadership research as they did on management science. As leadership theory developed, researchers moved away from studying the traits of the leader and placed emphasis on what he or she did—the leader's style of leadership. A major breakthrough occurred when Lewin (1951) and White and Lippitt (1960) isolated common leadership styles. Later, these styles came to be called authoritarian, democratic, and laissez-faire.

The following behaviors characterize *authoritarian* leaders:

- Strong control is maintained over the work group.
- Others are motivated by coercion.
- Others are directed with commands.
- Communication flows downward.
- Decision making does not involve others.
- Emphasis is on difference in status ("I" and "you").
- Criticism is punitive.

Authoritarian leadership results in well-defined group actions that are usually predictable, reducing frustration in the work group and giving members a feeling of security. Productivity is usually high, but creativity, self-motivation, and autonomy

Display 3.2	**Characteristics of a Leader**	
Intelligence	Personable	Ability
Knowledge	Adaptability	Able to enlist cooperation
Judgement	Creativity	Interpersonal skills
Decisiveness	Cooperativeness	Tact
Oral fluency	Alertness	Diplomacy
Emotional Intelligence	Self-confidence	Prestige
Independence	Personal integrity	Social participation
	Emotional balance and control	Nonconformity

are reduced. Authoritarian leadership, useful in crisis situations, is frequently found in very large bureaucracies, such as the armed forces.

Democratic leaders are characterized by the following:

- Less control is maintained.
- Economic and ego awards are used to motivate.
- Others are directed through suggestions and guidance.
- Communication flows up and down.
- Decision making involves others.
- Emphasis is on "we" rather than "I" and "you."
- Criticism is constructive.

Democratic leadership, appropriate for groups that work together for extended periods, promotes autonomy and growth in individual workers. This type of leadership is particularly effective when cooperation and coordination between groups are necessary. Because many people must be consulted, democratic leadership takes more time and, therefore, may be frustrating for those who want decisions made rapidly. Studies have shown that democratic leadership is less efficient quantitatively than authoritative leadership.

The *laissez-faire leader* is characterized by the following behaviors:

- Permissiveness, with little or no control.
- Motivation by support when requested by the group or individuals.
- Provision of little or no direction.
- Communication upward and downward flow among members of the group.
- Decision making dispersed throughout the group.
- Emphasis on the group.
- Criticism withheld.

Because it is nondirected leadership, the laissez-faire leadership style can be frustrating; group apathy and disinterest can occur. However, when all group members are highly motivated and self-directed, this leadership style can result in much creativity and productivity. Laissez-faire leadership is appropriate when problems are poorly defined and brainstorming is needed to generate alternative solutions.

A person's leadership style has a great deal of influence on the climate and outcome of the work group. For some time, theorists believed that leaders had a predominant leadership style and used it consistently. During the late 1940s and early 1950s, however, theorists began to believe that most leaders did not fit a textbook picture of any one style, but rather fell somewhere on a continuum between authoritarian and laissez-faire. They also came to believe that leaders moved dynamically along the continuum in response to each new situation. This recognition was a forerunner to what is known as situational or contingency leadership theory.

Situational and Contingency Leadership Theories

The idea that leadership style should vary according to the situation or the employees involved was first suggested almost a hundred years ago by Mary

Learning Exercise 3.4

What's Your Leadership Style?
Define your leadership style. Ask those who work with you if in their honest opinion this is indeed your leadership style. What style of leadership do you work best under? What leadership style best describes your present or former managers?

Parker Follett. Follett was one of the earliest management consultants and among the first to view an organization as a social system of contingencies. Her ideas, published in a series of books between 1896 and 1933, were so far ahead of their time that they did not gain appropriate recognition in the literature until the 1970s. Follett (1926) stressed the need for "integration," which involved finding a solution that satisfied both sides without having one side dominate the other. Her "law of the situation," which said that the situation should determine the directives given after allowing everyone to know the problem, was contingency leadership in its humble origins.

Fiedler's (1967) contingency approach reinforced these findings, suggesting that no one leadership style is ideal for every situation. Fiedler felt that the interrelationships between the group's leader and its members were most influenced by the manager's ability to be a good leader. The task to be accomplished and the power associated with the leader's position also were cited as key variables.

In contrast to the continuum from autocratic to democratic, Blake and Mouton's (1964) grid showed various combinations of concern or focus that managers had for or on productivity, tasks, people, and relationships. In each of these areas, the leader–manager may rank high or low, resulting in numerous combinations of leadership behaviors. Various formations can be effective depending on the situation and the needs of the worker.

Hersey and Blanchard (1977) also developed a situational approach to leadership. Their tri-dimensional leadership effectiveness model predicts which leadership style is most appropriate in each situation based on the level of the followers' maturity. As people mature, leadership style becomes less task focused and more relationship oriented.

Tannenbaum and Schmidt (1958) built on the work of Lewin and White, suggesting that managers need varying mixtures of autocratic and democratic leadership behavior. They believed that the primary determinants of leadership style should include the nature of the situation, the skills of the manager, and the abilities of the group members.

CONTEMPORARY THEORIES OF LEADERSHIP

Although situational and contingency theories added necessary complexity to leadership theory and continue to be applied effectively by managers, by the late

1970s, theorists began arguing that effective leadership depended on an even greater number of variables. These variables included organizational culture, the values of the leader and the followers, the work, the environment, the influence of the leader–manager, and the complexities of the situation. Efforts to integrate these variables are apparent in contemporary interactional and transformational leadership theories.

Interactional Leadership Theories

The basic premise of *interactional theory* is that leadership behavior is generally determined by the relationship between the leader's personality and the specific situation. Schein (1970) was the first to propose a model of humans as complex beings whose working environment was an open system to which they responded. A *system* may be defined as a set of objects, with relationships between the objects and between their attributes. A system is considered open if it exchanges matter, energy, or information with its environment. Schein's model, based on systems theory, had the following assumptions:

- People are very complex and highly variable. They have multiple motives for their actions. For example, a pay raise might mean status to one person, security to another, and both to a third.
- People's motives do not stay constant but change over time.
- Goals can differ in various situations. For example, an informal group's goals may be quite distinct from a formal group's goals.
- A person's performance and productivity are affected by the nature of the task and by his or her ability, experience, and motivation.
- No single leadership strategy is effective in every situation.

To be successful, the leader must diagnose the situation and select appropriate strategies from a large repertoire of skills. Hollander (1978) was among the first to recognize that both leaders and followers have roles outside the leadership situation and that both may be influenced by events occurring in their other roles. With leader and follower contributing to the working relationship and both receiving something from it, Hollander saw leadership as a dynamic two-way process. According to Hollander, a leadership exchange involves three basic elements:

- The leader, including his or her personality, perceptions, and abilities
- The followers, with their personalities, perceptions, and abilities
- The situation within which the leader and the followers function, including formal and informal group norms, size, and density

Leadership effectiveness, according to Hollander, requires the ability to use the problem-solving process; maintain group effectiveness; communicate well; demonstrate leader fairness, competence, dependability, and creativity; and develop group identification.

Greenleaf (1977) coined the term *servant leadership*. In more than four decades of working as Director of Leadership Development at AT&T, he noticed that most successful managers lead in a different way from traditional managers. The managers he termed servant leaders put serving others, including employees, customers, and the community, as their first priority. These successful managers shared certain defining qualities, including:

* The ability to listen on a deep level and to truly understand
* The ability to keep an open mind and hear without judgment
* The ability to deal with ambiguity, paradoxes, and complex issues
* The belief that honestly sharing critical challenges with all parties and asking for their input is more important than personally providing solutions
* Being clear on goals and good at pointing the direction without giving orders
* The ability to serve, help, and teach first, and then lead
* Always thinking before reacting
* Choosing words carefully so as not to damage those being led
* The ability to use foresight and intuition
* Seeing things whole and sensing relationships and connections

More recently Greenleaf's work has attracted new attention, especially in the healthcare industry. Scholars are showing an interest in adapting Greenleaf's work to explore the importance of values and trust in work relationships, and the impact that values, leadership, and trust have on work productivity and organizational climate (Bennett, 2001).

One of the pioneering leadership theorists of this time was Kanter (1977) who developed the theory that the structural aspects of the job shape a leader's effectiveness. She postulated that the leader becomes empowered through both formal and informal systems of the organization. A leader must develop relationships with a variety of people and groups within the organization in order to maximize job empowerment and be successful. The three major work empowerment structures within the organization are opportunity, power, and proportion. Kanter asserts these work structures have the potential to explain differences in leader responses, behaviors, and attitudes in the work environment.

Ouchi (1981) was a pioneer in introducing interactional leadership theory in his application of Japanese-style management to corporate America. *Theory Z,* the term Ouchi used for this type of management, is an expansion of McGregor's Theory Y and supports democratic leadership. Characteristics of Theory Z include consensus decision making, fitting employees to their jobs, job security, slower promotions, examining the long-term consequences of management decision making, quality circles, guarantee of lifetime employment, establishment of strong bonds of responsibility between superiors and subordinates, and a holistic concern for the workers. Ouchi was able to find components of Japanese-style management in many successful American companies. In the 1990s, Theory Z lost favor with many management theorists. Although Theory Z is more comprehensive than many of the earlier theories, it too neglects some of the variables that influence leadership effectiveness. It has the same shortcomings as situational theories in inadequately recognizing the dynamics of the interaction between worker and leader.

Nelson and Burns (1984) suggested that organizations and their leaders have four developmental levels and that these levels influence productivity and worker satisfaction. The first of these levels is *reactive*. The reactive leader focuses on the past, is crisis-driven, and is frequently abusive to subordinates. In the next level, *responsive*, the leader is able to mold subordinates to work together as a team, although the leader maintains most decision-making responsibility. At the *proactive* level, the leader and followers become more future-oriented and hold common driving values. Management and decision making are more participative. At the last level, *high-performance teams* (associated with maximum productivity) and worker satisfaction are apparent.

Brandt's (1994) interactive leadership model suggests that leaders develop a work environment that fosters autonomy and creativity through valuing and empowering followers. This leadership *affirms the uniqueness of each individual*, motivating them to *contribute their unique talents to a common goal*. The leader must accept the responsibility for quality of outcomes and quality of life for followers. Brandt states that this type of leadership affords the leader greater freedom while simultaneously adding to the burdens of leadership. The leader's responsibilities increase because priorities cannot be limited to the organization's goals, and authority confers not only power, but also responsibility and obligation. The leader's concern for each worker decreases the need for competition and fosters an atmosphere of collegiality, freeing the leader from the burden of having to resolve follower conflicts. Leaders in this model would understand what Drucker (1992) meant by his belief that leadership is a responsibility rather than a rank or privilege.

Wolf, Boland, and Aukerman (1994) also emphasized an interactive leadership model in their creation of a *collaborative practice matrix*. This matrix highlights the framework for the development and ongoing support of relationships between and among professionals working together. The *social architecture* of the work group is emphasized, as is how expectations, personal values, and interpersonal relationships affect the ability of leaders and followers to achieve the vision of the organization.

Kanter (1989) perhaps best summarized the work of the interactive theorists by her assertion that title and position authority were no longer sufficient to mold a work force where subordinates are encouraged to think for themselves, and instead managers must learn to work synergistically with others.

Transformational Leadership

A noted scholar in the area of leader–follower interactions, Burns (1978) was among the first to suggest that both leaders and followers have the ability to raise each other to higher levels of motivation and morality. Identifying this concept as transformational leadership, Burns maintained that there are two types of leaders in

> **Learning Exercise 3.5**
>
> **Which Theory Do You Identify With?**
> There are many theories of how the work environment, the leader, and the worker all interact together. Which of the above interactional theorists most closely reflects your views on what happens in the workplace to influence leadership effectiveness?
> **Assignment:** Research one of these theorists in greater depth. Use Internet resources or the library for your research. Either write a short essay on the individual or share your findings in class.

Vision is the essence of transformational leadership. Vision implies the ability to picture some future state and describe it to others so they will begin "to share the dream." This new shared vision provides the energy required to move an organizational unit toward the future.

management. The traditional manager, concerned with the day-to-day operations, was termed a *transactional leader;* the manager, on the other hand, who is committed, has a vision, and is able to empower others with this vision was termed a *transformational leader*. A composite of the two different types of leaders is shown in **Table 3.1.**

Wolf et al. (1994) define transformational leadership as "an interactive relationship, based on trust, that positively impacts both the leader and the follower. The purposes of the leader and follower become focused, creating unity, wholeness and collective purpose" (p. 38). The high-performing transformational leader demonstrates a strong commitment to the profession and the organization and is willing to tackle obstacles using group learning. This self-confidence comes from a strong sense of being in control. These transformational leaders also are able to create synergistic environments that enhance change. Change occurs because the transformational leader's futuristic focus values creativity and innovation. The transformational leader also holds organizational culture, behaviors, and values in high regard, perpetuating these values and behaviors in the staff (Wolf, Boland, & Aukerman, 1994).

Tyrrell (1994) identifies *visioning* as a mark of the transformational leader, stating that "nurses at all levels are expected to demonstrate leadership in setting direction for nursing practice, and that visionary leadership allows nurses to create

Table 3.1 Comparing Transactional and Transformational Leaders

Transactional Leader	Transformational Leader
Focuses on management tasks	Identifies common values
Is a caretaker	Is committed
Uses trade-offs to meet goals	Inspires others with vision
Does not identify shared values	Has long-term vision
Examines causes	Looks at effects
Uses contingency reward	Empowers others

Table 3.2 Leadership Theorists and Theories

Theorist	Theory
Aristotle	Great man theory
Lewin and White	Leadership styles
Follett	Law of the situation
Fiedler	Contingency leadership
Blake and Mouton	Task versus relationship in determining leadership style
Hersey and Blanchard	Situational leadership theory
Tannenbaum and Schmidt	Situational leadership theory
Selznick	Leadership as part of the organization
Kanter	Formal and informal organizational structures influence leaders empowerment
Greenleaf	Servant leadership
Burns	Transactional and transformational leadership
Tyrrell	Visioning in transformational leadership
Gardner	The integrated leader–manager

a picture of an ideal future. In sharing these visions, the transformational leader empowers staff to find common ground and a sense of connection" (p. 93).

Although the transformational leader is held as the current ideal, many management theorists, including Bass, Avoliio, and Goodheim (1987) and Dunham and Klafehn (1990), sound a warning about transformational leadership. Although transformational qualities are highly desirable, they must be coupled with the more traditional transactional qualities of the day-to-day managerial role. Both sets of characteristics need to be present in the same person in varying degrees. According to Bass et al., the transformational leader will fail without traditional management skills.

Bennis (1989) sounds a different warning about the quest for transformational leadership in his assertion that "there is an unconscious conspiracy in contemporary society that prevents leaders—no matter what their original vision—from taking charge and making changes" (p. xii). Bennis elaborates by pointing out that entrenched bureaucracy and a commitment to the status quo undermine leaders and that tensions between individual rights and the common good discourage the emergence of leaders. It is critical, then, to remember that the organization and the environment play a critical role in the development and support of the transformational and transactional leadership skills of its employees. The relationship must be symbiotic. **Table 3.2** summarizes the development of leadership theory presented in this chapter.

LEADERSHIP AND MANAGEMENT FOR NURSING'S FUTURE

Seemingly insurmountable problems, a lack of resources to solve those problems, and individual apathy have been and will continue to be issues nurse leaders–managers face. The downsizing of much of corporate America has resulted in a redesign of organizations. However, redesigned organizations will fail unless management is first reengineered. If managers fail to change their mindsets, attitudes, and behaviors, then the restructuring will not be successful.

Effective leadership is one of the most elusive keys to organizational success. Snow (2001) asks that nurses examine leadership development in other industries and states that nursing lags behind many other industries in teaching and supporting research-based leadership theory that is linked to performance. She maintains that successful companies put a premium on the importance of leadership and do a better job of selecting and developing their leaders. For example Snow (2001) says successful companies:

- Are more satisfied with the quality of their leadership.
- Place more value on leadership development.
- Are less tolerant of inappropriate leadership behaviors.
- More frequently use competency models and developmental programs in selecting and advancing their leaders.
- Have leaders who are perceived as possessing emotional intelligence.

Becoming better leader–managers begins with a basic understanding of what leadership is and how these skills can best be developed. The problem is that the skills needed to be an effective leader are dynamic and change constantly in response to the rapidly changing world in which we live. It is clear by looking at the evolution of leadership theory that what is considered effective or desirable leadership has changed virtually from decade to decade. Servant leadership, transformational leadership, interactional leadership theories, the learning organization, and reengineering management have been some of the recent ideas and theories to define and explain the complex role of the successful leader–manager. Will these strategies still be considered the answer to our problems in the next 10 years? The answer to this question is, probably not.

New Leadership Concepts

Already in the 21st century several new leadership concepts have emerged including the leader–manager's need for emotional intelligence as a means to achieve organizational goals.

Emotional Intelligence

Emotional intelligence (EI) is the process of regulating both feelings and expressions. Organizationally desired emotions are considered the standards of behavior that indicate which emotions are appropriate in each relationship and how these emotions should be publicly expressed or displayed. Theorists studying EI posit that it is a critical ingredient of leaders, which enables them to build a cooperative and effective team. Leaders with EI possess the ability to identify emotions in themselves and others, use emotions in their thought processes, manage emotions in themselves and others, and understand and reason with emotions (Vitello-Cicciu, 2003).

Cultural Bridges

A new role of leader–managers as a *cultural bridge* has become a requirement as our society becomes more diverse. The leader–manager must become culturally sensitive and assist staff when cultural misunderstandings occur. These misunderstandings and miscommunications can occur with patients, among staff members, and practicing physicians. Among other things, culture may affect how we motivate individuals, determine what patients want to be told, and how much is understood (de Ruiter and Saphiere, 2001).

Influence of Followers on Leaders

Leaders need to be aware of their followers' influence. Citing numerous recent news events (corporate fraud, the Challenger disaster, etc.) Offermann (2004) demonstrates how followers influence leaders in both positive and negative ways. There is no guarantee that followers will not mislead leaders, but adhering to certain principles will guard against this happening. By keeping vision and values front and center, cultivating truth tellers, honoring one's intuition, making sure people around you are allowed to disagree, setting a good ethical climate and delegating appropriately, the leader creates an atmosphere in which follower influence will result in positive and rather than negative outcomes (Offermann, 2004).

Recognition and Management of Flaws

Kellerman (2004) maintains that in this age of leadership development, theorists have concluded that leaders are always good, when in reality, flawed leaders are to be found everywhere. There is a need to remind ourselves that leaders are like the rest of us. Leaders may be deceitful and trustworthy, greedy and generous, cowardly and brave. To assume that all good leaders are good people is foolhardy and makes us blind to the human condition. It is only when we recognize and manage our failings that leaders achieve greatness (Kellerman, 2004). Future leadership theory may well focus on why leaders behave badly and why followers continue to follow bad leaders.

Concepts and Questions for Future Leadership

Obviously much is to be learned about the complexities of leadership. Porter-O'Grady (2003) states that the changing times have given leaders a more demanding and vital role to play in health care. The future raises many questions that remain to be answered:

> The challenging and changing healthcare system requires that all nurses use all the resources available to them to develop their leadership skills.

- If societal, group, organizational, and individual values conflict, what goals or objectives should guide the leader and his or her followers?
- What other variables that we have not even begun to consider may yet be a critical factor in understanding leadership?
- Must all followers be empowered? Should all followers be empowered?
- What safeguards should be used so that "shared vision" does not represent "group think," whereby all group members think alike?
- Can and should leader accountability be formalized? If so, how?

Gardner (1990) states, "We have barely scratched the surface in our efforts toward leadership development. In the mid-21st century, people will look back on our present practices as primitive" (p. xv). It is imperative, then, that nurse leader–managers not only actively pursue leadership development, but also make every effort possible to remain current in their understanding and application of contemporary leadership principles.

Kerfoot (2000) expands on this idea by stating that healthcare organizations have been *managing* only well enough to maintain the status quo, but have not been *leading* to build new models of supporting healthcare environments. New models must be developed in which the destiny of the organization is shared so that both the individual and the organization grow.

INTEGRATING LEADERSHIP AND MANAGEMENT SKILLS

In examining leadership and management, it becomes clear that these two concepts have a symbiotic or synergistic relationship. For managers and leaders to function at their greatest potential, the two must be integrated. Every nurse is a leader and manager at some level, and the nursing role requires leadership and management skills. The need for visionary leaders and effective managers in nursing precludes the option of stressing one role over the other. Because rapid, dramatic change will continue in nursing and the healthcare industry, it has grown increasingly important for nurses to develop skill in leadership roles and management functions. **Display 3.3** identifies distinguishing traits of the integrated leader–manager.

Display 3.3	**Characteristics of an Integrated Leader–Manager**

Nurses must strive for the integration of leadership characteristics throughout every phase of the management process. Six distinguishing traits of integrated leader–managers include the following:

1. They think longer term. They are visionary and futuristic. They consider the effect that decisions will have years from now as well as immediately.
2. They look outward, toward the larger organization. They do not become narrowly focused. They understand how their unit or department fits into the bigger picture.
3. They influence others beyond their own group. Effective leader–managers rise above an organization's bureaucratic boundaries.
4. They emphasize vision, values, and motivation. They understand intuitively the unconscious and often non-rational aspects of interactions with others. They are very sensitive to others and to differences in each situation.
5. They are politically astute. They can cope with conflicting requirements and expectations from their many constituencies.
6. They think in terms of change and renewal. The traditional manager accepts the structure and processes of the organization, but the leader–manager examines the ever-changing reality of the world and seeks to revise the organization to keep pace.

Source: Gardner, J. W. (1990). *On leadership.* New York: The Free Press.

Leadership and management skills can and should be integrated as they are learned. This union can best occur by (1) using experiential learning exercises designed to increase whole-brain thinking, (2) demonstrating the leadership component in all management functions, and (3) using a scientific approach to problem solving.

❋ Key Concepts

- Three primary forms of leadership styles have been identified: *authoritarian, democratic,* and *laissez-faire.*
- Research has shown that the leader–manager must assume a variety of leadership styles, depending on the needs of the worker, the task to be performed, and the situation or environment. This is known as *situational* or *contingency leadership theory.*
- Management and leadership have distinct differences and similarities and overlapping skills.
- There is a critical need for leadership development in nursing.
- *Leadership* is a process of persuading and influencing others toward a goal and is composed of a wide variety of roles.
- Early leadership theories focused on the traits and characteristics of leaders.
- *Servant leadership* is a leadership model that puts serving others as the first priority.
- Contemporary research focuses more on leadership as a process of influencing others within an organizational culture and the interactive relationship of the leader and follower.
- The basic premise of *interactional theory* is that leadership behavior is generally determined by the relationship between the leader's personality and the specific situation.
- The manager who is committed, has a vision, and is able to empower others with this vision is termed a *transformational leader.*
- The traditional manager, concerned with the day-to-day operations, is called a *transactional leader.*
- Transformational leaders and followers have the ability to raise each other to higher levels of motivation and morality.
- The organization and the environment play critical roles in the development and support of the transformational and transactional leadership skills of its employees.
- Integrating leadership skills with the ability to carry out management functions is necessary if an individual is to become an effective leader–manager.
- A new emerging role for a leader–manager is the role of cultural bridge.
- *Emotional intelligence* is required by leader–managers in order to enhance their success.

More Learning Exercises and Applications

These exercises may be discussed individually or in groups, or used as written assignments.

 Learning Exercise 3.6

When Culture and Policy Clash
You are the nurse manager of a medical unit. Recently your unit admitted a 16-year-old East Indian boy, newly diagnosed with type 2 (insulin-dependent) diabetes. The nursing staff has been interested in his case and has found him a delightful young man, very polite and easygoing. However, his family has been coming in increasing numbers and bringing him food that he should not have.

The nursing staff have come to you on two occasions and complained about the family's noncompliance with visiting hours and unauthorized food. Normally the nursing staff on your unit has tried to develop a culturally sensitive nursing care plan for patients with special cultural needs, so their complaints have taken you by surprise.

Yesterday two of the family members visited you and complained about hospital visitor policies and what they took to be rudeness by two different staff members. You spent time talking to the family and when they left they seemed agreeable and understanding.

Last night one of the staff nurses told the family that according to hospital policy only two members could stay (this is true) and if the other family members did not leave she would call hospital security. This morning the boy's mother and father suggest that they will take him home if this matter is not resolved. The patient's diabetes is still not controlled and you feel it would be unwise for this to happen.
Assignment: Divide into groups. Develop a plan of action for solving this problem. First select three desired objectives for solving the problem and then proceed to determine what you would do that would enable you to meet your objectives.

 Learning Exercise 3.7

Delineating Management Functions and Leadership Roles
Examine the scenario in Learning Exercise 3.6. How would you divide the management functions and leadership roles in this situation? For example you might say that having the nurse manager adhere to hospital policy was a management function and that counseling staff was a leadership role.
Assignment: List at least five management functions and five leadership roles that you could also delineate in this scenario. Share these with your group.

Learning Exercise 3.8

What's Your Emotional Intelligence Level?
Do you feel that you have emotional intelligence? Do you express appropriate emotions, such as empathy when taking care of patients? Are you able to identify your own emotions when you are in an emotionally charged situation?
Assignment: Describe a recent emotional experience. Write a short report (two to four paragraphs) on how you responded in this experience. Were you able to read the emotions on the other individuals involved? How did you respond and were you later able to reflect on this incident?

Web Links

Leadership case studies
http://www.fau.edu/nli/
Nursing Leadership Institute. It offers many nursing links to leadership.

Leader values
http://www.leader-values.com/Guests/Lead23.htm
Presents Bennis' insights on effective leadership, the distinction between leaders and managers, and the mistakes leaders can make.

The clinical nurse leader role
http://www.mapnp.org/library/ldrship/ldrship.htm
Overview of leadership in organizations.

References

Bass, B. M., Avoliio, B. J., & Goodheim, L. (1987, Jan.). Biography and the assessment of transformational leadership at the world-class level. *Journal of Management*, 7–19.
Bednash, G. (2003). Leadership redefined. *Policy, Politics & Nursing Practice, 4*(4), 257–258.
Bennett, J. L. (2001). Trainers as leaders of learning. *Training & Development, 55*(3), 42–46.
Bennis, W. (1989). *Why leaders can't lead.* San Francisco: Jossey-Bass.
Bennis, W. (2001). In Crainer, S. An interview with Warren Bennis, accessed 07/03/2001 at *http://www.managementskills.co.uk/articles/ ap98-bennis.htm*
Brandt, M. A. (1994). Caring leadership: Secret and path to success. *Nursing Management, 25*(8), 68–72.
Burns, J. M. (1978). *Leadership.* New York: Harper & Row.
Chapin, F. S. (1924). Socialized leadership. *Social Forces, 3*, 57–60.
de Ruiter, H. & Saphiere, D. H. (2001). Nurse leaders as cultural bridges. *Journal of Nursing Administration, 31*(9), 418–423.
Drucker, P. F. (1992). *Managing for the future: The 1990s and beyond.* New York: Truman Talley/Dutton.
Dunham, J., & Klafehn, K. A. (1990). Transformational leadership and the nurse executive. *Journal of Nursing Administration, 20*(4), 28–34.
Fiedler, F. (1967). *A theory of leadership effectiveness.* New York: McGraw-Hill.

Follett, M. P. (1926). The giving of orders. In H. C. Metcalf (Ed.), *Scientific foundations of business administration.* Baltimore: Williams & Wilkins.

Gardner, J. W. (1990). *On leadership.* New York: The Free Press.

Glasser, A. (1994). *The control theory manager.* New York: Harper Business.

Greenleaf, R. K. (1977). *Servant leadership: A journey in the nature of legitimate power and greatness.* New York: Paulist.

Hersey, P., & Blanchard, K. (1977). *Management of organizational behavior: Utilizing human resources* (3rd ed.). Englewood Cliffs, NJ: Prentice Hall.

Hollander, E. P. (1978). *Leadership dynamics: A practical guide to effective relationships.* New York: The Free Press.

Kanter, R. M. (1977). *Men and Women of the Corporation.* New York: Basic Books.

Kanter, R. M. (1989). The new managerial work. *Harvard Business Review, 67*(6), 85–92.

Kellerman, B. (2004). Leadership, warts and all. *Harvard Business Review, 82*(1), 40–45.

Kerfoot, K. (2000). Leadership: Creating a shared destiny. *Nursing Economic$, 18*(5), 263–264.

Lewin, K. (1951). *Field theory in social sciences.* New York: Harper & Row.

McGregor, D. (1960). *The human side of enterprise.* New York: McGraw-Hill.

Nelson, L., & Burns, F. (1984). High-performance programming: A framework for transforming organizations. In J. Adams (Ed.), *Transforming work* (pp. 225–242). Alexandria, VA: Miles River Press.

Offermann, L. R. (2004). When followers become toxic. *Harvard Business Review, 82*(1), 55–60.

Ouchi, W. G. (1981). *Theory Z: How American business can meet the Japanese challenge.* Reading, MA: Addison-Wesley.

Porter-O'Grady, T. (2003). A different age for leadership. *Journal of Nursing Administration, 33*(3), 173–178.

Schein, E. H. (1970). *Organizational psychology* (2nd ed.). Englewood Cliffs, NJ: Prentice-Hall.

Snow, J. L. (2003). Looking beyond nursing for clues to effective leadership. *Journal of Nursing Administration, 31*(9), 440–443.

Tannenbaum, R., & Schmidt, W. (1958). How to choose a leadership pattern. *Harvard Business Review, 36,* 95–102.

Tourangeau, A. E. (2003). Building nurse leader capacity. *Journal of Nursing Administration, 33*(12), 614–638.

Trent, B. A. (2003). Leadership myths. *Reflections on Nursing leadership, 29*(3), 8–9.

Tyrrell, R. A. (1994). Visioning: An important management tool. *Nursing Economic$, 12*(2), 93–95.

Vitello-Cicciu, J. M. (2003). Exploring emotional intelligence. *Journal of Nursing Administration, 33*(4), 203–210.

White, R. K., & Lippitt R. (1960). *Autocracy and democracy: An experimental inquiry.* New York: Harper & Row.

Wolf, G. A., Boland, S., & Aukerman, M. (1994). A transformational model for the practice of professional nursing. Part II. *Journal of Nursing Administration, 24*(5), 38–46.

Bibliography

Authier, P. (2001). Quality leadership: A balancing act. *Nursing Management, 32*(2), 14.

Bennis, W. G. (2004). The seven ages of the leader. *Harvard Business Review, 82*(1), 46–53.

Boswell, J. (2001). The missing link. *Nursing Management, 32*(5), 34.

Coutu, D. (2004). Putting leaders on the couch. *Harvard Business Review, 82*(1), 65–71.

Hill, K. S. (2003). Development of leadership competencies as a team. *Journal of Nursing Administration, 33*(12), 639–642.

Kerfoot, K. (2001). The leader as synergist. *Nursing Economic$, 19*(1), 29.

Kleinman, C. S. (2003). Leadership roles, competencies, and education. *Journal of Nursing Administration, 33*(9), 451–455.

Russell, G. & Scobie, K. (2003). Vision 2020, Part 1, Profile of the future nurse leader. *Journal of Nursing Administration, 33*(6), 324–336.

Russell, G. & Scobie, K. (2003). Vision 2020, Part 2, Educational preparation for the future nurse manager. *Journal of Nursing Administration, 33*(7/8), 404–409.

Upenieks, V. V. (2002). What constitutes successful nurse leadership? A qualitative approach utilizing Kanter's theory of organizational behavior. *Journal of Nursing Administration, 33*(12), 622–632.

Woods, N. F. (2003). Leadership—Not for just a few! *Policy, Politics & Nursing Practice, 4*(4), 255–256.

CHAPTER

4

Ethical Issues

*In some significant respects, moral distress
is embedded in the historical and structural
fabric of the nursing profession.*

—Hamric (2000, p. 200)

Unit 2 examines ethical, social, legal, and legislative issues affecting leadership and management as well as professional advocacy. This chapter focuses on applied ethical decision making as a critical leadership role for managers. Chapter 5 examines the impact of legislation and the law on leadership and management, and Chapter 6 focuses on advocacy for patients and for the nursing profession.

Ethics is the systematic study of what a person's conduct and actions ought to be with regard to self, other human beings, and the environment; it is the justification of what is right or good and the study of what a person's life and relationships ought to be, not necessarily what they are.

> Ethics is the systematic study of what a person's conduct and actions ought to be with regard to self, other human beings, and the environment; it is the justification of what is right or good and the study of what a person's life and relationships ought to be, not necessarily what they are.

Applied ethics requires application of normative ethical theory to everyday problems. The normative ethical theory for each profession arises from the purpose of the profession. The values and norms of the nursing profession, therefore, provide the foundation and filter from which ethical decisions are made. The nurse manager, however, has a different ethical responsibility than the clinical nurse and does not have as clearly defined a foundation to use as a base for ethical reasoning.

Because management is a discipline and not a profession, it does not have a defined purpose, such as medicine or the law; therefore, it lacks a specific set of norms to guide ethical decision making. Instead, the organization reflects norms and values to the manager, and the personal values of managers are reflected through the organization. The manager's ethical obligation is tied to the organization's purpose, and the purpose of the organization is linked to the function it fills in society and the constraints society places on it. Therefore, the responsibilities of the nurse manager emerge from a complex set of interactions. Society helps define the purposes of various institutions, and the purposes, in turn, help ensure that the institution fulfills specific functions. However, the specific values and norms in any particular institution determine the focus of its resources and shape its organizational life. The values of people within institutions influence actual management practice. In reviewing this set of complex interactions, it becomes evident that arriving at appropriate ethical management decisions is a difficult task.

Not only is nursing management ethics distinct from clinical nursing ethics, it is also distinct from other areas of management. Although there are many similar areas of responsibility between nurse managers and non-nurse managers, many leadership roles and management functions are specific to nursing. These differences require the nurse manager to deal with unique obligations and ethical dilemmas that are not encountered in non-nursing management.

In addition, because personal, organizational, subordinate, and consumer responsibilities differ, there is great potential for nursing managers to experience intrapersonal conflict about the appropriate course of action. *Moral uncertainty* occurs "when one is unsure what moral principles or values apply in an ethical conflict, or even if there is an ethical or moral problem" (Raines, 2000, p. 30). *Moral distress* occurs when one knows the right thing to do, but institutional or other constraints make it difficult to pursue the desired course of action" (p. 30). *Moral anguish, moral distress*, and *moral compromise* are also terms that have been used to refer to the emotional and psychological aspects of ethical dilemmas experienced by nurses.

Multiple advocacy roles and accountability to the profession further increase the likelihood that all nurse managers will be faced with ethical dilemmas in their practice. Hamric (2001) calls this "being in the middle." Nurses are often placed in situations where they are expected to be agents for patients, physicians, and the organization simultaneously, all of which may have conflicting needs, wants, and goals. "It is not unusual that moral uncertainty is first experienced and escalates to moral distress as patients' rights are not respected or as institutional constraints are applied and nurses feel unable to act on their moral choices and judgments" (Hamric, 2000, p. 199).

To make appropriate ethical decisions, the manager must use a professional approach that eliminates trial and error and focuses on proven decision-making models or problem-solving processes. Using a systematic approach allows managers to make better decisions and increases the probability that they will feel good about the decisions they have made. The systematic approaches presented in this chapter include ethical frameworks and principles and theoretical problem-solving and decision-making models. Leadership roles and management functions involved in management ethics are shown in **Display 4.1**.

Display 4.1 | **Leadership Roles and Management Functions Associated with Ethics**

Leadership Roles
1. Is self-aware regarding own values and basic beliefs about the rights, duties, and goals of human beings.
2. Accepts that some ambiguity and uncertainty must be a part of all ethical decision making.
3. Accepts that negative outcomes occur in ethical decision making despite high-quality problem solving and decision making.
4. Demonstrates risk taking in ethical decision making.
5. Role models ethical decision making, which is congruent with the American Nurses Association Code of Ethics and Interpretive Statements, as well as Professional Standards.
6. Clearly communicates expected ethical standards of behavior.

Management Functions
1. Uses a systematic approach to problem solving or decision making when faced with management problems with ethical ramifications.
2. Identifies outcomes in ethical decision making that should always be sought or avoided.
3. Uses established ethical frameworks to clarify values and beliefs.
4. Applies principles of ethical reasoning to define what beliefs or values form the basis for decision making.
5. Is aware of legal precedents that may guide ethical decision making and is accountable for possible liabilities should they go against the legal precedent.
6. Continually reevaluates the quality of own ethical decision making, based on the process of decision making or problem solving used.
7. Recognizes and rewards ethical conduct of subordinates.
8. Takes appropriate action when subordinates use unethical conduct.

ETHICAL DILEMMAS

Individual values, beliefs, and personal philosophy play a major role in the moral or ethical decision making that is part of the daily routine of all managers. How do managers decide what is right and what is wrong? What does the manager do if no right or wrong answer exists? What if all solutions generated seem wrong?

Ethical dilemmas can be defined as situations in which one must choose between two or more undesirable alternatives. Raines (2000) states an ethical dilemma occurs when two or more clear moral principles apply in a situation, that support mutually inconsistent courses of action. Similarly, Curtin (1982) maintains that for a problem to be an ethical dilemma, it must have three characteristics. First, the problem cannot be solved using only empirical data. Second, the problem must be so perplexing that deciding what facts and data need to be used in making the decision is difficult. Third, the results of the problem must affect more than the immediate situation; there should be far-reaching effects.

Remember that the way managers approach and solve ethical dilemmas is influenced by their values and basic beliefs about the rights, duties, and goals of all human beings. Self-awareness, then, is a vital leadership role in ethical decision making, just as it is in so many other aspects of management.

No rules, guidelines, or theories exist that cover all aspects of the ethical dilemmas that managers face. Indeed, the individual who must solve the dilemma is the only person who can ascertain if actions taken were congruent with personal values. Quinn and Smith (1987) state, however, that "In the end, ethical individuals must be prepared to live with a certain amount of ambiguity and uncertainty. The professional who accepts uncertainty in practice situations avoids the paralysis that comes from postponing action until all information is available" (p. 53). However, they also assert that "Although there is value in learning to tolerate uncertainty, there is a point at which excessive tolerance amounts to neglect of professional and ethical commitments" (p. 53). To tolerate uncertainty at all times and under all circumstances is to ignore the value of knowledge and dismiss the ability to think critically.

Critical thinking occurs when the manager is able to engage in an orderly process of ethical problem solving to determine the rightness or wrongness of courses of action. Learning systematic approaches to ethical decision making and problem solving reduces personal bias, facilitates decision making, and lets managers feel more comfortable about decisions they have made.

> Many nurses have difficulty solving ethical problems in clinical practice because they have erroneously been led to believe that ethical decision making is simply a matter of intuition or good character, rather than a body of knowledge that can be learned and applied.

ETHICAL PROBLEM SOLVING AND DECISION MAKING

Hamric (2002) suggests that many nurses have difficulty solving ethical problems in clinical practice because they have erroneously been led to believe that ethical decision making is simply a matter of intuition or good character, rather than a body of knowledge that can be learned and applied. Ethical concepts and their utility in clinical practice must be taught as well as the problem-solving skills that are a part of all decision making. Much of the difficulty people have in making ethical decisions can be attributed to a lack of formal education about problem solving.

Pitfalls in Problem Solving and Decision Making

Because problem solving and decision making were discussed in Chapter 1, only a brief review is included here. Trial-and-error decision making helps some managers learn to make good decisions, but much is left to chance. The cost of poor ethical decisions is measured in terms of human and fiscal resources. Another error made by managers in ethical problem solving is using the outcome of the decision as the sole basis for determining the quality of the decision making. Although decision makers should be able to identify desirable and undesirable outcomes, these alone cannot be used to assess the quality of the problem solving. Many variables affect outcome, and some of these are beyond the control or foresight of the problem solver. Even the most ethical courses of action can have undesirable and unavoidable consequences. The quality of ethical problem solving should be evaluated in terms of the process used to make the decision. If a structured approach to problem solving is used, data gathering is adequate, and multiple alternatives are analyzed, even with a poor outcome, the manager should accept that the best possible decision was made at that time with the information and resources available.

> If a structured approach to problem solving is used, data gathering is adequate, and multiple alternatives are analyzed, even with a poor outcome, the manager should accept that the best possible decision was made at that time with the information and resources available.

The Traditional Problem-Solving Process

Although not recognized specifically as an ethical problem-solving model, one of the oldest and most frequently used tools for problem solving is the traditional problem-solving process. This process, which was discussed in Chapter 1, consists of seven steps, with the actual decision being made at step five (**Display 4.2**). Although many individuals use at least some of these steps in their decision making, they frequently fail to generate an adequate number of alternatives or to evaluate the results—two essential steps in the process.

The Nursing Process

Another problem-solving model not specifically designed for ethical analysis but appropriate for it, is the nursing process. Most nurses are aware of the nursing process and the cyclic nature of its components of assessment, diagnosis, planning,

---

Display 4.2	**Steps of the Traditional Problem-Solving Process**

1. Identify the problem.
2. Gather data to analyze the causes and consequences of the problem.
3. Explore alternative solutions.
4. Evaluate the alternatives.
5. Select the appropriate solution.
6. Implement the solution.
7. Evaluate the results.

Learning Exercise 4.1

A Nagging Uneasiness

You are a nurse on a pediatric unit. One of your patients is a 15-month-old girl with a diagnosis of failure to thrive. The mother has stated that the child appears emotional, cries a lot, and does not like to be held. You have been taking care of the toddler for 2 days since her admission, and she has smiled and laughed and held out her arms to everyone. She has eaten well. Yet, there is something about the child's reaction to the mother's boyfriend that bothers you. The child appears to draw away from him when he visits. The mother is very young and seems to be rather immature but appears to care for the child.

This is the second hospital admission for this child. Although you were not on duty for the first admission six weeks ago, you check the records and see that the child was admitted with the same diagnosis. While you are on duty today, the child's father, who lives several hundred miles away, calls and inquires about her condition. He requests that the child be hospitalized until the weekend (it is Wednesday) so that he can "check things out." He tells you that he believes the child is mistreated. He says he also is concerned about his ex-wife's 4-year-old child from another marriage and is attempting to gain custody of that child in addition to his own child. From what little the father said, you are aware that the divorce was very bitter and that the mother has full custody.

You talk with the physician at length. He says that after the last hospitalization, he requested that the community health agency and Child Protective Services call on the family. Their subsequent report to him was that the 4-year-old appeared happy and well and that the 15-month-old appeared clean, although underweight. There was no evidence to suggest child abuse. However, the community health agency plans to continue following the children. He says the mother has been good about keeping doctor appointments and has kept the children's immunizations up to date. The pediatrician proceeds to write an order for discharge. He says that although he also feels somewhat uneasy, continued hospitalization is not justified, and the state medical aid will not pay for additional days.

When the mother and her boyfriend come to pick the child up, the child clings to you and refuses to go to the boyfriend. She also is very reluctant to go to the mother. All during the discharge, you are extremely uneasy. When you see the car drive away, you feel very upset.

After returning to the unit, you talk with your supervisor, who listens carefully and questions you at length. Finally she says, "It seems as if you have nothing concrete on which to act and are only experiencing feelings. I think you would be risking a lot of trouble for yourself and the hospital if you acted rashly at this time. Accusing people with no evidence and making them go through a traumatic experience is something I would hesitate to do."

You leave the supervisor's office still troubled. She did not tell you that you must do nothing, but you believe she would disapprove of further action on your part. The doctor also felt strongly that there was no reason to do more than was already being done. The child will be followed by community health nurses. Perhaps the disgruntled ex-husband was just trying to make trouble for his ex-wife and her new boyfriend. You would certainly not want anyone to have reported you or created problems regarding your own children. You remember how often your 5-year-old bruised himself when he was that age. He often looked like an abused child. You go about your duties and try to shake off your feeling. What should you do?

Assignment:

1. Solve the case in small groups using the traditional problem-solving process. Identify the problem and several alternative solutions to solving this ethical dilemma. What should you do and why? What are the risks? How does your value system play a part in your decision? Justify your solution.

2. Assume this was a real case. Twenty-four hours after the child's discharge, she is readmitted with critical head trauma. Police reports indicate that the child suffered multiple skull fractures after being thrown up against the wall by her mother's boyfriend. The child is not expected to live. Does knowing the outcome change how you would have solved the case? Does the outcome influence how you feel about the quality of your group's problem solving?

implementation, and evaluation (**Figure 4.1**). However, most nurses do not recognize its use as a decision-making tool. The cyclic nature of the process allows for feedback to occur at any step. It also allows the cycle to repeat until adequate information is gathered to make a decision. It does not, however, require clear problem identification. Learning Exercise 4.2 shows how the nursing process might be used as an ethical decision-making tool.

Figure 4.1 The nursing process.

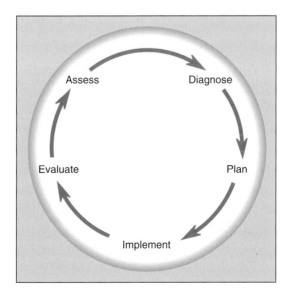

Learning Exercise 4.2

One Applicant Too Many

The reorganization of the public health agency has resulted in the creation of a new position of community health liaison. A job description has been written, and the job opening has been posted. As the chief nursing executive of this agency, it will be your responsibility to select the best person for the position. Because you are aware that all hiring decisions have some subjectivity, you want to eliminate as much personal bias as possible. Two people have applied for the position; one of them is a close personal friend. How will you proceed?

Analysis:

Assess: As the nursing executive, you have a responsibility to make personnel decisions as objectively as you can. This means that the hiring decision should be based solely on which employee is best qualified for the position. You do recognize, however, that there may be a personal cost in terms of the friendship.

Diagnose: You diagnose this problem as a potential intrapersonal conflict between your obligation to your friend and your obligation to your employer.

Plan: You must plan how you are going to collect these data. The tools you have selected are applications, résumés, references, and personal interviews.

Implement: Both applicants are contacted and asked to submit résumés and three letters of reference from recent employers. In addition, both are scheduled for structured formal interviews with you and two of the board members of the agency. Although the board members will provide feedback, you have reserved the right to make the final hiring decision.

Evaluate: As a result of your plan, you have discovered that both candidates meet the minimal job requirements. One candidate, however, clearly has higher-level communication skills, and the other candidate (your friend) has more experience in public health and is more knowledgeable regarding the resources in your community. Both employees have complied with the request to submit résumés and letters of reference; they are of similar quality.

Assess: Your assessment of the situation is that you need more information to make the best possible decision. You must assess whether strong communication skills or public health experience and familiarity with the community would be more valuable in this position.

Plan: You plan how you can gather more information about what the employee will be doing in this newly created position.

Implement: If the job description is inadequate in providing this information, it may be necessary to gather information from other public health agencies with a similar job classification.

Evaluate: You now believe that excellent communication skills are essential for the job. The candidate who had these skills has an acceptable level of public health experience and seems motivated to learn more about the community and its resources. This means that your friend will not receive the job.

Assess: Now you must assess whether a good decision has been made.

Plan: You plan to evaluate your decision in six months, basing your criteria on the established job description.

Implement: You are unable to implement your plan because this employee resigns unexpectedly four months after she takes the position. Your friend is now working in a similar capacity in another state. Although you correspond infrequently, the relationship has changed as a result of your decision.

Evaluate: Did you make a good decision? This decision was based on a carefully thought-out process, which included adequate data gathering and a weighing of alternatives. Variables beyond your control resulted in the employee's resignation, and there was no apparent reason for you to suspect that this would happen. The decision to exclude or minimize personal bias was a conscious one, and you were aware of the possible ramifications of this choice. The decision making appears to have been appropriate.

The MORAL Decision-Making Model

Crisham (1985) developed a model for ethical decision making incorporating the nursing process and principles of biomedical ethics. This model is especially useful in clarifying ethical problems that result from conflicting obligations. This model is represented by the mnemonic MORAL, representing the following:

M—*Massage the dilemma.* Collect data about the ethical problem and who should be involved in the decision-making process.

O—*Outline options.* Identify alternatives, and analyze the causes and consequences of each.

R—*Review criteria and resolve.* Weigh the options against the values of those involved in the decision. This may be done through a weighting or grid.

A—*Affirm position and act.* Develop the implementation strategy.

L—*Look back.* Evaluate the decision making.

The Murphy and Murphy Approach to Ethical Decision Making

Murphy and Murphy (1976) have also developed a systematic approach to ethical decision making:

- Identify the problem.
- Identify why the problem is an ethical problem.
- Identify the people involved in the ultimate decision.
- Identify the role of the decision maker.
- Consider the short- and long-term consequences of each alternative.
- Make the decision.

- Compare the decision with the decision maker's philosophy of ethics.
- Follow up on the results of the decision to establish a baseline for future decision making.

This type of systematic decision making differs from problem-solving models already discussed because it does not attempt to solve the underlying problem. It does, however, require the person to make a decision. Specifically geared toward ethical decision making, this approach helps clarify the basic beliefs and values of the people involved. Learning Exercise 4.3 should help you understand how the Murphy and Murphy approach could be used in making a human resource management decision with ethical ramifications.

Learning Exercise 4.3

Little White Lies

Sam is the nurse recruiter for a metropolitan hospital that is experiencing an acute nursing shortage. He has been told to do or say whatever is necessary to recruit professional nurses so the hospital will not have to close several units. He also has been told that his position will be eliminated if he does not produce a substantial number of applicants in the nursing career days to be held the following week. Sam loves his job and is the sole provider for his family. Because many organizations are experiencing severe personnel shortages, the competition for employees is keen. After his third career day without a single prospective applicant, he begins to feel desperate. On the fourth and final day, Sam begins making many promises to potential applicants regarding shift preference, unit preference, salary, and advancement that he is not sure he can keep. At the end of the day, Sam has a lengthy list of interested applicants but also feels a great deal of intrapersonal conflict. What can Sam do?

Analysis:

1. *Identify the problem.* In a desperate effort to save his job, Sam finds he has taken action that has resulted in high intrapersonal value conflict. Sam must choose between making promises he can't keep and losing his job.
2. *Identify why the problem is an ethical problem.* This is an ethical problem because it involves personal values and beliefs, has far-reaching implications for all involved, and presents several alternatives for decision making that are equally desirable or undesirable.
3. *Identify the people involved in the ultimate decision.* Sam has the ultimate responsibility for knowing his values and acting in a manner that is congruent with his value system. The organization is, however, involved in the value conflict in that its values and expectations conflict with Sam's. Sam and the organization have some type of responsibility to these applicants, although the exact nature of this responsibility is one of the values in conflict.
4. *Identify the role of the decision maker.* Because this is Sam's problem and an intrapersonal conflict, he must decide the appropriate course of action. His primary role is to examine his values and act in accordance with them.

5. *Consider the short- and long-term consequences of each alternative.*
   Alternative 1—Quit his job immediately. This would prevent future intrapersonal conflict provided that Sam becomes aware of his value system and behaves in a manner consistent with that value system in the future. It does not, however, solve the immediate conflict about the action Sam has already taken. This action takes away Sam's livelihood.
   Alternative 2—Do nothing. Sam could choose not to be accountable for his own actions. This will require Sam to rationalize that the philosophy of the organization is, in fact, acceptable or that he has no choice regarding his actions. Thus, the responsibility for meeting the needs and wants of the new employees is shifted to the hospital. Although Sam will have no credibility with the new employees, there will be only a negligible impact on his ability to recruit at least on a short-term basis. Sam will continue to have a job and be able to support his family.
   Alternative 3—If, after value clarification, Sam has determined that his values conflict with the hospital's directive to do or say whatever is needed to recruit employees, he could approach his superior and share these concerns. Sam should be very clear about what his values are and to what extent he is willing to compromise them. He also should include in this meeting what, if any, action should be taken to meet the needs of the new employees. Sam must be realistic about the time and effort usually required to change the values and beliefs of an organization. He also must be aware of his bottom line if the organization is not willing to provide a compromise resolution.
   Alternative 4—Sam could contact each of the applicants and tell them that certain recruitment promises may not be possible. However, he will do what he can to see that the promises are fulfilled. This alternative is risky. The applicants will probably be justifiably suspicious of both the recruiter and the organization, and Sam has little formal power at this point to fulfill their requests. This alternative also requires a time and energy commitment by Sam and does not prevent the problem from recurring.
6. *Make the decision.* Sam chose alternative 3.
7. *Compare the decision with the decision maker's philosophy of ethics.* In value clarification, Sam discovered that he valued truth telling. Alternative 3 allows Sam to present a recruiting plan to his supervisor that includes a bottom line that this value will not be violated.
8. *Follow up on the results of the decision to establish a baseline for future decision making.* Sam approached his superior and was told that his beliefs were idealistic and inappropriate in an age of severe worker shortages. Sam was terminated. Sam did, however, believe he made an appropriate decision. He did become self-aware regarding his values and attempted to communicate these values to the organization in an effort to work out a mutually agreeable plan. Although Sam was terminated, he knew that he could find some type of employment to meet immediate fiscal needs. Sam also used what he had learned in this decision-making process, in that he planned to evaluate more carefully the recruitment philosophy of the organization in relation to his own value system before accepting another job.

ETHICAL FRAMEWORKS FOR DECISION MAKING

In addition to theoretical problem-solving and decision-making models, managers may use *ethical frameworks* to guide them in solving ethical dilemmas. These frameworks do not solve the ethical problem but assist the manager in clarifying personal values and beliefs. Four of the most commonly used ethical frameworks are utilitarianism, duty-based reasoning, rights-based reasoning, and intuitionism (**Table 4.1**).

Using an ethical framework of *utilitarianism* encourages the manager to make decisions based on what provides the greatest good for the greatest number of people. In doing so, the needs and wants of the individual are diminished. Utilitarianism also suggests that the end can justify the means. For example, a manager using a utilitarian approach might decide to use travel budget money to send many staff to local workshops rather than to fund one or two people to attend a national conference. Another example would be an insurance program that meets the needs of many but refuses coverage for expensive organ transplants. In Learning Exercise 4.3, the organization used utilitarianism to justify lying to employee applicants because their hiring would result in good for many employees by keeping several units in the hospital open.

Duty-based reasoning is an ethical framework that says that some decisions must be made because there is a duty to do something or to refrain from doing something. In Learning Exercise 4.2, the supervisor feels a duty to hire the most qualified person for the job, even if the personal cost is high.

Rights-based reasoning is based on the belief that some things are a person's just due (i.e., each individual has basic claims, or entitlements, with which there should be no interference). Rights are different from needs, wants, or desires. In Learning Exercise 4.3, Sam believed that all people had the right to truth and, in fact, that he had the duty to be truthful. The supervisor in Learning Exercise 4.2 believed that both applicants had the right to fair and impartial consideration of their application.

The *intuitionist framework* allows the decision maker to review each ethical problem or issue on a case-by-case basis, comparing the relative weights of goals, duties, and rights. This weighting is determined primarily by intuition—what the decision

Table 4.1 Ethical Frameworks

Framework	Basic Premise
Utilitarian (Teleological)	Provide the greatest good for the greatest number of people
Rights-based (Deontological)	Individuals have basic inherent rights that should not be interfered with
Duty-based (Deontological)	A duty to do something or to refrain from doing something
Intuitionist (Deontological)	Each case weighed on a case-by-case basis to determine relative goals, duties, and rights

maker believes is right for that particular situation. Recently, some ethical theorists have begun questioning the appropriateness of intuitionism as an ethical decision-making framework because of the potential for subjectivity and bias. All of the cases solved in this chapter have involved some degree of decision making by intuition.

PRINCIPLES OF ETHICAL REASONING

Deontological theories arise from the intent of the action that the decision maker takes. Duty-based, rights-based, and intuitionist ethical reasoning derive their framework from deontological theory. *Teleological theories* are used to support utilitarianism. These are theories that support decisions that favor the common good. Both teleological and deontological theorists have developed a group of moral principles that are used for ethical reasoning. These principles of ethical reasoning further explore and define what beliefs or values form the basis for decision making. The most fundamental universal principle is respect for people. The major ethical principles stemming from this basic principle are discussed in **Display 4.3.**

> The most fundamental universal ethical principle is respect for people.

Autonomy (Self-Determination)

A form of personal liberty, *autonomy* also is called freedom of choice or accepting the responsibility for one's choice. The legal right of self-determination supports this moral principle. The use of progressive discipline recognizes the autonomy of the employee. The employee, in essence, has the choice to meet organizational expectations or to be disciplined further. If the employee's continued behavior warrants termination, the principle of autonomy says that the employee has made the choice to be terminated by virtue of his or her actions, not the manager's.

Bosek, Savage, Shaw, and Renella (2001) maintain that autonomy has become one of the most important ethical principles to be protected in healthcare decision making and has resulted in various policies and legislation regarding the role

Display 4.3	Ethical Principles

Autonomy: Promotes self-determination and freedom of choice
Beneficence: Actions are taken in an effort to promote good
Non-maleficence: Actions are taken in an effort to avoid harm
Paternalism: One individual assumes the right to make decisions for another
Utility: The good of the many outweighs the wants or needs of the individual
Justice: Seek fairness; treat "equals" equally and treat "unequals" according to their differences
Veracity: Obligation to tell the truth
Fidelity: Need to keep promises
Confidentiality: Keep privileged information private

of surrogate decision makers. Therefore, nurse managers must be cognizant of the ethical component present whenever an individual's decisional capacity is in question. To take away a person's right to self-determination is a serious but sometimes necessary action.

Beneficence (Doing Good)

This principle states that the actions one takes should be done in an effort to promote good. The concept of *nonmaleficence*, which is associated with *beneficence*, says that if one cannot do good, then one should at least do no harm. For example, if a manager uses this ethical principle in planning performance appraisals, he or she is much more likely to view the performance appraisal as a means of promoting employee growth.

Bosek (2001), however, feels that nonmaleficence (i.e., to do no harm) is not a passive act but requires action. In the prior example of nonmaleficence reasoning, the nurse manager's first priority when planning the performance appraisal would be to do no harm. Bosek feels that nonmaleficence should be the fundamental ethical principle for every nursing action.

Paternalism

This principle is related to beneficence in that one person assumes the authority to make a decision for another. Because *paternalism* limits freedom of choice, most ethical theorists believe paternalism is justified only to prevent a person from coming to harm. Unfortunately, some managers use the principle of paternalism in subordinates' career planning. In doing so, managers assume they have greater knowledge of what an employee's short- and long-term goals should be than the employee does.

Utility

This principle reflects a belief in utilitarianism—what is best for the common good outweighs what is best for the individual. Utility justifies paternalism as a means of restricting individual freedom. Managers who use the principle of utility need to be careful not to become so focused on production that they become less humanistic.

Justice (Treating People Fairly)

This principle states that equals should be treated equally and unequals should be treated according to their differences. This principle is frequently applied when there are scarcities or competition for resources or benefits. The manager who uses the principle of *justice* will work to see that pay raises reflect performance and not just time of service.

Truth Telling (Veracity)

This principle is used to explain how people feel about the need for truth telling or the acceptability of deception. A manager who believes deception is morally acceptable if it is done with the objective of beneficence may tell all rejected job applicants that they were highly considered, whether they had been or not.

Learning Exercise 4.4

Are Some More Equal Than Others?
Research suggests that individuals with health insurance in this country
have better access to healthcare services and better healthcare outcomes
than those who do not have insurance. This does not mean, however, that
all individuals with health insurance receive "equal treatment." Medicaid
recipients (the financially indigent) often complain that while they have
public insurance, many private providers refuse to accept them as
patients. Patients enrolled in managed care suggest that their treatment
options are more limited than traditional private insurance, because of
the use of gatekeepers, required authorizations, and queuing. Even individuals with private insurance suggest that co-payments and out-of-pocket
costs for deductibles place the cost of care beyond the reach of many.
Assignment: Using the ethical principle of justice, determine whether
health care in this country should be a right or a privilege. Are the uninsured and the insured "unequals" that should be treated according to their
differences? Does the type of health insurance one has also create a system
of unequals? If so, are they being treated according to their differences?

Fidelity (Keeping Promises)

Fidelity refers to the moral obligation that individuals should be faithful to their
commitments and promises (Veatch and Fry, 2000). Breaking a promise is believed
by many ethicists to be wrong regardless of the consequences. In other words, even
if there were no far-reaching negative results of the broken promise, it is still wrong
because it would render the making of any promise meaningless. However, there
are times when keeping a promise (fidelity) may not be in the best interest of the
other party, as discussed below under confidentiality.

Hamric (2001) suggests that it is helpful to view the "nurse in the middle" phenomenon from a fidelity perspective. Although nurses have multiple fidelity duties
(to patient, physician, organization, profession, and self) which at times may conflict, the ANA Code of Ethics is clear that one duty "trumps" all others, namely the
nurse's commitment to the patient.

Confidentiality (Respecting Privileged Information)

The obligation to observe the privacy of another and to hold certain information in
strict confidence is a basic ethical principle and is a foundation of both medical and
nursing ethics. Indeed, confidentiality was deemed so important that the federal
government implemented privacy laws regarding access to patient health information in the Health Insurance Portability and Accountability Act (HIPAA) of 1996.
(See Chapter 5.) However, as in deception, there are times when the presumption
against disclosing information must be overridden. For example, healthcare managers are required by law to report certain cases, such as drug abuse in employees,
elder abuse, and child abuse.

Learning Exercise 4.5

Family Values

You are the evening-shift charge nurse of the PACU. You have just admitted a 32-year-old woman who was thrown from the passenger seat of a vehicle two hours ago. She had been rushed to the emergency room and subsequently to surgery, where cranial burr holes were completed and an intracranial monitor was placed. No further cranial exploration was attempted, because the patient had extensive and massive neurologic damage. She will probably not survive your shift. The plan is to hold her in recovery for one hour and, if she is still alive, transfer her to the intensive care unit.

Shortly after receiving the patient in the PACU, you are approached by the evening house supervisor, who says that the patient's sister is pleading to be allowed into the recovery room. Normally, visitors are never allowed in the recovery room, but occasionally exceptions are made. Tonight, the recovery room is empty except for this patient. You decide to bend the rules and allow the young woman's sister into the recovery room. The visiting sister is near collapse; it is obvious that she was the driver of the vehicle. As the visitor continues to speak to the comatose patient, her behavior and words make you begin to wonder if she is indeed the sister.

Within 15 minutes, the house supervisor returns and states, "I have made a terrible mistake. The patient's family just arrived, and they say that the visitor we just allowed into the PACU is not a member of the family but is the patient's lover. They are very angry and demand that this woman not be allowed to see the patient."

You approach the visitor and confront her in a kindly manner regarding the information you have just received. She looks at you with tears streaming down her face and says, "Yes, it is true. Mary and I have been together for six years. Her family disowned her because of it, but we were everything to each other. She has been my life, and I have been hers. Please, please let me stay. I will never see her again. I know the family will not allow me to attend the funeral. I need to say my good-byes. Please let me stay. It is not fair that they have the legal right to be family when I have been the one to love and care for Mary."

Assignment: You must decide what to do. Recognize that your own value system will play a part in your decision. List several alternatives that are available to you. Identify which ethical frameworks or principles most affected your decision making.

ANA CODE OF ETHICS AND PROFESSIONAL STANDARDS

Another tool that managers can use for guidance in ethical problem solving is a *professional code of ethics*. A code of ethics is a set of principles, established by a profession, to guide the individual practitioner. The first code of ethics for nurses was adopted by the American Nurses Association (ANA) in 1950 and has been revised many times since then.

The most recent revision, the 2001 Code of Ethics for Nurses, departs from previous versions in several important ways (Daly, 2002). The newest code returns to the use of the term *patient* rather than *client* because patient more accurately reflects what the majority of nurses do, care for individuals with health problems. The code also explicitly details the nurse's most fundamental accountability is to the patient, whether an individual, family, group, or community (No. 2). The 2001 code also addresses the responsibility of the nurse for assuring that the environment they work in is safe, even in an era of cutting costs and reduced revenues (No. 6). Finally, there is a new provision (No. 5) that addresses duties of the nurse to him or herself (Daly, 2002).

Professional codes of ethics do not have the power of law. They do, however, function as a guide to the highest standards of ethical practice for nurses. The American Nurses Association Code of Ethics for Nurses (2001) is shown in **Display 4.4.**

Another document that may be helpful specifically to the nurse manager in creating and maintaining an ethical work environment is *The Scope and Standards for Nurse Administrators*. These standards are also used as the baseline for determining

> Professional codes of ethics function as a guide to the highest standards of ethical practice for nurses.

Display 4.4	**American Nurses Association Code of Ethics for Nurses**

The ANA House of Delegates approved these nine provisions of the new *Code of Ethics for Nurses* at its June 30, 2001, meeting in Washington, D.C. In July 2001, the Congress of Nursing Practice and Economics voted to accept the new language of the interpretive statements resulting in a fully approved revised *Code of Ethics for Nurses with Interpretive Statements*.

1. The nurse, in all professional relationships, practices with compassion and respect for the inherent dignity, worth, and uniqueness of every individual, unrestricted by considerations of social or economic status, personal attributes, or the nature of health problems.
2. The nurse's primary commitment is to the patient, whether an individual, family, group, or community.
3. The nurse promotes, advocates for, and strives to protect the health, safety, and rights of the patient.
4. The nurse is responsible and accountable for individual nursing practice and determines the appropriate delegation of tasks consistent with the nurse's obligation to provide optimum patient care.
5. The nurse owes the same duties to self as to others, including the responsibility to preserve integrity and safety, to maintain competence, and to continue personal and professional growth.
6. The nurse participates in establishing, maintaining, and improving healthcare environments and conditions of employment conducive to the provision of quality health care and consistent with the values of the profession through individual and collective action.
7. The nurse participates in the advancement of the profession through contributions to practice, education, administration, and knowledge development.
8. The nurse collaborates with other health professionals and the public in promoting community, national, and international efforts to meet health needs.
9. The profession of nursing, as represented by associations and their members, is responsible for articulating nursing values, for maintaining the integrity of the profession and its practice, and for shaping social policy.

Display 4.5	**Standards of Practice for Nurse Administrators**

Standard 11. Ethics
The nurse administrator's decisions and actions are based on ethical principles.

Measurement Criteria
1. Advocates on behalf of recipients of services and personnel.
2. Maintains privacy, confidentiality, and security of patient/client/resident, staff, and organization data.
3. Adheres to the Code of Ethics for Nurses with Interpretive Statements (ANA, 2001).
4. Assures compliance with regulatory and professional standards, as well as integrity in business practices.
5. Fosters a nondiscriminatory climate in which care is delivered in a manner sensitive to sociocultural diversity.
6. Assures a process to identify and address ethical issues within nursing and the organization.

Source: American Nurses Association. (2004). *Scope and standards for nurse administrators* (2nd ed.). Washington, D.C.: American Nurses Publishing.

eligibility for magnet status for acute care hospitals (see Chapter 12). *The Scope and Standards for Nurse Administrators*, revised in 2004, specifically delineates professional standards in management ethics and these are shown in **Display 4.5**.

ETHICAL DIMENSIONS IN LEADERSHIP AND MANAGEMENT

The need for ethical decisions occurs in every phase of the management process and many of the case studies in this book have an ethical component that must be considered in the problem solving. See examples in **Display 4.6.**

Display 4.6	**Ethical Issues and Questions for the Reader**

Most units in this book could appropriately include a section on ethical issues, such as the following:

Unit 3
• At what point do the needs of the organization become more important than those of the individual worker?
• Should employees ever be coerced into changing their stated values so they more closely align with the organization's values?
• How can managers fairly allocate resources when virtually all resources are limited?

Display 4.6	**Ethical Issues and Questions for the Reader**

Unit 4
- Should quality or cost be the final determinant when selecting the most appropriate type of patient care delivery system?
- Should LVNs/LPNs be allowed to function in the primary nursing role?
- How should the manager protect patients from an inadequate primary nurse?
- When should the manager step outside the chain of command?
- Which should be more important to the organization—human relations or productivity?
- Which is more corrupting—power or powerlessness?

Unit 5
- At what point does short staffing become unsafe?
- Should shift scheduling be used as a means of reward and punishment?
- Is seducing employees from other agencies ever ethical?
- How far can the truth be stretched in recruitment advertising before it becomes deceptive?
- Should preemployment testing be required as a condition of employment?
- Is it ethical for employees to take a position in an organization if they know they are planning to leave in a short time?
- Is it ever justified for an employee to lie in an interview?
- Who has the responsibility for socializing the new graduate into the professional nursing role: the nursing school, the hospital, or is it a joint process?
- What commitment does the organization have to the nurse who is reentering the profession after not practicing for many years?
- Should an employee's orientation be continued indefinitely until he or she feels ready to function autonomously?

Unit 6
- To whom do managers owe their primary allegiance: the organization or their subordinates?
- When is it appropriate to use money as the primary motivator?
- If employees are producing at acceptable or higher levels, what new rewards and incentives should be introduced?
- Is it ethical to promote union organizers to management to reduce the possibility of union formation?
- Is affirmative action hiring to compensate for past discrimination ethically justifiable, or does it promote reverse discrimination?
- Is it ethical for nurses to strike?
- Should the national nursing organization also be a collective bargaining agent?

Unit 7
- Is it necessary for each employee to be assisted to achieve at optimal levels? Can the manager be selective in determining which employees are assisted to reach optimal productivity?
- At what point does the power to evaluate the work of others become dangerous?
- Should the individual be allowed total self-determination in short- and long-term career planning?
- Is it ethical to promote or transfer a less qualified person to keep a valuable employee on a unit?

(display continues on page 86)

Display 4.6	**Ethical Issues and Questions for the Reader**

- Does the organization have an obligation to reemploy the chemically impaired employee who seeks rehabilitation?
- When does the employee's right to privacy regarding drug or alcohol use stop and the manager's right to that information begin?
- Is it ever ethical to file a grievance against another person for the purpose of harassment?
- Can discipline administered in anger ever be fair?
- In pursuing beneficence, is it more appropriate to discipline marginal employees progressively or to terminate them?

The bottom line is that concerns about ethical conduct in American institutions are rampant. Indeed, many believe it has become the norm. Governmental agencies, both branches of Congress, the stock exchange, oil companies, savings and loan institutions, and the U.S. armed forces have all experienced problems with unethical conduct. Many members of society wonder what has gone wrong. Nurse managers, then, have a responsibility to create a climate in their organizations in which ethical behavior is not only the norm but also the expectation.

In an era of markedly limited physical, human, and fiscal resources, however, nearly all decision making by nurse managers will involve some ethical component. Indeed, the following forces ensure that ethics will become an even greater dimension in management decision making in the future: increasing technology, regulatory pressures, competitiveness among healthcare providers; national nursing shortages; reduced fiscal resources; spiraling costs of supplies and salaries; and the public's increasing distrust of the healthcare delivery system and its institutions.

Separating Ethical and Legal Decision Making

Although they are not the same, separating legal and ethical issues is sometimes difficult. Legal controls are generally clear and philosophically impartial; ethical controls are much more unclear and individualized. In many ethical issues, courts have made a decision that may guide managers in their decision making. Often, however, these guidelines are not comprehensive or differ from the manager's own philosophy. Managers must be aware of established legal standards and cognizant of possible liabilities and consequences for actions that go against the legal precedent.

Legal precedents are frequently overturned later and often do not keep pace with the changing needs of society. Additionally, certain circumstances may favor an illegal course of action as the "right" thing to do. If a man were transporting his severely ill wife to the hospital, it might be morally correct for him to disobey traffic laws. Therefore, the manager should think of the law as a basic standard of conduct, whereas ethical behavior requires a greater examination of the issues involved.

The manager may confront several particularly sensitive legal/ethical issues, including termination or refusal of treatment, durable power of attorney, abortion, sterilization, child abuse, and human experimentation. Most healthcare organizations have legal counsel to assist managers in making decisions in such sensitive areas.

Many hospitals also have ethics committees to assist with problem solving in ethical issues. *Clinical ethics committees* are usually organized around patient health issues such as end of life concerns, whereas *organizational ethics committees* address the overall health of the facility itself (Angelucci, 2003). These ethics committees typically are multidisciplinary and are organized to consciously and reflectively consider significant and often difficult or ambiguous value issues related to patient care or organizational activities (Angelucci, 2003). In doing so, these committees promote, advocate, and protect patient rights; maximize benefit and minimize harm; establish a moral care standard; and enhance care delivery quality (Center for Bioethics, 2002).

The manager must consult with others when solving sensitive legal and ethical questions because a person's own value system may preclude examining all possible alternatives. Because legal aspects of management decision making are so important, Chapter 5 is devoted exclusively to this topic.

Creating an Ethical Work Environment

Perhaps the most important thing a manager can do to create an ethical work environment is to role model ethical behavior. Other important interventions, however, include encouraging staff to openly discuss ethical issues they face daily in their practice. This allows subordinates to gain greater perspective on complex issues and provides a mechanism for peer support. Raines (2000) also suggests the following proactive strategies for creating an ethical work environment and for reducing ethics stress:

- Start a nursing ethics library or nursing ethics journal club in the workplace.
- Sponsor a nursing ethics committee and/or nursing research committee as a counterpart to the interdisciplinary ethics committee and/or institutional review board.
- Support a nursing ethics grand rounds and plan for interdisciplinary participation.
- Provide all staff an annual educational program that uses current issues for case discussion.
- Circulate a nursing ethics article of the month to all units and encourage brief discussion at staff meetings or clinical rounds.
- Do a biannual survey of staff to assess what ethical issues they are facing most frequently or having most difficulty resolving.
- Send representatives from your nursing staff to other similar healthcare organizations to find out what their staff do related to ethical issues, ethics committees, nursing policies, educational programs, etc.
- If there are no staff nurse representatives on the agency's ethics committee or institutional review board, take a nurse manager or staff nurse to the regular meeting.

INTEGRATING LEADERSHIP ROLES AND MANAGEMENT FUNCTIONS IN ETHICS

Leadership roles in ethics focus on the human element involved in ethical decision making. Leaders are self-aware regarding their values and basic beliefs about the rights, duties, and goals of human beings. As self-aware and ethical people, they role model confidence in their decision making to subordinates. They also are realists and recognize that some ambiguity and uncertainty must be a part of all ethical decision making. Leaders are willing to take risks in their decision making despite the fact that negative outcomes can occur with quality decision making.

In ethical issues, the manager is often the decision maker. Because ethical decisions are so complex and the cost of a poor decision may be high, management functions focus on increasing the chances that the best possible decision will be made at the least possible cost in terms of fiscal and human resources. This usually requires that the manager become expert at using systematic approaches to problem solving or decision making, such as theoretical models, ethical frameworks, and ethical principles. By developing expertise, the manager can identify universal outcomes that should be sought or avoided.

The integrated leader–manager recognizes that ethical issues pervade every aspect of leadership and management. Rather than being paralyzed by the complexity and ambiguity of these issues, the leader–manager seeks counsel as needed, accepts his or her limitations, and makes the best possible decision at that time with the information and resources available.

☀ Key Concepts

- *Ethics* is the systematic study of what a person's conduct and actions ought to be with regard to self, other human beings, and the environment; it is the justification of what is right or good, and the study of what a person's life and relationships ought to be—not necessarily what they are.
- In an era of markedly limited physical, human, and fiscal resources, nearly all decision making by nurse managers involves some ethical component. Multiple advocacy roles and accountability to the profession further increase the likelihood that managers will be faced with ethical dilemmas in their practice.
- Many systematic approaches to ethical problem solving are appropriate. These include the use of theoretical problem-solving and decision-making models, ethical frameworks, and ethical principles.
- Outcomes should never be used as the sole criterion for assessing the quality of ethical problem solving, because many variables affect outcomes that have no reflection on whether the problem solving was appropriate. Quality instead, should be evaluated both by the outcome and the process used to make the decision. If a structured approach to problem solving is used, data gathering is adequate, and multiple alternatives are analyzed, then, regardless of the outcome, the manager should feel comfortable that the best possible decision was made at that time with the information and resources available.
- Four of the most commonly used ethical frameworks for decision making are *utilitarianism, duty-based reasoning, rights-based reasoning*, and *intuitionism*. These frameworks do not solve the ethical problem but assist individuals involved in the problem solving to clarify their values and beliefs.
- Principles of ethical reasoning explore and define what beliefs or values form the basis for our decision making. These principles include *autonomy, beneficence, nonmaleficence, paternalism, utility, justice, fidelity, veracity*, and *confidentiality*.

- Professional *codes of ethics* and *standards for practice* are a guide to the highest standards of ethical practice for nurses.
- Sometimes it is very difficult to separate legal and ethical issues, although they are not the same. Legal controls are generally clear and philosophically impartial. Ethical controls are much more unclear and individualized.

More Learning Exercises and Applications

Learning Exercise 4.6

The Impaired Employee

Beverly, a 35-year-old full-time nurse on the day shift, has been with your facility for 10 years. There have been rumors that she has been coming to work under the influence of alcohol. Staff members have reported the smell of alcohol on her breath, unexcused absences from the unit, and an increase in medication errors. Although the unit supervisor suspects Beverly is chemically impaired, she has been unable to observe directly any of these behaviors.

After arriving at work last week, the supervisor walked into the nurses' lounge and observed Beverly covertly drinking from a dark-colored flask in her locker. She immediately confronted Beverly and asked her if she was drinking alcohol while on duty. Beverly tearfully admitted that she was drinking alcohol but stated this was an isolated incident and begged her to forget it. She promised never to consume alcohol at work again.

In an effort to reduce the emotionalism of the event and to give herself time to think, the supervisor sent Beverly home and scheduled a conference with her for later in the day. At this conference, Beverly was defensive and stated, "I do not have a drinking problem, and you are overreacting." The supervisor shared data that she had gathered supporting her impression that Beverly was chemically impaired. Beverly offered no explanation for these behaviors. The plan for Beverly was a 2-week suspension without pay and the requirement that she attend three alcohol support group meetings before returning to work. She also was informed that failure to do so and further evidence of intoxication while on duty would result in immediate termination.

Beverly again became very tearful and begged the supervisor to reconsider. She stated that she was the sole provider for her four small children and that her frequent sick days had taken up all available vacation and sick pay. The supervisor stated that she believed her decision was appropriate and again encouraged Beverly to seek guidance for her drinking. Four days later, the supervisor read in the newspaper that Beverly committed suicide the day after this meeting.

Assignment: Evaluate the problem solving of the supervisor. Would your actions have differed if you were the manager? Are there conflicting legal and ethical obligations? To whom does the manager have the greatest obligation: patients, subordinates, or the organization? Could the outcome have been prevented? Does this outcome reflect on the quality of the problem solving?

Learning Exercise 4.7

Everything Is Not What It Seems

You are a perinatal unit coordinator at a large teaching hospital. In addition to your management responsibilities, you have been asked to fill in as a member of the hospital promotion committee, which reviews petitions from clinicians for a step-level promotion on the clinical specialist ladder. You believe you could learn a great deal on this committee and could be an objective and contributing member.

The committee has been convened to select the annual winner of the Outstanding Clinical Specialist Award. In reviewing the applicant files, you find that one file from a perinatal clinical specialist contains many overstatements and several misrepresentations. You know for a fact that this clinician did not accomplish all that she has listed, because she is a friend and close colleague. She did not, however, know that you would be a member of this committee and thus would be aware of this deception.

When the entire committee met, several members commented on this clinician's impressive file. Although you were able to dissuade them covertly from further considering her nomination, you are left with many uneasy feelings and some anger and sadness. You recognize that she did not receive the nomination and thus there is little real danger regarding the deceptions in the file being used inappropriately at this time. However, you will not be on this committee next year and that if she were to submit an erroneous file again, she could, in fact, be highly considered for the award. You also recognize that, even with the best of intentions and the most therapeutic of communication techniques, confronting your friend with her deception will cause her to lose face and will probably result in an unsalvageable friendship. Even if you did confront her, there is little you could do to stop her from doing the same in future nomination processes, other than formally reporting her conduct.

Assignment: Determine what you will do. Do the potential costs outweigh the potential benefits? Be realistic about your actions.

Learning Exercise 4.8

The Valuable Employee
Gina has been the supervisor of a 16-bed intensive care unit/critical care unit (ICU/CCU) in a 200-bed urban hospital for eight years. She is respected and well liked by her staff. Her staff retention level and productivity are higher than any other unit in the hospital. For the last six years, Gina has relied heavily on Mark, her permanent charge nurse on the day shift. He is bright and motivated and has excellent clinical and management skills. Mark seems satisfied and challenged in his current position, although Gina has not had any formal career planning meetings with him to discuss his long-term career goals. It would be fair to say that Mark's work has greatly increased Gina's scope of power and enhanced the reputation of the unit.

Recently, one of the physicians approached Gina about a plan to open an outpatient cardiac rehabilitation program. The program will require a strong leader and manager who is self-motivated. It will be a lot of work but also provides many opportunities for advancement. He suggests that Mark would be an excellent choice for the job, although he has given Gina full authority to make the final decision.

Gina is aware that Lynn, a bright and dynamic staff nurse from the open-heart surgery floor, also would be very interested in the job. Lynn has been employed at the hospital for only one year but has a proven track record and would probably be very successful in the job. In addition, there is a staffing surplus right now on the open-heart surgery floor because two of the surgeons have recently retired. It would be difficult and time-consuming to replace Mark as charge nurse in the CCU/ICU.

Assignment: What process should this supervisor pursue to determine who should be hired for the position? Should the position be posted? When does the benefit of using transfers or promotions as a means of reward outweigh the cost of reduced productivity?

Learning Exercise 4.9

To See or Not to See

For the last few days you have been taking care of Mr. Cole, a 28-year-old patient with end-stage cystic fibrosis. You have developed a caring relationship with Mr. Cole and his wife. They are both aware of the prognosis of the disease and realize Mr. Cole has only a short time left to live. When Dr. Jones made rounds with you this morning, she told the Coles that Mr. Cole could be discharged today if his condition remains stable. They were both excited about the news because they had been urging the doctor to let him go home to enjoy his remaining time surrounded by things he loves.

When you take Mr. Cole's discharge orders to his room to review his medications and other treatments, you see Mrs. Cole assisting Mr. Cole as he coughs up bright red blood. When you confront them, they both beg you not to tell the doctor or chart the incident because this is the first time this has happened. They believe it is their right to go home and let Mr. Cole die surrounded by his family. They say they know that they can leave the hospital against medical advice (AMA) and go home, but if they do, their insurance will not pay for home care.

Assignment: What is your duty in this case? What are Mr. Cole's rights? Is it ever justifiable to withhold information from the physician? Will you chart the incident, and will you report the incident to anyone? Solve this case, and justify your decision using ethical principles.

Web Links

The Center for Ethics & Human Rights, sponsored by the American Nurses Association (2004)

http://www.nursingworld.org/ethics/index.htm

Established in 1990, this center is devoted to the study of ethics and nursing, including issue updates and policy development.

Canadian Bioethics Society

http://www.bioethics.ca/english

Home page of the Canadian Bioethics Society, this site includes a discussion of why there is an increased interest in bioethics as well as links to bioethics sites.

John Dossetor Health Ethics Centre, University of Alberta (last updated November 2003)

http://www.ualberta.ca/BIOETHICS/

An interdisciplinary center committed to working in the area of health ethics.

International Code of Ethics (International Council of Nurses)

http://www.icn.ch/abouticn.htm

The ICN Code of Ethics for Nurses, revised in 2000, is a guide for action based on social values and needs. The Code has served as the standard for nurses worldwide since it was first adopted in 1953 (available in English, French, and Spanish).

Markkula Center for Applied Ethics (2003)
http://www.scu.edu/ethics/practicing/decision/framework.html
The ethics center of Santa Clara University suggests a framework for ethical decision making as well as provides links on the scope of ethics or moral philosophy, on alternative frameworks for ethical decision making, and on ethical relativism.

References

American Nurses Association. (2004). *Scope and standards for nurse administrators* (2nd ed.). Washington, D.C.: American Nurses Publishing.

American Nurses Association. (2001). *Code of ethics for nurses with interpretive statements.* Washington, D.C.: American Nurses Publishing.

Angelucci, P. (June 2003). Ethics committees: Guidance through gray areas. *Nursing Management, 34*(6), 30–33.

Bosek, M. S. D. (2001). Reaffirming a primary commitment to nonmaleficence. *Healthcare Law, Ethics and Regulation, 3*(2), 31–34.

Bosek, M. S. D., Savage, T. A., Shaw, L. A., & Renella, C. (2001). When surrogate decision-making is not straightforward. *Healthcare Law, Ethics and Regulation, 3*(2), 47–57.

Center for Bioethics. (2002, October 9). University lecture at University of Minnesota. Ethics committees: The consultation process.

Crisham, P. (1985). MORAL: How can I do what is right? *Nursing Management, 16*(3).

Curtin, L. (1982). Ethics in nursing administration. In A. Marriner (Ed.), *Contemporary nursing management.* St. Louis: C. V. Mosby.

Daly, B. J. (2002). Moving forward: A new code of ethics. *Nursing Outlook, 50* (3), 97–99.

Hamric, A. B. (2000). Moral distress in everyday ethics. *Nursing Outlook, 48*(5), 199–201.

Hamric, A. B. (2001). Reflections on begin in the middle. *Nursing Outlook, 49*(6), 254–257.

Hamric, A. B. (2002). Bridging the gap between ethics and clinical practice. *Nursing Outlook, 50*(5), 176–178.

Murphy, M., & Murphy, J. (1976). Making ethical decisions—Systematically. *Nursing, 76*(6), 13–14.

Quinn, C. A., & Smith, M. D. (1987). *The professional commitment: Issues and ethics in nursing.* Philadelphia: W. B. Saunders.

Raines, M. L. (2000). Ethical decision making in nurses. *JONA's Healthcare Law, Ethics, and Regulation, 2*(1), 29–41.

Veatch, R. M., & Fry, S. T. (2000). *Case studies in nursing ethics* (2nd ed.). Boston: Jones & Bartlett.

Bibliography

Carson, W., & Franklin, P. (2001). Workplace advocacy. *American Journal of Nursing, 101*(2), 55–57.

Cooper, R. W. (2002). Key ethical issues encountered in healthcare organizations: Perceptions of nurse executives. *Journal of Nursing Administration, 32*(6), 331–337.

Daly, G. (2000). Ethics and economics. *Nursing Economic$, 18*(4), 194–202.

Donnelly, P. J. (2000). Ethics and cross-cultural nursing. *Journal of Transcultural Nursing, 11*(2), 119–127.

Grace, P. J. (2001). Professional advocacy: Widening the scope of accountability. *Nursing Philosophy, 2*(2), 151–163.

Haddad, A. (2003). Ethics in action. Fess up to patients? *RN, 66*(9), 27–28, 30, 55.

Hamric, A. B. (2001). Ethics development for clinical faculty. *Nursing Outlook, 49*(3), 115–117.

Hyatt, L. (2000). Does your organization have a conscience? *Nursing Homes Long-Term Care Management, 49*(4), 14–17.

Jaeger, S. M. (2001). Teaching healthcare ethics: The importance of moral sensitivity for moral reasoning. *Nursing Philosophy, 2*(2), 131–143.

Johnstone, M. (2000). Informed consent and the betrayal of patient's rights. *Australian Nursing Journal, 8*(2), 40–42.

Lachman, V. D. (2002). Organizational ethics need not be an oxymoron. *Patient Care Management, 18*(3), 1, 4–6.

Mariano, C. (2001). Holistic ethics. *American Journal of Nursing, 101*(1), 24A–27.

Miller, S. H., & Cohen, M. Z. (2000). The measure of advocacy. *American Journal of Nursing, 100*(1), 61–64.

Milton, C. L. (2003). Response to Volker's column: nursing theoretical frameworks —An ethic for nursing service. *Nursing Science Quarterly, 16*(3), 212–213.

New edition of ICN classic provides a key tool for ethical decision-making world-wide. (2003). *Journal of Advanced Nursing, 41*(5), 421.

Salladay, S. A. (2003). Ethical problems. Conflict of interest: Prescription for trouble. *Nursing ,33*(6), 65.

Schwartz, E. (2000). Thinking about moral questions. *Creative Nursing, 6*(3), 10–12.

Volker, D. L. (2003). Ethical issues. Is there a unique nursing ethic? *Nursing Science Quarterly, 16*(3), 207–211.

Watson, J. (July-September 2003). Love and caring: Ethics of face and hand—An invitation to return to the heart and soul of nursing and our deep humanity. *Nursing Administration Quarterly, 27*(3), 197–202.

White, G. B. (2000). What we may expect from ethics and the law. *American Journal of Nursing, 100*(10), 114–118.

5

Legal and Legislative Issues

Your best protection against malpractice is to know the circumstances where you're most at risk, then make sure you avoid any mistakes when functioning in them.

—Nursing Malpractice, 2003, p. 7

Chapter 4 presented ethics as an internal control of human behavior and nursing practice. Therefore, ethics has to do with actions people should take, not necessarily actions they are legally required to take. On the other hand, ethical behavior written into law is no longer just desired; it is mandated. This chapter focuses on the external controls of legislation and law. Since the first mandatory Nurse Practice Act was passed in New York in 1938, nursing has been legislated, directed, and controlled to some extent.

The primary purpose of law and legislation is to protect the patient and the nurse. Laws and legislation define the scope of acceptable practice and protect individual rights. Nurses who are aware of their rights and duties in legal matters are better able to protect themselves against liability or loss of professional licensure.

This chapter is divided into five sections. The first section presents the primary sources of law and how each affects nursing practice. The nurse's responsibility to be proactive in establishing and revising laws affecting nursing practice is emphasized. The next section presents the types of legal cases in which nurses may be involved and differentiates between the burden of proof and the consequences if found guilty in each type. The next section identifies specific doctrines used by the courts to define legal boundaries for nursing practice. The role of state boards in professional licensure and discipline is examined. The fourth section deals with the components of malpractice for the individual practitioner and the manager or supervisor. Legal terms are defined. The last section in this chapter deals with issues such as informed consent, medical records, intentional torts, the Patient Self Determination Act, the Good Samaritan Act, and the Health Information Protection and Portability Act (HIPAA).

This chapter is not meant to be a complete legal guide to nursing practice. There are many excellent legal textbooks and handbooks that accomplish that function. The primary function of this chapter is to emphasize the widely varying and rapidly changing nature of laws and the responsibility that each manager has to keep abreast of legislation and laws affecting both nursing and management practice. Leadership roles and management functions inherent in legal and legislative issues are shown in **Display 5.1.**

SOURCES OF LAW

The U.S. legal system can be somewhat confusing because there are not only four sources of the law, but also parallel systems at the state and federal levels. The sources of law include constitutions, statutes, administrative agencies, and court decisions. A comparison is shown in **Table 5.1.**

A *constitution* is a system of fundamental laws or principles that governs a nation, society, corporation, or another aggregate of individuals. The purpose of a constitution is to establish the basis of a governing system for the future and the present. The U.S. Constitution establishes the general organization of the federal government and grants and limits its specific powers. Each state also has a constitution that establishes the general organization of the state government and grants and limits its powers.

Display 5.1	Leadership Roles and Management Functions Legal and Legislative Issues

Leadership Roles of the Nurse

1. Serves as a role model by providing nursing care that meets or exceeds accepted standards of care.
2. Updates knowledge and skills in the field of practice and seeks professional certification to increase expertise in a specific field.
3. Reports substandard nursing care to appropriate authorities following established chain of command.
4. Fosters nurse–patient relationships that are respectful, caring, and honest, thus reducing the possibility of future lawsuits.
5. Creates an environment that encourages and supports cultural diversity and sensitivity.
6. Prioritizes patient rights and patient welfare first in decision making.
7. Demonstrates vision, risk taking, and energy in determining appropriate legal boundaries for nursing practice, thus defining what nursing is and should be in the future.

Management Functions of the Nurse

1. Increases knowledge regarding sources of law and legal doctrines that affect nursing practice.
2. Delegates to subordinates wisely, looking at the manager's scope of practice and that of the individuals he or she supervises.
3. Understands and adheres to institutional policies and procedures.
4. Minimizes the risk of product liability by assuring that all staff are appropriately oriented to the appropriate use of equipment and products.
5. Monitors subordinates to ensure they have a valid, current, and appropriate license to practice nursing.
6. Uses foreseeability of harm in delegation and staffing decisions.
7. Increases staff awareness of intentional torts and assists them in developing strategies to reduce their liability in these areas.
8. Provides educational and training opportunities for staff on legal issues affecting nursing practice.
9. Monitors whether employees are practicing within their scope of competence.

The second source of law is *statutes*—laws that govern. Legislative bodies, such as the U.S. Congress, state legislatures, and city councils, make these laws. Statutes are officially enacted (voted on and passed) by the legislative body and compiled into codes, collections of statutes, and ordinances. The 51 nurse practice acts representing the 50 states and the District of Columbia are examples of statutes. These nurse practice acts define and limit the practice of nursing, stating what constitutes authorized practice as well as what exceeds the scope of authority. Although nurse practice acts may vary among states, all must be consistent with provisions or statutes established at the federal level.

Administrative agencies, the third source of law, are given authority to act by the state legislative body and create rules and regulations that enforce statutory laws. For example, state boards of nursing are administrative agencies set up to implement and enforce the state nurse practice act by writing rules and regulations and

Table 5.1 Sources of Law

Origin of Law	Use	Involvement with Nursing Practice
The Constitution	The highest law in the United States; interpreted by the U.S. Supreme Court; gives authority to other three sources of the law.	Little direct involvement in the area of malpractice.
Statutes	Also called *statutory law* or *legislative law;* laws passed by the state or federal legislators and signed by the president or governor.	Before 1970s, very few state or federal laws dealt with malpractice. Since the malpractice crisis, many statutes affect malpractice.
Administrative agencies	The rules and regulations established by appointed agencies of the executive branch of the government (governor or president).	Some of these agencies, such as the National Labor Relations Board or health and safety boards, can affect nursing practice.
Court decisions	Also called *tort law;* this is court mode law and the courts interpret the statutes and set precedents; in the United States, there are two levels of court: trial court and appellate court.	Most malpractice law is addressed by the courts.

by conducting investigations and hearings to ensure the law's enforcement. Administrative laws are valid only to the extent that they are within the scope of the authority granted to them by the legislative body.

The fourth source of law is *court decisions.* Judicial or decisional laws are made by the courts to interpret legal issues that are in dispute. Depending on the type of court involved, judicial or decisional law may be made by a single justice, with or without a jury, or by a panel of justices. Generally, initial trial courts have a single judge or magistrate, intermediary appeal courts have three justices, and the highest appeal courts have nine justices.

TYPES OF LAWS AND COURTS

Although most nurses worry primarily about being sued for malpractice, they may actually be involved in three different types of court cases: criminal, civil, and administrative (see **Table 5.2**). The court in which each is tried, the burden of proof required for conviction, and the resulting punishment differ with each.

Table 5.2 Types of Laws and Courts		
Type	**Burden of Proof Required for Guilty Verdict**	**Likely Consequences of a Guilty Verdict**
Criminal	Beyond a reasonable doubt	Incarceration, probation, fines
Civil	Based on a preponderance of the evidence	Monetary damages
Administrative	Clear and convincing standard	Suspension or loss of licensure

In *criminal* cases, the individual faces charges generally filed by the state or federal attorney general for crimes committed against an individual or society. In criminal cases, the individual is always presumed to be innocent, unless the state is able to prove the defendant's guilt beyond a reasonable doubt (Brent, 2003). Incarceration and even death are possible consequences for being found guilty in criminal matters. Nurses found guilty of intentionally administering fatal doses of drugs to patients would likely be charged in a criminal court.

In *civil* cases, one individual sues another monetarily to compensate for a perceived loss. The burden of proof required to be found guilty in a civil case is described as a *preponderance of the evidence*. In other words, the judge or jury must believe that it was more likely than not that the accused was responsible for the injuries of the complainant. Consequences of being found guilty in a civil suit are monetary. Most malpractice cases are tried in civil court.

In *administrative* cases, an individual is sued by a state or federal governmental agency assigned the responsibility of implementing governmental programs (Brent, 2003). State boards of nursing are one such governmental agency. When an individual violates the state nursing practice act, the board of nursing may seek to revoke licensure or institute some form of discipline. The burden of proof in these cases varies from state to state, but generally is considered to be the "clear and convincing standard" (Brent, 2003). When the clear and convincing standard is not used, the preponderance of the evidence standard may be used. Clear and convincing is a higher burden of proof than preponderance of evidence but significantly lower than beyond a reasonable doubt.

LEGAL DOCTRINES AND THE PRACTICE OF NURSING

Two important legal doctrines frequently guide all three courts in their decision making. The first of these, *stare decisis*, means "let the decision stand." *Stare decisis* uses precedents as a guide for decision making. This doctrine gives nurses insight into ways the court has previously fixed liability in given situations. However, the nurse must avoid two pitfalls in determining if *stare decisis* should apply to a given situation.

The first is that the previous case must be within the jurisdiction of the court hearing the current case. For example, a previous Florida case decided by a state

Learning Exercise 5.1

Both Guilty and Not Guilty?
Think of celebrated cases where defendants have been tried in both civil and criminal courts. What were the verdicts in both cases? If the verdicts were not the same, analyze why this happened. Do you agree that taking away an individual's personal liberty by incarceration should require a higher burden of proof than assessing them monetary damages?

Then do a literature search to see if you can find cases where a nurse faced both civil and administrative charges. Were you able to find cases where the nurse was found guilty in a civil court but did not lose his or her license? Did you find the opposite?

court does not set precedent for a Texas appellate court. Although the Texas court may model its decision after the Florida case, it is not compelled to do so. The lower courts in Texas, however, would rely on Texas appellate decisions.

The other pitfall is that the court hearing the current case can depart from the precedent and set a landmark decision. Landmark decisions generally occur because societal needs have changed, technology has become more advanced, or following the precedent would further harm an already injured person. *Roe v Wade*, the 1973 landmark decision to allow a woman to seek and receive a legal abortion during the first two trimesters of pregnancy, is an example. Given changes in societal views about abortion, this precedent may change again in the future.

The second doctrine that guides courts in their decision making is *res judicata*, which means a "thing or matter settled by judgment." It applies only when a competent court has decided a legal dispute and when no further appeals are possible. This doctrine keeps the same parties in the original lawsuit from retrying the same issues that were involved in the first lawsuit.

When using doctrines as a guide for nursing practice, the nurse must remember that all laws are fluid and subject to change. Laws cannot be static; they must change to reflect the growing autonomy and responsibility desired by nurses. It is critical that each nurse be aware of and sensitive to rapidly changing laws and legislation that affect his or her practice. The nurse also must recognize that state laws may differ from federal laws and that legal guidelines for nursing practice in the organization may differ from state or federal guidelines.

Boundaries for practice are defined in the nurse practice act of each state. These acts are general in most states to allow for some flexibility in the broad roles and varied situations in which nurses practice. Because this allows for some interpretation, many employers have established guidelines for nursing practice in their own organization. These guidelines regarding scope of practice cannot, however, exceed the requirements of the state nursing practice acts. Managers need to be aware of their organization's specific practice interpretations and ensure that subordinates are aware of the same and follow established practices. All nurses must understand the legal controls for nursing practice in their state.

PROFESSIONAL NEGLIGENCE

Historically, physicians were the healthcare provider most likely to be held liable for nursing care. As nurses have gained authority and autonomy, they have assumed responsibility, accountability, and liability for their own practice. As roles have expanded, nurses have begun performing duties traditionally reserved for medical practice. As a result of an increased scope of practice, many nurses now carry individual malpractice insurance. This is a double-edged sword. Nurses need malpractice insurance because of their expanded roles, but they also incur a greater likelihood of being sued if they have malpractice insurance, since injured parties will always seek damages from as many individuals with financial resources as possible.

Because of the enhanced role of nurses and the increased number of insured nurses, liability suits seeking damages from nurses as individuals have increased tremendously over the past few decades. From 1998 to 2001, for instance, the National Practitioner Data Bank reveals that the number of malpractice payments made by nurses increased from 253 to 413 and the trend shows no sign of stopping (Croke, 2003).

In all liability suits, there is a plaintiff and a defendant. In malpractice cases, the *plaintiff* is the injured party and the *defendant* is the professional who is alleged to have caused the injury. *Negligence* has been defined as the omission to do something that a reasonable person, guided by the considerations that ordinarily regulate human affairs, would do or as doing something that a reasonable and prudent person would not do. *Reasonable and prudent* generally means the average judgment, foresight, intelligence, and skill that would be expected of a person with similar training and experience. *Malpractice*—the failure of a person with professional training to act in a reasonable and prudent manner—also is called professional negligence. Five elements must be present for a professional to be held liable for malpractice (**Table 5.3**).

First, a *standard of care* must have been established that outlines the level or degree of quality considered adequate by a given profession. Standards of care outline the duties a defendant has to a plaintiff, or a nurse to a patient. These standards represent the skills and learning commonly possessed by members of the profession and generally are the minimal requirements that define an acceptable level of care. Standards of care, which guarantee patients safe nursing care, include organizational policy and procedure statements, job descriptions, and student guidelines. Guidelines for standards of care are shown in **Display 5.2.**

Second, after the standard of care has been established, it must be shown that the standard was violated—there must have been a *breach of duty*. This breach is shown by calling other nurses who practice in the same specialty area as the defendant to testify as expert witnesses.

Third, the nurse must have had the knowledge or availability of information that not meeting the standard of care could result in harm. This is called *foreseeability of harm*. If the average, reasonable person in the defendant's position could have anticipated the plaintiff's injury as a result of his or her actions, then the plaintiff's injury was foreseeable. Being ignorant is not a justifiable excuse, but

> Being ignorant is not a justifiable excuse, but not having all the information in a situation may impede one's ability to foresee harm.

Table 5.3 Components of Professional Negligence

Elements of Liability	Explanation	Example: Giving Medications
1. Duty to use due care (defined by the standard of care)	The care that should be given under the circumstances (what the reasonably prudent nurse would have done)	A nurse should give medications accurately, completely, and on time.
2. Failure to meet standard of care (breach of duty)	Not giving the care that should be given under the circumstances	A nurse fails to give medications accurately, completely, or on time.
3. Forseeability of harm	The nurse must have reasonable access to information about whether the possibility of harm exists	The drug handbook specifies that the wrong dosage or route may cause injury.
4. A direct relationship between failure to meet the standard of care (breach) and injury can be proved	Patient is harmed because proper care is not given	Wrong dosage causes patient to have a convulsion.
5. Injury	Actual harm results to patient	Convulsion or other serious complication occurs.

not having all the information in a situation may impede one's ability to foresee harm. An example might be a charge nurse who assigned another registered nurse (RN) to care for a critically ill patient. The assigned RN makes a medication error that injures the patient in some way. If the charge nurse had reason to believe that the RN was incapable of adequately caring for the patient or if the charge nurse failed to provide adequate supervision, foreseeability of harm is apparent, and the charge nurse also could be held liable. If the charge nurse was available as needed and had good reason to believe that the RN was fully capable, he or she would likely not be held liable.

Several recent malpractice cases have hinged on whether the nurse was persistent enough in attempting to notify healthcare providers of changes in a patient's condition or convincing healthcare providers of the seriousness of a patient's condition (Nursing Malpractice, 2003). Because the nurse has foreseeability of harm in these situations, the nurse who is not persistent can be held liable for failing to intervene because the intervention was below what was expected of him or her as a patient advocate.

The fourth element is that *failure to meet the standard of care must have the potential to injure the patient.* There must be a provable correlation between improper care and injury to the patient.

| Display 5.2 | **Guidelines for Standards of Care** |

1. Recognize that all professions have standards of care. Standards are the minimal level of expertise that may be delivered to the patient; they are a starting point for greater expectations.
2. Standards of care may be externally or internally set. The nurse is responsible for both categories of standards, those set by forces outside of nursing and those set by the role of nursing.
3. Standards of care can be found in the following:
   a. The state nurse practice act
   b. Published standards of professional organizations and specialty practice groups, such as the American Association of Critical Care Nurses or the Association of Operating Room Nurses
   c. Federal agency guidelines and regulations
   d. Hospital policy and procedure manuals
   e. The nurse's job descriptions
4. The nurse is accountable for all standards of care as they pertain to his or her profession. To remain competent and skillful, the nurse is encouraged to read professional journals and to attend pertinent continuing education and in-service programs.
5. Standards of care are determined for the judicial system by expert witnesses. Such people testify to the prevailing standards in the community—a standard that all nurses are accountable for matching and exceeding—thus ensuring that patients receive quality, competent nursing care.

Reprinted with permission from Guido, G. W. (1988). *Legal issues in nursing: A sourcebook for practice.* Norwalk, CT: Appleton & Lange.

The final element is that *actual patient injury* must occur. This injury must be more than transitory. The plaintiff must show that the action of the defendant directly caused the injury and that the injury would not have occurred without the defendant's actions. It is important to remember here, however, that not taking action is an action. Nurses can be held liable even if the patient injures him or herself because the nurse did not appropriately safeguard the patient from harm (Nursing Malpractice, 2003).

AVOIDING MALPRACTICE CLAIMS

Interactions between nurses and patients that are less businesslike and more personal are more satisfying to both. It has been shown that despite technical competence, nurses who have difficulty establishing positive interpersonal relationships with patients and their families are at greater risk of being sued. Caring and professional communication has been shown repeatedly to be a major reason people do not sue, despite adequate grounds for a successful lawsuit. The importance of working to create respectful, honest, and positive nurse–patient relationships cannot be underestimated (Cady, 2000).

Allegations of nursing negligence also cross all work settings. Although acute care facilities continue to be the primary site of such allegations for nurses (60%),

Learning Exercise 5.2

Who's Guilty? You Decide

You are a surgical nurse at Memorial Hospital. At 4 PM, you receive a female patient from the PACU. She has had a total hip replacement. You note that the hip dressings are saturated with blood but are aware that total hip replacements frequently have some postoperative oozing from the wound. There is an order on the chart to reinforce the dressing as needed, and you do so. When you next check the dressing at 6 PM, you find the reinforcements saturated and drainage on the bed linen. You call the physician and tell her that you believe the patient is bleeding too heavily. The physician reassures you the amount of bleeding you have described is not excessive but encourages you to continue to monitor the patient closely. You recheck the patient's dressings at 7 PM and 8 PM. You again call the physician and tell her that the bleeding still looks too heavy. She again reassures you and tells you to continue to watch the patient closely. At 10 PM, the patient's blood pressure becomes nonpalpable and she goes into shock. You summon the doctor and she comes immediately. **Assignment:** What are the legal ramifications of this case? Using the components of professional negligence outlined in Table 5.3, determine who in this case is guilty of malpractice. Justify your answer. At what point in the scenario should each character have altered his or her actions to reduce the probability of a negative outcome?

long-term care facilities represent 18% of such claims and psychiatric facilities represent another 8% (Croke, 2003). Advanced practice nurses face 9% of such claims and home health agencies represent 2%.

Croke (2003) identifies several factors that have contributed to the increasing number of malpractice cases against nurses. These are shown in **Display 5.3.** Crooke goes on to say that there are six major categories of negligence issues that prompt most malpractice suits. These include a failure to follow standards of care, failure to use equipment in a responsible manner, failure to communicate, failure to document, failure to assess and monitor, and failure to act as a patient advocate.

Display 5.3	**Factors Contributing to the Increase in Malpractice Cases for Nurses**

- Increased delegation to unlicensed assistive personnel
- Early discharge of patients
- The nursing shortage and downsizing
- Advances in technology
- Increased autonomy and responsibility of hospital nurses
- Better informed consumers
- Expanded legal definitions of liability

Source: Croke, E. M. (2003). Nurses, negligence, and malpractice. *American Journal of Nursing 103*(9), 54–64.

Nurses can, however, reduce their risk of being sued successfully for malpractice if they do the following:

- Practice within the scope of the nurse practice act
- Observe agency policies and procedures
- Model practice after established practice standards
- Always put patient rights and welfare first
- Be aware of relevant law and legal doctrines and combine such with the biological, psychological, and social sciences that form the basis of all rational nursing decisions
- Practice within the area of individual competence
- Upgrade technical skills consistently by attending continuing education programs and seeking specialty certification
- Purchase professional liability insurance and understand fully the limits of the individual policy

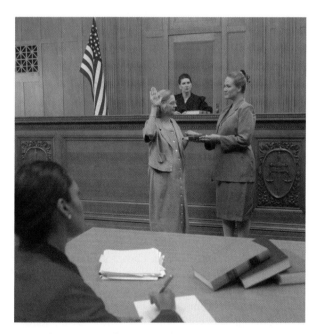

More than ever before, nurses need be concerned about malpractice. Protective measures include observing confidentiality, continuously updating skills, following institutional guidelines and protocols, documenting meticulously, and obtaining malpractice insurance.

Learning Exercise 5.3

Discussing Lawsuits and Liability
In small groups, discuss the following questions:
1. Do you believe there are unnecessary lawsuits in the healthcare industry? What criteria can be used to distinguish between appropriate and unnecessary lawsuits?
2. Have you ever advised a friend or family member to sue to recover damages you believed they suffered as a result of poor-quality health care? What motivated you to encourage them to do so?
3. Do you think you will make clinical errors in judgment as a nurse? If so, what types of errors should be considered acceptable (if any) and what types are not acceptable?
4. Do you believe the recent national spotlight on medical error identification and prevention will encourage the reporting of medical errors when they do occur?

EXTENDING THE LIABILITY

In recent years, the concept of *joint liability*, in which the nurse, physician, and employing organization are all held liable, has become the current position of the legal system. This probably more accurately reflects the higher level of accountability now present in the nursing profession. Before 1965, nurses were rarely held accountable for their own acts, and hospitals were usually exempt due to charitable immunity. However, following precedent-setting cases in the 1960s, employers are now held liable for the nurse's acts under a concept known as *vicarious liability*. One form of vicarious liability, called *respondeat superior*, means "the master is responsible for the acts of his servants." The theory behind the doctrine is that an employer should be held legally liable for the conduct of employees whose actions he or she has a right to direct or control.

The difficulty in interpreting *respondeat superior* is that many exceptions exist. The first and most important exception is related to the state in which the nurse practices. In some states, the *doctrine of charitable immunity* applies, which holds that a charitable (nonprofit) hospital cannot be sued by a person who has been injured as a result of a hospital employee's negligence. Thus, liability is limited to the individual employee.

Another exception to *respondeat superior* occurs when the state or federal government employs the nurse. The common-law rule of *governmental immunity* provides that governments cannot be held liable for the negligent acts of their employees while carrying out government activities. Some states have changed this rule by statute, however, and in these particular jurisdictions, *respondeat superior* continues to apply to the acts of nurses employed by the state government.

Nurses must remember that the purpose of *respondeat superior* is not to shift the burden of blame from the employee to the organization, but rather to share the blame, increasing the possibility of larger financial compensation to the injured party.

Some nurses erroneously assume that they do not need to carry malpractice insurance because their employer will in all probability be sued as well and thus will be responsible for financial damages. Under the doctrine of *respondeat superior*, any employer required to pay damages to an injured person because of an employee's negligence may have the legal right to recover or be reimbursed that amount from the negligent employee.

Nurses must also understand the concept of personal liability, which says that every person is liable for his or her own conduct. The law does not permit a wrongdoer to avoid legal liability for his or her own wrongdoing, even though someone else also may be sued and held legally liable. For example, if a manager directs a subordinate to do something that both know to be improper, the injured party can recover damages against the subordinate, even if the supervisor agreed to accept full responsibility for the delegation at the time. In the end, each nurse is always held liable for his or her own negligent practice.

Managers are not automatically held liable for all acts of negligence on the part of those they supervise, but they may be held liable if they were negligent in the supervision of those employees at the time they committed the negligent acts. Sheehan (2001) states that nurses remain responsible for all delegated tasks and are legally and professionally responsible for directing and supervising the activities of other staff. Liability for negligence is generally based on the manager's failure to determine which of the patient needs can be assigned safely to a subordinate, or the failure to supervise a subordinate adequately for the assigned task. Both the abilities of the staff member and the complexity of the task assigned must be considered when determining the type and amount of direction and supervision warranted.

Hospitals have also been found liable for assigning personnel who were unqualified to perform duties as shown by their evaluation reports. Managers, therefore, need to be cognizant of their responsibilities in assigning and appointing personnel, because they could be found liable for ignoring organizational policies or for assigning employees duties that they are not capable of performing. In such cases, though, the employee must provide the supervisor with the information that he or she is not qualified for the assignment. The manager does have the right to reassign employees as long as they are capable of discharging the anticipated duties of the assignment.

In addition, there has been a push to have more in-depth background checks when healthcare employees are hired, with some states already mandating such checks. In addition, federal legislation has recently been introduced along these lines. At present, except in a few states, personnel directors in hospitals (those making hiring decisions) are required to request information from the National Practitioner Data Bank only for those individuals who seek clinical privileges and many states even require nursing students to be fingerprinted before they are allowed to work with vulnerable populations. In the future, hiring someone without an adequate background check, who later commits a crime involving a patient, could be another area of liability for the manager. This is an example of the type of pending legislation with which a manager must keep abreast, so that if it becomes law, its impact on future management practices will be minimized.

Learning Exercise 5.4

Understanding Limitations and Risks
Have you ever been directed in your nursing practice to do something that you believed might be unsafe or that you felt inadequately trained or prepared to do? What did you do? Would you act differently if the situation occurred now? What risks are inherent in refusing to follow the direct orders of a physician or superior? What are the risks of performing a task you believe may be unsafe?

INCIDENT REPORTS

Incident reports are records of unusual or unexpected incidents that occur in the course of a patient's treatment. Because attorneys use incident reports to defend the health agency against lawsuits brought by patients, the reports are generally considered confidential communications and cannot be subpoenaed by patients or used as evidence in their lawsuits in most states. (Be sure, however, you know the law for the state in which you practice as this does vary.) However, incident reports that are inadvertently disclosed to the plaintiff are no longer considered confidential and can be subpoenaed in court. Thus, a copy of an incident report should not be left in the chart. In addition, no entry should be made in the patient's record about the existence of an incident report. The chart should, however, provide enough information about the incident or occurrence that appropriate treatment can be given.

INTENTIONAL TORTS

Torts are legal wrongs committed against a person or property, independent of a contract, that render the person who commits them liable for damages in a civil action. Whereas professional negligence is considered to be an unintentional tort, assault, battery, false imprisonment, invasion of privacy, defamation, and slander are intentional torts. *Intentional torts* are a direct invasion of someone's legal rights. Managers are responsible for seeing that their staff are aware of and adhere to laws governing intentional torts. In addition, the manager must clearly delineate policies and procedures about these issues in the work environment.

Nurses can be sued for assault and battery. *Assault* is conduct that makes a person fearful and produces a reasonable apprehension of harm and *battery* is an intentional and wrongful physical contact with a person that entails an injury or offensive touching (Nursing Malpractice, 2003). Unit managers must be alert to patient complaints of being handled in a rough manner or complaints of excessive force in restraining patients. In fact, performing any treatment without patient permission or without receiving an informed consent might constitute both assault and battery. In addition, many battery suits have been won based on the use of restraints when dealing with confused patients.

The use of physical restraints also has led to claims of *false imprisonment*. False imprisonment describes any unlawful confinement within fixed boundaries and this confinement can be produced by physical, emotional, or chemical means (Nursing Malpractice, 2003). Practitioners are liable for false imprisonment when they unlawfully restrain the movement of their patients. Physical restraints should be applied only with a physician's direct order. Likewise, the patient who wishes to sign out against medical advice should not be held against his or her will. This tort also is frequently applicable to involuntary commitments to mental health facilities. Managers in mental health settings must be careful to institutionalize patients in accordance with all laws governing commitment. Finally, false imprisonment by chemical confinement occurs when drugs are given, not for their therapeutic value, but to keep a patient within an institution (Nursing Malpractice).

Another intentional tort is defamation. *Defamation* is communicating to a third party false information that injures a person's reputation; causes economic damage; diminishes the esteem, respect, goodwill, or confidence that others have for the person; or causes adverse, derogatory, or unpleasant opinions of him (Nursing Malpractice, 2003). Being truthful reduces the risk of charges of defamation, however, "truth is no defense against charges of invasion of privacy, breach of confidentiality, or inflicting emotional distress" (p. 11).

OTHER LEGAL RESPONSIBILITIES OF THE MANAGER

Managers also have some legal responsibility for the quality control of nursing practice at the unit level, including such duties as reporting dangerous understaffing, checking staff credentials and qualifications, and carrying out appropriate discipline. Austin (2001*a*) reports that healthcare facilities may also be held responsible for seeing to it that staff members know how to operate equipment safely.

Likewise, standards of care as depicted in policies and procedures may pose a liability for the nurse if such policies and procedures are not followed. In such cases, the manager is responsible for auditing and providing follow-up interventions (or for delegating this aspect of practice to someone else) if the standard of care is not met. The chain of command in reporting inadequate care by a physician is another area where management liability may occur if employees do not learn and follow proper protocols. Both Austin (2001*b*) and Warlick (2000) feel that managers have a responsibility to see that written protocols, policies, and procedures are followed in order to reduce liability. Additionally, the manager, like all professional nurses, is responsible for reporting improper or substandard medical care, child and elder abuse, and communicable diseases as specified by the Centers for Disease Control and Prevention.

Individual nurses also may be held liable for *product liability*. When a product is involved, negligence does not have to be proved. This strict liability is a somewhat gray area of nursing practice. Essentially, strict liability holds that a product may be held to a higher level of liability than a person. In other words, if it can be proved that the equipment or product had a defect that caused an injury, then liability would be debated in court using all the elements essential for negligence, such as duty or breach. Therefore, equipment and other products fall within the scope of nursing responsibility. In general, if they are aware that equipment is faulty, nurses have a duty to refuse to use the equipment. If the fault in the equipment is not readily apparent, risks are low that the nurse will be found liable for the results of its use.

Informed Consent

Many nurses erroneously believe they have obtained informed consent when they witness a patient's signature on a consent form for surgery or procedure. Strictly speaking, *informed consent* (outlined in **Display 5.4**) is obtained only after the patient receives full disclosure of all pertinent information regarding the surgery or procedure and only if they understand the potential benefits and risks associated with doing so (Dunn, 2000). The information must be provided in language the patient can understand and should be provided by the individual who will be performing the procedure. Generally, this is a physician (Dunn). Patients must also be invited to ask questions. In witnessing the patient's signature to the consent form, the nurse's ethical obligation is to be sure the patient has been fully informed and does understand.

> Informed consent is obtained only after the patient receives full disclosure of all pertinent information regarding the surgery or procedure and only if they understand the potential benefits and risks associated with doing so.

Only a competent adult can legally sign a document to show informed consent. To be considered competent, the patient must be capable of understanding the nature and consequences of the decision and communicating the decision. Spouses or other family members cannot legally sign unless there is an approved guardianship or conservatorship or unless they hold a durable power of attorney for health care. If the patient is under age 16 (18 in some states), a parent or guardian must generally give consent (Dunn, 2000).

Display 5.4	Guidelines for Informed Consent

The person(s) giving consent must fully comprehend:
a. The procedure to be performed
b. The risks involved
c. Expected or desired outcomes
d. Expected complications or side effects that may occur as a result of treatment
e. Alternative treatments that are available

Consent may be given by:
a. A competent adult
b. A legal guardian or individual holding durable power of attorney
c. An emancipated, married minor
d. Mature minor (varies by state)
e. Parent of a minor child
f. Court order

In an emergency, the physician can invoke *implied consent*, in which the physician states in the progress notes of the medical record that the patient is unable to sign but that treatment is immediately needed and is in the patient's best interest. Usually, another physician must validate this type of implied consent.

Nurses frequently seek *express consent* from patients by witnessing patients sign a standard consent form. In express consent, the role of the nurse is to be sure that the patient has informed consent and to seek remedy if the patient does not.

Informed consent does pose ethical issues for nurses. Although nurses are obligated to provide teaching and to clarify information given to patients by their physicians, nurses must be careful not to give new information that contradicts or conflicts with information given by the physician, thus interfering in the physician–patient relationship. The nurse is not responsible for explaining the procedure to be done; rather the nurse's role is to advocate for patients by preserving their dignity, identifying their fears, determining their level of understanding and approval of the care to be given, and protecting their rights (Dunn, 2000). At times, this can be a cloudy issue both legally and ethically.

Medical Records

One source of information people seek to help them make decisions about their health care is their medical record. Nurses have a legal responsibility for accurately

Learning Exercise 5.5

Is It Really Informed Consent?
You are a staff nurse on a surgical unit. Shortly after reporting for duty, you make rounds on all your patients. Mrs. Jones is a 36-year-old woman scheduled for a bilateral salpingo-oophorectomy and hysterectomy. In the course of the conversation, Mrs. Jones comments that she is glad that she will not be undergoing menopause as a result of this surgery. She elaborates by stating that one of her friends had surgery that resulted in "surgical menopause" and that it was devastating to her. You return to the chart and check the surgical permit and doctor's progress notes. The operating room permit reads "bilateral salpingo-oophorectomy and hysterectomy," and it is signed by Mrs. Jones. The physician has noted "discussed surgery with patient" in his progress notes.

You return to Mrs. Jones' room and ask her what type of surgery she is having; she states, "I'm having my uterus removed." You phone the physician and relate your information to the surgeon. He says, "Mrs. Jones knows that I will take out her ovaries if necessary; I've discussed it with her. She signed the permit. Now, please get her ready for surgery—she is the next case."

Assignment: Discuss what you should do at this point. Why did you select this course of action? What issues are involved here? Be able to discuss legal ramifications of this case.

recording appropriate information in the patient's medical record. The alteration of medical records can result in license suspension or revocation.

Although the patient owns the information in that medical record, the actual record belongs to the facility that originally made the record and is storing it. Although patients must have reasonable access to their records, the method for retrieving the record varies greatly from one institution to another. Generally, a patient who wishes to inspect his or her records must make a written request and pay reasonable clerical costs to make such records available. The healthcare provider generally permits such inspection during business hours within several working days of the inspection request. Nurses should be aware of the procedure for procuring medical records for patients at the facilities where they work. Often a patient's attempt to procure medical records results from a lack of trust or a need for additional teaching and education. Cady (2000) maintains that a frequent reason that patients give for filing a malpractice suit is that they did not understand the information given to them. Nurses can do a great deal to reduce this confusion and foster an open, trusting relationship between the patient and his or her healthcare providers.

> A frequent reason that patients give for filing a malpractice suit is that they did not understand the information given to them.

The Patient Self Determination Act (PSDA)

The Patient Self Determination Act (PSDA), enacted in 1991, required healthcare organizations that received federal funding to provide education for staff and patients on issues concerning treatment and end-of-life issues. This education included the use of *advanced directives* where written instructions regarding end-of-life care are completed by competent individuals, to be implemented should they become incapacitated in the future (Shapiro & Bowles, 2002).

Although the PSDA requires acute-care facilities to document on the medical record whether a patient has an advance directive and to provide written information to patients who do not, there is nothing in the statute regarding the training for those who provide information (Shapiro & Bowles, 2002). Therefore, the intent of the statute may be lost or misinterpreted if staff members charged with providing information are neither knowledgeable nor comfortable with the subject (Shapiro & Bowles). A review of the literature suggests that this is the case with the majority of registered nurses (Shapiro & Bowles).

Good Samaritan Laws

Good Samaritan laws state that healthcare providers are protected from potential liability if they volunteer their nursing skills away from the workplace, provided that actions taken are not grossly negligent. The focus of Good Samaritan laws, however, is limited to emergencies and does not cover nonemergent care or advice given to family, friends, and neighbors, even if unpaid (Brooke, 2003).

Most states have Good Samaritan laws to encourage healthcare providers to help victims in an emergency, although protection under these laws varies tremendously from state to state. In some states, the law grants immunity to RNs but does not protect LVNs/LPNs. Other states offer protection to anyone who offers

Learning Exercise 5.6

Mrs. Brown's Chart

Mrs. Brown has been diagnosed as having invasive cancer. She has been having daily radiation treatments. Her husband is a frequent visitor and seems to be a devoted husband. They are both very interested in her progress and prognosis. Although they have asked many questions and you have given truthful answers, you know little because the physician has not shared much with the staff. Today, you walk into Mrs. Brown's room and find Mr. Brown sitting at Mrs. Brown's bedside reading her chart. The radiation orderly had inadvertently left the chart in the room when Mrs. Brown returned from x-ray.

Assignment: Identify several alternatives that you have. Discuss what you would do and why. Is there a problem here? What follow-up is indicated? Attempt to solve this problem on your own before reading the sample analysis that follows.

Analysis: The nurse needs to determine the most important goal in this situation. Possible goals include (1) getting the chart away from Mr. Brown as soon as possible, (2) protecting the privacy of Mrs. Brown, (3) gathering more information, or (4) becoming a patient advocate for the Browns.

In solving the case, it is apparent that not enough information has been gathered. Mr. Brown now has the chart, and it seems pointless to take it away from him. Usually the danger in patients' families reading the chart lies in the direction of their not understanding the chart and thereby obtaining confusing information or a patient's privacy being invaded because the patient has not consented to family members' access to the chart.

Using this as the basis for rationale, the nurse should use the following approach:

- Clarify that Mr. Brown has Mrs. Brown's permission to read the chart by asking her directly.
- Ask Mr. Brown if there is anything in the chart that he did not understand or anything that he questioned. You may even ask him to summarize what he has read. Clarify the things that are appropriate for the nurse to address, such as terminology, procedures, or nursing care.
- Refer questions that are inappropriate for the nurse to answer to the physician, and let Mr. Brown know that you will help him in talking with the physician regarding the medical plan and prognosis.
- After talking with Mr. Brown, the nurse should request the chart, and place it in the proper location. The incident should be reported to the immediate supervisor.
- The nurse should follow through by talking with the physician about the incident and Mr. Brown's concerns and by assisting the Browns to obtain the information they have requested.

Conclusion: The nurse first gathered more information before becoming the adversary or advocate. It is possible that the Browns had only simple questions to ask and that the problem was a lack of communication between staff and their patients, rather than a physician–patient communication deficit. Legally, patients have a right to understand what is happening to them, and that should be the basis for the decisions in this case.

assistance, even if they do not have a health background (Brooke, 2003). Still other states (Vermont and Minnesota) *require* individuals at an emergency to render aid to someone who's "exposed to grave physical harm" (Brooke, p. 46). Nurses should be familiar with the Good Samaritan laws in their states.

Health Insurance Portability and Accountability Act (HIPAA) of 1996

Another area of the law that nurses must understand is the right to confidentiality. Unauthorized release of information or photographs in medical records may make the person who discloses the information civilly liable for invasion of privacy, defamation, or slander. Written patient authorization to release information is needed to allow such disclosure. Many nurses have been caught unaware by the telephone call requesting information about a patient's condition. It is extremely important that the nurse not give out unauthorized information, regardless of the urgency of the person making the request. Likewise, managers must ensure that unauthorized people do not have access to patient charts or medical records and that unauthorized people are not allowed to observe procedures.

Privacy and Confidentiality

Efforts to preserve patient confidentiality increased tremendously with the passage of the *Health Insurance Portability and Accountability Act (HIPAA) of 1996* (also known as the Kassebaum-Kennedy Act). HIPAA gave Congress a deadline of August 1999 to pass legislation protecting the privacy of health information and to improve the portability and continuity of health insurance coverage. When this did not happen, the Department of Health and Human Services (DHHS) stepped in and issued the appropriate regulations (Charters, 2003). The first version of the privacy rule was issued in December 2000 under the Clinton administration, but it was modified by the Bush administration before it was ever implemented (HHS Privacy, 2002). The latest version of the privacy rule (Standards for Privacy of Individually Identifiable Health Information) was published in the Federal Register in 2002 (Charters, 2003).

Simplifying Communication and Healthcare Delivery

HIPAA essentially represents two areas for implementation. The first is the *Administrative Simplification Plan* and the second is the *Privacy Rules*. The Administrative Simplification Plan is directed at restructuring the coding of health information to simplify the digital exchange of information among healthcare providers and to improve the efficiency of healthcare delivery (Follansbee, 2002). The Privacy Rules are directed at ensuring strong privacy protections for patient without threatening access to care.

Compliance with the rules for transactions and code sets for large health plans (annual receipts in excess of $5 million) were effective as of October 2002, although a one-year extension was available from the Centers for Medicare and Medicaid. Compliance with the privacy act portion of HIPAA was required by April 14, 2003. The only exception was small health plans (fewer than 50 members), which had until April 14, 2004, to comply (Charters, 2003).

Privacy Rule

The Privacy Rule applies to three primary *covered entities* (CE): health plans, health-care clearinghouses, and healthcare providers. It also covers all patient records and other individually identifiable health information used or disclosed by a CE in any form (electronic, paper, or oral) (Maddox, 2002). Although there are many components to HIPAA, key components of the Privacy Rule are that direct treatment providers must make a good faith effort to obtain written acknowledgement of the notice of privacy rights and practices from patients. In addition, healthcare providers must disclose protected health information to patients requesting their own information or when oversight agencies request the data (HHS Privacy, 2002). Reasonable efforts must be taken, however, to limit the disclosure of personal health information to the minimum information necessary in order to complete the transaction.

There are situations, however, when limiting the information is not required. For example, minimum information is not required for treatment purposes since it is clearly better to have too much information than too little. The HIPAA Privacy Rule also requires that written authorization is needed before protected health information can be used for marketing purposes, such as selling lists of enrollees to third parties (Charters, 2003). The rule exempts face-to-face encounters or communication offering a nominal value promotional gift.

Implications for Nurses

Because of the complexity of the HIPAA regulations, it is not expected that a nursing manager would be responsible for compliance alone. Instead it is most important that the manager work with the administrative team to develop compliance procedures. It is equally important that managers remain cognizant of ongoing changes to the guidelines and be aware of how rules governing these issues may differ in the state in which they are employed. Some provisions of the Privacy Rules mention "reasonable efforts" towards achieving compliance. It is important to realize that being reasonable is provision specific and does not apply to achieving compliance with the entire Privacy Rules. Enforcement of HIPAA falls to the Office of Civil Rights (2003), which states it is taking a "cooperative" approach in helping covered entities achieve compliance.

Staff nurses are also impacted by HIPAA. Follansbee (2002) suggests that while part of HIPAA is directed at technology, the majority will involve changes in policies and procedures. Thus, all healthcare organizations have had to identify more accurately their security priorities and goals.

LEGAL CONSIDERATIONS OF MANAGING A DIVERSE WORKFORCE

Currently, minorities constitute about one quarter of the labor force, with a significant growth in the number of Hispanic, Asian, and African American employees expected over the next two decades. As will be discussed in later chapters, a primary area of diversity is language, including word meanings, accents, or dialects. Problems arising from this could be misunderstanding or reluctance to ask questions. Staff from cultures in which assertiveness is not promoted may find it difficult to disagree with or question others. How the manager handles these manifestations of cultural diversity is of major importance. If the manager's response is seen as discriminatory, the employee may file a complaint with one of the state or federal agencies that oversee civil rights or equal opportunity enforcement. Such things as overt or subtle discrimination are prohibited by Title VII (Civil Rights Act of 1964). Managers have a responsibility to be fair and just. Lack of promotions and unfair assignments may occur with minority employees just because they are different.

In addition, English-only rules in the workplace may be viewed as discriminatory under Title VII. Such rules may not violate Title VII if employers require English only during certain periods of time. Even in these circumstances, the employees must be notified of the rules and how they are to be enforced.

Clearly, managers should be taught how to deal sensitively and appropriately with an increasingly diverse workforce. Enhancing self-awareness and staff awareness of personal cultural biases, developing a comprehensive cultural diversity program, and role modeling cultural sensitivity are some of the ways that managers can effectively avoid many legal problems associated with discriminatory issues. However, it is hoped that future goals for the manager would go beyond compliance with Title VII and move toward understanding of and respect for other cultures.

> Licensure is a privilege and not a right.

PROFESSIONAL VERSUS INSTITUTIONAL LICENSURE

In general, a *license* is a legal document that permits a person to offer special skills and knowledge to the public in a particular jurisdiction, when such practice would otherwise be unlawful. Licensure establishes standards for entry into practice, defines a scope of practice, and allows for disciplinary action. Currently, licensing for nurses is a responsibility of state boards of nursing or state boards of nurse examiners, which also provide discipline as necessary. The manager, however, is responsible for monitoring that all licensed subordinates have a valid, appropriate, and current license to practice.

Licensure is a privilege and not a right. All nurses must safeguard this privilege by knowing the standards of care applicable to their work setting. Deviation from that standard should be undertaken only when nurses are prepared to accept the consequences of their actions, both in terms of liability and loss of licensure.

Nurses who violate specific norms of conduct, such as securing a license by fraud, performing specific actions prohibited by the nurse practice act, exhibiting unprofessional or illegal conduct, performing malpractice, or abusing alcohol or drugs, may have their licenses suspended or revoked by the licensing boards in all states. Frequent causes of license revocation are shown in **Display 5.5**.

Typically, suspension and revocation proceedings are administrative. Following a complaint, the board of nursing completes an investigation. The majority of these investigations reveal no grounds for discipline. If the investigation supports the need for discipline, nurses are notified of the charges and allowed to prepare a defense. At the hearing, which is very similar to a trial, the nurse is allowed to present evidence. Based on the evidence, an administrative law judge makes a recommendation to the state board of nursing, which makes the final decision. The entire process, from complaint to final decision may take up to two years.

| Display 5.5 | **Common Causes of Professional Nursing License Suspension or Revocation** |

- Professional negligence
- Practicing medicine or nursing without a license
- Obtaining a nursing license by fraud or allowing others to use your license
- Felony conviction for any offense substantially related to the function or duties of a registered nurse
- Participating professionally in criminal abortions
- Not reporting substandard medical or nursing care
- Providing patient care while under the influence of drugs or alcohol
- Giving narcotic drugs without an order
- Falsely holding oneself out to the public or to any healthcare practitioner as a "nurse practitioner"

Some professionals have advocated shifting the burden of licensure, and thus accountability, from individual practitioners to an institution or agency. Proponents for this move believe that *institutional licensure* would provide more effective use of personnel and greater flexibility. Most professional nursing organizations oppose this move strongly because they believe it has the potential for diluting the quality of nursing care.

An alternative to institutional licensure has been the development of *certification programs* by the ANA. By passing specifically prepared written examinations, nurses are able to qualify for certification in most nurse practice areas. This voluntary testing program represents professional organizational certification. In addition to ANA certification, other specialties, such as cardiac care, offer their own certification examinations. Many nursing leaders today strongly advocate professional certification as a means of enhancing the profession.

INTEGRATING LEADERSHIP ROLES AND MANAGEMENT FUNCTIONS IN LEGAL AND LEGISLATIVE ISSUES

Legislative and legal controls for nursing practice have been established to clarify the boundaries of nursing practice and to protect patients. The leader uses established legal guidelines to role model nursing practice that meets or exceeds accepted standards of care. Leaders also are role models in their efforts to expand expertise in their field and to achieve specialty certification. Perhaps the most important leadership roles in law and legislation are those of vision, risk taking, and energy. The leader is active in professional organizations and groups that define what nursing is and what it should be in the future. This is an internalized responsibility that must be adopted by many more nurses if the profession is to be a recognized and vital force in the political arena.

Management functions in legal and legislative issues are more directive. Managers are responsible for seeing that their practice and the practice of their subordinates are in accord with current legal guidelines. This requires that managers have a working knowledge of current laws and legal doctrines that affect nursing practice. Because laws are not static, this is an active and ongoing function. The manager has a legal obligation to uphold the laws, rules, and regulations affecting the organization, the patient, and nursing practice.

Managers have a responsibility to be fair and nondiscriminatory in dealing with all members of the workforce, including those whose culture differs from their own. The effective leader goes beyond merely preventing discriminatory charges and instead strives to develop sensitivity to the needs of a culturally diverse staff.

The integrated leader–manager reduces the personal risk of legal liability by creating an environment that prioritizes patient needs and welfare. In addition, caring, respect, and honesty as part of nurse–patient relationships are emphasized. If these functions and roles are truly integrated, the risk of patient harm and nursing liability is greatly reduced.

☀ Key Concepts

- *Sources of law* include constitutions, statutes, administrative agencies, and court decisions.
- The burden of proof for guilt and the subsequent punishment differs significantly between *criminal*, civil, and *administrative* courts.
- *Nurse practice acts* define the scope of nursing practice in each state.
- Professional organizations generally espouse standards of care that are higher than those required by law. These voluntary controls often are forerunners of legal controls.
- Legal doctrines such as *stare decisis* and *res judicata* frequently guide courts in their decision making.
- Licensing nurses is a responsibility of state boards of nursing or state boards of nurse examiners. These boards also provide discipline as necessary.
- Some professionals advocate shifting the burden of licensure, and thus accountability, from individual practitioners to institutions or agencies. Many professional nursing organizations oppose this move.
- *Malpractice* or *professional negligence* is the failure of a person with professional training to act in a reasonable and prudent manner. Five components must be present for an individual to be found guilty of malpractice.
- Employers can be held liable for an employee's acts under the concept of *vicarious liability*. Every person, however, is liable for his or her own tortuous conduct.
- Managers are not automatically held liable for negligence on the part of subordinates, but they may be held liable if they were negligent in supervising those employees when the negligent acts were committed.
- Assault, battery, false imprisonment, invasion of privacy, defamation, and slander are intentional torts.
- Consent can be *informed, implied* or *expressed.* Nurses must understand the differences between these types of consents and use the appropriate one.

- Although patients own the information in a medical record, the actual record belongs to the facility that originally made it and is storing it.
- It has been shown that despite good technical competence, nurses who have difficulty establishing positive interpersonal relationships with patients and their families are at greater risk of being sued for malpractice.
- Nurses should be aware how laws such as Good Samaritan immunity or legal access to incident reports are implemented in the states in which they live.
- New legislation pertaining to confidentiality (HIPAA) and patient rights (PSDA) continue to shape nurse–patient interactions in the healthcare system.

More Learning Exercises and Applications

 Learning Exercise 5.7

Where Does Your Responsibility Lie?
Mrs. Shin is a 68-year-old patient with liver cancer. She has been admitted to the oncology unit at Memorial Hospital. Her admitting physician has advised chemotherapy, even though he believes it has little chance of working. The patient asks her doctor, in your presence, if there is an alternative treatment to chemotherapy. He replies, "Nothing else has proved effective. Everything else is quackery, and you would be wasting your money." After he leaves, the patient and her family ask you if you know anything about alternative treatments. When you indicate that you do have some current literature available, they beg you to share your information with them.
Assignment: What do you do? What is your legal responsibility to your patient, the doctor, and the hospital? Using your knowledge of the legal process, the nurse practice act, patients' rights, and legal precedents (look for the case *Tuma v. Board of Nursing*, 1979), explain what you would do, and defend your decision.

Learning Exercise 5.8

Legal Ramifications of Exceeding One's Duties
You have been the evening charge nurse in the emergency room at
Memorial Hospital for the last two years. Besides yourself, you have two
LVNs and four RNs working in your department. Your normal staffing is to
have two RNs and one LVN on duty Monday through Thursday and one
LVN and three RNs on during the weekend.

It has become apparent that one of the LVNs, Maggie, resents the
recently imposed limitations of LVN duties, because she has had 10 years
of experience in nursing, including a tour of duty as a medic in Iraq. The
emergency room physicians admire her and are always asking her to assist
them with any major wound repair. Occasionally, she has exceeded her
job description as an LVN in the hospital, although she has done nothing
illegal of which you are aware. You have given her satisfactory performance evaluations in the past, even though everyone is aware that she
sometimes acts like a "junior physician." You also suspect that the physicians sometimes allow her to perform duties outside her licensure, but
you have not investigated this or actually seen it yourself.

Tonight, you come back from supper and find Maggie suturing a
deep laceration while the physician looks on. They both realize you are
upset, and the physician takes over the suturing. Later, the doctor
comes to you and says, "Don't worry! She does a great job, and I'll take
the responsibility for her actions." You are not sure what you should
do. Maggie is a good employee, and taking any action will result in
unit conflict.
Assignment: What are the legal ramifications of this case? Discuss what
you should do, if anything. What responsibility and liability exist for the
physician, Maggie, and yourself? Use appropriate rationale to support
your decision.

Learning Exercise 5.9

To Float or Not to Float?

You have been an obstetrical staff nurse at Memorial Hospital for 25 years. The obstetrical unit census has been abnormally low lately, although the patient census in other areas of the hospital has been extremely high. When you arrive at work today, you are told to float to the thoracic surgery critical care unit. This is a highly specialized unit, and you feel ill prepared to work with the equipment on the unit and the type of critically ill patients who are there. You call the staffing office and ask to be reassigned to a different area. You are told that the entire hospital is critically short-staffed, that the thoracic surgery unit is four nurses short, and that you are at least as well equipped to handle that unit as the other three staff who also are being floated. Now your anxiety level is even higher. You will be expected to handle a full RN patient load. You also are aware that more than half the staff on the unit today will have no experience in thoracic surgery. You consider whether to refuse to float. You do not want to place your nursing license in jeopardy, yet you feel conflicting obligations.

Assignment: To whom do you have conflicting obligations? You have little time to make this decision. Outline the steps you use to reach your final decision. Identify the legal and ethical ramifications that may result from your decision. Are they in conflict?

Web Links

Ethics in Medicine—Informed Consent:
http://eduserv.hscer.washington.edu/bioethics/topics/consent.html
Provides a definition and elements of informed consent, including when it is appropriate to have patient participation in decision making and guidelines for obtaining informed consent.

Managed Care and Patient Privacy (last updated March 10, 2003):
http://www.managedcareandpatientprivacy.com/
Collection of newspaper articles dealing with managed care and patient privacy issues.

Confidentiality of Health Information (HIPPA)
http://www.hhs.gov/ocr/hipaa/
View the Department of Health and Human Services recommendations on the confidentiality of individual identifiable health information.

Nursing & Healthcare Directories on: The Nursefriendly Nursing Malpractice Case Studies By Date
http://www.lopez1.com/lopez/clinical.cases/nursing.malpractice.cases.by.date.htm
Provides brief summary of precedent cases involving nurses in malpractice cases and includes URL addresses to more comprehensive legal summaries.

University of Cincinnati, College of Law- Legal Resources for the Nurse Paralegal (May 2003)

http://www.law.uc.edu/library/nurse.pdf

Provides a comprehensive bibliography for the nurse paralegal.

Ethics in Medicine—University of Washington School of Medicine: Advance Directives

http://eduserv.hscer.washington.edu/bioethics/topics/advdir.html

Provides information about advance directives, durable power of attorney as well as case studies discussing the need for both.

References

Austin, S. (2001*a*). Proper equipment use makes or breaks care. *Nursing Management, 32*(6), 16.

Austin, S. (2001*b*). Policies or procedures: Friend or foe? *Nursing Management, 32*(3), 22.

Brent, N. (2003, fall). Standard of proof in cases involving nurses: One standard does not fit all. *Nursing Spectrum Student Career Fitness Guide.* pp. 36–38.

Brooke, P. S. (2003). How good a Samaritan should you be? *Nursing 2003, 33*(6), 46–47.

Cady, R. F. (2000). The legal forum. *Journal of Nursing Administration's Healthcare Law, Ethics, and Regulation, 2*(4), 110.

Charters, K. G. (2003). HIPAA's latest privacy rule. *Policy, Politics, & Nursing Practice, 4*(1), 75–78.

Croke, E. M. (2003). Nurses, negligence, and malpractice. *American Journal of Nursing 103*(9), 54–64.

Dunn, D. (2000). Exploring the gray areas of informed consent. *Nursing Management, 31*(7), 21–25.

Follansbee, N. M. (2002). Implications of the information portability and accountability act. *Journal of Nursing Administration, 32*(1), 42–47.

HHS privacy rule's marketing provisions criticized by Kennedy as not strong enough. (2002). *Federal News, 10,* 1115–1117.

Maddox, P. J. (2002). HIPAA: Update on rule revisions and compliance requirements. *Nursing Economic$, 20*(2), 88–92.

Nursing malpractice: Understanding the risks. [Special issue]. (2003, June). *Travel Nursing 2003.* 7–12.

Office of Civil Rights (last revised August 2003). HIPAA. Available at http://www.hhs.gov/ocr/hipaa/. Accessed January 7, 2004.

Shapiro, J. D. & Bowles, K. (2002). *Journal of Nursing Administration, 32*(10), 503–508.

Sheehan, J. P. (2001). UAP delegation: A step-by-step process. *Nursing Management, 32*(4), 22.

Warlick, D. T. (2000). Negligence goes to the top. *Nursing Management, 31*(6), 22–24.

Bibliography

Austin, S. (2000). Staffing: Know your liability. *Nursing Management, 31*(7), 19.

Bower, F. L. & McCullough, C. S. (2000). Restraint use in acute care settings. Can it be reduced? *Journal of Nursing Administration, 30*(12), 592–598.

Byerly, R. T., Carpenter, J. E., & Davis, J. (2001). Managed care and the evolution of patient rights. *Journal of Nursing Administration's Healthcare Law, Ethics, and Regulation, 3*(2), 58–67.

Calfee, B. E., & Follows, J. M. (2000). Legal questions. *Nursing, 30*(12), 82–84.

Cohen, S. M. (2000). Patient confidentiality. *American Journal of Nursing, 100*(9), 24HH–27HH.

False claims action. (2001). *Nursing Homes Long Term Care Management, 50*(5), 22–27.

Gebbie, K. M., & Heinrich, J. (2001). Privacy: The patient's right. *American Journal of Nursing, 101*(6), 69–71.

Guglielmo, W. (2002). Do Good Samaritan laws protect you in the hospital? *Medical Economics, 79*(9), 95–96.

Lee, N. G. (2000). Proving nursing negligence. *American Journal of Nursing, 100*(11), 55–57.

Murer, M. J. (2001). Ten resolutions to minimize liability. *Nursing Homes Long Term Care Management, 50*(4), 64–68.

No restraints allowed: Legalities and realities. (2004). *Nursing 2004, 34*(1), 54–55.

Parsons, L. C. (2002). Protecting patient rights: A nursing responsibility. *Policy, Politics & Nursing Practice, 3*(3), 274–278.

Simpson, R. L. (2001). How can we keep private data private? *Nursing Management, 32*(5), 12–14.

White, G. B. (2000). Informed consent. *American Journal of Nursing, 100*(9), 83.

White, G. B. (2000). What we may expect from ethics and the law. *American Journal of Nursing, 100*(10), 114–118.

Patient, Subordinate, and Professional Advocacy

To see what is right, and not do it, is want of courage, or of principle.

—*Confucius*

Advocacy—helping others to grow and fulfill their potential—is a critically important leadership role. Many of the leadership skills that are described in this book, such as risk taking, vision, self-confidence, ability to articulate needs, and assertiveness, are used in the advocacy role. Management skills are also needed to be an effective advocate.

Nurse leader–managers often find themselves in the role of advocate for their patients, subordinates, and the profession. The actions of an advocate are to inform others of their rights and to ascertain that they have sufficient information on which to base their decisions. The term advocacy actually comes from the Latin word *advocatus*, which means "one summoned to give evidence" (Blais, Hayes, Kozier, Erb, 2002, p. 61). The goals then of the advocate are to inform, enhance autonomy, and respect the decisions of others.

Advocacy, in fact, has been recognized as one of the most vital and basic roles of the nursing profession since the time of Florence Nightingale. The role, however, is complex. Nurses may act as advocates by helping others make informed decisions, by acting as an intermediary in the environment, or by directly intervening on the behalf of others (Blais et al., 2002).

> ➤ Nurses may act as advocates by either helping others make informed decisions, by acting as an intermediary in the environment, or by directly intervening on behalf of others.

This chapter will examine the processes through which advocacy is learned as well as the ways in which leader–managers can advocate for their patients, subordinates, and the profession. Specific suggestions for interacting with legislators and the media to influence health policy are included. Leadership roles and management functions essential for advocacy are shown in **Display 6.1.**

BECOMING AN ADVOCATE

Foley, Minick, and Kee (2002) suggest that although advocacy is assumed to be an inherent part of all nursing curricula and is present in all clinical practice settings, the nursing literature contains little description of how nurses learn the advocacy role. Indeed, in research conducted by Foley et al., participants suggested that being committed to protect and care for others was a core family or community value that reflected who they were as individuals and that it was not deeply rooted in any learning process. Other study participants, however, stated that they learned advocating practices by watching how other nurses interacted with patients and by talking with the nurses about what they did. Still other participants reported that advocacy skills were gained as a result of the increased self-confidence they gained from working with mentors who provided a supportive environment for gaining experience. Regardless of how advocacy is learned, there are nursing values central to advocacy. These values emphasize caring, autonomy, respect, and empowerment. (See **Display 6.2.**)

PATIENT ADVOCACY

Standard V, number 3, of the American Nurses Association (ANA) Standards of Professional Performance in Clinical Practice (1998) states that the nurse acts as a patient advocate and assists patients in developing skills so that they can advocate

Display 6.1 **Leadership Roles and Management Functions Associated with Advocacy**

Leadership Roles
1. Creates a climate where advocacy and its associated risk-taking are valued.
2. Seeks fairness and justice for individuals who are unable to advocate for themselves.
3. Seeks to strengthen patient and subordinate support systems to encourage autonomous, well-informed decision making.
4. Influences others by providing information necessary to empower them to act autonomously.
5. Assertively advocates on behalf of patients and subordinates when an intermediary is necessary.
6. Participates in professional nursing organizations and other groups that seek to advance the profession of nursing.
7. Role models proactive involvement in healthcare policy through both formal and informal interactions with the media and legislative representatives.

Management Functions
1. Gives subordinates and patients adequate information to make informed decisions.
2. Assures that provider's rights and values do not infringe upon patient's rights and values.
3. Seeks appropriate consultation when advocacy results in intrapersonal or interpersonal conflict.
4. Promotes and protects the workplace safety and health of subordinates and patients.
5. Encourages subordinates to bring forth concerns about the employment setting and seeks impunity for whistleblowers.
6. Demonstrates the skills needed to interact appropriately with the media and legislators regarding nursing and healthcare issues.
7. Is aware of current legislative efforts affecting nursing practice and organizational and unit management.

Display 6.2 **Nursing Values Central to Advocacy**

1. Each individual has a right to autonomy in deciding what course of action is most appropriate to meet his or her healthcare goals.
2. Each individual has a right to hold personal values and to use those values in making their own healthcare decisions.
3. All individuals should have access to the information they need to make informed decisions and choices.
4. The nurse must act on behalf of patients who are unable to advocate for themselves.
5. Empowerment of patients and subordinates to make decisions and take action on their own is the essence of advocacy.

Learning Exercise 6.1

Values and Advocacy
How important a role do you believe advocacy to be in nursing? Do you believe your willingness to assume this role is a learned value? Were the values of caring and service emphasized in your family and community when you were growing up? Have you identified any role models in nursing who actively advocate for patients, subordinates, or the profession? What strategies might you use as a new nurse, to impart the need for advocacy to your peers and to the student nurses who work with you?

for themselves. Patient advocacy is necessary because disease almost always results in decreased independence, loss of freedom, and interference with the ability to make choices autonomously. Benner (2003, p. 375) concurs, arguing that being a "good" practitioner means more than just examining patient rights; it requires being moved by the patient's plight and responding to the patient as a person. Thus, advocacy becomes the foundation and essence of nursing, and nurses have a responsibility to promote human advocacy.

Managers also must advocate for patients with regard to distribution of resources and the use of technology. The advances in science and limits of financial resources have created new problems and ethical dilemmas. For example, although diagnosis-related groupings may have eased the strain on government fiscal resources, they have created ethical problems such as patient dumping, premature patient discharge, and inequality of care. See **Display 6.3.**

Display 6.3	**Common Areas Requiring Nurse–Patient Advocacy**

1. End of life decisions
2. Technological advances
3. Healthcare reimbursement
4. Access to health care
5. Provider–patient conflicts regarding expectations and desired outcomes
6. Withholding of information or blatant lying to patients
7. Insurance authorizations, denials, and delays in coverage
8. Medical errors
9. Patient information disclosure (privacy and confidentiality)
10. Patient grievance and appeals processes
11. Cultural and ethnic diversity and sensitivity
12. Respect for patient dignity
13. Informed consent
14. Incompetent healthcare providers
15. Complex social problems including AIDS, teenage pregnancy, violence, poverty
16. Aging population

First- and middle-level managers are in the best position to advocate for patients affected by such problems. Benner (2003) states:

> Meeting patients and their families and recognizing their concerns about health care comprise the everyday ethical comportment of the practitioner. Patients and families, while encouraged to become empowered and take more responsibility for their health, are often vulnerable due to lack of knowledge of health care or due to crisis and reduced capacities. Thus, ethically and legally, healthcare workers are expected to act in the best interests of patients (p. 374).

It is important, however, for the patient advocate to be able to differentiate between controlling patient choices (domination and dependence) and in assisting patient choices (allowing freedom). "When appropriate assessments are conducted, nurses care in ways that offer support, expanding patient possibilities, and engendering independence—thus advocacy. In contrast, nurses who impose their values and opinions on patients limit patient's possibilities and create situations of domination and dependence" (Foley et al., 2002, p. 185). It is essential that patients have at least mutual responsibilities in decision making.

> It is important, however, for the patient advocate to be able to differentiate between controlling patient choices (domination and dependence) and assisting patient choices (allowing freedom).

Learning Exercise 6.2

Considering Culture

You are a staff nurse on a medical unit. One of your patients, Mr. Dau, is a 56-year-old Hmong immigrant to the United States. He has lived in this country for four years and became a citizen two years ago. His English is marginal, although he understands more than he can verbalize. He was admitted to the hospital with sepsis resulting from urinary tract infection. His condition is now stable.

Today, Mr. Dau's physician informed him that his CT scan shows a large tumor in his prostate that is likely cancer. She wants to do immediate follow-up testing and surgical resection of the tumor to relieve his symptoms of hesitancy and urinary retention. She tells him that although the tumor is probably cancerous, she believes it will respond well to traditional cancer treatments. Her expectation is that Mr. Dau should recover fully.

One hour later, when you go in to check on Mr. Dau, you find him sitting on his bed, with his suitcase packed, waiting for a ride home. He informs you that he is checking out of the hospital. He states that he believes he can make himself better at home with herbs and through prayers by the Hmong "faith healer." He concludes by telling you that "if he is meant to die, that there is little anyone can do." When you reaffirm the hopeful prognosis reported by his physician that morning, Mr. Dau says, "She is just trying to give me false hope. I need to go home and prepare for my death."

Assignment: What should you do? How can you best advocate for this patient? Is the problem a lack of information? How does culture play a role in the patient's decision? Can paternalism be justified in this case?

Patient Rights

The legislative controls of nursing practice primarily protect the rights of patients. Until the 1960s, patients had few rights; in fact, patients often were denied basic human rights during a time when they were most vulnerable. In 1973, however, the American Hospital Association published its first Patient Bill of Rights, which was revised in 1992 (**Display 6.4**). Many healthcare organizations and states have passed a bill of rights for patients since that time.

Display 6.4	A Patient's Bill of Rights

1. The patient has the right to considerate and respectful care.
2. The patient has the right to and is encouraged to obtain from physicians and their direct caregivers relevant, current, and understandable information concerning diagnosis, treatment, and prognosis.
3. The patient has the right to make decisions about the plan of care prior to and during the course of treatment and to refuse a recommended treatment or plan of care to the extent permitted by law and hospital policy and to be informed of the medical consequences of this action. In case of such refusal, the patient is entitled to other appropriate care and services that the hospital provides or transfer to another hospital. The hospital should notify patients of any policy that might affect patient choice within the institution.
4. The patient has the right to have an advance directive (such as a living will, health care proxy, or durable power of attorney for health care) concerning treatment or designating a surrogate decision maker with the expectation that the hospital will honor the intent of that directive to the extent permitted by law and hospital policy.
5. The patient has the right to every consideration of privacy. Case discussion, consultation, examination, and treatment should be conducted so as to protect each patient's privacy.
6. The patient has the right to expect that all communications and records pertaining to his/her care will be treated as confidential by the hospital, except in cases such as suspected abuse and public health hazards when reporting is permitted or required by law. The patient has the right to expect that the hospital will emphasize the confidentiality of this information when it releases it to any other parties entitled to review information in these records.
7. The patient has the right to review the records pertaining to his/her medical care and to have the information explained or interpreted as necessary, except when restricted by law.
8. The patient has the right to expect that, within its capacity and policies, a hospital will make reasonable response to the request of a patient for appropriate and medically indicated care and services. The hospital must provide evaluation, service, and/or referral as indicated by the urgency of the case. When medically appropriate and legally permissible, or when a patient has so requested, a patient may be transferred to another facility. The institution to which the patient is to be transferred must first have accepted the patient for transfer. The patient must also have the benefit of complete information and explanation concerning the need for, risks, benefits, and alternatives to such a transfer.
9. The patient has the right to ask and to be informed of the existence of business relationships among the hospital, educational institutions, other health care providers, or payers that may influence the patient's treatment and care.

(display continues on page 130)

Display 6.4   A Patient's Bill of Rights

10. The patient has the right to consent to or decline to participate in proposed research studies or human experimentation affecting care and treatment or requiring direct patient involvement, and to have those studies fully explained prior to consent. A patient who declines to participate in research or experimentation is entitled to the most effective care that the hospital can otherwise provide.
11. The patient has the right to expect reasonable continuity of care when appropriate and to be informed by physicians and other caregivers of available and realistic patient care options when hospital care is no longer appropriate.
12. The patient has the right to be informed of hospital policies and practices that relate to patient care, treatment, and responsibilities. The patient has the right to be informed of available resources for resolving disputes, grievances, and conflicts, such as ethics committees, patient representatives, or other mechanisms available in the institution. The patient has the right to be informed of the hospital's charges for services and available payment methods.

Source: American Hospital Association (1973, Last Revised 1992). "A patient's bill of rights."

A *bill of rights* that has become law or state regulation has the most legal authority because it provides the patient with legal recourse. A bill of rights issued by healthcare organizations and professional associations is not legally binding but may influence federal or state funding and certainly should be considered professionally binding. However, although there has been significant progress in the field of patient rights since 1960, Byerly, Carpenter, and Davis (2001) note that there is still no comprehensive federal legislation directed to the granting and protection of patient rights.

Today, patients are more assertive and involved in their health care. They have more information to review when looking at treatment options and are demanding to be participants in decisions about their health care. The patient's right to information and participation in medical care decisions has led to conflicts in the areas of informed consent and access to medical records. Although the manager has a responsibility to see that all patient rights are met in the unit, the areas that are particularly sensitive involve the right to privacy and personal liberty, both guaranteed by the Constitution.

SUBORDINATE ADVOCACY

Standard V of the ANA Scope and Standards for Nurse Administrators (2004) suggests that nurse administrators should advocate for subordinates as well as patients. *Subordinate advocacy* is a neglected concept in management theory but an essential part of the leadership role. In this area of advocacy, the manager must help subordinates resolve ethical problems and live with the solutions at the unit level. Angelucci (2003) suggests that managers have an obligation to assist staff in dealing with ethical issues. She maintains that nurse–managers must advocate for their staff through the following steps:

- Invite collaborative decision making
- Listen to staff needs

- Get to know staff personally
- Take time to understand the challenges faced by the staff in delivering care
- Face challenges and solve problems together
- "Go to bat" for staff when needed

Managers must recognize what subordinates are striving for and the goals and values subordinates consider appropriate. The leader–manager should be able to guide subordinates toward actualization while defending their right to autonomy. To help nurses deal with ethical dilemmas in their practice, nurse–managers should establish and utilize appropriate support groups, ethics committees, and channels for dealing with ethical problems.

Another critical part of subordinate advocacy is *workplace advocacy*. In workplace advocacy, the manager works to see that the work environment is both safe and conducive to professional and personal growth for subordinates. Occupational health and safety must be assured by interventions such as reducing worker exposure to needle sticks or blood and body fluids. Subordinates should also be able to have the expectation that their work hours and schedules will be reasonable, that staffing ratios will be adequate to support safe patient care, that wages will be fair and equitable, and that nurses will be allowed participation in organizational decision making. When these working conditions do not exist, managers must advocate to higher levels of the administrative hierarchy to correct the problems.

Top- and middle-level managers can advocate for subordinates in a different way. For example, when the healthcare industry has faced the crisis of inadequate human resources and nursing shortages, many organizations have made quick, poorly

Learning Exercise 6.3

How Can You Best Advocate?
You are a unit supervisor in a skilled nursing facility. One of your aides, Martha Greenwald, recently reported that she suffered a "back strain" several weeks ago when she was lifting an elderly patient. She did not report the injury at the time because she did not think it was serious. Indeed, she finished the remainder of her shift and has performed all of her normal work duties since that time.

Today, Martha reports that she has just left her physician's office and that he has advised her to take four to six weeks off from work to fully recover from her injury. He has also prescribed physical therapy and electrical nerve stimulation for chronic pain. Martha is a relatively new employee, so she has not yet accrued enough sick leave to cover her absence. She asks you to complete the paperwork for her absence and the cost of her treatments to be covered as a work-related injury.

When you contact the Worker's Compensation case manager for your facility, you learn that the claim will be investigated; however, with no written or verbal report of the injury at the time it occurred, that there is great likelihood the claim will be rejected.

Assignment: How best can you advocate for this subordinate?

thought-out decisions to find short-term solutions to a long-term and severe problem. New workers have been recruited at a phenomenally high cost, yet the problems that caused high worker attrition have not been solved. Top- and middle-level managers must advocate for subordinates in solving problems and making decisions about how best to use limited resources. These decisions must be made carefully, following a thorough examination of the political, social, economic, and ethical costs.

Top- and middle-level managers must also be willing to advocate for *whistle-blowers*, who speak out about organizational practices they believe may be harmful or inappropriate. Subordinates want the assurance that if they are acting within the scope of their expertise that they will be able to speak up through appropriate channels without fear of retaliation (Green & Jordan, 2002). While whistle-blower protection has been advocated for at the federal level and has passed in some states, many employees are reluctant to report unsafe conditions for fear of retaliation. Nurses should check with their state association to assess the status of whistle blower protection in their state (Green & Jordan).

> Top- and middle-level managers must also be willing to advocate for *whistle-blowers* who speak out about organizational practices they believe may be harmful or inappropriate.

PROFESSIONAL ADVOCACY

Managers also must be advocates for the nursing profession. This type of advocacy is described by Quinn and Smith (1987):

> Choosing to enter a profession amounts to voluntarily biting off a chunk of the human condition. The professional chooses to become involved (with expertise and commitment) in an area of human life in which important elements of human welfare are at stake and in which people must depend on experts. In making that choice, the professional becomes committed to living with and wrestling with the problem of professional issues and sometimes unavoidable consequences (p. 55).

Joining a profession requires making a very personal decision to involve oneself in a system of roles that is socially defined. Thus, entry into a profession involves a personal and public promise to serve others with the special expertise that a profession can provide and that society legitimately expects it to provide.

> A professional commitment means that people cannot shrink from their duty to question and contemplate problems that face the profession.

Professional issues are always ethical issues. When nurses find a discrepancy between their perceived role and society's expectations, they have a responsibility to advocate for the profession. At times, individual nurses believe the problems of the profession are too big for them to make a difference. A professional commitment means that people cannot shrink from their duty to question and contemplate problems that face the profession. They cannot afford to become powerless or helpless or claim that one person cannot make a difference. Often, one voice is all it takes to raise the consciousness of colleagues within a profession.

If nursing is to advance as a profession, practitioners and managers must broaden their sociopolitical knowledge base to understand better the bureaucracies in which they live. This includes speaking out on consumer issues, continuing and expanding attempts to influence legislation, and increasing membership on governmental health policy-making boards and councils. Only then will nurses be able to influence the tremendous problems facing society today in terms of the homeless, teenage pregnancy, drug and alcohol abuse, inadequate health care for the poor and elderly, and medical errors. These are essential advocacy roles for the profession.

There are many ways for the profession and individual nurses to advocate social issues. For example, the ANA has advocated for more diversity in nursing (Gonzalez, 1999). A leadership role would be one that supports and advocates for diversity within an organization. Other issues the ANA and its constituent member associations have been working to bring attention to include the impact of the current nursing shortage on the quality of care; staffing ratios; and working conditions for nurses, including mandatory overtime. Indeed, in April 2002, the ANA and more than 60 partner organizations issued a report entitled *Nursing's Agenda for the Future*, which detailed the complex factors leading to and exacerbating the current nursing shortage.

Blakeney (2003) suggests that other organizations outside of nursing are also stepping forward to bring these issues to the attention of the public, media, and policy makers. For example, in July 2002, the U.S. Department of Health and Human Services released a report, *Projected Supply, Demand, and Shortages of Registered Nurses: 2000–2020*. In August 2002, the Joint Commission on Accreditation of Healthcare Organizations released *Health Care at the Crossroads: Strategies for Addressing the Evolving Nursing Crisis*. In addition, Johnson and Johnson Health Care Systems, Inc. launched a $20 million campaign in February 2002 to attract more people to nursing and to increase awareness of the value of the nursing profession in society and America's health care system (Nursing Shortage, 2002).

 Learning Exercise 6.4

Write It Down. What Would You Change?
List five things you would like to change about nursing or the healthcare system. Prioritize the changes you have identified. Write a one-page essay about the change you believe is most needed. Identify the strategies you could use individually and collectively as a profession to make the change happen. Be sure you are realistic about the time, energy, and fiscal resources you have to implement your plan.

Nursing's Advocacy Role in Legislation and Public Policy

A distinctive feature of American society is the manner in which citizens can participate in the political process. People have the right to express their opinions about issues and candidates by voting. People also have relatively easy access to lawmakers and policy makers and can make their individual needs and wants known. Theoretically, then, any one person can influence those in policy-making positions. In reality, this rarely happens; policy decisions are generally focused on group needs or wants.

Reutter and Williamson (2000) argue that one of the most effective strategies for improving the health and welfare of a population is by advocating for its healthcare policy. "Nurses at all levels of practice must create and develop strategies to promote and increase the participation of registered nurses in the political process and healthcare policy decision making" (Greipp, 2002, p. 35).

Nurses who participate in professional organizations are integral in determining whether voluntary or legal controls represent what nursing is and should be.

The need for organized group efforts by nurses to influence legislative policy has long been recognized in this country. In fact, the first state associations were organized expressly for unifying nurses to influence the passage of state licensure laws. *Political action committees* (PACs) of the Congress of Industrial Organizations attempt to persuade legislators to vote in a particular way. Lobbyists of the PAC may be members of a group interested in a particular law or paid agents of the group that wants a specific bill passed or defeated. Nursing must become more actively involved with PACs to influence healthcare legislation and PACs provide one opportunity for small donors to feel like they are making a difference.

In addition, professional organizations generally espouse standards of care that are higher than those required by law. Voluntary controls often are forerunners of legal controls. Nurses who participate in professional organizations are integral in determining whether voluntary or legal controls represent what nursing is and should be.

Currently, nursing lobbyists in our nation's capitol are influencing legislation on quality, access to care issues, patient and health worker safety, healthcare restructuring, direct reimbursement for advanced practice nurses, and funding for nursing education. Representatives of the American Nurse's Association regularly attend and provide testimony for meetings of the U.S. Department of Health and Human Services (DHHS), the Department of Health, the National Institutes of Health (NIH), Occupational Safety and Health Administration (OSHA), and the White House to be sure that the "nursing perspective" is heard in health policy issues (Huston, 1998).

As a whole, the nursing profession has not yet recognized the full potential of collective political activity. Nurses must exert their collective influence and make their concerns known to policy makers before they can have a major impact on political and legislative outcomes. Because they have been reluctant to become politically involved, nurses have failed to have a strong legislative voice in the past. Legislators and policy makers generally are more willing to deal with nurses as a group rather than as individuals; thus, joining and supporting professional organizations allow nurses to become active in lobbying for a stronger nurse practice act or for the creation or expansion of advanced nursing roles.

In addition to active participation in national nursing organizations, nurses can influence legislation and health policy in many ways. Nurses who want to be directly involved can lobby legislators either in person or by letter. This process may seem intimidating to the new nurse; however, many books and workshops are available that deal with the subject and a common format is used.

Personal letters are more influential than form letters and the tone should be formal but polite. The letter should also be concise (no more than one page). Be sure to address the legislator properly by title. Establish your credibility early in the letter as both a constituent and as a healthcare expert. State your reason for writing the letter in the first paragraph and refer to the specific bill you are writing about. Then state your position on the issue and give personal examples as necessary to support your position. Offer your assistance as a resource person for additional information. Then, sign the letter, including your name and contact information. Remember too to be persistent and to write legislators repeatedly who are undecided on an issue. **Display 6.5** displays a format common to letters written to legislators.

Display 6.5	Exemplar: A Letter to Your Legislator

March 15, 2005

The Honorable John Doe
Member of the Senate
State Capitol, Room _____
City, State, Zip Code

Dear Senator Doe,

I am a registered nurse and member of the American Nurses Association (ANA). I am also a constituent in your district. I am writing in support of SB XXX, which requires the establishment of minimum RN staffing ratios in acute care facilities. As a staff nurse on an oncology unit in our local hospital, I see first-hand the problems that occur when staffing is inadequate to meet the complex needs of acutely ill patients: medical errors, patient and nurse dissatisfaction, workplace injuries, and perhaps most importantly, the inability to spend adequate time with and comfort patients who are dying.

I have enclosed a copy of a recent study conducted by John Smith and published in the January 2005 edition of *Nurses Today*. This article details the positive impact of legislative staffing ratio implementation on patient outcomes as measured by medication errors, patient falls, and nosocomial infection rates.

I strongly encourage you to vote for SB XXX when it is heard by the Senate Business and Professions Committee next week. Thank you for your ongoing concern with nursing and healthcare issues and for your past support of legislation to improve healthcare staffing. Please feel free to contact me if you have any questions or would like additional information

Respectfully,

Nurse Nancy

Nurse Nancy, R.N., B.S.N.
Street,
City, State, Zip Code
Phone number including area code
Email address

 Learning Exercise 6.5

Realistic Advocacy for the Nursing Profession
Do you belong to your state nursing organization or student nursing organization? Why or why not? Make a list of six other things you could do to advocate for the profession. Be specific. Is your list realistic in terms of your energy and commitment to nursing?

Other nurses may choose to monitor the progress of legislation, count congressional votes, and track specific legislator's voting intents as well as past voting records. Still other nurses may choose join *network groups* where colleagues meet to discuss professional issues and pending legislation.

For nurses interested in a more indirect approach to professional advocacy, their role may be to influence and educate the public about nursing and the nursing agenda to reform health care. This may be done by speaking with professional and community groups about healthcare and nursing issues and by interacting directly with the media. Never underestimate the influence a single nurse may have even in writing letters to the editor of local newspapers, or by talking about nursing and healthcare issues with friends, family, neighbors, teachers, clergy, and civic leaders.

Nursing's Role in the Media

Although nurses have the greatest knowledge about nursing issues, too few are willing to interact with the media about vital nursing and healthcare issues. This is especially unfortunate because both the media and the public place a high trust in nurses and want to hear about healthcare issues from a nursing perspective.

Many nurses avoid media exposure because they believe they lack the expertise to do so or because they lack self-confidence. The reality is that "nurses possess tremendous amounts of knowledge, clinical experience, and intellectual and communication skills that can contribute to and expand the dialogue and debate surrounding healthcare issues and subsequent decision making" (Greipp, 2002, p. 35), and self-confidence is usually simply a matter of being prepared for the task at hand.

Trossman (2003) suggests that nurses can ease into the spokesperson role by first presenting information on a hot healthcare topic in a group setting where they already feel comfortable. Nurses should also complete media training programs to increase their self-confidence in working with journalists. Regardless, the first few media interactions will likely be stressful, just like any new task or learning. Trossman, however, offers the following basic tips to help nurses navigate media waters (**Display 6.6**):

Display 6.6	Tips for Interacting with the Media

1. Be prepared or at least as prepared as possible given a reporter's deadline. This means researching the topic if there is time, knowing up-to-date information, and knowing three or four facts or figures that can be cited about pertinent issues.
2. Stick to three or four key points that will drive home your message and repeat them during the interview.
3. Make it easy for the media by providing them with clear, concise information and by meeting reporter's deadlines.
4. Stay on track by sticking to predetermined points, using phrases such as "I think the important point is...." Also avoid repetition of any negative language a reporter might pick up on and instead focus on solutions or strategies to solve problems.
5. Don't be afraid to say that you do not have enough information or expertise to answer a question. Be sure not to guess when factual data is needed.

Learning Exercise 6.6

Preparing for a Media Interview

You are the staffing coordinator for a medium-sized community hospital in California. Minimum staffing ratios were implemented in January 2004. While this has represented an even greater challenge in terms of meeting your organization's daily staffing needs, you believe the impetus behind the legislative mandate was sound. You also are a member of the state nursing association that sponsored this legislation and wrote letters of support for its passage. Your hospital and the state hospital association fought unsuccessfully against the passage of minimum staffing ratios.

The local newspaper contacted you this morning and wants to interview you about staffing ratios in general as well as how these ratios are impacting the local hospital. You approach your CNO and she tells you to go ahead and do the interview if you want, but to remember that you are a representative of the hospital.

Assignment: Assume that you have agreed to participate in the interview.

1. How might you go about preparing for the interview?
2. Identify three or four factual points you can state during the interview as your sound bites. What would be your primary points of emphasis?
3. Is there a way to reconcile any potential conflict between your personal feelings about staffing ratios and those of your employer? How would you respond if asked directly by the reporter to comment about whether staffing ratios are a good idea?

The bottom line is that "stories about healthcare are hot" right now and nurses need to respond "when the iron is hot" (Trossman, 2003, p. 69) to advocate both for their profession and for the patients they serve.

INTEGRATING LEADERSHIP ROLES AND MANAGEMENT FUNCTIONS IN ADVOCACY

Nursing leaders and managers recognize they have an obligation not only to advocate for the needs of their patients, subordinates, and themselves at a particular time, but also to be active in furthering the goals of the profession. To accomplish all these types of advocacy, nurses must value autonomy and empowerment.

The leadership roles and management functions, however, to achieve advocacy with patients, subordinates, and for the profession differ greatly. Advocating for patients requires that the manager create a work environment that recognizes patient's needs and goals as paramount. This means creating a work culture where patients are respected, well informed, and empowered. The leadership role required to advocate for patients is often one of risk taking, particularly when advocating for a patient may be in direct conflict with provider or institutional goals. Leaders must also be willing to accept and support patient choices that may be different from their own.

Advocating for subordinates requires that the manager create a safe and equitable work environment where employees feel valued and appreciated. When working conditions are less than favorable, the manager is responsible for relaying these concerns to higher levels of management and advocating for needed changes. The same risk taking that is required in patient advocacy is a leadership role in subordinate advocacy, since subordinate needs and wants may be in conflict with the organization. There is always a risk that the organization will view the manager advocate as a troublemaker, but this does not provide an excuse for managers to be complacent in this role. Managers also must advocate for subordinates in creating an environment where ethical concerns, needs, and dilemmas can be openly discussed and resolved.

Advocating for the profession requires the nurse manager be informed and involved in all legislation affecting the unit, organization, and the profession. The manager also must be an astute handler of public relations and demonstrate skill in working with the media. It is the leader, however, who proactively steps forth to be a role model and active participant in educating the public and improving health care through the political process.

☀ Key Concepts

- *Advocacy* is helping others to grow and self-actualize and is a leadership role.
- Managers, by virtue of their many roles, must be advocates for patients, subordinates, and the profession.
- It is important for the patient advocate to be able to differentiate between controlling patient choices (domination and dependence) and in assisting patient choices (allowing freedom).
- Since the 1960s, the NLN, the American Hospital Association, and many states have passed *bills of rights for patients*. Although these are not legally binding, they can be used to guide professional practice.
- In *workplace advocacy*, the manager works to see that the work environment is both safe and conducive to professional and personal growth for subordinates.
- Professional issues are ethical issues. When nurses find a discrepancy between their perceived role and society's expectations, they have a responsibility to advocate for the profession.
- If nursing is to advance as a profession, practitioners and managers must broaden their sociopolitical knowledge base to understand better the bureaucracies in which they live.
- Because legislators and policy makers are more willing to deal with nurses as a group rather than as individuals, joining and actively supporting professional organizations allows nurses to have a greater voice in healthcare and professional issues.
- Nurses need to exert their collective influence and make their concerns known to policy makers before they can have a major impact on political and legislative outcomes.
- Nurses have great potential to educate the public and influence policy through the media as a result of the public's high trust in nurses and because the public wants to hear about healthcare issues from a nursing perspective.

More Learning Exercises and Applications

 Learning Exercise 6.7

Ethics and Advocacy

You are a new graduate staff nurse in a home health agency. One of your patients is a 23-year-old male with acute schizophrenia who was just released from the local county, acute care, behavioral healthcare facility, following a 72-hour hold. He has no insurance. His family no longer has contact with him and he is unable to hold a permanent job. He is non-compliant in taking his prescription drugs for schizophrenia. He is home-less and has been sleeping and eating intermittently at the local homeless shelter; however, they recently asked him not to return, since he is increasingly agitated and at times, violent. He calls you today and asks you "to help him with the voices in his head."

You approach the senior RN case manager in the facility for help in identifying options for this individual to get the behavioral healthcare services he needs. She suggests that you tell the patient to go to "Maxwell's Mini Mart," a local convenience store, at 3 P.M. today and to wait by the counter. Then she tells you that you should contact the police at 2:55 P.M. and tell them that Maxwell's Mini Mart is being robbed by your patient, so that he will be arrested. She states that "she does this with all of her uninsured mental health patients, since the state Medicaid program offers only limited mental health services and the state penal system provides full mental health services for the incarcerated." She goes on to say that the mini-mart owner and the police are aware of what she is doing and support the idea since it is the only way "patients really have a chance of getting better." She ends the conversation by saying, "I know you are a new nurse and don't understand how the real world works, but the reality is that this is the only way I can advocate for patients like this and you need to do the same for your patients."

Assignment:

1. Will you follow the advice of the senior RN case manager?
2. If not, how else might you advocate for this patient?
3. What are the legal, ethical, and advocacy implications of this case?

 Learning Exercise 6.8

Letter Writing in Advocacy

Identify three legislative bills affecting nursing that are currently being considered either in committee, the House of Representatives, or the Sen-ate. Select one and draft a letter to your state assemblyperson or senator regarding your position on the bill.

Learning Exercise 6.9

Determining Nursing's Entry Level

Grandfathering is the term used to grant certain people working within the profession for a given period of time, or prior to a deadline date, a privilege of applying for a license without meeting normal requirements such as taking the licensing examination. Grandfathering clauses have been used to allow licensure for wartime nurses—those with on-the-job training and expertise—even though they did not graduate from an approved school of nursing.

Some professional nursing organizations are once again proposing that the BSN become the entry-level requirement for professional nursing. Some have suggested, as a concession to current ADN and diploma-prepared nurses, that all nurses who have passed the state board of registered nursing licensure examination before the new legislation, regardless of educational preparation or experience, would retain the title of professional nurse. Non-baccalaureate nurses after that time would be unable to use the title professional nurse.

Assignment: Talk about this issue in a group. Do you believe the BSN-as-entry-level proposal advocates the advancement of the nursing profession? Is grandfathering conducive to meeting this goal? Would you personally support both of these proposals? Does the long-standing internal dissension about making the BSN the entry level into professional nursing reduce nursing's status as a profession? Do lawmakers or the public understand this dilemma or care about it?

Learning Exercise 6.10

How Would You Proceed?

You are an RN case manager for a large insurance company. Sheila Johannsen is a 34-year-old mother of two small children. She was diagnosed with advanced, metastatic breast cancer six months ago. Traditional chemotherapy and radiation seem to have slowed the spread of the cancer, but the prognosis is not good.

Sheila contacted you this morning to report that she has been in contact with a physician at one of the most innovative medical centers in the country. He told her that she might benefit from an experimental gene therapy treatment; however, she is ineligible for participation in the free clinical trials since her cancer is so advanced. The cost for the treatment then is approximately $150,000. Sheila states that she does not have the financial resources to pay for the treatment and begs you "to do whatever you can, to get the insurance company to pay. Otherwise, she will die."

You know that your insurance company almost always disallows the cost of experimental treatments. You also know that even with the experimental treatment, Sheila's probability of a cure is minimal.

Assignment: Decide how you will proceed. How can you best advocate for this patient?

Web Links

ANA-PAC
http://www.nursingworld.org/gova/federal/gfederal.htm
This American Nurses Association web page has a large selection of political action sites to choose from.

ANA—National Awards Program
http://www.ana.org/about/honaward/staff.htm
This American Nurses Association web page details the award criteria and includes nomination forms for the Staff Nurse Advocate of the Year Award. The Staff Nurse Advocacy Award was established in 1998 to recognize excellence in individual staff nurses who provide direct patient care in all practice settings and who have advocated for their patients.

David L. Bazelon Center for Mental Health Law
http://www.bazelon.org/about/index.htm
This center is one of the nation's leading advocates for people with mental disabilities, with precedent setting litigation outlawing institutional abuse and providing protections against arbitrary confinement.

Electronic Policy Network
http://movingideas.org/
A source for current public policy issues, including healthcare policy. Provides search engine for current policy issues.

Foundation for Informed Medical Decision Making
http://www.fimdm.org/index.html
The primary mission of the Foundation for Informed Medical Decision Making (FIMDM) is to strengthen the role patients play in selecting treatments for their medical conditions. The site includes a bibliography as well as helpful links.

Sigma Theta Tau International: Media Guide to Health Care Experts (1999–2004)
http://www.nursingsociety.org/media/ME_intro.html
Source for healthcare experts from various medical specialties and practices who are willing to interact with the media.

Iroquois Healthcare Alliance—Representing Healthcare Providers in Upstate New York (2004)
http://www.iroquois.org/advocacy.htm
Provides sample electronic letters that can be sent to legislators and government officials regarding multiple pending healthcare bills. Includes links to determine current government officials who will vote on pending legislation.

References
American Hospital Association. (1973, last revised 1992). "A patient's bill of rights." Available at http://web.carroll.edu/msmillie/bioethics/patbillofrights.htm. Accessed October 14, 2004.
American Nurses Association. (1998). *Standards of clinical nursing practice* (2nd edition). Washington, D.C.: American Nurses Publishing.

American Nurses Association. (2004). *Scope and standards for nurse administrators* (2nd ed.) Washington, D.C.: American Nurses Publishing.

Angelucci, P. (2003). Ethics committees: Guidance through gray areas. *Nursing Management, 34*(6), 30–33.

Benner, P. (2003). Current controversies in critical care. Enhancing patient advocacy and social ethics. *American Journal of Critical Care, 12*(4), 374–375.

Blais, K. K., Hayes, J. S., Kozier, B. & Erb, G. (2002). *Professional nursing practice* (4th ed.). Upper Saddle River, NJ: Prentice Hall.

Blakeney, B. (2003, January). Addressing the nursing shortage. *American Journal of Nursing. Career Guide 2003* (Part 2 of 2). 16.

Byerly, R. T., Carpenter, J. E., & Davis, J. (2001). Managed care and the evolution of patient rights. *Journal of Nursing Administration's Healthcare Law, Ethics, & Regulation, 3*(2), 58–67.

Foley, B. J., Minick, M.P., & Kee, C.C. (2002). How nurses learn advocacy. *Journal of Nursing Scholarship, 34*(2), 181–186.

Gonzalez, R. (1999). ANA advocates more diversity in nursing. *American Journal of Nursing, 99*(11), 24.

Green , A., & Jordan, C. B. (2002). Workplace advocacy and workplace issues. In Cherry, B. & Jacob, S. R. (Eds.). *Contemporary nursing. Issues, trends, & management* (2nd ed.). St. Louis: Mosby.

Greipp, M.E. (2002). Forces driving healthcare policy decisions. *Policy, Politics, & Nursing Practice, 3*(1), 35–42.

Huston, C. (1998). We're not in Kansas anymore: Shaping a new and better healthcare system. *Revolution: Journal of Nurse Empowerment, 8*(3/4), 44–45.

Nursing shortage: Johnson & Johnson campaign aims to increase awareness, generate interest. (2002). *Nursing Economics, 20*(2), 93–95.

Quinn, C. A., & Smith, M. D. (1987). *The professional commitment: Issues and ethics in nursing.* Philadelphia: W. B. Saunders.

Reutter, L., & Williamson, D. (2000). Advocating healthy public policy: Implications for baccalaureate nursing education. *Journal of Nursing Education, 39*, 21–26.

Trossman, S. (2003). Media relations 101. *American Journal of Nursing, 103*(1), 69–70.

Bibliography

Allen, J. E. (2003, July 21). Alone in the ER: People receiving invasive or lifesaving treatment often want loved ones present, but many hospitals limit access. *Los Angeles Times,* pp. F3.

Bass, M. (2003). Oncology nurses' perceptions of their role in resuscitation decisions. *Professional Nurse, 18*(12), 710–713.

Bell, S. (2003). CAN addressing professional advocacy. *Arizona Nurse, 56*(5), 3.

Center for American Nurses. (2003). Background on workplace advocacy initiatives at the national level. *Prairie Rose, 72*(3), 10.

Des Jardin, K. E. (2001). Political involvement in nursing—Politics, ethics, and strategic action. (Second article in a two-part series). *AORN Journal, 74*(5), 613–615, 617–618, 621–626.

Dinsdale, P. (2000). Robust research is key to nurses' political influence. *Nursing Standard, 14*(31), 7.

Ecker, H. A. (2003). Washington watch. Politics and responsibility: Lend your voice and make a difference in the 2004 elections—and beyond. *American Journal of Nursing, 103*(11), 29.

Fletcher, M. (2002). Mortgages for nurses? Political will lacking in shortage solution. *Canadian Nurse, 98*(9), 9.

Grace, P. J. (2001). Professional advocacy: Widening the scope of accountability. *Nursing Philosophy, 2*(2), 151–162.

Kaiser reverses on transplant denial for HIV-positive patient. (2003). *AIDS Policy Law, 18*(20), 2.

Mason, D. J. (2002). Invisible nurses: Media neglect is one cause of the nursing shortage. *American Journal of Nursing, 102*(8), 7.

Paniagua, H. (2003). Developing practice nurses' political voice. *Journal of Practical Nursing, 14*(1), 34–37.

Reutter, L. & Duncan, S. (2002). Preparing nurses to promote health-enhancing public policies. *Policy, Politics, & Nursing Practice, 3*(4), 294–305.

Schoeter, K. (2003). May the force be with you: Nurses need to break the bonds of their dependency and become empowered so they can stand up for their patients' wishes. *Surgical Services Management, 9*(4), 6–8.

Steele, S. (2003). Analyzing and promoting issues in health policy: Nurse manager's perspective. *Nursing Economic$, 21*(2), 80–83.

Ulmer, B. C. (2000). President's message. Professional advocacy. *AORN Journal, 72*(1), 9–11.

Zavadsky, M. (2003). Expert advice: Insights & innovations from top industry professionals. How to change public policy. *EMS Insider, 30*(11), 6–7.

CHAPTER

7

The Planning Hierarchy and Strategic Planning

In the absence of clearly defined goals, we are forced to concentrate on activity and ultimately become enslaved by it.

—Chuck Conradt

Planning is deciding in advance what to do; who is to do it; and how, when, and where it is to be done. All planning involves choice: a necessity to choose from among alternatives. This implies that planning is a proactive and deliberate process. It is a function required of all managers so that personal, as well as organizational, needs and objectives can be met. This cyclic process allows for unity of goals, continuity of energy expenditure (human and fiscal resources), and the opportunity to minimize uncertainty and chance. This process also directs attention to the objectives of the organization and provides the manager with a means of control.

Adequate planning encourages the best use of resources. In effective planning, the manager must identify short- and long-term goals and changes that need to be undertaken to ensure that the unit will continue to meet its goals.

Identifying short- and long-term goals requires leadership skills, such as vision and creativity. It is impossible to plan what cannot be dreamed or envisioned. Likewise, planning requires flexibility and energy, two other leadership characteristics. Planning is critically important to and precedes all other management functions. Without adequate planning, the management process will fail.

Unit 3 focuses on several aspects of planning, including the planning hierarchy, strategic planning, planned change, short-term planning, time management, fiscal planning, and career planning. This chapter deals with skills needed by the leader–manager to implement the planning hierarchy and strategic planning. In addition, the leadership roles and management functions involved in developing, implementing, and evaluating that hierarchy are discussed (**Display 7.1**).

PROACTIVE PLANNING

Planning has a specific purpose and is one approach to strategy making. Planning represents specific activities that lead to achievement of objectives; therefore, planning is purposeful and proactive. Proactive planning minimizes risks and uncertainty, provides the leader–manager with a means of control, and encourages the best possible use of resources.

Planning has traditionally been oriented toward the present or future. Although there has been some crossover between types of planning within organizations, there is generally an orientation toward one of four planning modes: reactive planning, inactivism, preactivism, or proactive planning.

Reactive planning occurs *after* a problem exists. Because there is dissatisfaction with the current situation, planning efforts are directed toward returning the organization to a previous, more comfortable state. Frequently, in reactive planning, problems are dealt with separately without integration with the whole organization. Because it is done in response to a crisis, reactive planning can lead to hasty decisions and mistakes.

Inactivism is another type of conventional planning. Inactivists consider the status quo as the stable environment and they spend a great deal of energy preventing change and maintaining conformity. When changes do occur in this type of organization, they occur slowly and incrementally.

Display 7.1	**Leadership Roles and Management Functions Associated with the Planning Hierarchy and Strategic Planning**

Leadership Roles

1. Assesses the organization's internal and external environment in forecasting and identifying driving forces and barriers to strategic planning
2. Demonstrates visionary, innovative, and creative thinking in organizational and unit planning, thus inspiring proactive rather than reactive planning
3. Influences and inspires group members to be actively involved in long-term planning
4. Periodically completes value clarification to increase self-awareness
5. Encourages subordinates toward value clarification by actively listening and providing feedback
6. Communicates and clarifies organizational goals and values to subordinates
7. Encourages subordinates to be involved in policy formation, including developing, implementing, and reviewing unit philosophy, goals, objectives, policies, procedures, and rules
8. Is receptive to new and varied ideas
9. Role models proactive planning methods to subordinates

Management Functions

1. Is knowledgeable regarding legal, political, economic, and social factors affecting healthcare planning
2. Demonstrates knowledge of and uses appropriate techniques in both personal and organizational planning
3. Provides opportunities for subordinates, peers, competitors, regulatory agencies, and the general public to participate in planning
4. Coordinates unit-level planning to be congruent with organizational goals
5. Periodically assesses unit constraints and assets to determine available resources for planning
6. Develops and articulates a unit philosophy that is congruent with the organization
7. Develops and articulates unit goals and objectives that reflect unit philosophy
8. Develops and articulates unit policies, procedures, and rules that operationalize unit objectives
9. Periodically reviews unit philosophy, goals, policies, procedures, and rules and revises them to meet the unit's changing needs
10. Actively participates in organizational strategic planning, defining and operationalizing, such strategic plans on the unit level

A third planning mode is *preactivisim*. Preactive planners utilize technology to accelerate change and are future-oriented. Unsatisfied with the past or present, preactivists do not value experience and believe the future is always preferable.

The last planning mode is *interactive* or *proactive* planning. Planners who fall into this category consider the past, present, and future and attempt to plan the future of their organization rather than react to it. Proactive planning is dynamic. Adaptation is considered to be a key requirement in proactive planning because

Proactive planning is done in anticipation of changing needs.

the environment around us changes so frequently. Proactive planning is done in anticipation of changing needs or to promote growth within an organization. Proactive planning is required of all leader–managers so that personal as well as organizational needs and objectives are met.

Learning Exercise 7.1

What is Your Planning Style?
Individually write a plan for the current year. How would you describe your planning? Which type of planner are you? Write a brief essay that describes your planning style. Use specific examples then share your insights in a group.

THE PLANNING HIERARCHY

There are many types of planning; in most organizations, these plans form a hierarchy, with the plans at the top influencing all the plans that follow. As depicted in the pyramid in **Figure 7.1,** the hierarchy broadens at lower levels, representing an increase in the number of planning components. In addition, planning components at the top of the hierarchy are more general and lower components are more specific.

VISION AND MISSION STATEMENTS

The purpose or *mission statement* is a brief statement identifying the reason that an organization exists, while its future aim or function is often written as a *vision statement*. A mission statement identifies the organization's constituency and addresses its

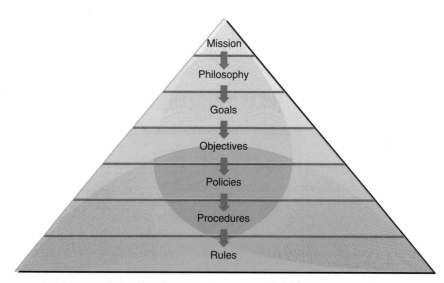

Figure 7.1 The planning hierarchy.

Display 7.2	County Hospital's Mission Statement

County Hospital is a tertiary care facility and provides comprehensive, holistic care to all state residents who seek treatment. The purpose of County Hospital is to combine high-quality, holistic health care with the provision of learning opportunities for students in medicine, nursing, and allied health sciences. Research is encouraged to identify new treatment regimens and to promote high-quality health care for generations to come.

position regarding ethics, principles, and standards of practice. An example of a mission statement for County Hospital, a teaching hospital, appears in **Display 7.2.**

An appropriate vision statement for County Hospital would be: To become an exemplar for health care in the region. Vision statements are always future oriented while mission statements provide the foundation for organizational planning.

The mission statement is of highest priority in the planning hierarchy because it influences the development of an organization's philosophy, goals, objectives, policies, procedures, and rules. Managers employed by County Hospital would have two primary goals to guide their planning: (1) to provide high-quality, holistic care and (2) to provide learning opportunities for students in medicine, nursing, and allied health sciences. To meet these goals, adequate fiscal and human resources would have to be allocated for preceptorships and clinical research. In addition, an employee's performance appraisal would examine the worker's performance in terms of organizational and unit goals.

THE ORGANIZATION'S PHILOSOPHY STATEMENT

The *organizational philosophy* flows from the purpose or mission statement and delineates the set of values and beliefs that guide all actions of the organization. It is the basic foundation that directs all further planning toward that mission. Tuck, Harris, and Baliko (2000) maintain that the values and principles set forth in the philosophy provide the parameters for decision making in determining what is critical to an organization. A statement of philosophy can usually be found in policy manuals at the institution or is available on request. A philosophy that might be generated from County Hospital's mission statement appears in **Display 7.3.**

The organizational philosophy provides the basis for developing nursing philosophies at the unit level and for nursing service as a whole. Written in conjunction with the organizational philosophy, the nursing service philosophy should address fundamental beliefs about nursing and nursing care; the quality, quantity, and scope of nursing services; and how nursing specifically will meet organizational goals. Frequently, the nursing service philosophy draws on the concepts of holistic care, education, and research. The sample nursing service philosophy (shown in **Display 7.4**) builds on County Hospital's mission statement and organizational philosophy.

The unit philosophy, adapted from the nursing service philosophy, specifies how nursing care provided on the unit will correspond with nursing service and

| Display 7.3 | County Hospital's Statement of Philosophy |

The board of directors, medical and nursing staff, and administrators of County Hospital believe that human beings are unique, due to different genetic endowments, personal experiences in social and physical environments, and the ability to adapt to biophysical, psychosocial, and spiritual stressors. Thus, each patient is considered a unique individual, with unique needs. Identifying outcomes and goals, setting priorities, prescribing strategy options, and selecting an optimal strategy will be negotiated by the patient, physician, and healthcare team.

As unique individuals, patients provide medical, nursing, and allied health students invaluable diverse learning opportunities. Because the board of directors, medical and nursing staff, and administrators believe that the quality of health care provided directly reflects the quality of the education of its future healthcare providers, students are welcomed and encouraged to seek out as many learning opportunities as possible. Because high-quality health care is defined by and depends on technological advances and scientific discovery, County Hospital encourages research as a means of scientific inquiry.

| Display 7.4 | County Hospital's Nursing Service Philosophy |

The philosophy of nursing at County Hospital is based on respect for the individual's dignity and worth. We believe all patients have the right to receive effective nursing care. This care is a personal service that is based on patients' needs and their clinical disease or condition. Recognizing the obligation of nursing to help restore patients to the best possible state of physical, mental, and emotional health and to maintain patients' sense of spiritual and social well-being, we pledge intelligent cooperation in coordinating nursing service with the medical and allied professional practitioners. Understanding the importance of research and teaching for improving patient care, the nursing department will support, promote, and participate in these activities. Using knowledge of human behavior, we shall strive for mutual trust and understanding between nursing service and nursing employees to provide an atmosphere for developing the fullest possible potential of each member of the nursing team. We believe that nursing personnel are individually accountable to patients and their families for the quality and compassion of the patient care rendered and for upholding the standards of care as delineated by the nursing staff.

organizational goals. This congruency in philosophy, goals, and objectives between the organization, nursing service, and unit is shown in **Figure 7.2.**

Although unit-level managers have limited opportunity to help develop organizational philosophy, they are active in determining, implementing, and evaluating the unit philosophy. In formulating this philosophy, the unit manager incorporates knowledge of the unit's internal and external environments and an understanding of the unit's role in meeting organizational goals. The manager must understand the planning hierarchy and be able to articulate ideas in writing. Leader–managers also must be visionary, innovative, and creative in

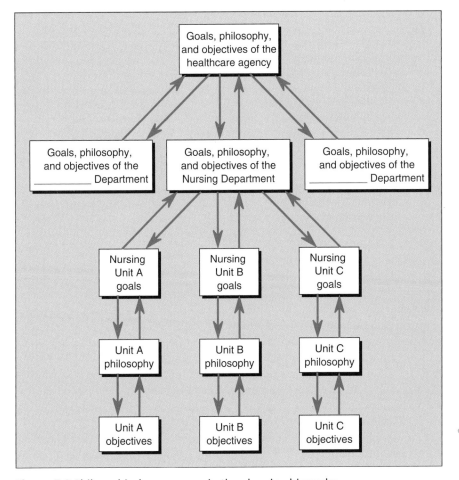

Figure 7.2 Philosophical congruence in the planning hierarchy.

A philosophy that is not or cannot be implemented is useless.

identifying unit purposes or goals so that the philosophy not only reflects current practice, but also incorporates a view of the future.

Statements of philosophy, in general, can be helpful only if they truly direct the work of the organization toward a specific purpose. A working philosophy is evident in a department's decisions, in its priorities, and in its accomplishments. Hegyvary (2000) maintains that organizations, individuals, managers, and leaders accomplish and prioritize those things that they believe in. It is the things that individuals believe in that get done in an organization.

A person should be able to identify exactly how the organization is implementing their stated philosophy by observing members of the staff, reviewing the budgetary priorities, and talking to consumers of health care. The decisions made in an organization make the philosophy visible to all—no matter what is espoused on paper. A philosophy that is not or cannot be implemented is useless.

Learning Exercise 7.2

Develop a Philosophy Statement

Recover, Inc., a fictitious for-profit home health agency, provides complete nursing and supportive services for in-home care. Services include skilled nursing, bathing, shopping, physical therapy, occupational therapy, meal preparation, housekeeping, speech therapy, and social work. The agency provides around-the-clock care, seven days a week, to a primarily underserved rural area in northern California. The brochure the company publishes says that it is committed to satisfying the needs of the rural community and that it is dedicated to excellence.

Assignment: Based on this limited information, develop a brief philosophy statement that might be appropriate for Recover, Inc. Be creative and embellish information given in the learning exercise if appropriate.

SOCIETAL PHILOSOPHIES AND VALUES

Societies and organizations have philosophies or sets of beliefs that guide their behavior. These beliefs that guide behavior are called *values*. Values have an intrinsic worth for a society or an individual. Some strongly held American values are individualism, the pursuit of self-interest, and competition. Bennis (1989) states that American society has always been at war with itself: "We have always dreamt of community and democracy, but always practiced democracy and capitalism. We have celebrated innocence, but sought power" (p. 46). These values have profoundly affected healthcare policy formation and implementation. The result is a healthcare system that promotes structured inequalities. Despite spending over a trillion dollars on health care in 2004, over 45 million American citizens had no health insurance, and even more were underinsured.

Although values seem to be of central importance for healthcare policy development and analysis, public discussion of this crucial variable is often neglected. Instead, healthcare policy makers tend to focus on technology, cost-benefit analysis, and cost-effectiveness. Although this type of evaluation is important, it does not address the underlying values in this country that have led to unequal access to health care.

INDIVIDUAL PHILOSOPHIES AND VALUES

As discussed in Chapter 1, values have a tremendous impact on the decisions people make. For the individual, personal philosophies and values are shaped by the socialization processes experienced by that person. All people should carefully examine their value system and recognize the role it plays in how they make decisions and resolve conflicts, and even how they perceive things. Therefore, the nurse–leader must be self-aware and provide subordinates with learning opportunities or experiences that foster increased self-awareness.

Learning Exercise 7.3

Health Care at What Cost?

Both Canada and Germany have been held up as models in healthcare reform because they guarantee health care for all citizens. Although the United States spends more per capita than either Germany or Canada, many citizens do not have access to comprehensive, quality health care. Canadians receive hospitalization, doctor visits, and most dental care free of charge. Germany spends even less and provides a level of services similar to Canada, but with a very small co-payment for hospitalization. Unlike the emphasis on specialized care in the United States with limited choice of physicians, healthcare systems in Canada and Germany emphasize primary care, unlimited choice of physicians, free physician visits, and an emphasis on health promotion. With little financial incentive for physician specialization and a nationwide focus on health promotion, there are many more general practitioners per capita in Germany and Canada than in the United States.

At what cost is this health care offered? Canadians and Germans experience longer waits for some "high-tech" procedures, and the governments of those countries have limitations on the proliferation of technology. However, the United States continues to have a higher incidence of infant mortality and low birth weight than in either of these two countries and lower life expectancy at birth. Despite the highest spending as a percentage of gross domestic product, American consumers had the fewest number of physician visits and the shortest average hospital stay.

Assignment: In small groups, discuss the following: Do you agree or disagree that the United States healthcare system represents societal values of individualism, the pursuit of self-interests, and competition? Do you believe that U.S. citizens are willing to pay the costs required to pursue collectivism, cooperation, and equality in health care? Would you be willing to have fewer choices about your health care if access could be guaranteed to all? Do you believe the cost of universal coverage should be picked up by the consumer or by the employer? Recognize that both societal and individual values will affect your thinking.

At times, it is difficult to assess whether something is a true value. McNally (1980) identified the following four characteristics that determine a true value:

1. It must be freely chosen from among alternatives only after due reflection.
2. It must be prized and cherished.
3. It is consciously and consistently repeated (part of a pattern).
4. It is positively affirmed and enacted.

If a value does not meet all four criteria, it is a "value indicator." Most people have many value indicators but few true values. For example, many nurses assert that they value their national nursing organization, yet they do not pay dues or participate in the organization. True values require that the person take action, whereas value indicators do not. Thus, the value ascribed to the national nursing organization is a value indicator for these nurses and not a true value.

In addition, because our values change with time, periodic clarification is necessary to determine how our values may have changed. Values clarification includes examining values, assigning priorities to those values, and determining how they influence behavior so that one's lifestyle is consistent with prioritized values. Sometimes values change as a result of life's experiences or newly acquired knowledge. Most of the values we have as children reflect our parents' values. Later, peers and role models modify our values. Although they are learned, values cannot be forced on a person, because they must be internalized. However, restricted exposure to other viewpoints also limits the number of value choices a person is able to generate. Therefore, becoming more worldly increases a person's awareness of alternatives from which values are selected.

 Learning Exercise 7.4

Reflecting on Your Values
Using what you have learned about values, value indicators, and values clarification, answer the following questions. Take time to reflect on your values before answering.
1. List three or four of your basic beliefs about nursing.
2. Knowing what you know now, ask yourself, "Do I value nursing?" Was it freely chosen from among alternatives after appropriate reflection? Do you prize and cherish nursing? If you had a choice to do it over, would you still choose nursing as a career?
3. Are your personal and professional values congruent? Are there any values espoused by the nursing profession that are inconsistent with your personal values? How will you resolve resulting conflicts?

Occasionally, individual values are in conflict with those of the organization. Because the philosophy of an organization determines its priorities in goal selection and distribution of resources, nurses need to understand the organization's philosophy. For example, assume that a nurse is employed by County Hospital, which clearly states in its philosophy that teaching is a primary purpose for the hospital's existence. Consequently, medical students are allowed to practice endotracheal intubation on all people who die in the hospital, allowing the students to gain needed experience in emergency medicine. This practice disturbs the nurse a great deal; it is not consistent with his or her own set of values and thus creates great personal conflict.

Nurses who frequently make decisions that conflict with their personal values may experience confusion and anxiety. This intrapersonal struggle will lead ultimately to job stress and dissatisfaction, especially for the novice nurse who comes to the organization with inadequate values clarification. The choices nurses make about patient care are not merely strategic options; they are moral choices. When a nurse experiences cognitive dissonance between personal and organizational values, the result may be intrapersonal conflict and burnout.

When a nurse experiences cognitive dissonance between personal and organizational values, the result may be intrapersonal conflict and burnout.

As part of the leadership role, the manager should encourage all potential employees to read and think about the organization's mission statement or philosophy before accepting the job. The manager should give a copy of the philosophy to the prospective applicant before the hiring interview. The applicant also should be encouraged to speak to employees in various positions within the organization regarding how the philosophy is implemented at their job level. For example, a potential employee may want to determine how the organization feels about cultural diversity and what policies they have in place to ensure that patients from diverse cultures and languages have a mechanism for translation as needed. Finally, new employees should be encouraged to speak to community members about the institution's reputation for care. New employees who understand the organizational philosophy will not only have clearer expectations about the institution's purposes and goals, but will also have a better understanding of how they fit into the organization.

Although all nurses should have a philosophy compatible with their employer's, it is especially important for the new manager to have a value system consistent with the organization's. Institutional changes that closely align with the value system of the nurse–manager will receive more effort and higher priority than those that are not true values or that conflict with the nurse–manager's value system. It is unrealistic for managers to accept a position under the assumption that they can change the organization's philosophy to more closely match their personal philosophy. Such a change will require extraordinary energy and precipitate inevitable conflict because the organization's philosophy reflects the institution's historical development and the beliefs of those people who were vital in the institution's development. Nursing managers must recognize that closely held values may be challenged by current social and economic constraints and that philosophy statements must be continually reviewed and revised to ensure ongoing accuracy of beliefs.

GOALS AND OBJECTIVES

Goals and objectives are the ends toward which the organization is working. All philosophies must be translated into specific goals and objectives if they are to result in action. Thus, goals and objectives "operationalize" the philosophy.

A *goal* may be defined as the desired result toward which effort is directed; it is the aim of the philosophy. Although institutional goals are usually determined by the organization's highest administrative levels, there is increasing emphasis on including workers in setting organizational goals. Goals, much like philosophies and values, change with time and require periodic reevaluation and prioritization.

Goals, although somewhat global in nature, should be measurable and ambitious, but realistic. Goals also should clearly delineate the desired end-product. When goals are not clear, simple misunderstandings may be compounded, and communication may break down. Organizations usually set long- and short-term goals for services rendered; economics; use of resources, including people, funds, and facilities; innovations; and social responsibilities. **Display 7.5** lists sample goal statements.

Display 7.5   Sample Goal Statements

- All nursing staff will recognize the patient's need for independence and right to privacy and will assess the patient's level of readiness to learn in relation to his or her illness.
- The nursing staff will provide effective patient care relative to patient needs insofar as the hospital and community facilities permit through the use of care plans, individual patient care, and discharge planning, including follow-up contact.
- An ongoing effort will be made to create an atmosphere that is conducive to favorable patient and employee morale and that fosters personal growth.
- The performance of all employees in the nursing department will be evaluated in a manner that produces growth in the employee and upgrades nursing standards.
- All nursing units within County Hospital will work cooperatively with other departments within the hospital to further the mision, philosophy, and goals of the institution.

Although goals may direct and maintain the behavior of an organization, there are several dangers in using goal evaluation as the primary means of assessing organizational effectiveness. The first danger is that goals may be in conflict with each other, creating confusion for employees and consumers. For example, the need for profit maximization in healthcare facilities today may conflict with some stated patient goals or quality goals. The second danger with the goal approach is that publicly stated goals may not truly reflect organizational goals. Organizational goals can be a mask for individual unit or personal goals. The final danger is that because goals are global, it is often difficult to determine whether they have been met.

Objectives are similar to goals in that they motivate people to a specific end and, in addition, are explicit, measurable, observable or retrievable, and obtainable. Objectives, however, are more specific and measurable than goals because they identify how and when the goal is to be accomplished.

Goals usually have multiple objectives that are each accompanied by a targeted completion date. The more specific the objectives for a goal can be, the easier for all involved in goal attainment to understand and carry out specific role behaviors. This is especially important for the nurse–manager to remember when writing job descriptions; if there is little ambiguity in the job description, there will be little role confusion or distortion. Clearly written goals and objectives must be communicated to all those in the organization responsible for their attainment. This is a critical leadership role for the nurse–manager.

Objectives can focus either on the desired process or the desired result. *Process objectives* are written in terms of the method to be used, whereas *result-focused objectives* specify the desired outcome. An example of a process objective might be, "100% of staff nurses will orient new patients to the call-light system, within 30 minutes of their admission, by first demonstrating its appropriate use and then asking the patient to repeat said demonstration." An example of a result-focused objective might be, "All postoperative patients will perceive a decrease in their pain levels following the administration of parenteral pain medication." (The measurement of process and result-focused objectives is discussed further in Chapter 23.)

However, for the objectives to be measurable, they should have certain criteria. There should be a specific time frame in which the objectives are to be completed, and the objectives should be stated in behavioral terms, be objectively evaluated, and identify positive rather than negative outcomes.

As a sample objective, one of the goals at Mercy Hospital is, "All registered nurses will be proficient in the administration of intravenous fluids." Objectives for Mercy Hospital might include the following:

- All registered nurses will complete Mercy Hospital's course "IV Therapy Certification" within one month of beginning employment. The hospital will bear the cost of this program.
- Registered nurses scoring less than 70% on a comprehensive examination in "IV Therapy Certification" must attend the remedial four-hour course "Review of Basic IV Principles" not more than two weeks after the completion of "IV Therapy Certification."
- Registered nurses achieving a score of 70% or better on the comprehensive examination for "IV Therapy Certification" after completing "Review of Basic IV Principles" will be allowed to perform IV therapy on patients. The unit manager will establish individualized plans of remediation for employees who fail to achieve this score on the examination.

The leader–manager clearly must be skilled in determining and documenting goals and objectives. Prudent managers assess the unit's constraints and assets and determine available resources before developing goals and objectives. The leader must then be creative and futuristic in identifying how goals might best be translated into objectives and thus implemented. The willingness to be receptive to new and varied ideas is a tremendous leadership skill. In addition, well-developed interpersonal skills allow the leader to involve and inspire subordinates in goal setting. The final step in the process involves clearly writing the identified goals and objectives, communicating changes to subordinates, and periodically evaluating and revising goals and objectives as needed.

 Learning Exercise 7.5

Writing Goals and Objectives
Practice writing goals and objectives for County Hospital based on the mission and philosophy statements in this chapter. Identify three goals and three objectives to operationalize each of these goals.

POLICIES AND PROCEDURES

Policies are plans reduced to statements or instructions that direct organizations in their decision making. A policy is a statement of expectations that sets boundaries for action taking and decision making (Paige, 2003).

These comprehensive statements, derived from the organization's philosophy, goals, and objectives, explain how goals will be met and guide the general course

Display 8.1	**Leadership Roles and Management Functions in Planned Change**

Leadership Roles
1. Is visionary in identifying areas of needed change in the organization and the health-care system.
2. Demonstrates risk taking in assuming the role of change agent.
3. Demonstrates flexibility in goal setting in a rapidly changing healthcare system.
4. Anticipates, recognizes, and creatively problem solves resistance to change.
5. Serves as a role model to subordinates during planned change by viewing change as a challenge and opportunity for growth.
6. Role models high-level interpersonal communication skills in providing support for followers undergoing rapid or difficult change.
7. Demonstrates creativity in identifying alternatives to problems.
8. Demonstrates sensitivity to timing in proposing planned change.
9. Takes steps to prevent aging in the organization and to keep nursing current with the new realities of nursing practice.

Management Functions
1. Forecasts unit needs with an understanding of the organization's and unit's legal, political, economic, social, and legislative climate.
2. Recognizes the need for planned change and identifies the options and resources available to implement that change.
3. Appropriately assesses the driving and restraining forces when planning for change.
4. Identifies and implements appropriate strategies to minimize or overcome resistance to change.
5. Seeks subordinates' input in planned change and provides them with adequate information during the change process to give them some feeling of control.
6. Supports and reinforces the individual efforts of subordinates during the change process.
7. Identifies and uses appropriate change strategies to modify the behavior of subordinates as needed.
8. Periodically assesses the unit/department for signs of organizational aging and plans renewal strategies.

Display 8.1 delineates selected leadership roles and management functions necessary for leader–managers acting either in the change agent role or as a coordinator of the team.

THE DEVELOPMENT OF CHANGE THEORY

Most of the current research on change builds on the classic change theories developed by Kurt Lewin in the mid-20th century. Lewin (1951) identified three phases through which the change agent must proceed before a planned change becomes part of the system: unfreezing, movement, and refreezing.

In the *unfreezing stage,* the change agent unfreezes forces that maintain the status quo. Thus, people become discontented and aware of a need to change. Unfreezing is necessary because before any change can occur, people must believe the change is needed. Unfreezing occurs when the change agent convinces members of the group to change or when guilt, anxiety, or concern can be elicited. For effective change to occur, the change agent needs to have made a thorough and accurate assessment of the extent of and interest in change, the nature and depth of motivation, and the environment in which the change will occur. Change should be implemented only for good reasons. Because human beings have little control over many changes in their lives, the change agent must remember that people need a balance between stability and change in the workplace. Change for change's sake subjects employees to unnecessary stress and manipulation.

 Learning Exercise 8.1

Unnecessary Change
Try to remember a situation in your own life that involved unnecessary change. Why do you think the change was unnecessary? What types of turmoil did it cause? Were there things a change agent could have done that would have increased unfreezing in this situation?

The second phase of planned change is *movement.* In movement, the change agent identifies, plans, and implements appropriate strategies, ensuring that driving forces exceed restraining forces. Whenever possible, change should be implemented gradually. Because change is such a complex process, it requires a great deal of planning and intricate timing. Recognizing, addressing, and overcoming resistance may be a lengthy process. Any change of human behavior, or the perceptions, attitudes, and values underlying that behavior, takes time. Therefore, any change must allow enough time for those involved to be fully assimilated in that change.

The last phase is *refreezing.* During the refreezing phase, the change agent assists in stabilizing the system change so it becomes integrated into the status quo. If refreezing is incomplete, the change will be ineffective and the pre-change behaviors will be resumed. For refreezing to occur, the change agent must be supportive and reinforce the individual adaptive efforts of those affected by the change. Because change needs at least three to six months before it will be accepted as part of the system, change should never be attempted unless the change agent can make a commitment to be available until the change is complete.

It is important to realize that refreezing does not eliminate the possibility of further improvements to the change. **Display 8.2** illustrates the change agent's responsibilities during the various stages.

Display 8.2	Stages of Change and Responsibilities of the Change Agent

Stage 1—Unfreezing
1. Gather data
2. Accurately diagnose the problem
3. Decide if change is needed
4. Make others aware of the need for change; often involves deliberate tactics to raise the group's discontent level; do not proceed to Stage 2 until the status quo has been disrupted, and the need for change is perceived by the others

Stage 2—Movement
1. Develop a plan
2. Set goals and objectives
3. Identify areas of support and resistance
4. Include everyone who will be affected by the change in its planning
5. Set target dates
6. Develop appropriate strategies
7. Implement the change
8. Be available to support others and offer encouragement through the change
9. Use strategies for overcoming resistance to change
10. Evaluate the change
11. Modify the change, if necessary

Stage 3—Refreezing
Support others so the change remains

Lippitt, Watson, and Westley (1958) built on Lewin's theories in identifying seven phases of planned change:

1. The patient must feel a need for change. Unfreezing occurs.
2. A helping relationship begins between the change agent and his or her patients. Movement begins.
3. The problem is identified and clarified. Data are collected.
4. Alternatives for change are examined. Resources are assessed.
5. Active modification or change occurs. Movement is complete.
6. Refreezing occurs as the change is stabilized.
7. The helping relationship ends, or a different type of continuing relationship is formed.

Murphy (1999), in a more contemporary model, suggests that there are four predictable stages that people pass through when exposed to any change: *resistance, confusion, exploration,* and *commitment.* There are predictable behaviors associated with each of these stages, and the most effective managers study these behaviors and are able to respond appropriately to get their team back on track toward the goals.

Display 8.3	**Ten Emotional Phases of the Change Process**

1. Equilibrium: Characterized by high energy and emotional and intellectual balance. Personal and professional goals are synchronized.
2. Denial: Individual denies reality of the change. Negative changes occur in physical, cognitive, and emotional functioning.
3. Anger: Energy is manifested by rage, envy, and resentment.
4. Bargaining: In an attempt to eliminate the change, energy is expended by bargaining.
5. Chaos: Characterized by diffused energy, feelings of powerlessness, insecurity, and loss of identity.
6. Depression: Defense mechanisms are no longer operable. No energy left to produce results. Self-pity apparent.
7. Resignation: Change accepted passively but without enthusiasm.
8. Openness: Some renewal of energy in implementing new roles or assignments that have resulted from the change.
9. Readiness: Willful expenditure of energy to explore new event. Physical, cognitive, and emotional reunification occurs.
10. Reemergence: Person again feels empowered and begins initiating projects and ideas.

Adapted from Perlman, D., & Takacs, G. J. (1990). The ten stages of change. *Nursing Management, 21*(4), 33–38.

Perlman and Takacs (1990), building on Lewin's work, identified 10 such behaviors or emotional phases in the change process (**Display 8.3**). The phases of equilibrium, denial, anger, and bargaining reflect Lewin's unfreezing phase; chaos, depression, and resignation, the movement phase; and openness, readiness, and reemergence, the refreezing phase. Regardless of the number of phases or their names, it is critical that the manager recognizes that organizations must consciously and constructively deal with the human emotions associated with all phases of planned change.

Quinn, Spreitzer, and Brown (2000) state that any real adaptive change can be achieved only by mobilizing people to make painful adjustments in their attitudes, work habits, and lives. They must "surrender their present selves and put themselves in jeopardy of becoming part of an emergent system. This process usually requires the surrender of personal control, the toleration of uncertainty, and the development of a new culture at the collective level and a new self at the individual level" (p. 147).

DRIVING AND RESTRAINING FORCES

Lewin also theorized that people maintain a state of status quo or equilibrium by the simultaneous occurrence of both driving and restraining forces operating within any field. The forces that push the system toward the change are *driving forces*, whereas the forces that pull the system away from the change are called *restraining forces*. Lewin's model maintained that for change to occur, the balance of driving and restraining forces must be altered. The driving forces must be increased or the restraining forces decreased.

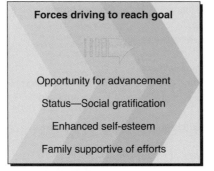
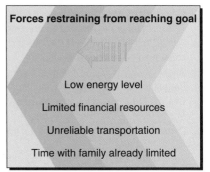

Figure 8.1 Driving and restraining forces.

Driving forces may include a desire to please one's boss, to eliminate a problem that is undermining productivity, to get a pay raise, or to receive recognition. Restraining forces include conformity to norms, an unwillingness to take risks, and a fear of the unknown. In **Figure 8.1,** the person wishing to return to school must reduce the restraining forces or increase the driving forces to alter the present state of equilibrium. There will be no change or action until this occurs. Therefore, creating an imbalance within the system by increasing the driving forces or decreasing the restraining forces is one of the tasks required for a change agent.

Learning Exercise 8.2

Making Change Possible
Identify a change that you would like to make in your personal life (such as losing weight, exercising daily, or stopping smoking). List the restraining forces keeping you from making this change. List the driving forces that make you want to change. Determine how you might be able to change the status quo and make the change possible.

Numerous factors affect successful implementation of planned change. Many good ideas are never realized because of poor timing or a lack of power on the part of the change agent. For example, both organizations and individuals tend to reject outsiders as change agents because they are perceived as having inadequate knowledge or expertise about the current status, and their motives often are not trusted. Therefore, there is less widespread resistance if the change agent is an insider. The outside change agent, however, tends to be more objective in his or her assessment, whereas the inside change agent is often influenced by a personal bias regarding how the organization functions.

Many good ideas are never realized because of poor timing or a lack of power on the part of the change agent.

Likewise, some greatly needed changes are never implemented because the change agent lacks sensitivity to timing. If the organization or the people within that organization have recently undergone a great deal of change or stress, any other change should wait until group resistance decreases.

CHANGE STRATEGIES

Three commonly used strategies for effecting change in others were described by Bennis, Benne, and Chinn (1969). The appropriate strategy for any situation depends on the power of the change agent and the amount of resistance expected from the subordinates. One of these strategies is to give current research as evidence to support the change. This group of strategies is often referred to as *rational–empirical strategies*. The change agent using this set of strategies assumes that resistance to change comes from ignorance or superstition (Quinn, Spreitzer, & Brown, 2000) and that humans are rational beings who will change when given factual information documenting the need for change. This type of strategy is used when there is little anticipated resistance to the change or when the change is perceived as reasonable.

Because peer pressure is often used to effect change, another group of strategies that uses group process is called *normative–re-educative strategies*. These strategies use group norms to socialize and influence people so change will occur. The change agent assumes humans are social animals, more easily influenced by others than by facts. This strategy does not require the change agent to have a legitimate power base. Instead, the change agent gains power by skill in interpersonal relationships. He or she focuses on noncognitive determinants of behavior, such as people's roles and relationships, perceptual orientations, attitudes, and feelings, to increase acceptance of change.

The third group of strategies, *power–coercive strategies*, are based on the application of power by legitimate authority, economic sanctions, or political clout of the change agent. These strategies include influencing the enactment of new laws and using group power for strikes or sit-ins. Using authority inherent in an individual position to effect change is another example of a power–coercive strategy. These strategies assume that people often are set in their ways and will change only when rewarded for the change or are forced by some other power–coercive method. Resistance is handled by authority measures; the individual must accept it or leave.

Often the change agent uses strategies from each of these three groups. An example would be the change agent who wants someone to stop smoking. The change agent might present the person with the latest research on cancer and smoking (the rational–empirical approach); at the same time, the change agent might have friends and family educate the person socially (normative–re-educative approach). The change agent also might refuse to ride in the car if the person smokes while driving (power–coercive approach). By selecting from each set of strategies, the manager increases the chance of successful change.

Learning Exercise 8.3

Using Change Strategies to Increase Sam's Compliance
You are a staff nurse in a home health agency. One of your patients, Sam Little, is a 38-year-old man with Type 1 diabetes. He has developed some loss of vision and had to have two toes amputated as consequences of his disease process. Sam's compliance with four times a day Accu-checks and sliding-scale insulin administration has never been particularly good, but he has been worse than usual lately. However, he does seem willing to follow a prescribed diabetic diet and has kept his weight to a desired level.

Sam's wife called you at the agency yesterday and asked you to work with her in developing a plan to increase Sam's compliance with his blood sugar monitoring and insulin administration. She said that Sam, while believing it "probably won't help," has agreed to meet with you to discuss such a plan.

Assignment: What change strategy or combination thereof (rational–empirical, normative–reeducative, power–coercive) do you believe has the greatest likelihood of increasing Sam's compliance? How could you use this strategy? Who would be involved in this change effort? What efforts might you undertake to increase the unfreezing so Sam is more willing to actively participate in such a planned change effort?

RESISTANCE: THE EXPECTED RESPONSE TO CHANGE

Resistance is recognized as a natural and expected response to change.

Because change disrupts the homeostasis or balance of the group, resistance should always be expected. The level of resistance generally depends on the type of change proposed. Technological changes encounter less resistance than changes that are perceived as social or that are contrary to established customs or norms. For example, nursing staff are more willing to accept a change in the type of intravenous pump to be used than a change regarding who is able to administer certain types of IV therapy. Nursing leaders also must recognize that subordinates' values, educational levels, cultural and social backgrounds, and experiences with change (positive or negative) will have a tremendous impact on their degree of resistance. It also is much easier to change a person's behavior than it is to change an entire group's behavior. Likewise, it is easier to change knowledge levels than attitudes.

In an effort to eliminate resistance to change in the workplace, managers historically used an autocratic leadership style with specific guidelines for work, an excessive number of rules, and a coercive approach to discipline. The resistance, which occurred anyway, was both covert (such as delaying tactics or passive–aggressive behavior) and overt (openly refusing to follow a direct command), and resulted in wasted managerial energy and time and a high level of frustration.

Today, resistance is recognized as a natural and expected response to change. Instead of wasting time and energy trying to eliminate opposition, contemporary managers immerse themselves in identifying and implementing strategies to minimize or manage this resistance to change. One such strategy is to encourage subordinates to

Display 8.4	**Common Responders and Responses to Change**

- Innovators: enthusiastic and thrive on change
- Early adopters: open and receptive to new ideas
- Early majority: adopt new ideas before the average person
- Late majority: skeptical of innovation and change
- Laggards: dedicated to tradition and the last to adopt a change
- Rejecters: openly oppose innovation and encourage others to also oppose change

Source: Bushy, A., & Kamphuis, J. (1993). Response to innovation: Behavioral patterns. *Nursing Management*, *24*(3), 62–64.

speak openly so options can be identified to overcome objections. Likewise, workers are encouraged to talk about their perceptions of the forces driving the planned change so the manager can accurately assess change support and resources.

Bushy and Kamphuis (1993) identified six behavioral patterns commonly seen in response to change: *innovators, early adopters, early majority, late majority, laggards*, and *rejecters* (see **Display 8.4**). Innovators are enthusiastic, energetic people who thrive on change and are almost obsessed with adventure. Described by some as disruptive radicals, they are able to effect change, often amidst controversy within the organization. Early adopters are open and receptive to new ideas but are less obsessed with seeking out changes than innovators. Early majority individuals adhere to the adage, "Be not the last to lay the old aside, nor the first by which the new is tried." Early majority individuals prefer the status quo but adopt new ideas shortly before the average person. Late majority individuals are followers, skeptical of innovation, and frequently express their negative views. Only after a majority of the organization accepts an innovation will the late majority favor it. Laggards, the last to adopt an innovation, are dedicated to tradition. They interact primarily with other traditionalists and are highly suspicious of innovations and innovators. Rejectors openly oppose innovation and actively encourage others to do so. Although covert in nature, their activities may completely immobilize the change process, the change agent, or the system, even to the extent of sabotaging an innovation.

Similarly, Pesut (2000) classifies individuals as either *crusaders* or *tradition bearers* in response to their propensity to seek change. Crusaders are change agents who

 Learning Exercise 8.4

What Is Your Attitude Toward Change?
Which behavioral pattern do you most commonly assume in response to change: innovator, early adopter, early majority, late majority, laggard, or rejecter? Is this behavioral pattern similar to your friends' and family's? Has your behavior always fit this pattern, or has the pattern changed throughout your life? If so, what life events have altered how you view and respond to change?

see problems in the present and want to make things better for the future. Tradition bearers are the preservers of what is best from the past and the present.

Perhaps the greatest factor contributing to the resistance encountered with change is a lack of trust between the employee and the manager or the employee and the organization. Workers want security and predictability. That's why trust erodes when the ground rules change, as the assumed "contract" between the worker and the organization is altered. Subordinates' confidence in the change agent's ability to manage change depends on whether they believe they have sufficient resources to cope with it. In addition, the leader–manager must remember that subordinates in an organization will generally focus more on how a specific change will affect their personal lives and status than on how it will affect the organization.

Heifetz and Laurie (2001) maintain that most followers want comfort, routine stability, and good problem solving. Change creates chaos and order is disturbed. Leaders must recognize this and continue to "push the walls" even as they meet resistance. Porter-O'Grady (2003) feels that this is the time of great challenge for the leader. The skills necessary to move reticent groups cannot be understated. The leader must use developmental, political, and relational expertise to ensure that needed change is not sabotaged.

PLANNED CHANGE AS A COLLABORATIVE PROCESS

Often times, the change process begins with a few people who meet to discuss their dissatisfaction with the status quo, and an inadequate effort is made to talk with anyone else in the organization. This approach virtually guarantees that the change effort will fail. People abhor "information vacuums," and when there is no ongoing conversation about the change process, gossip usually fills the void. These rumors are generally much more negative than anything that is actually happening.

Whenever possible, all those who may be affected by a change should be involved in planning for that change. Ayers (2002) suggests that the empirical picture that is emerging is that communication and organizational change processes are inextricably linked. When change agents fail to communicate with the rest of the organization, they prevent people from understanding the principles that guided the change, what has been learned from prior experience, and why compromises have been made. Research by Knox and Irving (1997) found that communication about the goals and progression of organizational change by healthcare executives was the most important factor for subordinate managers in ensuring a successful change effort. The importance of being perceived as a legitimate and informed participant in the change process was critical to their role success.

Likewise, subordinates affected by the change should thoroughly understand the change and how it affects them as individuals. Good, open communication throughout the process can reduce resistance. Leaders must ensure that group members share perceptions about what change is to be undertaken, who is to be involved and in what role, and how the change will directly and indirectly affect each person in the organization.

The easiest way for the manager to ensure that subordinates share this perception is to involve them in the change process. When information and decision making are shared, subordinates feel that they have played a valuable role in the change. Change agents and the elements of the system—the people or groups within it—must openly develop goals and strategies together. All must have the opportunity to define their interest in the change, their expectation of its outcome, and their ideas on strategies for achieving change.

It is not always easy to attain grassroots involvement in planning efforts. Even when managers communicate that change is needed and that subordinate feedback is wanted, the message often goes unheeded. Some people in the organization may need to hear a message repeatedly before they hear, understand, and believe the message. If the message is one they do not want to hear, it may take even longer for them to come to terms with the anticipated change.

THE LEADER–MANAGER AS A ROLE MODEL DURING PLANNED CHANGE

Leader–managers must act as role models to subordinates during the change process. The leader–manager must attempt to view change positively and to impart this view to subordinates. It is critical that managers not view change as a threat. Instead, it should be viewed as a challenge and the chance or opportunity to do something new and innovative. Porter-O'Grady (2003) suggests that these dramatically changing times in the practice of nursing have given leaders a more demanding role in health care, and that the manager's behavior is the single most important factor in how people in the organization accept change. Presently, the need for change is so important in healthcare organizations and in the nursing profession that Porter-O'Grady says leaders should accelerate disruptive change as a vehicle for making sure change occurs.

The leader has two responsibilities in facilitating change in nursing practice. First, leader–managers must be actively engaged in change in their own work and role model this behavior to staff. Secondly, leaders must be able to assist staff members make the needed change requirements in their work. For a change to become part of the organization, staff must internalize it. One way to assist staff with internalization is to show a relationship between the process of change and outcome, when this can be measured then the evidence to support the change is convincing (Porter-O'Grady, 2003).

Managers must believe that they can make a difference. This feeling of control is probably the most important trait for thriving in a changing environment. Friends, family, and colleagues should be used as a support network for managers during change. Likewise, managers should learn to recognize their own stress signals during change and take appropriate steps when the stress level becomes too high.

ORGANIZATIONAL AGING: CHANGE AS A MEANS OF RENEWAL

Organizations progress through developmental stages, just as people do—birth, youth, maturity, and aging. As organizations age, structure increases to provide greater control and coordination. The young organization is characterized by high energy, movement, and virtually constant change and adaptation. Aged organizations have established "turf boundaries," function in an orderly and predictable fashion, and are focused on rules and regulations. Change is limited. Other characteristics of aged organizations include hierarchical structures and bureaucratic processes that are resistant to change (Ayers, 2002).

It is clear that organizations must find a critical balance between stagnation and chaos, between birth and death. In the process of maturing, workers within the organization can become prisoners of procedures, forget their original purposes, and allow means to become the ends. Gardner (1990) argues that organizations must be *ever renewing*. The ever-renewing organization is infant-like—curious and open to new experience and change. Gardner says that the only way to conserve an organization is to keep it changing. Without change, the organization may stagnate and die.

The other term Gardner uses to describe the aged organization is *organizational dry rot*. Gardner states that organizational dry rot can be prevented by having effective programs for the recruitment and development of young talent; providing a hospitable organizational environment that fosters individuality; building in provisions for self-criticism by providing an atmosphere in which uncomfortable questions can be raised; and being forward-thinking. The organization needs to keep foremost what it is going to do, not what it has done.

ORGANIZATIONAL CHANGE ASSOCIATED WITH NONLINEAR DYNAMICS

Most organizations frequently experience stability followed by intense transformation. Some later organizational theorists feel that Lewin's refreezing to establish equilibrium should not be the focus of contemporary organizational change. Ayers (2002) maintains that when change was predictable and rare in the industrial age, Lewin's theory worked well for organizations. However, during the information age of the 21st century, change is unforeseeable and ever present. In the past, organizations have looked at change and organizational dynamics as linear, both occurring in steps and sequential, but some theorists maintain that the world is so unpredictable that the dynamics are nonlinear and do not occur in any order (Wagner and Huber, 2003).

Chaos Theory

Because of the rapidly changing nature of health care and healthcare organizations, long-term outcomes are unpredictable, resulting in the potential for chaos (Thietart & Forgues, 1995). The basic tenets of *chaos theory* are that organizations can no longer rely on rules, policies, and hierarchies, or afford to be inflexible; and that small changes in the initial conditions of a system can drastically affect the long-term behavior of that system (Wagner & Huber, 2003). Organizations are open systems operating in a complex environment that changes rapidly and much of the change is unpredictable. "The richness of the interactions among parts and between the system and its environment allows the system as a whole to undergo spontaneous self-organization" (McDaniel, 1998, p. 356).

System thinking refers to the need for both individuals and organizations to understand how each is an open system with constant input from both visible and invisible interactions. Senge (1990) maintains that the dialogue necessary in system thinking promotes both organizational and individual learning. Organizations that use this learning approach to deal with constant change are often referred to as *learning organizations* (Senge). *Continuous learning* as a concept of organizational philosophy promotes adaptation to change within the organization.

Complex Adaptive Systems Change Theory

Highly unstable environmental conditions require today's organizations to deal with change in a manner that allows for constant fluidity and continuous renewal (Ayers, 2003). A contemporary approach to changing organizations, which is quite different from traditional change, is Olson and Eoyang's (2001) theory of *complex adaptive systems* (CAS). The authors say that the self-organizing nature of human interactions in a complex organization leads to surprising effects. Rather than focusing on the macro level of the organization system, complexity theory suggests that most powerful change processes occur at the micro level where relationships, interactions, and simple rules shape emerging patterns. Olson and Eoyang summarize the main features of the CAS approach to change as follows:

- Change should be achieved through connections between change agents, instead of from the top-down.
- There should be an adaptation during the change to uncertainty instead of trying to predict stages of development.
- Goals, plans, and structures should be allowed to emerge instead of depending on clear, detailed plans and goals.
- Value differences should be amplified instead of focusing on consensus.
- Self-similarity should be created instead of differences between levels of change.
- Success should be regarded as a matter of fit with the organizational environment instead of focusing on one-dimensional success measurement.

IS THE NURSING PROFESSION IN NEED OF RENEWAL?

This is a time of changing nursing practice, a change that often creates crisis when nurses try to defend existing models of practice instead of embracing change.

Learning Exercise 8.5

Young or Old Organization?
Reflect on the organization in which you work or the nursing school you attend. Do you believe this organization has more characteristics of a young or aged organization and do you believe that nonlinear dynamics is at work in the organization? Diagram on a continuum from birth to death where you feel this organization would fall. What efforts has this organization taken to be ever renewing? What further efforts could be made? Do you agree or disagree that most organizations change unpredictably? Can you support your conclusions with examples?

Porter-O'Grady (2003) posits that the profession must examine and adapt to the changing context of nursing practice. The traditional realities are:

- institutional based care
- process oriented
- procedurally driven
- based on mechanical and manual intervention
- provider driven
- treatment based
- late-stage intervention
- based on vertical clinical relationships

According to Porter-O'Grady the emerging realities of nursing practice for this century will be the following:

- mobility based or multisettings
- outcome driven
- best-practice oriented
- technology and minimal-invasive intervention
- user driven
- health based
- early intervention
- based on horizontal clinical relationships

Perhaps there is no greater need for the leader, at this point in the changing profession, than to be the catalyst for change. Many people attracted to the profession now find that their values and traditional expectations no longer fit as they once did. It is the leader's role to help the staff turn around and confront the opportunities and challenges of the realties of emerging nursing practice: to create enthusiasm and passion for renewing the profession; to embrace the change of locus of control, which now belongs to the healthcare consumer; and to engage a new social context for nursing practice.

INTEGRATING LEADERSHIP ROLES AND MANAGEMENT FUNCTIONS IN PLANNED CHANGE

It should be clear that leadership and management skills are necessary for successful planned change to occur. The manager must understand the planning process and planning standards and be able to apply both to the work situation. The manager, then, is the mechanic who implements the planned change.

The leader, however, is the inventor or creator. Leaders today are forced to plan in a chaotic healthcare system that is changing at a frenetic pace. Out of this chaos, leaders must identify trends and changes that may affect their organizations and units and proactively prepare for these changes. Thus, the leader must retain a big-picture focus while dealing with each part of the system. In the inventor or creator role, the leader displays such traits as flexibility, confidence, tenacity, and the ability to articulate vision through insights and versatile thinking.

Both leadership and management skills are necessary in planned change. The change agent fulfills a management function when identifying situations where change is necessary and appropriate and when assessing the driving and restraining forces affecting the plan for change. The leader is the role model in planned change; he or she is open and receptive to change and views change as a challenge and an opportunity for growth. Perhaps the most critical element in successful planned change is the change agent's leadership skills—interpersonal communication, group management, and problem-solving skills.

☀ Key Concepts

- Change should not be viewed as a threat but as a challenge or the chance to do something new and innovative.
- Change should be implemented only for good reason.
- Because change disrupts the homeostasis or balance of the group, resistance should be expected as a natural part of the change process.
- The level of resistance to change generally depends on the type of change proposed. Technological changes encounter less resistance than changes that are perceived as social or that are contrary to established customs or norms.
- Perhaps the greatest factor contributing to the resistance encountered with change is a lack of trust between the employee and the manager or the employee and the organization.
- It is much easier to change a person's behavior than it is to change an entire group's behavior. It also is easier to change knowledge levels than attitudes.
- Change should be planned and thus implemented gradually, not sporadically or suddenly.
- Those who may be affected by a change should be involved in planning for it. Likewise, workers should thoroughly understand the change and its effect on them.
- The feeling of control is critical to thriving in a changing environment.
- Friends, family, and colleagues should be used as a network of support during change.
- The change agent has the leadership skills of problem solving and decision making and has good interpersonal skills.
- In contrast to planned change, *change by drift* is unplanned or accidental.
- Historically, many of the changes that have occurred in nursing or have affected the profession are the results of change by drift.
- People maintain status quo or equilibrium when both *driving* and *restraining* forces operating within any field simultaneously occur. For change to happen, this balance of driving and restraining forces must be altered.
- Organizations are preserved by change and constant renewal. Without change, the organization may stagnate and die.
- Some modern theorists believe that change is unpredictable, occurs at random, and small changes can effect the entire organization.

More Learning Exercises and Applications

Learning Exercise 8.6

Implementing Planned Change in a Family Planning Clinic
You are an Hispanic RN who has recently received a two-year grant to establish a family planning clinic in an impoverished, primarily Hispanic area of a large city. The project will be evaluated at the end of the grant to determine whether continued funding is warranted. As project director, you have the funding to choose and hire three healthcare workers. You will essentially be able to manage the clinic as you see fit.

The average age of your patients will be 14 years, and many come from single-parent homes. In addition, the population with which you will be working has high unemployment, high crime and truancy levels, and great suspicion and mistrust of authority figures. You are aware that many restraining forces exist that will challenge you, but you feel strongly committed to the cause. You believe that the exorbitantly high teenage pregnancy rate and maternal and infant morbidity can be reduced.

Assignment:
1. Identify the restraining and driving forces in this situation.
2. Identify realistic short- and long-term goals for implementing such a change. What can realistically be accomplished in two years?
3. How might the project director use hiring authority to increase the driving forces in this situation?
4. Is refreezing of the planned change possible so that changes will continue if the grant is not funded again in 2 years?

Learning Exercise 8.7

Retain the Status Quo or Implement Change?
Assume that morale and productivity are low on the unit where you are the new manager. In an effort to identify the root of the problem, you have been meeting informally with staff to discuss their perceptions of unit functioning and to identify sources of unrest on the unit. You believe that one of the greatest factors leading to unrest is the limited advancement opportunity for your staff nurses. You have a fixed charge nurse on each shift. This is how the unit has been managed for as long as everyone can remember. You would like to rotate the charge nurse position but are unsure of your staff's feelings about the change.

Assignment: Using the phases of change identified by Lewin, identify the actions you could take in unfreezing, movement, and refreezing. What are the greatest barriers to this change? What are the strongest driving forces?

Learning Exercise 8.8

How Would You Handle This Response to Change?
You are the unit manager of a cardiovascular surgical unit. The work station on the unit is small, dated, and disorganized. The unit clerks have complained for some time that the chart racks on the counter above their desk are difficult to reach, that staff frequently impinge on their work space to discuss patients or to chart, that the call-light system is antiquated, and that supplies and forms need to be relocated. You ask all eight of your shift unit clerks to make a "wish list" of how they would like the work station to be redesigned for optimum efficiency and effectiveness.

Construction is completed several months later. You are pleased that the new work station incorporates what each unit clerk included in his or her top three priorities for change. There is a new revolving chart rack in the center of the work station, with enhanced accessibility to both staff and unit clerks. A new state-of-the-art call-light system has been installed. A small, quiet room has been created for nurses to chart and conference, and new cubbyholes and filing drawers now put forms within arm's reach of the charge nurse and unit clerk.

Almost immediately, you begin to be barraged with complaints about the changes. Several of the unit clerks find the new call-light system's computerized response system overwhelming and complain that patient lights are now going unanswered. Others complain that with the chart rack out of their immediate work area, charts can no longer be monitored and are being removed from the unit by physicians or left in the charting room by nurses. One unit clerk has filed a complaint that she was injured by a staff member who carelessly and rapidly turned the chart rack. She refuses to work again until the old chart racks are returned. The regular day-shift unit clerk complains that all the forms are filed backward for left-handed people and that after 20 years, she should have the right to put them the way she likes it. Several of the nurses are complaining that the work station is "now the domain of the unit clerk" and that access to the telephones and desk supplies is limited by the unit clerks. There have been some rumblings that several staff members believe that you favored the requests of some employees over others.

Today, when you make rounds at change of shift, you find the day-shift unit clerk and charge nurse involved in a heated conversation with the evening-shift unit clerk and charge nurse. Each evening, the charge nurse and unit clerk reorganize the work station in the manner that they believe is most effective, and each morning, the charge nurse and unit clerk put things back the way they had been the prior day. Both believe that the other shift is undermining their efforts to "fix" the work station organization and that their method of organization is the best. Both groups of workers turn to you and demand that you "make the other shift stop sabotaging our efforts to change things for the better."

Assignment: Despite your intent to include subordinate input into this planned change, resistance is high and worker morale is plummeting. Is the level of resistance a normal and anticipated response to planned change? If so, would you intervene in this conflict? How? Was it possible to have reduced the likelihood of such a high degree of resistance?

Learning Exercise 8.9

Old and New Roles of Nursing Practice
Examine the old and new realities of nursing practice as identified on p.184.
Assignment: In a small group discuss the old and new roles of nursing practice. In your observations, based on your nursing school clinical experiences, theory based classes, and watching other nurses in their roles, what type of nursing practice do you see being practiced? Give specific examples. Are the practice models in evidence provider driven or user driven? Is the nursing practice process oriented or outcome driven? As an organization do you believe nursing would be classified as a) an aging organization, b) in constant motion and ever renewing, or c) a closed system that does not respond well to change?

Web Links

Orlikowski, W. J., & Hofman, D. An Improvisational Model of Change Management
http://ccs.mit.edu/papers/CCSWP191/CCSWP191.html
The Case of Groupware Technologies: Massachusetts Institute of Technology, Sloan School of Management. Examines a dynamic and variable "improvisational" approach to technological change in which the major steps of change are defined in advance and the organization then strives to implement these changes in a specified period of time.

Kurt Lewin
http://muskingum.edu/%7Epsychology/psycweb/history/lewin.htm
Biography, overview of planned change theory, timeline of his theoretical developments, and bibliography.

Kurt Lewin Institute homepage
http://www.psy.vu.nl/kli
Describes the institute's mission, training program, and current research.

References

Ayers, D. F. (2002). Developing climates for renewal in the community college: A case study of dissipative self-organization. *Community College Journal of research and practice, 26*, 165–185.
Bednash, G. (2003). Leadership redefined. *Policy, Politics, & Nursing Practice, 4*(4), 257–258.
Bennis, W., Benne, K., & Chinn, R. (1969). *The planning of change* (2nd ed.). New York: Holt, Rinehart, & Winston.

Bushy, A., & Kamphuis, J. (1993). Response to innovation: Behavioral patterns. *Nursing Management, 24*(3), 62–64.

Dye, C. F. (2000). *Leadership in healthcare. Values at the top*. Chicago: Health Administration Press.

Gardner, J. W. (1990). *On leadership*. New York: The Free Press.

Heifetz, R. & Laurie, D. (2001). The work of leadership. *Harvard Business Review, 79*, (11), 121–130.

Knox, S., & Irving, J. A. (1997). Nurse manager perceptions of healthcare executive behaviors during organizational change. *Journal of Nursing Administration, 27*(11), 33–39.

Lewin, K. (1951). *Field theory in social sciences*. New York: Harper & Row.

Lewis, L. K. (1999). Disseminating information and soliciting input during planned organizational change. *Management Communication Quarterly, 13*(1), 43.

Lippitt, R., Watson, J., & Westley, B. (1958). *The dynamics of planned change*. New York: Harcourt, Brace & World.

McDaniel, R. R. (1998). Strategic leadership: A view from quantum and chaos theories. In W. J. Duncan, P. Ginter & L. Swayne (Eds.). *Handbook of health care management*. Oxford, England: Basil Blackwell Publishing.

Murphy, S. (1999). Mindshift for managers: Change is inevitable, growth is optional. *Home Health Care Management and Practice, 11*(2), 6–14.

Olson, E. E., & Eoyang, G. H. (2001*). Facilitating Organization Change: Lessons from Complexity Science*. San Francisco: Jossey-Bass/Pfeiffer.

Perlman, D., & Takacs, G. J. (1990). The ten stages of change. *Nursing Management, 21*(4), 33–38.

Pesut, D. (2000). Crusaders and tradition bearers. *Nursing Outlook, 48*(6), 262.

Porter-O'Grady, T. (2003). A different age for leadership part 2: New rules, new roles. *Journal of Nursing Administration, 33*(3), 173–178.

Quinn, R. E., Spreitzer, G. M., & Brown, M. V. (June 2000). Changing others through changing ourselves. *Journal of Management Inquiry, 9*(2), 147–165.

Scobie, K. B. & Russell, G. (2003). Vision 2020, Part I: Profile of the future nurse leader. *Journal of Nursing Administration, 33*(6), 324–330.

Senge, P. M. (1990). *The Fifth Discipline*. New York: Doubleday.

Thietart, R. A., & Forgues, B. (1995). Chaos theory organization. *Organization Science,* 6(1), 19–31.

Trent, B. A. (2003). Leadership myths. *Reflections on Nursing Leadership, 29*(3), 8–9.

Wagner, C. M., & Huber, D. L. (2003). Catastrophe and nursing turnover: Nonlinear models. *Journal of Nursing Administration, 33*(9), 486–492.

Bibliography

Bozak, M. G. (2003). Using Lewin's force field analysis in implementing a nursing information system. *Computers, Informatics, Nursing, 21*(2), 80–87.

Hallowell, B. (2003). Leadership and management. Tips on transforming an organization. *Healthcare Financial Management, 57*(8), 64–65.

Hill, J. E. (2003). New directions in nursing management. *Journal of Nursing Management,* 11(1), 4–5.

Hilz, L. M. (2000). The informatics nurse specialist as change agent: Application of innovation-diffusion theory. *Computers in Nursing, 18*(6), 272–281.

Jost, S. G. (2000). An assessment and intervention strategy for managing staff needs during change. *Journal of Nursing Administration, 30*(1), 34–40.

Lam, S. S. K., & Schaubroeck, J. (2000). A field experiment testing front-line opinion leaders as change agents. *Journal of Applied Psychology, 85*(6), 987.

McCarthy, A., Hegney, D., & Pearson, A. (2000). The perceptions of rural nurses towards role change within the context of organizational change. *Australian Journal of Advanced Nursing, 17*(4), 21–28.

Mee, C. L. (2003). Research, change, and reap the rewards. *Nursing, 33*(11), 6.

Navarra, T. (March 6, 2000). Perspectives in leadership. A recipe for becoming a change agent. *Nursing Spectrum* (New York/New Jersey Metro Edition), 12A(5), 6–7.

Parse, R. R. (2003). Reflections on change. *Illuminations, 11*(3/4), 1.

Sproat, S. B. (2003). Using organizational artifacts to influence change. *Journal of Nursing Administration, 31*(11), 524–526.

Szarmach, R. (2000). President's message: Are you a change agent for the future? *Surgical Technologist, 32*(8), 3.

Time Management

The "too much to do and not enough time to do it" phenomenon is rampant.

—Polly Gerber Zimmermann

Another part of the planning process is *short-term planning*. This operational planning focuses on achieving specific tasks. Short-term plans involve a period of one hour to three years and are usually less complex than strategic or long-range plans. Short-term planning may be done annually, bimonthly, weekly, daily, or even hourly.

Previous chapters examined the need for prudent planning of resources, such as money, equipment, supplies, and labor. Time is an equally important resource. If managers are to direct employees effectively and maximize other resources, they must first be able to find the time to do so. *Time management* is making optimal use of available time. Because time is a finite and valuable resource, learning to use it wisely requires both leadership skills and management functions. The leader–manager must initiate an analysis of how time is managed on the unit level, involve team members and gain their cooperation in maximizing time use, and guide work to its conclusion and successful implementation.

There is a close relationship between time management and stress. Managing time appropriately is one method to reduce stress and increase productivity. The current status of health care, both the nursing shortage and decrease in funding, has resulted in many healthcare organizations trying to do more with less. The effective use of time

---

Display 9.1   Leadership Roles and Management Functions in Time Management

Leadership Roles

1. Is self-aware regarding personal blocks and barriers to efficient time management as well as how one's own value system influences one's own use of time and the expectations of followers.
2. Functions as a role model, supporter, and resource person to subordinates in setting priorities.
3. Assists followers in working cooperatively to maximize time use.
4. Prevents and/or filters interruptions that prevent effective time management.
5. Role models flexibility in working cooperatively with other people whose primary time management style is different.
6. Presents a calm and reassuring demeanor during periods of high unit activity.

Management Functions

1. Appropriately prioritizes day-to-day planning to meet short-term and long-term unit goals.
2. Builds time for planning into the work schedule.
3. Analyzes how time is managed on the unit level using job analysis and time-and-motion studies.
4. Eliminates environmental barriers to effective time management for unit staff.
5. Handles paperwork promptly and efficiently and maintains a neat work area.
6. Breaks down large tasks into smaller ones that can more easily be accomplished by unit members.
7. Utilizes appropriate technology to facilitate timely communication and documentation.
8. Discriminates between inadequate staffing and inefficient use of time when time resources are inadequate to complete assigned tasks.

management tools therefore, becomes even more important to enable managers to meet personal and professional goals. Good time management skills allow an individual to spend time on things that matter. Leadership roles and management functions needed for effective time management are included in **Display 9.1.**

THREE BASIC STEPS IN TIME MANAGEMENT

There are three basic steps to time management (**Figure 9.1**). The first step requires that time be set aside for planning and establishing priorities. The second step entails completing the highest-priority task (as determined in step 1) whenever possible and finishing one task before beginning another. In the final step, the person must reprioritize the tasks to be accomplished based on new information received. Because this is a cyclic process, all three steps must be accomplished sequentially.

Unfortunately, two mistakes common to novice managers are underestimating the importance of a daily plan and not allowing adequate time for planning. Daily planning is essential if the manager is to manage by efficiency rather than by crisis. The old adage "fail to plan—plan to fail" is timeless. Managers may believe they are unproductive if they sit at their desk designing the plan of care for the day, rather than accomplishing a specific task. Without adequate planning, however, the manager finds getting started difficult and begins to manage by crisis. In addition, there

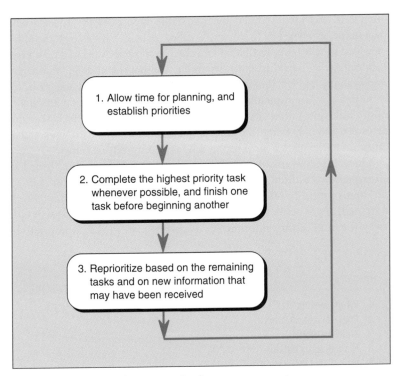

Figure 9.1 The three basic steps in time management.

can be no sense of achievement at day's end if the goals for the day have not been clearly delineated.

Planning takes time; it requires the ability to think, analyze data, envision alternatives, and make decisions. Setting aside time at the beginning of each day to plan the day allows the manager to spend time on high-priority tasks. During this planning time, the manager should review short-term, intermediate, and long-term goals and determine what progress will be made toward these goals. Sometimes the manager does allow time for planning but has problems accurately predicting the length of time it will take to complete an activity.

Priority Setting and Procrastination

Because managers are inundated with many requests for their time and energy, the next step in time management is prioritizing. Priority setting is perhaps the most critical skill in good time management, because all actions we take have some type of relative importance.

Vacarro (2001) suggests there are five priority-setting traps. The first is "whatever hits first." This trap occurs when an individual simply responds to things as they happen rather than thinking first and then acting. The second trap is the "path of least resistance." In this trap, the individual makes an erroneous assumption that it is always easier to do a task personally and fails to delegate appropriately. The third trap is the "squeaky wheel." In this trap, the individual falls prey to those who are most vocal about their urgent requests. Compounding the trap is that the individual often feels a need to respond to the time frame imposed by the "squeaky wheel," rather than his or her own. The fourth trap is called "default." In this trap, the individual feels obligated to take on tasks that no one else has come forward to do. To keep this from happening, the individual must determine whether the undone job is truly his or her responsibility and whether it serves to accomplish his or her stated goals. The last trap is "inspiration." In inspiration, individuals wait until they become "inspired" to accomplish a task. Some necessary tasks will never be inspiring, and the wise manager recognizes that the only thing that will complete these tasks is hard work and appropriate attention to the matter (see **Display 9.2** for priority-setting traps).

One simple means of prioritizing what needs to be accomplished is to divide all requests into three categories: "don't do," "do later," and "do now." The "don't do" items probably reflect problems that will take care of themselves, are already outdated, or are better accomplished by someone else. The manager either throws away the unnecessary information or passes it on to the appropriate person in a

Display 9.2	**Five Priority-Setting Traps**

1. Whatever hits first
2. Path of least resistance
3. Squeaky wheel
4. Managing by default
5. Waiting for inspiration

timely fashion. In either case, the manager removes unneeded clutter from his or her work area.

Some "do later" items reflect trivial problems or those that do not have immediate deadlines; thus, they may be procrastinated. *Procrastination* means to put off something until a future time, to postpone, or to delay needlessly. Bakunas (2001) states that procrastination is a major problem that can shrink productivity, undermine self-esteem, and affect a career. It is also a difficult problem to solve because it rarely results from a single cause and can involve a combination of dysfunctional attitudes, rationalizations, and resentment. Indeed, Bakunas maintains that the major causes of procrastination are performance anxiety, low frustration tolerance, resentment of working conditions, escapism, over-preparation, overworking, poor working conditions, over-commitment, and rationalizing.

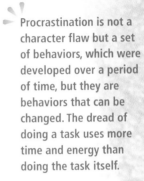

Procrastination **is not a** character flaw **but a set** of behaviors, **which were** developed over **a period** of time, **but they are** behaviors that **can be** changed. The dread of doing a task uses **more** time and energy **than** doing the task itself.

Learning Exercise 9.1

Targeting Personal Procrastination
Spend a few moments reflecting on the last two weeks of your life. What are the things that you put off doing? Do these things form a pattern? For instance, do you always put off writing a school paper until the last minute? Do you wait to do certain tasks at work until you cannot avoid the task any longer?
Assignment: Write a one-page essay on at least two things that you procrastinate and then develop two strategies for breaking each of these habits.

Although managers should selectively procrastinate, they should not avoid a task because it is overwhelming or unpleasant. Before setting "do later" items aside, the manager must be sure that large projects have been broken down into smaller projects and that a specific time line and plan for implementation are in place. The plan should include short-term, intermediate, and final deadlines. Likewise, a manager cannot ignore items without immediate time limits forever and must make a definite time commitment in the near future to address these requests.

The "do now" requests most commonly reflect a unit's day-to-day operational needs. These requests may include daily staffing needs, dealing with equipment shortages, meeting schedules, conducting hiring interviews, and giving performance appraisals. "Do now" requests also may represent items that had been put off earlier.

In prioritizing all the "do now" items, the manager may find preparing a written list helpful. Remember, however, that a list is a plan, not a product and that the creation of the list is not the final goal. The list is a planning tool. Although the manager may use monthly or weekly lists, a list also can assist in coordinating daily operations. This daily list, however, should not be longer than what can be realistically accomplished in one day; otherwise, it demotivates instead of assisting the manager. In addition, although the manager must be cognizant of and plan for routine tasks, it is not always necessary to place them on the list because they may only distract attention from other priority tasks. Lists should allow adequate time for each task and have blocks of time built in for the unexpected.

Learning Exercise 9.2

Creating Planning Lists
Do you make a daily plan to organize what needs to be done? Mentally or on paper, develop a list of five items that must be accomplished today. Prioritize that list. Now make a list of five items that must be done this week. Prioritize that list also.

Periodically, the manager should review lists from prior days to see what was not accomplished or completed. If a task appears on a list for several successive days, the manager must reexamine it and assess why it was not accomplished. Some projects need to be removed from the list. A project may not be accomplished because it was not broken down into manageable tasks. For example, many well-meaning people begin thinking about completing their tax returns in early January but feel overwhelmed by a project that cannot be accomplished in one day. If preparing a tax return is not broken down into several smaller tasks with intermediate deadlines, it may be almost perpetually procrastinated.

Learning Exercise 9.3

Making Big Projects Manageable
Masikiewicz (2000) states that the best way to get big projects done is to break them down, with mini-deadlines that you set yourself. Think of the last major paper you wrote for a class. Did you set short-term and intermediate deadlines? Did you break the task down into smaller tasks to eliminate a last-minute crisis? What short-term and intermediate deadlines have you set to accomplish major projects that have been assigned to you this quarter or semester?

The manager must remember that because the list is a planning tool, there must be some flexibility in its implementation. In fact, the last step in time management is reprioritizing. Often the manager's priorities or list will change during a day, week, or longer because new information is received. If the manager does not take time to reprioritize after each major task is accomplished, other priorities set earlier may no longer be accurate.

In addition, no amount of planning can prevent an occasional crisis. If a crisis does occur, the individual may need to set aside the original priorities for the day and reorganize, communicate, and delegate a new plan reflecting the new priorities associated with the unexpected event causing the crisis.

MANAGING TIME AT WORK

Being overwhelmed by work and time constraints leads to increased errors, the omission of important tasks, and general feelings of stress and ineffectiveness. Although some people seem to be "naturals" with time management, the skill is learned and improves with practice.

All workers need to allow time for daily planning to appropriately manage time at work. Examples of the types of plans a charge nurse might make in day-to-day planning include staffing schedules, patient care assignments, coordination of lunch and work break schedules, and interdisciplinary coordination of patient care. Examples of an acute care staff nurse's day-to-day planning might include determining how reports will be given and received; the timing and method used for initial patient assessments; the coordination of medication administration, treatments, and procedures; and the organization of documentation of the day's activities.

Some staff nurses appear disorganized in their efforts to care for patients. Usually, this disorganization results from poor planning. Planning occurs first in the management process because the ability to be organized develops from good planning. During planning, there should be time to think about how plans will be translated into action. The planner must pause and decide how people, activities, and materials are going to be put together to carry out the objectives. The following suggestions using industrial engineering principles may assist the staff nurse in planning work activities:

- Gather all the supplies and equipment that will be needed before starting an activity. Breaking a job down mentally into parts before beginning the activity may help the staff nurse identify what supplies and equipment will be needed to complete the activity.
- Group activities that are in the same location. If you have walked a long distance down a hallway, attempt to do several things there before going back to the nurses' station. If you are a home health nurse, group patient visits geographically when possible to minimize travel time and maximize time with patients.
- Use time estimates. For example, if you know an intermittent intravenous medication (IV piggyback) will take 30 minutes to complete, then use that time estimate for planning some other activity that can be completed in that 30-minute window of time.
- Document your nursing interventions as soon as possible after an activity is completed. Waiting until the end of the workday to complete necessary documentation increases the risk of inaccuracies and incomplete documentation.
- Always strive to end the workday on time. Although this is not always possible, delegating appropriately to others and making sure that the workload goal for any given day is reasonable are two strategies that will accomplish this goal.

Like staff nurses, unit managers need to coordinate how their duties will be carried out and devise methods to make work simpler and more efficient. Often this includes simple tasks, such as organizing how supplies are stored or determining the most efficient lunch and break schedules for staff. The goal in planning work and activities is to facilitate greater productivity and satisfaction. Daily planning

Learning Exercise 9.4

Setting Daily Priorities

Assume that you are the RN leader of a team with one LVN and one nursing assistant on the 7 AM to 3 PM shift at an acute care hospital. The three of you are responsible for providing total care to 10 patients. Prioritize the following list of 10 things you need to accomplish this morning. Use a 1 for the first thing you will do and a 10 for the last. Be prepared to provide rationale for your priorities.

___Check medication cards/sheets against the rand or kardex

___Listen to night shift report 0700–0720

___Take brief walking rounds to assess the night shift report and to introduce yourself to patients

___Hang four 0900 IV medications

___Set up the schedule for breaks and lunch among your team members

___Give 0845 preop on patient going to surgery at 0900

___Pass 0830 breakfast trays

___Meet with team members to plan schedule for the day and to clarify roles

___Read charts of patients who are new to you

___Check 0600 blood sugar lab results for 0730 insulin administration

---

actions that may help the unit manager identify and utilize time as a resource most efficiently might include:

- At the start of each workday, identify key priorities to be accomplished that day. Identify what specific actions need to be taken to accomplish those priorities and in what order they should be done. Also identify specific actions that should be taken to meet ongoing, long-term goals.
- Determine the level of achievement you expect for each prioritized task. Is a maximizing or "satisficing" approach more appropriate or more reasonable for each of the goals you have identified?
- Assess the staff assigned to work with you. Assign work that must be delegated to staff members who are both capable and willing to accomplish the priority task you have identified. Be sure you have clearly expressed any expectations you may have about how and when a delegated task must be completed. (Delegation will be discussed further in Chapter 20.)
- Review the short- and long-term plans of the unit regularly. Include colleagues and subordinates in identifying unit problems or concerns so they can be fully involved in planning for needed change.
- Plan ahead for meetings. Prepare and distribute agendas in advance.
- Allow time at several points throughout the day and at the end of the day to assess progress in meeting established daily goals and to determine if unanticipated events have occurred or if new information has been received that may have altered your original plan. Setting new priorities or adjusting priorities to reflect ever-changing work situations is an ongoing reality for the unit manager.

Taking Breaks

Taking regularly scheduled breaks from work is important as breaks allow the worker to refresh both physically and mentally. Planning for periodic breaks from work during the workday is an integral part of an individual's time and task management. In Strongman and Burt's (2000) studies of students, hunger/thirst, boredom, feeling tired, lack of concentration, and mental exhaustion were identified most commonly as the reasons given for taking breaks. Many more reasons were given for taking breaks from mental tasks than from physical tasks, and participants believed that breaks should be taken sooner and more often from mental work than from physical work. Interestingly, those students who took shorter breaks, more often, tended to perform at higher levels. Clearly, the working nurse who often faces both physical and mental stress in the workplace must factor time for breaks into his or her daily plan.

Kriegel (2002) says that when individuals are overworked, they must recognize that longer hours on the job do not necessarily produce the desired outcomes. Most people's knee-jerk response to pressure is to run harder and faster but Kriegel maintains that working longer at a rushed pace not only increases the potential for stress and burnout but also results in more mistakes. Taking a 15-minute daily time out to think creatively about how to achieve work objectives is recommended.

> A passionate 90% of work effort is more effective than a panicked 110%. —*R. Kriegel.*

Dealing with Interruptions

All managers experience interruptions. Lower-level managers experience more interruptions than higher-level managers. This occurs in part because first- and middle-level managers are more involved in daily planning than higher-level managers and thus directly interact with a greater number of subordinates. In addition, many lower-level managers do not have a quiet workspace or clerical help to filter interruptions. Frequent work interruptions result in situational stress and lowered job satisfaction. Managers need to develop skill in preventing interruptions that prevent effective time management.

Lancaster (1984) identified 10 external time-wasters that keep managers from accomplishing their "do now" and "do later" lists. These external time-wasters are listed in **Display 9.3.** Several of these items are discussed in previous chapters; others are discussed in later chapters.

Time Wasters

Three time-wasters warrant special attention here. The first of the three is socializing. Although socializing can help workers meet relationship needs or build power, it can tremendously deter productivity. People can be discouraged from taking up a manager's time with idle chatter in several ways.

1. Don't make yourself overly accessible. Make it easy for people to ignore you. Try not to "work" at the nursing station if this is possible. If charting is to be done, sit with your back to others. If you have an office, close the door. Have people make appointments to see you. All these behaviors will discourage casual socializers.

Display 9.3	**External Time-Wasters**

1. Telephone interruptions
2. Socializing
3. Meetings
4. Lack of information
5. Poor communication
6. Lack of feedback
7. Lack of adequately described policies and procedures
8. Incompetent coworkers
9. Poor filing system
10. Paperwork and reading

Lancaster, J. (1984). Making the most of every minute: Reminders for nursing leaders. In M. S. Berger, D. Elhart, S. Firsich, S. Jordan, & S. Stone (Eds.), *Management for nurses.* St. Louis: C. V. Mosby.

2. Interrupt. When someone is rambling on without getting to the point, break in and say gently, "Excuse me. Somehow I'm not getting your message. What exactly are you saying?"
3. Avoid promoting socialization. Having several comfortable chairs in your office, a full candy dish, and posters on your walls that invite comments encourage socializing in your office.
4. Be brief. Watch your own long-winded comments, and stand up when you are finished. This will signal an end to the conversation.
5. Schedule long-winded pests. If someone has a pattern of lengthy chatter and manages to corner you on rounds or at the nurse's station, say, "I can't speak with you now, but I'm going to have some free time at 11 AM. Why don't you see me then?" Unless the meeting is important, the person who just wishes to chat will not bother to make a formal appointment.
6. If you would like to chat and have the time to do so, use coffee breaks and lunch hours for socializing.

The other external time-wasters that a manager must conquer are paperwork overload and a poor filing system. Managers are generally inundated with paper clutter, including organizational memos, staffing requests, quality assurance reports, incident reports, and patient evaluations. Because paperwork is often redundant or unnecessary, the manager needs to become an expert at handling it. Whenever possible, incoming correspondence should be handled the day it arrives; it should either be thrown away or filed according to the date to be completed. Try to address each piece of correspondence only once.

An adequate filing system also is invaluable to handling paper overload. Keeping correspondence organized in easily retrievable files rather than disorganized stacks saves time when the manager needs to find specific information. The manager also may want to consider increased use of computerization and electronic mail to reduce the paper use and to increase response time in time-sensitive communication.

Personal Time Management

Personal time management refers in part to the knowing of self. Self-awareness is a leadership skill. Managing time is difficult if a person is unsure of his or her priorities for time management, including personal short-term, intermediate, and long-term goals. These goals give structure to what should be accomplished today, tomorrow, and in the future. However, goals alone are not enough; a concrete plan with time lines is needed. Plans outlined in manageable steps are clearer, more realistic, and attainable. By being self-aware and setting goals accordingly, people determine how their time will be spent. If goals are not set, others often end up deciding how a person should spend his or her time.

Think for a moment about last week. Did you accomplish all you wanted to accomplish? How much time did you or others waste? In your clinical practice, did you spend your time hunting for supplies and medicines instead of teaching your patient about his or her diabetes? Morgenstern (2000) maintains that we should first analyze our work and time management efforts and then develop strategies that attack our problems because we each waste time differently.

Too often, irrelevant decisions and insignificant activities take priority over real purposes. Clearly, work redesign, clarification of job descriptions, or a change in the type of care delivery system may alleviate some of these problems. However, the same general principle holds: Professional nurses who are self-aware and have clearly identified personal goals and priorities have greater control over how they expend their energy and what they accomplish.

Hansten and Washburn (1998) suggest that there are three primary areas of practice that consume the time of the professional registered nurse: professional, technical, and amenity care. Professional practice refers to implementation of the nursing process—the ability to make assessments, plan care, effectively coordinate the efforts of the healthcare team, and evaluate their effect. Technical practice includes technical or psychomotor tasks such as venous cannulation, catheterizations, and injections. Amenity care is more service-oriented, such as focusing on customer satisfaction by ensuring appetizing meals, aesthetic environmental surroundings, and friendliness of the staff. Although all three areas of practice are important, the professional role must be valued more highly and time allocated accordingly in determining work priorities. Hansten and Washburn (1998) suggest that "by realizing your part in the determination of what needs to be done, you are allowing yourself the time to practice the professional component of nursing—the implementation of the nursing process" (p. 185). The extensive knowledge and judgment of the registered nurse are key ingredients to planning and delivering quality nursing care.

Monochronic and Polychronic Time Management Styles

In addition to being self-aware regarding the values that influence how people prioritize the use of their time, people must be self-aware regarding their general tendency to complete tasks in isolation or in combination. Davidhizar, Giger, and Turner (1994) suggest that most people have tendencies toward either a monochronic or

Learning Exercise 9.5

A Busy Day at the Public Health Agency

You work in a public health agency. It is the agency's policy that at least one public health nurse is available in the office every day. Today is your turn to remain in the office. From 1 PM to 5 PM, you will be the public health nurse at the scheduled immunization clinic; you hope to be able to spend some time finishing your end-of-month reports, which are due at 5 PM. The office stays open during lunch; you have a luncheon meeting with a Cancer Society group from noon to 1 PM today. The RN in the office is to serve as a resource to the receptionist and handle patient phone calls and drop-ins. In addition to the receptionist, you may delegate appropriately to a clerical worker. However, the clerical worker also serves the other clinic nurses and is usually fairly busy. While you are in the office today trying to finish your reports, the following interruptions occur:

8:30 AM: Your supervisor, Anne, comes in and requests a count of the diabetic and hypertensive patients seen in the last month.

9:00 AM: An upset patient is waiting to see you about her daughter who just found out she is pregnant.

9:00 AM: Three drop-in patients are waiting to be interviewed for possible referral to the chest clinic.

9:30 AM: The public health physician calls you and needs someone to contact a family about a child's immunization.

9:30 AM: The dental department drops off 20 referrals and needs you to pull charts of these patients.

10:00 AM: A confused patient calls to find out what to do about the bills he has received.

10:45 AM: Six families have been waiting since 8:30 AM to sign up for food vouchers.

11:45 AM: A patient calls about her drug use; she doesn't know what to do. She has heard about Narcotics Anonymous and wants more information now.

Assignment: How would you handle each interruption? Justify your decisions. Don't forget lunch for yourself and the two office workers.

Note: Attempt your own solution before reading the possible solution presented in the back of this book.

polychronic time management style. People with a *monochronic style* prefer to do one thing at a time, whereas people with the *polychronic style* typically do two or more things simultaneously. Monochronic people tend to begin and finish projects on time, have clean and organized desks as a result of handling each piece of paperwork only once, and are highly structured. Polychronic people tend to change plans, borrow and lend things frequently, emphasize relationships rather than tasks, and build longer-term relationships.

It is important to recognize one's own preferred time management style and to be self-aware about how this orientation may affect your interaction with others in the

Learning Exercise 9.6

Realistic Prioritizing

You are an RN providing total patient care to four patients on an orthopedic unit during the 7 AM to 3 PM shift. Given the following patient information, prioritize your activities for the shift in eight one-hour blocks of time. Be sure to include time for reports, planning your day's activities, breaks, and lunch. Be realistic about what you can accomplish. What activities will you delegate to the next shift? What overall goals have guided your time management? What personal values or priorities were factors in setting your goals?

101A—Ms. Jones, 84 years old. Fractured left hip secondary to fall at home. Disoriented since admission, especially at night. Soft restraints in use. Moans frequently. Being given IV pain medication every 2 hours prn. Vital signs and checks for circulation, feeling, and movement in toes ordered every 2 hours. Scheduled for surgery at 1030. Preoperative medications scheduled for 0930 and 1000. Consent yet to be signed. Family members will be here at 0800 and have expressed questions about the surgery and recovery period. Patient to return from surgery at approximately 1430. Will require postoperative vital signs every 15 minutes.

101B—Ms. Wilkins, 26 years old. Compound fracture of the femur with postoperative fat emboli, now resolved. 10-lb Buck's traction. Has been in the hospital three weeks. Very bored and frustrated with prolonged hospitalization. Upset about roommate who calls out all night and keeps her from sleeping. Wants to be moved to new room. Has also requested to have hair washed during bath today. Has IV running at 100 cc/h. IV antibiotic piggybacks at 0800 and 1200. Oral medications at 0800, 0900, and 1200.

102A—Mr. Jenkins, 47 years old. T-6 quadriplegic due to diving accident 14 years ago. Two days postoperative above-knee amputation due to osteomyelitis. Cultures show methicillin-resistant Staphylococcus aureus. Strict wound isolation. Has been hospitalized for two weeks. Expressing great deal of anger and frustration to anyone who enters room. IV site red and puffy. IV needs to be restarted. Dressing change of operative site ordered daily. Heat lamp treatments ordered b.i.d. to small pressure sores on coccyx. IV antibiotic piggybacks at 0800, 1000, 1200, and 1400. Main IV bag to run out at 1000. 0600 lab work results to be called to physician this morning. Needs total assistance in performing activities of daily living, such as bathing and feeding self.

103A—Mr. Novak, 19 years old. Severe tear of rotator cuff in left shoulder while playing football. One day postoperative rotator cuff repair. Very quiet and withdrawn. Refusing pain medication, which has been ordered every two hours prn. Says he can handle pain and does not want to "mess up his body with drugs." He wants to be recruited into professional football after this semester. Nonverbal signs of grimacing, moaning, and inability to sleep suggest moderate pain is present. Physician states that likelihood of Mr. Novak ever playing football again is very low but has not yet told patient. Girlfriend frequently in room at patient's bedside. IV infusing at 150 cc/h. IV antibiotics at 0800 and 1400. Has not had a bath since admission two days ago.

workplace. For example, an agency manager with a polychronic time management style may become frustrated and irritable when assigned to work with a department secretary with more monochronic tendencies. Both people risk frustration and conflict if they are unable to allow their coworker some discretion in how assigned work will be accomplished.

Personal Time-Wasters

A significant part of personal time management depends on self-awareness about how and when a person is most productive. Everyone avoids certain types of work or has methods of wasting time. Likewise, each person works better at certain times of the day or for certain lengths of time. Self-aware people schedule complex or difficult tasks during the periods when they are most productive and simpler or routine tasks during less productive times. Other personal or internal time-wasters are shown in **Display 9.4.**

Using a Time Inventory

Because most people have an inaccurate perception of the time they spend on a particular task or the total amount of time they are productive during the day, a *time inventory* may provide insight. A time inventory is shown in **Display 9.5.**

Because the greatest benefit from a time inventory is being able to objectively identify patterns of behavior, it may be necessary to maintain the time inventory for several days or even several weeks. It also may be helpful to repeat the time inventory annually to see if long-term behavior changes have been noted. Remember, there is no way to beg, borrow, or steal more hours in the day. If time is habitually used ineffectively, being a manager will be very stressful.

> The time we have is all the time available to us. Therefore, time often becomes our one real barrier because most other things are flexible.

Display 9.4	Internal Time-Wasters

1. Procrastination
2. Poor planning
3. Failure to establish goals and objectives
4. Failure to set objectives
5. Inability to delegate
6. Inability to say no
7. Management by crisis
8. Haste
9. Indecisiveness
10. Open-door policy

Display 9.5	Time Inventory

5:00 AM _____
6:00 AM _____
6:30 AM _____
7:00 AM _____
7:30 AM _____
8:00 AM _____
8:30 AM _____
9:00 AM _____
9:30 AM _____
10:00 AM _____
10:30 AM _____
11:00 AM _____
11:30 AM _____
12:00 PM _____
12:30 PM _____
1:00 PM _____
1:30 PM _____
2:00 PM _____
2:30 PM _____
3:00 PM _____
3:30 PM _____
4:00 PM _____
4:30 PM _____
5:00 PM _____
5:30 PM _____
6:00 PM _____
6:30 PM _____
7:00 PM _____
7:30 PM _____
8:00 PM _____
8:30 PM _____
9:00 PM _____
9:30 PM _____
10:00 PM _____
11:00 PM _____
12:00 PM _____
1:00 AM _____
2:00 AM _____
3:00 AM _____
4:00 AM _____

Learning Exercise 9.7

Writing a Personal Time Inventory
Use the time inventory shown in Display 9.5 to identify your activities for a 24-hour period. Record your activities on the time inventory on a regular basis. Be specific. Do not trust your memory. Star the periods of time when you were most productive. Circle periods of time you were least productive. Do not include sleep time. Was this a typical day for you? Could you have modified your activity during your least productive time periods? If so, how?

 ## INTEGRATING LEADERSHIP ROLES AND MANAGEMENT FUNCTIONS IN TIME MANAGEMENT

The leadership skills needed to manage time resources draw heavily on interpersonal communication skills. The leader is a resource and role model to subordinates in how to manage time. As has been stressed in other phases of the management process, the leadership skill of self-awareness also is necessary in time management. Leaders must understand their own value system, which influences how they use time and how they expect subordinates to use time.

The management functions inherent in using time resources wisely are more related to productivity. The manager must be able to prioritize activities of unit functioning to meet short- and long-term unit needs.

Successful leader–managers are able to integrate leadership skills and management functions; they accomplish unit goals in a timely and efficient manner in a concerted effort with subordinates. They also recognize time as a valuable unit resource and share responsibility for the use of that resource with subordinates. Perhaps most importantly, the integrated leader–manager with well-developed time management skills is able to maintain greater control over time and energy constraints in his or her personal and professional life.

☀ Key Concepts

- Because time is a finite and valuable resource, learning to use it wisely is essential for effective management.
- *Time management* can be reduced to three cyclic steps: (1) allow time for planning, and establish priorities; (2) complete the highest priority task, and, whenever possible, finish one task before beginning another; and (3) reprioritize based on remaining tasks and new information that may have been received.
- Setting aside time at the beginning of each day to plan the day allows the manager to spend appropriate time on high-priority tasks.
- Making lists is an appropriate tool to manage daily tasks. This list should not be any longer than what can realistically be accomplished in a day and must include adequate time to accomplish each item on the list and time for the unexpected.

- A common cause of *procrastination* is failure to break large tasks down into smaller ones so that the manager can set short-term, intermediate, and long-term goals.
- Lower-level managers have more interruptions in their work than higher-level managers. This results in situational stress and lowered job satisfaction.
- Managers must learn strategies to cope with interruptions from socializing.
- Because so much paperwork is redundant or unnecessary, the manager needs to develop expertise at prioritizing it and eliminating unnecessary clutter at the work site.
- An efficient filing system is invaluable to handling paper overload.
- Personal time management refers to "the knowing of self." Managing time is difficult if a person is unsure of his or her priorities, including personal short-term, intermediate, and long-term goals.
- Using a time inventory is one way to gain insight into how and when a person is most productive. It also assists in identifying internal time-wasters.

More Learning Exercises and Applications

Learning Exercise 9.8

Creating a Shift Time Inventory
You are a 3 PM to 11 PM shift coordinator for a skilled nursing facility. You are the only registered nurse on your unit this shift. All the other personnel assigned to work with you this evening are unlicensed. The unit census is 21. As the shift coordinator, your responsibility is to make shift assignments, provide needed patient treatments, administer intravenous medications, and coordinate the work of team members. The patients that you will need to administer treatments and/or medications to this evening include:

Room 101 A	Gina Adams	88 years old. Senile dementia. Resident for six years. Confused—strikes out at staff. Soft wrist restraints bilaterally. Has small Grade 2 decubitus ulcer on coccyx, which requires evaluation and dressing change each shift.
Room 102 B	Gus Taylor	64 years old. Diabetes. New resident. Bilateral AK amputee. Right amputation two weeks ago. Left amputation performed eight years ago. Needs stump dressing on right amputation site this shift. Has developed MRSA in wound site. Wound isolation protocol ordered. IV antibiotics due at 4 PM and 10 PM tonight. Accu-checks due at 4:30 PM and 9:00 PM with sliding-scale coverage.
Room 106A	Marvin Young	26 years old. Closed head injury five years ago. Resident since that time. Decerebrate posturing only. Does not follow commands. PEG feeding tube site red and inflamed; Dr. has not yet been notified. Needs feeding solution bag change this PM.

Room 107A	Sheila Abood	93 years old. Functional decline. Refusing to eat. Physician has written an order not to resuscitate in the event of cardiac or respiratory failure, but wants an intravenous line begun this PM to minimize patient dehydration. Family will also be here this PM and want to talk about their mother's status.
Room 109C	Tina Crowden	89 years old. Admit from local hospital, two weeks post-op left hip replacement. Anticipated length of stay—two weeks. Arrives by ambulance at 3:30 PM. Needs to have admission assessment and paperwork completed and care plan started.

Oral Medications Schedule
Room 101A—4 PM, 8 PM
Room 101B—4 PM, 8 PM
Room 102A—5 PM, 9 PM
Room 103B—4 PM, 10 PM
Room 104C—5 PM, 6 PM, 9 PM
Room 106B—6 PM, 9 PM
Room 108C—9 PM
Room 109C—5 PM, 6 PM, 8 PM, 9 PM

Assignment: Create a time inventory from 3:00 PM to 11:30 PM using one-hour blocks of time. Plan what activities you will do during each one-hour block. Be sure you start with the activities you have prioritized for the shift. Also, remember that you will be in shift report from 3:00 to 3:30 PM and from 11:00 to 11:30 PM and that you need to schedule a dinner break for yourself. Allow adequate time for planning and dealing with the unexpected. Compare the inventory you created with other students in your class. Did you identify the same priorities? Were you more focused on professional, technical, or amenity care? Is your plan more monochronic or polychronic in nature? Was the time inventory you created realistic? Is this a workload you believe you could handle?

Learning Exercise 9.9

Plan Your Day
It is October of your second year as coordinator of nursing management for the surgical department. A copy of your appointment calendar for Monday, October 27, follows.

You will review your unfinished business from the preceding Friday and look at the new items of business that have arrived on your desk this morning. (The new items follow the appointment calendar.) The unit ward clerk is usually free in the afternoon to provide you with one hour of clerical assistance, and you have a charge nurse on each shift to whom you may delegate.

1. Assign a priority to each item, with 1 being the most important and 5 being the least important.

2. Decide when you will deal with each item, being careful not to use more time than you have open on your calendar.
3. If the problem is to be handled immediately, explain how you will do this (e.g., delegated, phone call).
4. Explain the rationale for your decisions.

Monday, October 27

8:00 AM	Arrive at work
8:15 AM	Daily rounds with each head nurse in your area
8:30 AM	Continuation of daily rounds with head nurses
9:00 AM	Open
9:30 AM	Open
10:00 AM	Department Head meeting
10:30 AM	United Givers committee
11:00 AM	United Givers committee
11:30 AM	Open
Noon	Lunch
12:30 PM	Lunch
1:00 PM	Weekly meeting with administrator—Budget and annual report due
1:30 PM	Open
2:00 PM	Infection Control meeting
2:30 PM	Infection Control meeting continued
3:00 PM	Fire drill and critique of drill
3:30 PM	Fire drill and critique of drill continued
4:00 PM	Open
4:30 PM	Open
5:00 PM	Off duty

Correspondence

Item 1

From the desk of M. Jones, personnel manager
October 24
Dear Joan:

I am sending you the names of two new graduate nurses who are interested in working in your area. I have processed their applications; they seem well qualified. Could you manage to see them as early as possible in the week? I would hate to lose these prospective employees, and they are anxious to obtain definite confirmation of employment.

Item 2

From the desk of John Brown, purchasing agent
October 23
Joan:

We really must get together this week and devise a method to control supplies. Your area has used three times the amount of thermometer covers as any other area. Are you taking that many more temperatures? This is just one of the supplies your area uses excessively. I'm open to suggestions.

Item 3
Roger Johnson, MD, chief of surgical department
October 24
Ms. Kerr:
   I know you have your budget ready to submit, but I just remembered this week that I forgot to include an arterial pressure monitor. Is there another item that we can leave out? I'll drop by Monday morning, and we'll figure something out.

Item 4
October 23
Ms. Kerr:
   The following personnel are due for merit raises, and I must have their completed and signed evaluations by Tuesday afternoon: Mary Rocas, Jim Newman, Marge Newfield.
M. Jones, personnel manager

Item 5
Roger Johnson, MD, chief of surgical department
October 23
Ms. Kerr:
   The physicians are complaining about the availability of nurses to accompany them on rounds. I believe you and I need to sit down with the doctors and head nurses to discuss this recurring problem. I have some free time Monday afternoon.

Item 6
5 AM
Joan:
   Sally Knight (your regular night RN) requested a leave of absence due to her mother's illness. I told her it would be OK to take the next three nights off. She is flying out of town on the 9 AM commuter flight to San Francisco, so phone her right away if you don't want her to go. I felt I had no choice but to say yes.
Nancy Peters, night supervisor
   P.S. You'll need to find a replacement for her for the next three nights.

Item 7
To: Ms. Kerr
From: Administrator
Re: Patient complaint
Date: October 23
   Please investigate the following patient complaint. I would like a report on this matter this afternoon.

Dear Sir:
   My mother, Gertrude Boswich, was a patient in your hospital, and I just want to tell you that no member of my family will ever go there again.
   She had an operation on Monday, and no one gave her a bath for three days. Besides that, she didn't get anything to eat for two days, not even water. What kind of a hospital do you run anyway?
Elmo Boswich

Item 8
To: Joan Kerr
From: Nancy Newton, RN, head nurse
Re: Problems with x-ray department
Date: October 23
    We have been having problems getting diagnostic x-ray procedures scheduled for patients. Many times, patients have had to stay an extra day to get x-ray tests done. I have talked to the radiology chief several times, but the situation hasn't improved. Can you do something about this?

Item 9
To: All department heads
From: Store room
Re: Supplies
Date: October 23
    The storeroom is out of the following items: Toilet tissue, paper clips, disposable diapers, and pencils. We are expecting a shipment next week.

Telephone Messages

Item 10
    Sam Surefoot, Superior Surgical Supplies, Inc., returned your call at 7:50 AM on October 27. He will be at the hospital this afternoon to talk about problems with defective equipment received.

Item 11
    Donald Drinkley, Channel 32-TV, called at 8:10 AM on October 27 to say he will be here at 11:30 AM to do a feature story on the open-heart unit.

Item 12
    Lila Green, director of nurses at St. Joan's Hospital, called at 8:05 AM on October 24 about a phone reference on Jane Jones, RN. Ms. Jones has applied for a job there. Isn't that the one we fired last year?

Item 13
    Betty Brownie, Bluebird Troop 35, called at 8 AM on October 27 about the Bluebird troop visit to patients on Halloween with trick-or-treat candy. She will call again.

Learning Exercise 9.10

Avoiding Crises

Some people always seem to manage by crisis. The following scenarios depict situations that likely could have been avoided with better planning. Write down what could have been done to prevent the crisis. Then outline at least three alternatives to exist to deal with the problem, as it already exists.

- It is the end of your eight-hour shift. Your team members are ready to go home. You have not yet begun to chart on any of your six patients. Neither have you completed your intake/output totals or given patients the medications that were due one hour ago. The arriving shift asks you to give report now.
- You need to use the home computer to write your midterm essay, which is due tomorrow, but your mother is online doing the family's taxes, which must be mailed by midnight. The taxes will likely take several additional hours.
- Your computer hard drive crashes when you try to print your term paper, which is due tomorrow.
- An elderly, frail patient pulls out her intravenous line. You make six attempts, over a one-hour period, to restart the line but are unsuccessful. You have missed your lunch break and now must choose between taking time for lunch and finishing your shift on time.

 Web Links

Organizational skills: Are you ready for a change?
http://www.womensmedia.com/organize-goals-0200.htm
A women's resource for organizational skills.

Personal time management for busy managers
http://www.ee.ed.ac.uk/~gerard/Management/art2.html
This article looks at the basics of personal time management and describes how the manager can assume control of this basic resource.

Leadership Skills for Professionals Desktop Workshop
http://www.consultskills.com/contents.htm
Point to and click on the underlined name of the document you wish. Documents included under subsection strategy, setting priorities, and saying no.

References

Bakunas, B. (2001). Don't think about it tomorrow at Tara: Beat procrastination now! *Education Digest, 66*(6), 51–55.

Davidhizar, R., Giger, J. N., & Turner, G. (1994). Understanding monochronic and polychronic individuals in the workplace. *Clinical Nurse Specialist, 8*(329), 334–336.

Emmett, R. (2002). *The procrastinator's handbook: Mastering the art of doing it now.* New York: Walker & Co.

Hansten, R. I., & Washburn, M. J. (1998). *Clinical delegation skills: A handbook for professional practice.* Gaithersburg, MD: Aspen Publications.

Kriegel, R. (2002). *How to succeed in business without working so damm hard: Rethinking the rules, reinventing the game.* New York: Warner Books.

Lancaster, J. (1984). Making the most of every minute: Reminders for nursing leaders. In M. S. Berger, D. Elhart, S. Firsich, S. Jordan, & S. Stone (Eds.), *Management for nurses.* St. Louis, MO: C. V. Mosby.

Masikiewicz, M. (2000). Get ready, get set, get organized. *Career World, 29*(1), 6–11.

Morgenstern, J. (2000). *Time Management from the inside out: The foolproof system for taking control of your schedule and life.* New York: Henry Holt & Company.

Strongman, K. T., & Burt, C.D.B. (2000). Taking breaks from work: An exploratory inquiry. *Journal of Psychology, 134*(3), 229–243.

Vacarro, P. J. (2001). Five priority-setting traps. *Family practice management, 8*(4), 60.

Zimmermann, P. G. (2002). Nursing secrets: Managing our work life. *Emergency Nurse, 10*(4), 14–17.

Bibliography

Adams, D. (2001). Time management: Work and family. *Independent School, 60*(3), 14–21.

Adamson, B. J. (2001). Implications for tertiary education: Managerial competencies required of beginning practitioners in the health service sector. *Medical Teacher, 23*(2), 198–205.

Clarke, R. D. (2001). Too busy to work? *Black Enterprise, 31*(8), 63.

Gonzales, S. (2001). Get organized: Tips for de-cluttering your desk, office and computer. *EMS Manager and Supervisor, 3*(3), 3.

Humphrey, C. J. (2003). Productivity, time management—right! *Home Healthcare Nurse, 21*(6), 356.

Hymowitz, C. (2001, March 20). How some CEOs get the energy to work those endless days. *The Wall Street Journal,* p. B1.

Irons, L. M. (2003). Time valuing: A teaching strategy for time management. *American Journal of Health Education, 34*(3), 172–173.

Lister, P. (2001, March). Get organized! *Family Life,* 56–60.

Lundgren, S., & Segesten, K. (2001). Nurses' use of time in a medical-surgical ward with all RN staffing. *Journal of Nursing Management, 9*(1), 13–20.

Michaud, E. (2001, July). Get back 15 days of your life! *Prevention, 53,* 144.

Nicholls, J. (2001). The Ti-Mandi window: A time management tool for managers. *Industrial and Commercial Training, 33*(3), 104–109.

Pettiford, H. (2001). Time's a-wastin! *Black Enterprise, 31*(11), 322.

Schlabach, R. (2001). Too much to do. *Campus Life, 59*(8), 12.

Taigman, M., Shost, D. A. & DuGray, R. (2003). Time savers: 3 experts tackle a real-life management problem. *EMS Manager & Supervisor, 5*(4), 1–2r.

Tips from your peers. (2001). *Nursing Management, 32*(5), 24.

Yourdon, E. (2001). Finding time to think. *Computerworld, 35*(17), 39.

Fiscal Planning

Nurses are practicing caring in an environment where the economics and costs of health care permeate discussions and impact decisions.

—Marian C. Turkel

Scarce resources and soaring healthcare costs have strained all healthcare delivery systems. There has never been a time when healthcare organizations needed to operate more efficiently or be more aware of *cost containment*. Cost containment refers to effective and efficient delivery of services while generating needed revenues for continued organizational productivity. Cost containment is the responsibility of every healthcare provider, and the viability of most healthcare organizations today depends on their ability to use their fiscal resources wisely.

It is critical that unit managers have expertise in managing costs. Of all forms of planning, many managers often perceive fiscal planning as the most difficult. Although familiar with the basics of fiscal planning, unit managers may encounter difficulty with forecasting costs based on current and projected needs. Sometimes this occurs because the manager has had little formal education or training on budget preparation. Fiscal planning, like all types of planning, is a learned skill and improves with practice. It is essential that fiscal planning be included in nursing curricula and in management preparation programs.

Historically, nursing management played a limited role in determining resource allocation in healthcare institutions. Nurse–managers were given budgets without any rationale and were allowed limited input. In addition, because nursing was classified as a "non–income-producing service," nursing input was undervalued.

During the last 20 years, healthcare organizations have grown to recognize the importance of nursing input in fiscal planning, and unit managers in the 21st century are expected to be well versed in financial matters. Because nursing budgets generally account for the greatest share of the total expenses in healthcare institutions, participation in fiscal planning has become a fundamental and powerful tool for nursing.

An essential feature of fiscal planning is *responsibility accounting,* which means that each of an organization's revenues, expenses, assets, and liabilities is someone's responsibility. As a corollary, the person with the most direct control or influence on any of these financial elements should be held accountable for them. At the unit level, this accountability generally falls to the manager. The manager, then, should be an active participant in unit budgeting, have a high degree of control over what is included in the unit budget, receive regular data reports that compare actual expenses with budgeted expenses, and be held accountable for the financial results of the operating unit.

Because unit managers are involved in daily operations and see firsthand their unit's functioning, they generally have great expertise in forecasting patient census trends as well as supply and equipment needs for their units. Forecasting involves making an educated budget estimate using historical data.

The unit manager also can best monitor and evaluate all aspects of a unit's budget control. Like other types of planning, the unit manager also has a responsibility to communicate budgetary planning goals to staff. The more the staff understands the budgetary goals and the plans to carry out those goals, the more likely goal attainment is. Sadly, many nurses have little knowledge of the nursing budget model applied by their hospital system.

Fiscal planning uses many of the same concepts and rules that were discussed in earlier chapters. For example, just as each person's value system determines how personal resources are spent, fiscal planning reflects the philosophy, goals, and objectives of the organization.

Fiscal planning must be proactive, flexible, and clearly stated in measurable terms; include short- and long-term planning; and involve as many people as feasible in the budgetary process. This type of planning also requires vision, creativity, and a thorough knowledge of the political, social, and economic forces that shape health care. This chapter discusses the unit manager's role in fiscal planning, identifies types of budgets, and delineates the budgetary process. These roles and functions are outlined in **Display 10.1.**

Display 10.1	**Leadership Roles and Management Functions in Fiscal Planning**

Leadership Roles

1. Is visionary in identifying or forecasting short- and long-term unit needs, thus inspiring proactive rather than reactive fiscal planning.
2. Is knowledgeable about political, social, and economic factors that shape fiscal planning in health care today.
3. Demonstrates flexibility in fiscal goal setting in a rapidly changing system.
4. Anticipates, recognizes, and creatively problem solves budgetary constraints.
5. Influences and inspires group members to become active in short- and long-range fiscal planning.
6. Recognizes when fiscal constraints have resulted in an inability to meet organizational or unit goals and communicates this insight effectively, following the chain of command.
7. Ensures that patient safety is not jeopardized by cost containment.

Management Functions

1. Identifies the importance of and develops short- and long-range fiscal plans that reflect unit needs.
2. Articulates and documents unit needs effectively to higher administrative levels.
3. Assesses the internal and external environment of the organization in forecasting to identify driving forces and barriers to fiscal planning.
4. Demonstrates knowledge of budgeting and uses appropriate techniques to budget effectively.
5. Provides opportunities for subordinates to participate in relevant fiscal planning.
6. Coordinates unit-level fiscal planning to be congruent with organizational goals and objectives.
7. Accurately assesses personnel needs using predetermined standards or an established patient classification system.
8. Coordinates the monitoring aspects of budget control.
9. Ensures that documentation of patient's need for services and services rendered is clear and complete to facilitate organizational reimbursement.

BASICS OF BUDGETS

A *budget* is a plan that uses numerical data to predict the activities of an organization over a period of time, and it provides a mechanism for planning and control, as well as for promoting each unit's needs and contributions (Carruth, Carruth, & Noto, 2000). The budget's value is directly related to its accuracy; the more accurate the budget blueprint, the better the institution can plan the most efficient use of its resources. Because a budget is at best a prediction, a plan, and not a rule, fiscal planning requires flexibility, ongoing evaluation, and revision.

In the budget, expenses are classified as fixed or variable and either controllable or noncontrollable. *Fixed expenses* do not vary with volume, whereas *variable expenses* do. Examples of fixed expenses might be a building's mortgage payment or a manager's salary; variable expenses might include the payroll of hourly wage employees and the cost of supplies. *Controllable expenses* can be controlled or varied by the manager, whereas *noncontrollable expenses* cannot. For example, the unit manager can control the number of personnel working on a certain shift and the staffing mix; he or she cannot, however, control equipment depreciation, the number and type of supplies needed by patients, or overtime that occurs in response to an emergency. A list of the fiscal terminology that a manager needs to know is shown in **Display 10.2.**

> The desired outcome of budgeting is maximal use of resources to meet organizational short- and long-term needs.

Display 10.2	**Fiscal Terminology**

Acuity index—Weighted statistical measurement that refers to severity of illness of patients for a given time. Patients are classified according to acuity of illness, usually in one of four categories. The acuity index is determined by taking a total of acuities and then dividing by the number of patients.

Assets—Financial resources that a healthcare organization receives, such as accounts receivable.

Baseline data—Historical information on dollars spent, acuity level, patient census, resources needed, hours of care, and so forth. This information is used as basis on which future needs can be projected.

Break-even point—Point at which revenue covers costs. Most healthcare facilities have high fixed costs. Because per-unit fixed costs in a noncapitated model decrease with volume, health care facilities under this model need to maintain a high volume to decrease unit costs.

Capitation—A prospective payment system that pays health plans or providers a fixed amount per enrollee per month for a defined set of health services (Chang, Price, & Pfoutz, 2001).

Case mix—Type of patients served by an institution. A hospital's case mix is usually defined in such patient-related variables as diagnosis, personal characteristics, and patterns of treatment.

Cash flow—Rate at which dollars are received and dispersed.

Controllable costs—Costs that can be controlled or that vary. An example would be the number of personnel employed, the level of skill required, wage levels, and quality of materials.

(display continues on page 218)

Display 10.2	**Fiscal Terminology**

Cost–benefit ratio—Numerical relationship between the value of an activity or procedure in terms of benefits and the value of the activity's or procedure's cost. The cost–benefit ratio is expressed as a fraction.

Cost center—Smallest functional unit for which cost control and accountability can be assigned. A nursing unit is usually considered a cost center, but there may be other cost centers within a unit (orthopedics is a cost center, but often the cast room is considered a separate cost center within orthopedics).

Diagnosis-related groups (DRGs)—Rate setting prospective payment system used by Medicare to determine payment rates under 495 DRGs (Change et al., 2001). Each DRG represents a particular case type for which Medicare provides a flat dollar amount of reimbursement. This set rate may, in actuality, be higher or lower than the cost of treating the patient in a particular hospital.

Direct costs—Costs that can be attributed to a specific source, such as medications and treatments. Costs that are clearly identifiable with goods or service.

Fee-for-service (FFS) system—A reimbursement system under which insurance companies reimburse health care providers after the needed services are delivered.

Fixed budget—Style of budgeting that is based on a fixed, annual level of volume, such as number of patient-days or tests performed, to arrive at an annual budget total. These totals are then divided by 12 to arrive at the monthly average. The fixed budget does not make provisions for monthly or seasonal variations.

Fixed costs—Costs that do not vary according to volume. Examples of fixed costs are mortgage or loan payments.

For-profit organization—Organization in which the providers of funds have an ownership interest in the organization. These providers own stocks in the for-profit organization and earn dividends based on what is left when the cost of goods and of carrying on the business is subtracted from the amount of money taken in.

Full costs—Total of all direct and indirect costs.

Full-time equivalent (FTE)— Number of hours of work for which a full-time employee is scheduled for a weekly period. For example, 1.0 FTE = five eight-hour days of staffing, which equals 40 hours of staffing per week. One FTE can be divided in different ways. For example, two part-time employees, each working 20 hours per week, would equal 1 FTE. If a position requires coverage for more than five days or 40 hours per week, the FTE will be greater than 1.0 for that position. Assume a position requires seven-day coverage, or 56 hours; then the position requires 1.4 FTE coverage (56 divided by 40 = 1.4). This means that more than one person is needed to fill the FTE positions for a seven-day period.

Health maintenance organization—Originally, a prepaid organization that provided health care to voluntarily enrolled members in return for a preset amount of money on a per-person, per-month basis. With the increase in self-insured businesses or financial arrangements that do not include prepayment, this definition now generally includes two possibilities: a licensed health plan that places at least some of the providers at risk for medical expenses, and a health plan that utilizes designated (usually primary care) physicians as gatekeepers (although some HMOs do not) (Kongstvedt, 1997). Often referred to as a managed care organization (MCO).

Hours per patient-day (HPPD)—Hours of nursing care provided per patient per day by various levels of nursing personnel. HPPD are determined by dividing total production hours by the number of patients.

Display 10.2 Fiscal Terminology

Indirect costs—Costs that cannot be directly attributed to a specific area. These are hidden costs and are usually spread among different departments. Housekeeping services are considered indirect costs.

Managed care—Term used to describe a variety of healthcare plans designed to contain the cost of healthcare services delivered to members while maintaining the quality of care.

Medicaid—Federally assisted and state-administered program to pay for medical services on behalf of certain groups of low-income individuals. Generally, these people are not covered by Social Security. Certain groups of people (e.g, the elderly, blind, disabled, members of families with dependent children, and certain other children and pregnant women) also qualify for coverage if their incomes and resources are sufficiently low.

Medicare—Nationwide health insurance program authorized under Title 18 of the Social Security Act that provides benefits to people 65 years of age or older. Part A is the hospital insurance program. Part B is the supplementary medical insurance program. Part C (also known as Medicare + Choice) allows Medicare beneficiaries to opt out of the original Medicare program and instead receive services from alternative plans. Medicare coverage also is available to certain groups of people with catastrophic or chronic illness, such as patients with renal failure requiring hemodialysis, regardless of age.

Noncontrollable costs—Indirect expenses that you cannot usually control or vary. Examples might be rent, lighting, and depreciation of equipment.

Not-for-profit organization—This type of organization is financed by funds that come from several sources, but the providers of these funds do not have an ownership interest. Profits generated in the not-for-profit organization are frequently funneled back into the organization for expansion or capital acquisition.

Operating expenses—Daily costs required to maintain a hospital or healthcare institution.

Patient classification system—Method of classifying patients. Different criteria are used for different systems. In nursing, patients are usually classified according to severity of illness.

Preferred provider organization—Healthcare financing and delivery program with a group of providers, such as physicians and hospitals, who contract to give services on a fee-for-service basis. This provides financial incentives to consumers to use a select group of preferred providers and pay less for services. Insurance companies usually promise the preferred provider organization a certain volume of patients and prompt payment in exchange for fee discounts.

Production hours—Total amount of regular time, overtime, and temporary time. This also may be referred to as actual hours.

Prospective payment system (PPS)—A hospital payment system that sets payment rates before treatment begins (Chang et al., 2001).

Revenue—Source of income or the reward for providing a service to a patient.

Staffing distribution—Determination of number of personnel allocated per shift (e.g., 45% days, 35% evenings, and 20% nights). Hospitals vary on how staff are distributed.

Staffing mix—Ratio of RNs to other personnel (e.g., a shift on one unit might have 40% RNs, 40% LPNs/LVNs, and 20% other). Hospitals vary on their staffing mix policies.

Third-party payment system—a system of healthcare financing in which providers deliver services to patients, and a third party, or intermediary, usually an insurance company or a government agency, pays the bill (Chang et al., 2001).

(display continues on page 220)

Display 10.2	**Fiscal Terminology**

Turnover ratio—Rate at which employees leave their jobs for reasons other than death or retirement. The rate is calculated by dividing the number of employees leaving by the number of workers employed in the unit during the year and then multiplying by 100.

Variable costs—Costs that vary with the volume. Payroll costs are variable costs, for example.

Workload units—In nursing, workloads are usually the same as patient-days. For some areas, however, workload units might refer to the number of procedures, tests, patient visits, injections, and so forth.

Zero-based budgeting—Type of budgeting that begins at zero each year. That means that every dollar that is to be spent needs to be justified. Established costs are not automatically continued from one year to the next. This style of budgeting ensures that the activities aren't continued simply because they were carried out in the past. In zero-based budgeting, objectives are very important, and they are listed according to priority. Zero-based budgeting also indicates what will happen if an objective is eliminated and which objectives could be accomplished for less money.

Learning Exercise 10.1

Would You Accept This Gift?
One of the oncologists on your unit (Dr. Sam Jones) has offered to give you his old photocopier because his office is purchasing a new one. As a condition of acceptance, he requires that all the oncologists and radiologists be allowed to use the copier free of charge.

Assignment:
1. Justify acceptance or rejection of the gift. What influenced your choice?
2. What are the fixed and variable costs?
3. What are the controllable and noncontrollable costs?
4. How much control will you as a unit manager have over the use of the copier?

STEPS IN THE BUDGETARY PROCESS

The nursing process provides a model for the steps in budget planning:

1. The first step is to **assess** what needs to be covered in the budget. Historically, top-level managers frequently developed the budget for an institution without input from middle- or first-level managers. Because unit managers who participate in fiscal planning are more apt to be cost-conscious and better understand the institution's long- and short-term goals, budgeting today generally reflects input from all levels of the organizational hierarchy. Unit managers develop goals, objectives, and budgetary estimates with input from colleagues and subordinates. Budgeting is most effective when

all personnel using the resources are involved in the process. Managers, therefore, must be taught how to prepare a budget and must be supported by management throughout the budgeting process. A composite of unit needs in terms of manpower, equipment, and operating expenses can then be compiled to determine the organizational budget.

2. The second step is to develop a **plan.** The budget plan may be developed in many ways. A budgeting cycle that is set for 12 months is called a *fiscal-year budget.* This fiscal year, which may or may not coincide with the calendar year, is then usually broken down into quarters or subdivided into monthly, quarterly, or semiannual periods. Most budgets are developed for a one-year period, but a *perpetual budget* may be done on a continual basis each month so that 12 months of future budget data are always available. Selecting the optimal time frame for budgeting also is important; a budget that is predicted too far in advance has greater probability for error. If the budget is shortsighted, compensating for unexpected major expenses or purchasing capital equipment may be difficult.

3. The third step is **implementation.** In this step, ongoing monitoring and analysis occur to avoid inadequate or excess funds at the end of the fiscal year. In most healthcare institutions, monthly computerized statements outline each department's projected budget and any deviations from that budget. Each unit manager is accountable for budget deviations in his or her unit. Most units can expect some change from the anticipated budget, but large deviations must be examined for possible causes, and remedial action must be taken if necessary. Some managers artificially inflate their department budgets as a cushion against budget cuts from a higher level of administration. If several departments partake in this unsound practice, the entire institutional budget may be ineffective. If a major change in the budget is indicated, the entire budgeting process must be repeated. Top-level managers must watch for and correct unrealistic budget projections before they are implemented.

4. The last step is **evaluation.** The budget must be reviewed periodically and modified as needed throughout the fiscal year. With each successive year of budgeting, managers can more accurately predict their unit's budgetary requirements. Managers develop a more historical approach to budgeting as they grow more adept at predicting seasonal variations in the population they serve or in their particular institution.

TYPES OF BUDGETS

There are three major types of expenditures the unit manager is directly involved in with fiscal planning: personnel, operating, and capital budgets.

The Personnel Budget

The largest of the budget expenditures is the workforce or *personnel budget* because health care is *labor intensive.* To handle fluctuating patient census and acuity, managers need to develop a comprehensive variable budget (Kirkby, 2003). This requires the prudent manager to use historical data about unit census fluctuations in forecasting short- and long-term personnel needs. Likewise, a manager must monitor the personnel budget closely to prevent understaffing or overstaffing. As patient-days or volume decreases, managers must decrease personnel costs in relation to the decrease in volume.

In addition to numbers of staff, the manager must be cognizant of the staffing mix. The manager also must be aware of the institution's patient acuity so that the most economical level of nursing care that will meet patient needs can be provided. Although Unit Five discusses staffing, it is necessary to briefly discuss here how staffing needs are expressed in the personnel budget.

Most staffing is based on a predetermined standard. This standard may be addressed in hours per patient-day (medical units), visits per month (home health agencies), or minutes per case (the operating room). Because the patient census, number of visits, or cases per day never remains constant, the manager must be ready to alter staffing when volume increases or decreases. In addition, sometimes the population and type of cases change so that the established standard is no longer appropriate. For example, an operating room that begins to perform open-heart surgery would involve more nursing time per case; therefore, the standard (number of nursing minutes per case) would need to be adjusted. Normally, the standard is adjusted upward or downward once a year, but staffing is adjusted daily depending on the volume.

The standard formula for calculating *nursing care hours (NCH) per patient-day (PPD)* is shown in **Figure 10.1.** A unit manager in an acute care facility, might use

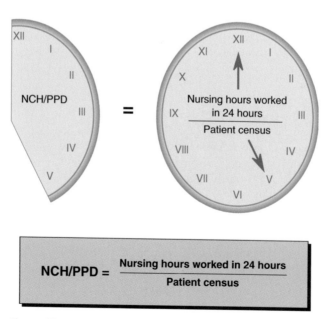

Figure 10.1 Standard formula for calculating nursing care hours (NCH) per patient-day (PPD).

this formula to calculate daily staffing needs. For example, assume that your budgeted nursing care hours are 6 NCH/PPD. You are calculating the NCH/PPD for today, January 31; at midnight, it will be February 1. The patient census at midnight is 25 patients. In checking staffing, you find the following information:

Shift	Staff on Duty	Hours Worked
11 PM (1/30) to 7 AM (1/31)	2 RNs	8 hours each
(last night)	1 LVN	8 hours
	1 CNA	8 hours
7 AM to 3 PM	3 RNs	8 hours each
	2 LVNs	8 hours each
	1 CNA	8 hours
	1 ward clerk	8 hours
3 PM to 11 PM	2 RNs	8 hours each
	2 LVNs	8 hours each
	1 CNA	8 hours
	1 ward clerk	8 hours
11 PM (1/30) to 7 AM (1/31)	2 RNs	8 hours each
(last night)	2 LVNs	8 hours each
	1 CNA	8 hours

Ideally you would use 12 midnight to 12 midnight to compute the NCH/PPD for January 31, but most staffing calculations based on traditional 8-hour shifts are made beginning at 11 PM and ending at 11 PM the following night. Therefore, in this case, it would be acceptable to figure the NCH/PPD for January 31 using numerical data from the 11 PM to 7 AM shift last night and the 7 AM to 3 PM and 3 PM to 11 PM shifts today. The first step in this calculation requires a computation of total nursing care hours worked in 24 hours (including the ward clerk's hours). This can be calculated by multiplying the total number of staff on duty each shift by the hours each worked in their shift. Each shift total then is added together to get the total number of nursing hours worked in all three shifts or 24 hours:

$$\text{Last night: 11 PM to 7 AM} \quad 4 \text{ staff @ 8 hours each} = 32 \text{ hours}$$
$$\text{7 AM to 3 PM} \quad 7 \text{ staff @ 8 hours each} = 56 \text{ hours}$$
$$\text{3 PM to 11 PM} \quad 6 \text{ staff @ 8 hours each} = 48 \text{ hours}$$
$$= 136 \text{ hours}$$

The nursing hours worked in 24 hours are 136 hours.

The second step in solving NCH/PPD requires that you divide the nursing hours worked in 24 hours by the patient census. The patient census in this case is 25. Therefore, 136 divided by 25 = 5.44.

The NCH/PPD for January 31 was 5.44, which is less than your budgeted NCH/PPD of 6.0. It would be possible to add up to 14 additional hours of nursing care in the next 24 hours and still maintain the budgeted nursing care hours standard. However, the unit manager must remember that the standard is flexible and that it would be necessary to assess the patient acuity and staffing mix to determine whether to add additional staff for February 1 and to determine what type of staff would be best and on what shift.

Learning Exercise 10.2

Calculating NCH/PPD

Calculate the NCH/PPD if the midnight census remained the same as on page 223, but use the following as the number of hours worked:

12 midnight to 12 noon	2 RNs	12 hours each
	2 LVNs	12 hours each
	1 CNA	12 hours
	1 ward clerk	5 hours
12 noon to 12 midnight	3 RNs	12 hours each
	2 LVNs	12 hours each
	1 CNA	12 hours
	1 ward clerk	11 hours

Now, calculate the NCH/PPD if the following staff were working.

12 midnight to 12 noon	3 RNs	12 hours each
	1 LVN	12 hours
12 noon to 12 midnight	2 RNs	12 hours each
	1 LVN	12 hours
	1 ward clerk	4 hours

The personnel budget includes actual worked time (also called *productive time* or *salary expense*) and time the organization pays the employee for not working (*nonproductive* or benefit time). Nonproductive time includes the cost of benefits, new employee orientation, employee turnover, sick and holiday time, and education time. For example, the average 8.5-hour shift includes a 30-minute lunch break and two 15-minute breaks. Thus, this employee would work 7.5 productive hours and have 1.0 hours of nonproductive time.

The Operating Budget

The *operating budget* is the second area of expenditure that involves all managers. The operating budget reflects expenses that change in response to the volume of service. Included in this budget are such daily expenses as the cost of electricity, repairs and maintenance, and supplies.

Next to personnel costs, supplies are the second most significant component in the hospital budget. Effective unit managers should be alert to the types and quantities of supplies used in their unit. They also should understand the relationship between supplies used in the unit and patient mix, occupancy rate, technology requirements, and types of procedures performed on the unit. There is great potential for cost savings with unused supplies from packs or trays and by reducing obsolete and slow-moving inventory, pilferage, the uncontrolled usage of supplies, and giveaways.

In addition, Contino (2002) advocates staff involvement with product evaluation. Some examples where staff involvement is essential is in examination of the cost-effectiveness of reusable versus disposable supplies and in adding products that make patient care more efficient (Contino). Other ways to cut supply costs might be in rental versus facility-owned equipment, stocking products on consignment, and *just-in-time* stockless inventory. Just-in-time ordering is a process where inventory is delivered to the organization by suppliers only when it is needed and then immediately before it is to be used.

Learning Exercise 10.3

Missing Supplies

You are a unit manager in an acute care hospital. You are aware that staff occasionally leave at the end of the shift with forgotten hospital supplies in their pockets. You remember how often as a staff nurse you would unintentionally take home rolls of adhesive tape, syringes, penlights, and bottles of lotion. Usually you remembered to return the items, but other times you did not.

Recently, however, your budget has shown a dramatic and unprecedented increase in missing supplies, including gauze wraps, blood pressure cuffs, stethoscopes, surgical instruments, and personal hygiene kits. Although this increase represents only a fraction of your total operating budget, you believe it is necessary to identify the source of their use. An audit of patient charts and charges reveals that these items were not used in patient care.

When you ask your charge nurses for an explanation, they reveal that a few employees have openly expressed that taking a few small supplies is, in effect, an expected and minor fringe benefit of employment. Your charge nurses do not believe that the problem is widespread, and they cannot objectively document which employees are involved in pilfering supplies. The charge nurses suggest that you ask all employees to document in writing when they see other employees taking supplies and then turn in the information to you anonymously for follow-up.

Because supplies are such a major part of the operating budget, you believe some action is indicated. You must determine what that action should be. Analyze your actions in terms of the desirable and undesirable effects on the employees involved in taking the supplies and those who are not. Is the amount of the fiscal debit in this situation a critical factor? Is it worth the time and energy that would be required to truly eliminate this problem?

The Capital Budget

The third type of budget used by managers is the *capital expenditure budget*. Capital budgets plan for the purchase of buildings or major equipment, which include equipment that has a long life (usually greater than five to seven years), is not used in daily operations and is more expensive than operating supplies. Capital budgets are composed of long-term planning, or a major acquisitions component, and a short-term budgeting component. The long-term major acquisitions component outlines future replacement and organizational expansion that will exceed one year. Examples of these types of capital expenditures might include the acquisition of a positron emission tomography imager or the renovation of a major wing in a hospital. The short-term component of the capital budget includes equipment purchases within the annual budget cycle, such as call-light systems, hospital beds, and medication carts.

Often the designation of capital equipment requires that the value of the equipment exceed a certain dollar amount. That dollar amount will vary from institution to institution, but $1,000 to $5,000 is common. Managers are usually required to complete specific capital equipment request forms either annually or semiannually and to justify their request.

COST-EFFECTIVENESS AS A UNIT MANAGER'S GOAL

The desired result of careful fiscal planning is *cost-effectiveness.* Cost-effective does not mean inexpensive; it means getting the most for your money, or that the product is worth the price. Buying a very expensive piece of equipment may be cost-effective if it can be shown that sufficient need exists for that equipment and that it was the best purchase to meet the need at that time. Cost-effectiveness takes into account factors such as anticipated length of service, need for such a service, and availability of other alternatives.

BUDGETING METHODS

Budgeting is frequently classified according to how often it is done and the base on which budgeting takes place. Three of the most common budgeting methods are incremental budgeting, also called flat-percentage increase budgeting, zero-based budgeting, and new performance budgeting.

Incremental Budgeting

Incremental or the *flat-percentage increase* method is the simplest method for budgeting. By multiplying current year expenses by a certain figure, usually the inflation rate or consumer price index, this method arrives at the budget for the coming year. Although this method is simple and quick and requires little budgeting expertise on the part of the manager, it is generally inefficient fiscally because there is no motivation to contain costs and no need to prioritize programs and services.

Zero-Based Budgeting

In comparison, managers who use *zero-based budgeting* must rejustify their program or needs every budgeting cycle. This method does not automatically assume that because a program has been funded in the past, it should continue to be funded. Thus, this budgeting process is labor intensive for nurse–managers.

Display 10.3	**Key Components of Decision Packages in Zero-Based Budgeting**

1. Listing of all current and proposed objectives or activities in the department
2. Alternative plans for carrying out these activities
3. Costs for each alternative
4. Advantages and disadvantages of continuing or discontinuing an activity

The use of a *decision package* to set funding priorities is a key feature of zero-based budgeting. Key components of decision packages are shown in **Display 10.3.**

The following is an example of a decision package for implementing a mandatory hepatitis B vaccination program at a nursing school.

- **Objective:** All nursing students will complete a hepatitis B vaccination series.
- **Driving forces:** Hepatitis B is a severely disabling disease that carries a significant mortality. According to the National Centers for Disease Control and Prevention (NCDC), student nurses are at high risk for infection by hepatitis B. This vaccination will greatly reduce that risk. The current vaccination series has been proven to have few serious side effects. The nursing school risks liability if it does not follow NCDC recommendations to have all high-risk groups vaccinated.
- **Restraining forces:** The vaccination series costs $175 per student. Some students do not want to have the vaccinations and believe requiring them to do so is a violation of free choice. It is unclear whether the school is liable if a student experiences a damaging side effect as a result of the vaccinations.
- **Alternative 1:** Require the vaccinations, but because the school of nursing cannot afford to pay for the cost of the series, require the students to pay for it. Advantage: No cost to the school. All students receive the vaccinations. Disadvantage: Many students cannot afford the cost of the vaccination and believe requiring it infringes on their right to control choices about their bodies.
- **Alternative 2:** Do not require the vaccination series. Advantage: No cost to anyone. Students have choice regarding whether to have the vaccinations and assume the responsibility of protecting their health themselves. Disadvantage: Some nursing students will be unprotected against hepatitis B while working in a high-risk clinical setting.
- **Alternative 3:** Require the vaccination series, but share the cost between the student and the school. Advantage: Decreased cost to students. All students would be vaccinated. Disadvantage: Costs and limited choice.

Decision packages and zero-based budgeting are advantageous because they force managers to set priorities and use resources most efficiently. This rather lengthy and complex method also encourages participative management because information from peers and subordinates is needed to analyze adequately and prioritize the activities of each unit.

Learning Exercise 10.4

Developing a Decision Package
Given the following objective, develop a decision package to aid you in fiscal priority setting.

Objective: To have reliable, economic, and convenient transportation when you enter nursing school in three months.

Additional Information: You currently have no car and rely on public transportation, which is inexpensive and reliable but not very convenient. Your current financial resources are limited, although you could probably qualify for a car loan if your parents were willing to cosign the loan. Your nursing school's policy states that you must have a car available to commute to clinical agencies outside the immediate area. You know that this policy is not enforced and that some students do carpool to clinical assignments.

Assignment: Identify at least three alternatives that will meet your objective. Choose the best alternative based on the advantages and disadvantages that you identify. You may embellish information presented in the case to help your problem solving.

New Performance Budgeting

The third method of budgeting, *new performance budgeting*, emphasizes accountability, efficiency, and economy by emphasizing outcomes and results instead of activities or outputs (Contino, 2001). Thus, the manager would budget as needed to achieve specific outcomes and would evaluate budgetary success accordingly. For example, a home health agency would set and then measure a specific outcome in a group of patients, such as diabetics, as a means of establishing and justifying a budget.

CRITICAL PATHWAYS

Critical pathways (also called *clinical pathways* and *care pathways*) are one method of planning, assessing, implementing, and evaluating the cost-effectiveness of patient care. Critical pathways are predetermined courses of progress that patients should be making after admission for a specific diagnosis or after a specific surgery. For example, a critical pathway for a specific diagnosis might suggest an average length of stay (ALOS) of four days, and that the patient should have certain interventions completed by certain points on the pathway (much like a PERT diagram; see page 35). Any patient's progress found not to be in compliance with the critical pathway prompts a *variance analysis* regarding why the critical pathway has been violated. De Luc (2000), in a study of two care pathways, found that the use of pathways made the staff focus on the clinical care they were providing and how it could be improved.

Although critical pathways can be used as a tool for monitoring quality of care, they can also be used as a fiscal planning tool. Once the cost of a pathway is known, analyzing the cost-effectiveness of the pathway as well as the associated cost variances is possible. Research suggests that critical pathways reduce the cost of care through reduced laboratory and radiology tests and by reducing length of stay (Renholm, Leino-Kilpi, & Suominen, 2002). Additionally, by using clinical and cost variance data, decisions on changing the pathway can be made with both clinical and financial outcome projections.

The advantage of critical pathways is that they do provide some means of standardizing medical care for patients with similar diagnoses. Their weakness, however, is the difficulties they pose in accounting for and accepting what are often justifiable differentiations between unique patients who have deviated from their pathway. Critical pathway documentation also poses one more paperwork and utilization review function in a system that is already overburdened with administrative costs.

HEALTHCARE REIMBURSEMENT

Historically, healthcare institutions have placed little or no emphasis on budgeting. When budgeting was done, incremental budgeting was used. Because insurance carriers reimbursed fully on virtually a limitless basis, there was not a great deal of motivation to save costs and budget effectively. Organizations found it unnecessary to justify costs or prove that their services met patient needs because they were not required to justify their charges. Reimbursement was based on costs incurred to provide the service (*fee-for-service*), with no ceiling placed on the amount that could be charged. Little attention was given to how the quest for increasingly high-quality care would affect healthcare costs.

The Prospective Payment System

During the 1960s, government assumed an increasingly significant role in healthcare reimbursement in this country with the advent of Medicare and Medicaid. Medicare is a federal government–sponsored health insurance program for the elderly (over age 65) and for certain groups of people with catastrophic or chronic illness, regardless of age. Medicaid is a federal–state cooperative health insurance plan directed primarily for the financially indigent.

With the advent of Medicare and Medicaid in the 1960s, whereby government reimbursed providers cost plus administrative fees, healthcare costs skyrocketed. As a result, the government began establishing regulations requiring organizations to justify the need for services and to monitor the quality of services. Healthcare providers were forced for the first time to submit budgets and justify costs. This new "big brother" surveillance and existence of external controls have had a tremendous effect on the industry.

The advent of *diagnosis-related groups* (DRGs) in the early 1980s added to the need for monitoring cost containment. DRGs were predetermined payment schedules that reflected historical costs for treatment of specific patient conditions. The first version of the DRG system included 383 categories. Approximately 500 DRGs or "product lines" have now been established. With DRGs, hospitals join the *prospective payment system* (PPS), whereby they receive a specified amount for

> With the advent of Medicare and Medicaid in the 1960s, whereby government reimbursed providers cost **plus** administrative fees, healthcare costs skyrocketed.

each Medicare patient's admission, regardless of the actual cost of care. Exceptions to this predetermined reimbursement occur when the provider can demonstrate that a patient's case is an *outlier*, meaning that the cost of providing care for that patient justifies extra payment.

As a result of the PPS and the need to contain costs, the length of stay for most hospital admissions has decreased greatly. Many argue, however, that quality standards have been lowered and that patients are being discharged before they are ready. The nurse–leader is responsible for recognizing when cost containment begins to impinge on patient safety and for taking appropriate action to guarantee at least the minimum standard of care. Chapter 23 further discusses the PPS and its impact on quality control.

The government again deeply affected healthcare administration in the United States in 1997 with the passage of the Balanced Budget Act (BBA). This health reform act contained numerous cost-containment measures, including reductions in provider payments for the traditional fee-for-service Medicare program participants. The bulk of the savings resulted from limiting the growth rates for hospital and physician payments. A second major source of savings was derived from restructuring the payment methods for rehabilitation hospitals, home health agencies, skilled nursing facilities, and outpatient services. The BBA also, for the first time, authorized payments to nurse practitioners for Medicare-provided services at 85% of the physician-fee schedule.

The ever-increasing impact of the federal government on how health care is delivered in the United States must be recognized. For the past decade, the federal government has been the largest purchaser of health care in America (Barton, 1999). Accompanying this funding is an increase in regulations for facilities treating these patients and a system that rewards cost containment. Healthcare providers are encountering financial crises as they attempt to meet unlimited healthcare needs and services with limited fiscal reimbursement. Competition has intensified, reimbursement levels have declined, and utilization controls have increased. Rapidly changing federal and state reimbursement policies make long-range budgeting and planning very difficult for healthcare facilities.

 Learning Exercise 10.5

Providing Care with Limited Reimbursement
You are the manager at a home health agency. One of your elderly patients has insulin-dependent diabetes. He has no family support. He speaks limited English and has little understanding of his disease. He lives alone. Your reimbursement from a government agency pays $90 per visit. Because this gentleman needs so much care, you find that the actual cost to your agency is $130 for each visit to him. What will be the impact to your agency if this patient is seen twice a week for three months? How can you recover the lost revenue? How can you make each visit less costly and still meet the needs of the patient?

THE MANAGED CARE MOVEMENT

Nearly 70 million Americans were enrolled in managed care health programs by the late 1990s. Broadly defined, *managed care* is a system that attempts to integrate efficiency of care, access, and cost of care. Common denominators of managed health care include panels of contracted providers, some type of limitation on benefits to subscribers who use noncontracted providers (unless authorized to do so), and some type of authorization system (Kongstvedt, 1997). Other key principles of managed care include the use of primary care physicians as "gatekeepers" to the healthcare system, a strong focus on prevention, a decreased emphasis on inpatient hospital care, the use of clinical practice guidelines for providers, selective contracting (whereby providers agree to lower reimbursement levels in exchange for patient population contracts), utilization review, the use of formularies to manage pharmacy care, and continuous quality monitoring and improvement.

Another frequent hallmark of managed care is *capitation*, whereby providers receive a fixed monthly payment regardless of what services are used by that patient during the month. If the cost of caring for a specific person is less than the capitated amount, the provider profits. If the cost is greater than the capitated amount, the provider suffers a loss. The goal, then, for capitated providers is to see that patients receive the essential services to stay healthy or to keep from becoming ill, but to eliminate unnecessary use of healthcare services. Critics of capitation argue that this reimbursement strategy leads to undertreatment of patients.

One of the most common types of managed care organizations (MCO) is the *health maintenance organization* (HMO). An HMO was originally defined as a prepaid organization that provided healthcare to voluntarily enrolled members in return for a preset amount of money on a per-person, per-month basis. With the increase in self-insured businesses or financial arrangements that do not include prepayment, this definition now generally includes two possibilities: (1) it is a licensed health plan that places at least some of the providers at risk for medical expenses, and (2) it is a health plan that utilizes designated (usually primary care) physicians as gatekeepers (although some HMOs do not) (Kongstvedt, 1997).

The Health Maintenance Organization Act of 1973 authorized spending $375 million over five years to set up and evaluate HMOs in communities across the country. Although HMOs were originally created as an alternative to traditional health insurance plans, some of the largest private insurers, including BlueCross BlueShield and Aetna, have created HMOs within their organization while maintaining their traditional indemnity plans.

In discussing HMOs, it is important to remember that there are different types of HMOs as well as different types of plans within HMOs that members may subscribe to. Several types of HMOs include: (1) *staff,* (2) *independent practice association (IPA),* (3) *group,* and (4) *network.* In staff HMOs, physician providers are salaried by the HMO and under direct control of the HMO. In IPA HMOs, the HMO contracts with a group of physicians through an intermediary to provide services for members of the HMO. In a group HMO, the HMO contracts directly with one independent physician group. In network HMOs, the HMO contracts with multiple independent physician group practices.

The types of plans available within HMOs typically vary according to the degree of provider choice available to enrollees. Two such plans include *point-of-service* (POS) and *exclusive provider organization* (EPO) options. In POS plans, the patient has the option, at the time of service, to select a provider outside the network, but pays a higher premium as well as a copayment (amount of money enrollees pay out of their pocket at the time a service is provided) for the flexibility to do so. In the EPO option, enrollees must seek care from the designated HMO provider or pay all of the cost out of pocket.

Another common type of MCO is the *preferred provider organization (PPO)*. PPOs render services on a fee-for-service basis but provide financial incentives to consumers (they pay less) when the preferred provider is used. Providers are motivated to become part of a PPO because it ensures them an adequate population of patients.

Although Medicare and Medicaid patients were historically excluded from managed care under the *free choice of physician rule*, these restrictions were lifted in the 1970s and 1980s, and these public programs began buying managed care insurance from private companies. As a result, 327 managed care plans participated in the Health Care Financing Administration (HCFA) risk contract program as of 1997, with each receiving a capitation payment equivalent to 95% of the average adjusted per capita cost (Reichard, 1997). The Health Care Financing Administration (HCFA) has recently been renamed and is now know as the Centers for Medicare and Medicaid.

MCOs receive reimbursement for Medicare-eligible patients based on a formula established by the Centers for Medicare and Medicaid, which looks at age, gender, geographic region, and the average cost per patient at a given age. Then the government gives itself a 5% discount and gives the rest to the MCO.

By 1996, 40% of Medicaid beneficiaries were enrolled in managed care, comprising more than 500 plans (Kaiser Commission on the Future of Medicaid, 1997). By 1998, all states but Alaska had waivers for their Medicaid beneficiaries to enroll in managed care plans (Barton, 1999).

A recent report, prepared by the University of California comparing fee-for-service with managed care for Medi-Cal (California's program for Medicaid) patients, suggests that managed care is a better system to improve access and health outcomes (California HealthCare Foundation, 2004). It is unclear at this time what the future of managed care will be. See **Display 10.4** for a history of healthcare reimbursement in the United States.

DRIVING AND RESTRAINING FORCES FOR THE MANAGED CARE MOVEMENT

Proponents of managed care argue that prepaid healthcare plans, such as those offered by HMOs, decrease healthcare costs between 10% and 40%, provide broader benefits for patients than under the traditional fee-for-service model, appropriately shift care from inpatient to outpatient settings, result in higher physician productivity, and have high enrollee satisfaction levels. Critics, however, suggest that participation in MCOs may result in a loss of existing physician–patient relationships, a limited

Display 10.4	**History of Healthcare Revenue Reimbursement in the United States**

Early 1930: Emergence of health insurance
Post WWII: Escalation of third-party payment for health care
1965: Medicare and Medicaid added to fee-for-service reimbursement programs
1970s: The rapid growth of HMOs begins
Early 1980s: Use of Diagnostic Related Groups and Preferred Provider Service
Late 1980s: Proliferation of the managed care and health maintenance operations (HMO)
1990 to present: The era of managed care and capitation

choice of physicians for consumers, a lower level of continuity of care, reduced physician autonomy, longer wait times for care, and consumer confusion about the many rules to be followed.

A common complaint heard from managed care subscribers is that services must be approved or authorized by a gatekeeper before services can be received or that second opinions must be obtained before surgery. Although this loss of autonomy is difficult for consumers accustomed to a fee-for-service system with few limits on choice and access, such utilization constraints are necessary due to *moral hazard*. Moral hazard refers to the propensity of insured patients to use more medical services than necessary because their insurance covers so much of the cost. Because the copayment is typically small for patients in managed care programs, the risk of moral hazard rises.

Another aspect complicating healthcare reimbursement, through the PPS, an HMO, or a PPO, is that clear and comprehensive documentation of the need for services and actual services provided is mandatory. Provision of service no longer guarantees reimbursement. Thus, the fiscal accountability of nurses goes beyond planning and implementing; it includes responsible recording and communication of activities.

Perhaps the most serious concerns about the advancement of managed care in this country are the change in the relationships among insurers, physicians, nurses, and patients. Apker's (2002) findings show that nurses held greater identification to their occupation than their employing organization. Significant factors influencing feelings were managed care changes and the effects of managed care on the nursing role.

The full impact on clinical judgment of tying physician and nursing salaries to bonuses, incentives, and penalties designed to reduce utilization of services and resources and increase profit is not known. As a result, a need for self-awareness regarding the values that guide individual professional nursing practice has never been greater.

THE FUTURE OF MANAGED CARE

Rosenbaum (1998) suggests that the transformation to managed care is one of the most important and complex changes ever to take place in the American healthcare system. "In less than a generation, a long-standing but relatively little-used model

Learning Exercise 10.6

How Does Policy Influence Your Decision?
You are the evening house supervisor of a small, private, rural hospital. In your role as house supervisor, you are responsible for staffing the upcoming shift and for troubleshooting any and all problems that cannot be handled at the unit level.

Because of legislative changes and reductions in federal monies being reimbursed to your facility over the last few years, the hospital has developed a policy that says that emergency care will be provided to indigent patients (patients who cannot pay for services) only when the patient needs immediate medical intervention and would not tolerate a transfer to county facilities, which are approximately 30 minutes away.

Tonight, you receive a call to come to the emergency room to handle a "patient complaint." When you arrive, you find a Hispanic woman in her mid-20s arguing vehemently with the emergency room charge nurse and physician. When you intercede, the patient introduces herself as Teresa Garcia and states, "There is something wrong with my father and they won't help him because we can't pay. They say we must go to the county hospital and the care he would get there will not be as good. If we had money, you would be willing to do something." The charge nurse intercedes by saying, "Teresa's father began vomiting about 2 hours ago and blacked out approximately 45 minutes ago, following a 14-hour drinking binge." The ER physician added, "Mr. Garcia's blood alcohol level is 0.25 (two and one-half times the level required to be declared legally intoxicated), and my baseline physical examination would indicate nothing other than he is drunk and needs to sleep it off. Besides, I have seen Mr. Garcia in the ER before, and it's always for the same thing. If he wants further treatment, it should be provided at the county facility."

Teresa persists in her pleas to you that "there is something different this time" and that she believes this hospital should evaluate her father further. She intuitively feels that something terrible will happen to her father if he is not cared for immediately. The ER physician becomes even angrier after this comment and states to you, "I am not going to waste my time and energy on someone who is just drunk, and I refuse to order any more expensive lab tests or x-rays on this patient. If you want something else done, you will have to find someone else to order it." With that, he walks off and returns to the examination room, where other patients are waiting to be seen. The ER nurse turns to look at you and is waiting for further directions.

Assignment: How will you handle this situation? Would your decision be any easier if there were no limitations in resource allocation? Are your values to act as an agent for the patient or the agency more strongly developed?

of healthcare financing and service delivery has become the healthcare norm" (p. 68). Instead of insurers and purchasers shouldering the financial risks of health care, a new model has emerged in which financing and service delivery have become integrated; health care is sold and controlled by large companies; and practitioners and institutions bear much of the financial risk for the cost of care (Rosenbaum, 1998).

Many nurse leaders are concerned that in the economic debate, the caring component of nursing has been lost. Furthermore, nurses have been slow to document the economic importance of a caring relationship between nurses and their patients (Turkel, 2001). Turkel says that initially in the Clinton healthcare reform proposal, nursing was identified as a key resource for maintaining quality while decreasing costs; however, over the past 10 years the healthcare environment has changed rapidly and pressure in terms of managed care and corporatization of health care has had a tremendous impact upon both nursing and hospitals. Nursing is entering a new reality for practice that is controlled by costs.

Managed care is not going to go away—at least, not any time soon. Although it permeates the current healthcare system, it remains unclear if managed care, as we know it today, will change significantly in the future. However, it is apparent that nurses in all roles need at least a basic understanding of healthcare costs and how reimbursement strategies directly and indirectly affect their practice. Only then will nurses be able to be active participants in the proactive and visionary fiscal planning required to survive in the current healthcare marketplace.

> Many nurse leaders are concerned that in the economic debate, the caring component of nursing has been lost.

INTEGRATING LEADERSHIP ROLES AND MANAGEMENT FUNCTIONS IN FISCAL PLANNING

Managers must understand fiscal terminology, be aware of their budgetary responsibilities, and be accountable to the organization for maintaining a cost-effective unit. The ability to forecast unit fiscal needs with sensitivity to the organization's economic, social, and legislative climate is a high-level management function. In budgeting, managers also must be able to articulate unit needs to ensure sufficient funds for adequate nursing staff, supplies, and equipment. Finally, managers must be skillful in the monitoring aspects of budget control.

Leadership skills allow the manager to involve in fiscal planning all people who will be affected by the plan. Other leadership skills required in fiscal planning include flexibility, creativity, and vision regarding future needs. The skilled leader is able to anticipate budget constraints and act proactively.

In contrast, many managers allow budget constraints to dictate alternatives. In an age of inadequate fiscal resources, the leader is creative in identifying alternatives to meet patient needs. The skilled leader, however, also ensures that cost containment does not jeopardize patient safety.

Leaders also are assertive, articulate people who ensure that their department's budgeting receives a fair hearing. Because leaders can delineate unit budgetary needs in an assertive, professional, and proactive manner, they generally obtain a fair distribution of resources for their unit.

❈ Key Concepts

- Fiscal planning, as in all types of planning, is a learned skill that improves with practice.
- Historically, nursing management played a limited role in determining resource allocation in healthcare institutions.
- Today, the nursing budget often accounts for the majority of the organization's total expenses.
- The desired outcome of budgeting is maximal use of resources to meet organizational short- and long-term needs.
- The budget's value to the institution is directly related to its accuracy.
- A budget is at best a forecast or prediction; it is a plan and not a rule. Therefore, a budget must be flexible and open to ongoing evaluation and revision.
- The largest expenditure is in workforce because health care is *labor intensive.*
- Most staffing is based on a predetermined standard that varies with each unit, department, organization, or service.
- Personnel budgets include actual worked time (productive time or salary expense) and time the organization pays the employee for not working (nonproductive or benefit time).
- The operating budget reflects expenses that flex up or down in a predetermined manner to reflect variation in volume of service provided.
- Capital budgets plan for the purchase of buildings or major equipment. This includes equipment that has a long life (usually greater than five years), is not used daily, and is more expensive than operating supplies.
- A budget that is predicted too far in advance is open to greater error. If the budget is shortsighted, compensating for unexpected major expenses or capital equipment purchases may be difficult.
- Managers must rejustify their program or needs every budgeting cycle in *zero-based budgeting.* Using a "*decision package*" to set funding priorities is a key feature of zero-based budgeting.
- With the advent of state and federal reimbursement for health care in the 1960s, providers were forced to submit budgets and costs to payers that more accurately reflected their actual cost to provide these services.
- With DRGs, hospitals join the prospective payment system (PPS), whereby they receive a specified amount for each Medicare patient's admission, regardless of the actual cost of care. Exceptions occur when the provider can demonstrate that a patient's case is an "outlier," meaning that the cost of providing care for that patient justifies extra payment.
- Key principles of managed care include the use of primary care physicians as "*gatekeepers*" to the healthcare system, a strong focus on prevention, a decreased emphasis on inpatient hospital care, the use of clinical practice guidelines for providers, selective contracting (whereby providers agree to lower reimbursement levels in exchange for patient population contracts), capitation, utilization review, the use of formularies to manage pharmacy care, and continuous quality monitoring and improvement.

- The types of plans available within HMOs typically vary according to the degree of provider choice available to enrollees. In *point-of-service* (POS) plans, the patient has the option, at the time of service, to select a provider outside the network, but pays a higher premium as well as copayment for the flexibility to do so. In the *exclusive provider organization* (EPO), enrollees must seek care from the designated HMO provider or pay all of the cost out of pocket.
- Managed care has altered the relationships among insurers, physicians, nurses, and patients, with providers today often having to assume a role as agent for the patient as well as agent of resource allocation for an insurance carrier, hospital, or particular practice plan.

More Learning Exercises and Applications

 Learning Exercise 10.7

Weighing Choices in Budget Spending

One of your goals as the unit manager of a critical care unit is to prepare all your nurses to be certified in advanced cardiac life support. You currently have five staff nurses who need this certification. You can hire someone to teach this class locally and rent a facility for $800; however, the cost will be taken out of the travel and education budget for the unit, and this will leave you short for the rest of the fiscal year. It also will be a time-consuming effort because you must coordinate the preparation and reproduction of educational materials needed for the course and make arrangements for the rental facility. A certification class also will be provided in the near future in a large city approximately 150 miles from the hospital. The cost per participant will be $200. In addition, there would be travel and lodging expenses.

Assignment: You have several decisions to make. Should the class be held locally? If so, how will you organize it? Are you going to require your staff to have this certification or merely highly recommend that they do so? If it is required, will the unit pay the costs of the certification? Will you pay the staff nurses their regular hourly wage for attending the class on regularly scheduled work hours? Can this certification be cost effective? Use group process in some way to make your decision.

Learning Exercise 10.8

How Will You Meet New Budget Restrictions?
You are the director of the local aging agency, which cares for ill and well elderly. You are funded by a private corporation grant, which requires matching of city and state funds. You have received a letter in the mail today from the state that says state funding will be cut by $20,000, effective in two weeks, when the state's budget year begins. This means that your private funding also will be cut $15,000, for a total revenue loss of $40,000. It is impossible at this time to seek alternative funding sources.

In reviewing your agency budget, you note that, as in many healthcare agencies, your budget is labor intensive. More than 80% of your budget is attributable to personnel costs, and you believe that the cuts must come from within the personnel budget. You may reduce the patient population that you serve, although you do not really want to do so. You briefly discuss this communication with your staff; no one is willing to reduce his or her hours voluntarily, and no one is planning to terminate his or her employment at any time in the near future.

Assignment: Given the following brief description of your position and each of your five employees, decide how you will meet the new budget restrictions. What is the rationale for your choice? What decision do you believe will result in the least disruption of the agency and of the employees in the agency? Should group decision making be involved in fiscal decisions such as this one? Can fiscal decisions such as this be made without value judgments?

Your position is project director. As the project director, you coordinate all the day-to-day activities in the agency. You also are involved in long-term planning, and a major portion of your time is allotted to securing future funding for the agency to continue. As the project director, you have the authority to hire and fire employees. You are in your early 30s and have a master's degree in nursing and health administration. You enjoy your job and believe you have done well in this position since you started four years ago. Your yearly salary as a full-time employee is $60,000.

Employee #1 is Mrs. Potter. Mrs. Potter has worked at the agency since it started seven years ago. She is an RN with 30 years experience working with the geriatric population in public health nursing, care facilities, and private duty. She plans to retire in seven years and travel with her independently wealthy husband. Mrs. Potter has a great deal of expertise she can share with your staff, although at times you believe she overshadows your authority because of her experience and your young age. Her yearly salary as a full-time employee is $50,000.

Employee #2 is Mr. Boone. Mr. Boone has BS degrees in both nursing and dietetics and food management. As an RN and RD, he brings a unique expertise to your staff, which is highly needed when dealing with a chronically ill and improperly nourished elderly population. In the six months since he joined your agency, he has proven to be a dependable, well-liked, and highly respected member of your staff. His yearly salary as a full-time employee is $44,000.

Employee #3 is Miss Barns. Miss Barns is the receptionist/secretary in the agency. In addition to all the traditional secretarial duties, such as typing, filing, and transcription of dictation, she screens incoming telephone calls and directs people who come to the agency for information. Her efficiency is a tremendous attribute to the agency. Her full-time yearly salary is $16,000.

Employee #4 is Ms. Lake. Ms. Lake is an LPN/LVN with 15 years of work experience in a variety of healthcare agencies. She is especially attuned to patient needs. Although her technical nursing skills are also good, her caseload frequently is more focused around elderly who need companionship and emotional support. She does well at patient teaching because of her outstanding listening and communication skills. Many of your patients request her by name. She is a single mother, supporting six children, and you are aware that she has great difficulty in meeting her personal financial obligations. Her full-time yearly salary is $30,000.

Employee #5 is Mrs. Long. Mrs. Long is an "elderly help aide." She has completed nurse aide training, although her primary role in the agency is to assist well elderly with bathing, meal preparation, driving, and shopping. The time Mrs. Long spends in performing basic care has decreased the average visit time for each member of your staff by 30%. She is widowed and believes that she needs this job to meet her social and self-esteem needs. Financially, her resources are adequate, and the money she earns is not a motivator for working. Mrs. Long works three days a week, and her yearly salary is $10,000.

Learning Exercise 10.9

Identifying, Prioritizing, and Choosing Program Goals

Jane is the supervisor of a small cardiac rehabilitation program. The program includes inpatient cardiac teaching and an outpatient exercise rehabilitation program. Because of limited reimbursement by third-party insurance payers for patient education, there has been no direct charge for inpatient education. Outpatient program participants pay $120/month to attend three one-hour sessions per week, although the revenue generated from the outpatient program still leaves an overall budget deficit for the program of approximately $1,200/month.

Today, Jane is summoned to the associate administrator's office to discuss her budget for the upcoming year. At this meeting, the administrator states that the hospital is experiencing extreme financial difficulties due to DRGs and the prospective payment system. He states that the program must become self-supporting in the next fiscal year, or services must be cut. On returning to her office, Jane decided to make a list of several alternatives for problem solving and to analyze each for driving and restraining factors. These alternatives include the following:

1. Implement a charge for inpatient education. This would eliminate the budget deficit, but the cost would probably have to be borne by the patient. (Implication: Only patients with adequate fiscal resources would select to receive vital education.)
2. Reduce department staffing. There are currently three staff members in the department, and it would be impossible to maintain the same level or quality of services if staffing were cut.
3. Reduce or limit services. The inpatient education program or educational programs associated with the outpatient program could be eliminated. These are both considered valuable aspects of the program.
4. The fee for the outpatient program could be increased. This could easily result in a decrease in program participation, because many outpatient program participants do not have insurance coverage for their participation.

Assignment: Identify at least five program goals, and prioritize them as you would if you were Jane. Based on the priorities you have established, which alternative would you select? Explain your choice.

Learning Exercise 10.10

Addressing Conflicting Values

You are a single parent of two children younger than five years and are currently employed as a pediatric office nurse. You enjoy your job, but your long-term career goal is to become a pediatric nurse practitioner, and you have been taking courses part time preparing to enter graduate school in the fall. Your application for admission has been accepted, and the next cycle for admissions will not be for another three years. Your recent divorce and assignment of sole custody of the children have resulted in a need for you to reconsider your plan.

Restraining Forces: You had originally planned to reduce your work hours to part time to allow time for classes and studying, but this will be fiscally impossible now. You also recognize that tuition and educational expenses will place a strain on your budget even if you continue to work full time. You have not looked into the availability of scholarships or loans and have missed the deadline for the upcoming fall. In addition, you have not yet overcome your anxiety and guilt about leaving your small children for even more time than you do now.

Driving Forces: You also recognize, however, that gaining certification as a pediatric nurse practitioner should result in a large salary increase over what you are able to make as an office nurse and that it would allow you to provide resources for your children in the future that you otherwise may be unable to do. You also recognize that although you are not dissatisfied with your current job, you have a great deal of ability that has gone untapped and that your potential for long-term job satisfaction is low.

Assignment: Fiscal planning always requires priority setting, and often this priority setting is determined by personal values. Priority setting is made even more difficult when there are conflicting values. Identify the values involved in this case. Develop a plan that addresses these value conflicts and has the most desirable outcomes.

Learning Exercise 10.11

How Would You Change This Budget?

Today is April 1, and you have received the following budget printout. Your charge nurses are requesting an additional RN on each shift since the acuity has increased dramatically over the last two years. Dr. Robb has requested two new continuous limb movement machines for the postoperative orthopedic patients on your unit at a cost of $3,000 each. In addition, you would like to attend a national orthopedics conference in New York in August at a projected cost of $1,500. The registration fee is $350 and is due now.

	Annual Budget	Expended in March	Expended Year to Date[*]	Amount Remaining
Personnel	300,000	25,000	175,000	125,000
Overtime	50,000	3,800	50,000	0
Supplies	18,000	1,500	13,500	4,500
Travel (personal)	2,200	0	1,700	500
Equipment	5,000	0	5,000	0
Staff development (personal)	1,000	200	800	200

[*]Fiscal year begins July 1

Assignment: How will you deal with these requests based on the budget printout? What expenses can and should be deferred to the new fiscal year? In what budgeting area were your previous projections most accurate? Most inaccurate? What factors may have contributed to these inaccuracies? Were they controllable or predictable?

Web Links

Medicare, Medicaid, and State Children's Health Insurance Program
http://www.cms.hhs.gov/
Introduces the Medicare, Medicaid, and the State Children's Health Insurance Program.

The Resource Directory for Older People
http://www.aoa.dhhs.gov
A cooperative effort of the National Institute on Aging and the Administration on Aging Agency for Health Care Policy.

U.S. Department of Health and Human Services
http://www.os.dhhs.gov
The United States government's principal agency for protecting the health of all Americans and providing essential human services.

Managed Care Magazine
http://www.managedcaremag.com
A guide for managed care executives and physicians covering capitation, compensation, and disease management.

Managed care/healthcare economics terms
http://www.amso.com/terms.html
A dictionary of terms common to managed care and healthcare economics discussions.

References

Apker, J. (2002). Communication: Improving RNs' organizational and professional identification in managed care hospitals. *Journal of Nursing Administration, 32*(2),106–114.

Barton, P. L. (1999). *Understanding the U.S. health services system.* Chicago: Health Administration Press.

California HealthCare Foundation. (2004). Preventing unnecessary hospitalizations in Medi-Cal: Comparing fee-for-service with managed care. Available at University of California San Francisco's Primary Care Research website: http://www.chcf.org/topics/medi-cal.

Carruth, A. K., Carruth, P. J., & Noto, E. C. (2000). Nurse managers flex their budgetary might. *Nursing Management, 31*(2), 16–17.

Chang, C. F, Price, S. A., & Pfoutz, S. K. (2001). *Economics and nursing: Critical professional issues.* Philadelphia: F. A. Davis Co.

Contino, D. S. (2001). Budget training: It's overdue. *Nursing Management, 32*(8), 16–17.

Contino, D. S. (2002). Breaking even: How low can you go? *Nursing Management, 33*(8), 11–15.

De Luc, K. (2000). Care pathways: An evaluation of their effectiveness. *Journal of Advanced Nursing, 32*(2), 485–496.

Kaiser Commission on the Future of Medicaid. (1997). *Medicaid and managed care.* Washington, D.C.: Kaiser Family Foundation.

Kirkby, M. P. (2003). Number crunching with variable budgets. *Nursing Management, 34*(3), 28–35.

Kongstvedt, P. R. (1997). *Essentials of managed care* (2nd ed.). Gaithersburg, MD: Aspen Publications, Inc.

Reichard, J. (Ed.). (1997). Briefly this week. *Medicine and Health, 50*(37), 4.

Renholm, M., Leino-Kilpi, H., & Suominen, T. (2002). Critical pathways: A systematic review. *Nursing Management, 32*(4), 196–202.

Rosenbaum, S. (1998). Negotiating the new health system: Purchasing publicly accountable managed care. *American Journal of Preventive Medicine, 14*(3S), 67–71.

Turkel, M. C. (2001). Struggling to find a balance: The paradox between caring and economics. *Nursing Administration Quarterly, 26*(1), 67–82.

Zarabozo, C., & LeMasurier, J. D. (1997). Chapter 26: Medicare and managed care. In P. R. Kongstvedt (Ed.), *Essentials of managed health care* (2nd ed.). Gaithersburg, MD: Aspen Publishers, Inc.

Bibliography

Adom, N. K., (2001). An expanded professional role: Increasing hospital reimbursement. *Journal of Nursing Administration, 31*(1), 7–8.

Angart, B. (2002). Surviving in stagnant industries. *The Journal of Corporate Renewal, 15*(2), 14.

Becker, D. S. (2000). Budget basics: 10 steps to create correct & comprehensive annual budgets. *EMS- Manager and Supervisor, 3*(4), 1–2.

Bell, S. E. (2003). Ethical climate in managed care organizations. *Nursing Administration Quarterly, 27*(2), 133–139.

Breser, C., & Kovner, C. T. (2001). Is there another nursing shortage? What the data tell us. *Nursing Outlook, 49*(1), 20–26.

Burke, R. J. (2001). Surviving hospital restructuring. *Journal of Nursing Administration, 31*(4), 169–172.

Carter, M. (2002). Rural nurse managers' use of a labor computer decision support system. *Nursing Economic$, 20*(5), 237–243.

Copeland, H. L. (2003). Managed care education for nurses: Practices and proposals. *Nursing Economic$ 21*(1), 24–30.

Fitzpatrick, M. A. (2002). Let's bring balance back to care. *Nursing Management, 33*(3), 56.

Harrison, F. G., & Kuhlemeier, K. A. (2001). How do skilled nursing rehabilitation managers track efficiency and costs? *Journal of Allied Health, 30*(1), 43–47.

Kiel, J. M. (2003). Electronic managed care: the utilization of information technology in a managed care environment. *Health Care Manager, 33*(1), 52–59.

Career Development

Every individual you hire for a leadership role should have the capability to grow into your role.

—Carolyn Hope Smeltzer

• Avoids obsolescence and builds new skills. Due to the rapid changes in the healthcare industry, especially in the areas of consumer demands and technology, employees may find that their skills have become obsolete. A successful career development program begins to retrain employees proactively, providing them with the necessary skills to remain current in their field and therefore valuable to the organization. Retraining also provides employees with an opportunity to survive downsizing.

Johnstone (2003) found that the main reason nurse–managers left their jobs was to seek career development elsewhere. Although no longer able to provide workers with jobs for life, organizations can offer skills to enable workers to thrive in chaos. Tuttas (2002) says that career development strategies to retain nurses in today's scarce market are essential. Some of the most basic career development programs, such as financial planning and general equivalency diploma (GED) programs can be the most rewarding programs for the staff.

> Career development strategies to retain nurses in today's scarce market are essential.

CAREER STAGES

Before managers can plan a successful career development program, they need to understand the normal career stages of individuals, because people require different types of development in different stages of their careers

McNeese-Smith (2000) suggests there are three different job stages among nurses: *entry, master,* and *disengagement.* Entry is the process of involvement, skill development, and increasing congruity between an individual's self-conception and his or her role in the job. Group membership follows a period of training, orientation, and supervision. If the employee is socialized appropriately, he or she begins to become an "insider."

Mastery begins with the new member having advanced beginner skills, possessing some job esteem, and moving toward seniority, expertise, and high esteem. This is a time of accomplishment, challenge, and a sense of purpose, and the individual often achieves a high enough level of expertise to be a role model to others. However, as the member gains experience and skills, his or her ideal concept of the position begins to decrease.

The last stage, disengagement, commences if the congruency and relationship between self-identity and job identity begins to decline. The focus of identity shifts to something else and the job no longer provides growth and a relevant sense of identity. Thus, the employee may become bored and indifferent to the job. Friends leave or are promoted, the system changes, and the future suggests increasing frustration as the employee can become confined at a level where performance and behavior steadily decline.

In McNeese-Smith's (2000) survey of 412 nurses in three hospitals, 13% identified themselves as being in the entry stage, with their average time on the job of 1.6 years. Sixty-two percent identified themselves as in the mastery stage, with an average of 7.2 years on the job, although the percentage of nurses in mastery was highest between two and three years on the job (83%) and tended to decrease with increased time on the job until reaching a low of 40% after 25 to 30 years on the job.

Twenty-four percent of nurses were in the disengagement stage, with an average of 9.86 years on the job. The percentage of nurses who reported disengagement increased from a low of 4% in the first six months to a high of 60% after 25 to 30 years on the job.

The implications for career development based on this study are enormous. Clearly, boredom and job indifference leading to disengagement increase with time in the same job. Thus, managers must offer support for a continuous, challenging career program for employees that includes support for advanced degrees and certification as well as specialty skills and job transfer.

> The percentage of nurses who reported disengagement increased from a low of 4% in the first six months to a high of 60% after 25 to 30 years on the job.

Learning Exercise 11.1

Exploring Career Stages
In a group, discuss the job stages described by McNeese-Smith. What stage most closely reflects your present situation? In what stages of their careers are nurses that you know (colleagues, managers, your nursing instructors)? Do you believe male and female nurses have similar or dissimilar career stages.

THE ORGANIZATION'S RESPONSIBILITY FOR CAREER MANAGEMENT

Both the manager and the individual staff member have responsibilities for career development. In addition to understanding the various stages of careers, managers should be able to differentiate between the organization's and the individual's responsibilities for career development. A list of both the individual and the organizational components of career development can be seen in **Display 11.3.**

Display 11.3 The Components of Career Development

Career Planning (Individual)
- Self-assess interests, skills, strengths, weaknesses, and values.
- Determine goals.
- Assess the organization for opportunities.
- Assess opportunities outside the organization.
- Develop strategies.
- Implement plans.
- Evaluate plans.
- Reassess and make new plans as necessary, at least biannually.

Career Management (Organizational)
- Integrate individual employee needs with organizational needs.
- Establish, design, communicate, and implement career paths.
- Disseminate career information.
- Post and communicate all job openings.
- Assess employees' career needs.
- Provide work experience for development.
- Give support and encouragement.
- Develop new personnel policies as necessary.
- Provide training and education.

Career management focuses on the responsibilities of the organization for career development. In career management, the organization creates career paths and advancement ladders. It also attempts to match position openings with appropriate people. This includes accurately assessing employees' performance and potential in order to offer the most appropriate career guidance, education, and training. Many of the organizational responsibilities outlined in Display 11.3 are discussed elsewhere in this book and therefore are only mentioned here. These organizational responsibilities include the following:

- **Integration of needs.** The human resources department, nursing division, nursing units, and education department must work and plan together to match job openings with the skills and talents of present employees.
- **Establishment of career paths.** Not only must career paths be developed, but they also must be communicated to the staff and implemented consistently. Although various career ladders have been present for some time, they are still not widely used. This problem is not unique to nursing. Even when healthcare organizations design and use a career structure, the system often breaks down once the nurse leaves that organization. For example, nurses at the level of clinical nurse 3 in one hospital will usually lose that status when they leave the organization for another position. When designing career paths, each successive job in each path should contain additional responsibilities and duties that are greater than the previous jobs in that path. Each successive job also must be related to and use previous skills. Once career paths are established, they must be communicated effectively to all concerned staff. What employees must do to advance in a particular path should be very clear.
- **Dissemination of career information.** The education department, human resources department, and unit manager are all responsible for sharing career information. Employees should not be encouraged to pursue unrealistic goals.
- **Posting of job openings.** Although this is usually the responsibility of the human resources department, the manager should communicate this information, even when it means that one of the unit staff may transfer to another area. Effective managers know who needs to be encouraged to apply for openings and who is ready for more responsibility and challenges.
- **Assessment of employees.** One of the benefits of a good appraisal system is the important information it gives the manager on the performance, potential, and abilities of all staff members. The use of long-term coaching will give managers insight into their employees' needs and wants so that appropriate career counseling will occur.
- **Provision of challenging assignments.** Planned work experience is one of the most powerful career development tools. This includes jobs that temporarily stretch employees to their maximum skill, temporary projects, assignment to committees, shift rotation, assignment to different units, or shift charge duties.
- **Giving support and encouragement.** Because excellent subordinates make managers' jobs easier, they are often reluctant to encourage these subordinates to move up the corporate ladder or to seek more challenging experiences outside the manager's span of control. Thus, many managers hoard

their talent. A leadership role requires that managers look beyond their immediate unit or department and consider the needs of the entire organization. Leaders recognize and share talent.

- **Development of personnel policies.** An active career development program often results in the recognition that certain personnel policies and procedures are impeding the success of the program. When this occurs, the organization should reexamine these policies and make necessary changes.
- **Provision of education and training.** The impact of education and training on career development and retention of subordinate staff was discussed previously. The need for organizations to provide for the development of leaders and managers is presented later in this chapter.

COMPETENCY ASSESSMENT AND SPECIALTY CERTIFICATION AS PART OF CAREER MANAGEMENT

Competency assessment and *professional specialty certification* are also a part of career management. Managers should appraise each employee's competency level as part of the performance appraisal process. This appraisal should lead to the development of a performance plan that outlines what the nurse must do to achieve desired competencies in his or her current position. Often, however, competency assessment as part of the performance appraisal process focuses on whether the employee has achieved required minimal competency levels to meet federal, state, or organizational standards. Competency assessment and goal setting in career planning should help the employee identify how to exceed these levels of competency as well as to identify competencies the employee may wish or need to achieve in the future. Thus, competency assessment and goal setting in career planning are more proactive, with the employee identifying areas of potential future growth and the manager assisting in identifying strategies that would help the employee achieve that goal.

Professional specialty certification is one way an employee can demonstrate advanced achievement of competencies. Professional associations grant specialty certification as a formal but voluntary process of demonstrating expertise in a particular area of nursing (Chitty, 2001). For example, the American Nurses Association established the ANA Certification Program in 1973 to provide tangible recognition of professional achievement in a defined functional or clinical area of nursing. The American Nurses Credentialing Center (ANCC) became its own corporation, a subsidiary of ANA, in 1991 and since then has certified more than 151,000 nurses throughout the United States and its territories in more than 30 specialty and advanced practice areas of nursing. A few of the other organizations offering specialty certifications for nurses are the American Association of Critical Care Nursing, the American Association of Nurse Anesthetists, the American College of Nurse Midwives, the Board of Certification for Emergency Nursing, and the Rehabilitation Nursing Certification Board.

While the role for nurses continues to evolve, ANCC has responded positively to the reconceptualization of certification and "Open Door 2000," a program that enables all qualified registered nurses, regardless of their educational preparation, to become certified in any of five specialty areas: gerontology, medical-surgical, pediatrics, perinatal, and psychiatric and mental health nursing.

LONG-TERM COACHING

Short-term coaching is a means to develop and motivate employees. It should be a spontaneous part of the experienced manager's repertoire. *Long-term coaching*, on the other hand, is a planned management action that occurs over the duration of employment. Savage (2001) suggests that it is, in essence, an organizational intervention focused at the individual level; that is, it is an intervention to help employees deal with their responses to organizational concerns or needs.

Because this form of coaching may cover a long period of time, it is frequently neglected unless the manager uses a systematic scheduling plan for coaching conferences and a form for documentation. Although long-term documentation has been used successfully to track an employee's deficiencies, documenting long-term coaching for career development has been less successful. Because employees and managers move frequently within an organization, the lack of record-keeping regarding employees' career needs has deterred nursing career development. In the present climate of organizational restructuring and downsizing, a manager's staff is even more in need of career coaching, and documentation of the career coaching takes on an even more important role.

Long-term coaching is a major step in building an effective team and an excellent strategy to increase productivity and retention. In fact, a survey of 100 executives from Fortune 1000 companies revealed a 53% increase in organizational productivity, a 61% rise in managerial job satisfaction, and a 39% increase in the managerial retention rate as a result of executive coaching (Manchester Inc., 2000).

Long-term coaching has some of the same attributes of a mentoring relationship but is less intense and is not limited to one or a few subordinates. In fact, *team coaching* (coaching as a group) is possible, but it is generally focused on a specific event or situation facing executive teams (Savage, 2001).

 Learning Exercise 11.2

Encouragement and Coaching to Move Toward Goals
In your employment have you ever had someone coach you in either a formal or informal way, to encourage you to develop your career? For example, has someone you worked for told you about career or educational opportunities? Have any companies you worked for offered tuition reimbursement? If so, how did you find out about such policies? Have you ever coached (something more than just encouraging) someone else to pursue educational or career goals? Share the answers to these questions in class.

THE STRUCTURED COACHING INTERVIEW

The effective manager has at least one coaching session with each employee annually, in addition to any coaching that may occur during the appraisal interview. Although some coaching should occur during the performance appraisal interview, additional coaching should be planned at a less stressful time. **Display 11.4** is an example of a long-term coaching progress form.

Curran (2003) suggests that there is a lack of career development programs in the healthcare arena and having such a program in place is one way to become the employer of choice. Succession planning through effective career coaching is one means to improve career development in the workplace (Smeltzer, 2002). This type of coaching has several vital components that are discussed in the following three phases:

1. **Gathering data.** One of the best methods of gathering data about employees is to observe their behavior. When managers spend time observing employees, they are able to determine who has good communication skills, is well organized, is able to use effective negotiating skills, and works collaboratively. Managers also should seek information about the employee's past work experience, performance appraisals, and educational experiences. Data also can include academic qualifications and credentials. Most of this information can be obtained by examining the personnel file. Finally, employees themselves are an excellent source of information that can assist the manager in the long-term coaching interview. All these sources of data should be reviewed before the coaching interview.

2. **What is possible?** As part of career planning, the manager should assess the department for possible changes in the future, openings or transfers, and potential challenges and opportunities. The manager should anticipate what type of needs lie ahead, what projects are planned, and what staffing and budget changes will occur. After carefully assessing the employee's profile and future opportunities, managers should consider each staff member and ask the following questions: How can this employee be helped so that he or she is better prepared to take advantage of the future? Who needs to be encouraged to return to school, to become credentialed, or to take a special course? Which employees need to be encouraged to transfer to a more challenging position, given more responsibility on their present unit, or moved to another shift? Managers are able to create a stimulating environment for career development by being aware of the uniqueness of their employees.

> Managers are able to create a stimulating environment for career development by being aware of the **uniqueness** of their employees.

3. **The coaching interview session.** The goals of the career development coaching interview are to help employees increase their effectiveness, see where potential opportunities in the organization lie, and advance their knowledge, skills, and experience. Many of the techniques and guidelines listed in the post-appraisal interview also are useful in the coaching interview. It is important not to intimidate employees when questioning them about their future and their goals. Although there is no standard procedure

Display 11.4 Sample Long-term Coaching Form

Name of employee _____

Name of supervisor _____

Date _____ Date of last coaching interview _____

1. What new challenges and responsibilities could be given to this employee that would utilize his or her special talents?

   _____

   _____

2. What events happening in the organization do you foresee affecting this employee? (Examples would be plans to go to an all-RN staff, changing the mode of patient care delivery, increasing emphasis on credentialing by the new CEO of the nursing division, changing the medication system, and changing the ratio of nonprofessionals to professionals for nurse staffing.)

   _____

   _____

3. How should the employee be preparing to meet new or changing expectations?

   _____

   _____

4. What specific suggestions and guidance for the future can you give this employee? (Examples would be taking specific courses to prepare for change, urging them to pursue an advanced degree, considering changing shifts, urging them to seek challenges outside of your unit, and suggesting that they apply for the next management opening.)

   _____

   _____

5. What specific organizational resources can you offer the employee?

   _____

   _____

6. What new information regarding this employee's long-term plans, aspirations, and potential have the perusal of the personnel record, your observations, and this interview given you?

   _____

   _____

7. Do the organizational and professional career plans held by the individual match your vision of his or her future? If not, how do they differ?

   _____

   _____

8. What developmental and professional growth has taken place since the last coaching session?

   _____

   _____

9. Date of next coaching interview _____

for conducting the interview, the main emphasis should be on employee growth and development. The manager can assist the employee in exploring future options. Coaching sessions give the manager a chance to discover potential future managers—employees who should then begin to be groomed for a future managerial role in subsequent coaching sessions.

Both the performance-appraisal interview and the coaching session provide opportunities to assist employees in the growth and development necessary for expanded roles and responsibilities. A major leadership role is the development of subordinate staff. This interest in the future of individual employees plays a vital role in retention and productivity.

Learning Exercise 11.3

Why Won't Beth Apply for Your Position?
You have been the evening charge nurse of a large surgical unit for the last four years. Each year, you perform a career development conference with all your licensed staff.

These sessions are held separately from the performance-appraisal interviews. You have been extremely pleased with the results of these conferences. Two of your LVNs/LPNs are now enrolled in an RN program. Several of the RNs from your unit have obtained advanced clinical positions, and many have returned to school. As a result of your encouragement and support, several of the nurses have taken charge positions on other units. You are proud of your ability to recognize talent and to perform successful career counseling.

This is the last time you will be performing career counseling, because you have resigned your position to return to graduate school. You have encouraged several of the staff to apply for your position but think one particular nurse, Beth, a 34-year-old woman, would be exceptional. She is extremely capable clinically, is very mature, is well respected by everyone, and has excellent interpersonal skills. Beth only works four days a week but has been invaluable to you in the four years since you have been charge nurse. However, Beth is one of the few nurses who has never acted on any of your suggestions at previous career-coaching interviews.

Last week, you had another coaching interview with Beth and told her of your plans. You urged her to apply for your position and told her you would recommend her to your supervisor, although you would not be making the final selection. Beth told you she would think about it, and today she told you that she does not wish to apply for the position. You are very disappointed and believe that perhaps you have failed in some way.

Assignment: Examine this scenario carefully. Make a list of the possible reasons that Beth declined the promotion. Be creative. Were the coaching sessions valuable or a waste of your time? Compare your findings with others in the group. After comparison, determine what influence, if any, values had on the development of the lists.

TRANSFERS

A *transfer* may be defined as a reassignment to another job within the organization. In a strict business sense, a transfer usually implies similar pay, status, and responsibility. Because of the variety of positions available for nurses in any healthcare organization, coupled with the lack of sufficient higher-level positions available, two additional terms have come into use. A *lateral transfer* describes one staff person moving to another unit, to a position with a similar scope of responsibilities, within the same organization. A *downward transfer* occurs when someone takes a position within the organization that is below his or her previous level. This frequently happens in health care. An example is when a charge nurse decides to learn another nursing specialty. For example, the nurse may step down from a charge position on a medical-surgical unit to a staff position in labor and delivery. It may be in a nurse's interest to consider a downward transfer because it often increases the chances of long-term career success. For example, a nurse's long-term career goal might be to hold a position in cardiac rehabilitation. The nurse determines that most of the cardiac rehabilitation staff are hired out of the hospital's critical care unit (CCU). Although this nurse has had previous experience in a cardiac care unit, he or she has not held that position in this organization. The nurse requests a downward transfer from an evening charge position on a surgical unit to day-shift staff nurse in the CCU. This transfer will provide the nurse with current experience in CCU and more exposure to the manager of the cardiac rehabilitation unit. In this example, a downward transfer increases the likelihood that the nurse's long-term goal will be realized.

Downward transfers also should be considered when nurses are experiencing periods of stress or role overload. Self-aware nurses often request such transfers. In some circumstances, the manager may need to intervene and use a downward transfer to alleviate temporarily a nurse's overwhelming stress.

Another type of transfer may accommodate employees in the later stages of their career. Managers often assist valuable employees who desire a reduced role in their careers to locate a position that will use their talents and still allow them a degree of status. These *accommodating transfers* generally allow someone to receive a similar salary but with a reduction in energy expenditure. For example, a long-time employee might be given a position as ombudsman to use his or her expertise and knowledge of the organization and at the same time assume a status position that is less physically demanding.

Inappropriate Transfers

One deterrent to successful career development is the inappropriate transfer. One method managers use to solve unit personnel problems is to transfer problem employees to another unsuspecting department. Such transfers are harmful in many ways. They contribute to decreased productivity, are demotivating for all employees, and are especially destructive for the employee who is transferred.

This is not to say that employees who do not "fit" in one department will not do well in a different environment. It is not uncommon for an employee to struggle in one department but improve his or her performance in a new department or unit. Before such transfers, however, both the manager and the employee must speak candidly with each other regarding the employee's capabilities and the manager's expectations. All types of transfers should be individually evaluated for appropriateness.

Learning Exercise 11.4

How Would You Handle This Transfer Request?
You are the manager of a surgical unit. Many novice nurses apply to your unit for the purpose of perfecting their basic skills before transferring to a specialty unit. Although this is somewhat frustrating to you, you recognize that you can do little about it.

The hospital policy dictates that nurses requesting another position must fill out a "request for transfer" form when they apply for the new position. This form, which must be completed by their current manager, contains information regarding when they can be released from their present position for the new position and a current appraisal of their work performance.

Today, you find another "request for transfer" form on your desk. However, when you read the name on the form, you feel a sense of relief rather than despair. The nurse requesting the transfer is one of your more difficult employees. Scott Powell is a very qualified nurse but he is frequently absent from work, is very critical of the other nurses' work performance, and is generally unpleasant to be around. During the two years he has worked on this unit, you have tried many different approaches in an effort to improve Scott's absenteeism and attitude. There would frequently be temporary improvement.

Scott has requested a transfer to the emergency room. His career goal is to be part of the flight rescue team. He certainly has the skills and intelligence to be part of this exciting and highly skilled group.

However, you believe that if you include all the negative aspects of Scott's performance, he may not be selected for the position. On one hand, you believe this job could be a turning point for Scott. It might be what he needs to overcome some of his work problems. On the other hand, the relief you feel at the possibility of transferring Scott off your unit indicates that there are some ethical issues present in this situation. **Assignment:** Decide what you should do about Scott Powell's request to transfer to the emergency room. Outline your plan. Be specific about the alternatives open to you and what course of action you will take.

PROMOTIONS

Promotions are reassignments to a position of higher rank. It is normal for promotions to include a pay raise. Most promotions include increased status, title changes, more authority, and greater responsibility. Because of the importance American society places on promotions, certain guidelines must accompany

Organizations often have poorly developed plans for handling promotions.

promotion selection to ensure that the process is fair and equitable. When position openings occur, they are often posted and filled hastily with little thought of long-term organizational or employee goals. This frequently results in negative personnel outcomes. To avoid this, the following elements should be determined in advance:

- **Recruitment from without or within.** There are obvious advantages and disadvantages to recruiting for promotions from within the organization. Recruiting from within, also called *succession management*, is less expensive and can help to develop employees to fill higher-level positions as they become vacant. It can also serve as a powerful motivation and recognition tool. There are advantages to recruiting from outside the organization, however. When promotions are filled with people outside the organization, it allows the organization to seek people with new ideas. This prevents the stagnation that often occurs when all promotions are filled from within. Regardless of what the organization decides, the policy should be consistently followed and communicated to all employees. Some companies recruit from within first and recruit from outside the organization only if they are unable to find qualified people from among their own employees.

- **Establishment of promotion and selection criteria.** Employees should know in advance what the criteria for promotion are and what selection method is to be used. Some organizations use an interview panel as a selection method to promote all employees beyond the level of charge nurse. Decisions regarding the selection method and promotion criteria should be justified with rationale. Additionally, employees need to know what place seniority will have in the selection criteria.

- **Identification of a pool of candidates.** When promotions are planned, as in succession management, there will always be an adequate pool of candidates identified and prepared to seek higher-level positions. A word of caution must be given regarding the zeal with which managers urge subordinates to seek promotions. The leader's role is to identify and prepare such a pool. It is not the manager's role to urge the employee to seek a position in a manner that would lead the employee to think that he or she was guaranteed the job or to unduly influence him or her in the decision to seek such a job. When employees actively seek promotions, they are making a commitment to do well in the new position. When they are pushed into such positions, the commitment to expend the energy to do the job well may be lacking. For many reasons, the employee may not feel ready, either due to personal commitments or because he or she feels inadequately educated or experienced.

- **Handling rejected candidates.** All promotion candidates who are rejected must be notified before the selected candidate. This is common courtesy. Candidates must be told of their nonselection in a manner that is not demotivating. They should be thanked for taking the effort to apply and, when appropriate, be encouraged to apply for future position openings.

Sometimes, employees should be told what deficiencies kept them from getting the position. For instance, employees should be told if they lack some educational component or work experience that would make them a stronger competitor for future promotions. This can be an effective way of encouraging career development.

- **How employee releases are to be handled.** Knowledge that the best candidate for the position currently holds a critical job or difficult position to fill should not influence decisions regarding promotions. Managers frequently find it difficult to release employees to another position within the organization. Policies regarding the length of time that a manager can delay releasing an employee should be written and communicated. On the other hand, some managers are so good at developing their employees that they frequently become frustrated because their success at career development results in constantly losing their staff to other departments. In such cases, higher-level management should reward such leaders and set release policies that are workable and realistic.

THE EMPLOYEE'S RESPONSIBILITY FOR CAREER PLANNING

Career planning is the subset of career development that represents individual responsibility. It includes evaluating one's strengths and weaknesses, setting goals, examining career opportunities, preparing for potential opportunities, and using appropriate developmental activities. Sensitive managers and progressive organizations can assist employees in career planning through long-term coaching. Various career-planning guides also can assist the person in career planning. Managers should encourage the use of such tools and make them available to their staff.

Career planning should be an ongoing, conscious, and deliberate process. To be a fully engaged professional requires commitment to personal and career development. Many novice professionals and most young people neglect to make long-term career plans. Career planning is often made easier when a career map is created to assist in developing a long-term master plan. Use the career guide shown in **Figure 11.1,** along with the steps in career planning outlined in Display 11.3, to assist with developing the personal plan described in Learning Exercise 11.5.

Learning Exercise 11.5

Developing a Realistic 20-Year Career Plan
Develop a 20-year career plan, taking into account the constraints of family responsibilities such as marriage, children, and aging parents. Have your career plan critiqued to determine its feasibility and if the time lines and goals are realistic.

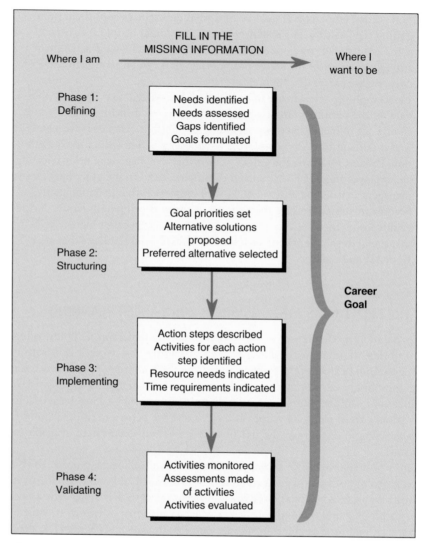

Figure 11.1 A career-planning guide for a professional nurse.

RÉSUMÉ PREPARATION

In addition to career mapping and self-assessment, the professional nurse is responsible for developing strategies that assist in realizing career goals. Such strategies include presenting a positive image by using good interviewing skills and a well-prepared résumé.

The Résumé

The résumé is an important screening tool used by employers for selection of applicants. Often résumés are attached to the application, but they serve a somewhat different purpose. The application is designed by the employer and serves the needs of the organization, whereas the applicant creates the résumé. Assessing one's own values, skills, and interests is an essential part of the résumé preparation process. Résumés should concentarte on what applicants like to do and what they do well.

When examining résumés, the selector must remember that applicants use the device to summarize their education and experience in the best possible light. Managers must look beyond the neat and well-prepared résumé and examine critical issues, such as length of time the applicant was employed in other positions and what positions were held. Developing as clear a picture of the recently graduated nurse with little work experience is more difficult.

Résumés are important as a career-planning tool. They also are used for promotion decisions; therefore, maintaining an accurate and current résumé becomes a career-planning necessity for the professional nurse.

Various acceptable styles and formats of résumés exist. However, because the résumé represents professionalism and is often used by recruiters as a summary of the applicant's qualifications, it must be professionally prepared, make an impression, and quickly capture the reader's attention. The following are guidelines for résumé preparation:

- The résumé should be typed in a format that is easy to read.
- The résumé should maximize strong points and minimize weakness.
- The style should reflect good grammar, correct punctuation, proper sentence structure, and simple, direct language.

The content of the résumé should consist of educational history; work experience; personal characteristics; membership in professional organizations; community involvement; awards, honors, and publications; professional objectives; health status; and license information. A sample résumé is shown in **Display 11.5.**

PREPARING A PROFESSIONAL PORTFOLIO

A *professional portfolio* can be described as a collection of materials that document a nurse's competencies and illustrate the expertise of the nurse. All nurses should maintain a portfolio to reflect their own professional growth. The portfolio is developed over time and does not replace a curriculum vitae or a résumé. Rather, it is used to reflect the professional development of a nurse during his or her career.

Oermann (2002) states that there are two types of professional portfolios, *best-work* and *growth* and *development*. Best-work portfolios are used for documentation for career ladder promotions, job applications, performance reviews, and other situations where others will review the portfolio.

Growth and development portfolios are designed for nurses to monitor their progress in meeting their own individual goals for professional and personal growth. This later portfolio is a working document to be used only by the individual nurse; however, should the nurse choose to do so, selected material can be used from the portfolio to be placed in the best-work portfolio that is shown to others (Oermann, 2002).

Display 11.5	Sample Résumé

SUSAN CARMEL GUEVARA
553-12-8456
628 Normal Street
Chico, CA 95928
(530) 555-3718

CAREER GOAL	To practice professional nursing within a progressive environment that will provide challenges and opportunities for personal and professional growth.
EDUCATION	Bachelor of Science in Nursing California State University, Chico May 2005 Public Health Certificate January 2000
GPA	3.18—overall 3.34—within major
HONORS	Sigma Theta Tau International Society of Nursing, Kappa Omicron Chapter. CSUC School of Nursing Scholarship Award. Selection of one of my papers by the Writing Across the Discipline project for publication in *An Expression of Nursing, A Journal of Student Writing in The School of Nursing*, 2004, Vol. 1.
RELATED EXPERIENCE	June 2002–Present Nurse Attendant, Memorial Hospital, Chico, CA Performed nursing assignments and various aspects of nursing care under the supervision and guidance of a registered nurse. (Job description available on request.) July 2004–Present Home health aide/respite worker for various agencies and individuals throughout the academic school years and summers.
REFERENCES	Available on request.

The individual needs to be selective in collecting best-work documentation, and only include those materials that illustrate competency and highlight achievement. Separate files for the following would be helpful:

- Formal education documentation including a curriculum vitae or résumé; copies of diplomas and state license numbers and certification of any specialty should be included.
- Continuing education documentation including programs attended and credits earned as well as learning outcomes of such programs.
- Performance documentation, including evaluations, position descriptions, reference letters, awards or commendations.
- Community service documentation, including committee or organizational membership.
- Professional nursing activities documentation, especially offices held or other type of participation.

Maintaining a professional portfolio avoids lost opportunities to save documents. It allows the nurse to always have readily available documentation when pursuing a promotion, considering a new position in a new agency, or when applying for another position in the present employment.

MANAGEMENT DEVELOPMENT

Management development is a planned system of training and developing people so they acquire the skills, insights, and attitudes needed to manage people and their work effectively within the organization. Management development is often referred to as *succession planning*.

With the flattening of organizational hierarchies and a rise in nurse–managers' responsibilities, it is vital to ensure that future nurse–managers have the competencies to succeed. Kleinman (2003) states, "The new healthcare leadership must possess synthesized competence that includes clinical health services and the management of these services from a business perspective" (p. 455).

Management development programs, as a part of career development, must be supported by top-level administration. The program also must be planned and systematically implemented. The program must include a means of developing appropriate attitudes through social learning theory and adequate management theoretical content.

Support for management development programs by the organization should occur in two ways. First, top-level management must do more than bear the cost of management development classes. They must create an organizational structure that allows managers to apply their new knowledge. Therefore, for such programs to be effective, the organization must be willing to practice a management style that incorporates sound management principles.

Secondly, training outcomes will be improved if nursing executives are active in planning and developing the program. Whenever possible, nursing administrators should teach some of the classes and, at the very least, make sure that the program supports top-management philosophy.

Just as nurses are required to be certified in critical care before they accept a position in a critical care unit, so too should nurses be required to take part in a management development program before their appointment to a management position.

Potential managers should be identified and groomed early. The first step in this process would be an appraisal of the present management team and an analysis of possible future needs. The second step would be the establishment of a training and development program. This would require decisions such as the following: How often should the formal management course be offered? Should outside educators be involved, or should in-house staff teach it? Who should be involved in teaching the didactic portion? Should there be two levels of classes, one for first-level and one for middle-level managers? Should the management development courses be open to all, or should people be recommended by someone from management? In addition to formal course content, what other methods should be used to develop managers? Should other methods be used, such as job rotation through an understudy system of pairing selected people with a manager and management coaching?

The inclusion of social learning activities also is a valuable part of management development. Management development will not be successful unless learners have ample chance to try out new skills. Providing potential managers with didactic management theory alone inadequately prepares them for the attitudes, skills, and insights necessary for effective management. Case studies, management games, transactional analysis, and sensitivity training also are effective in changing attitudes and increasing self-awareness. All these techniques appropriately use social learning theory strategies.

Smeltzer (2002) maintains that developing future managers and leaders needs to be viewed very broadly. That is, there is an obligation for current nurse leaders to develop future leader–managers even for positions that may not be in their institution. Present leaders will be rewarded when they see those, who they have helped develop, advance in their careers and in turn develop leadership and management skills in others.

INTEGRATING LEADERSHIP ROLES AND MANAGEMENT FUNCTIONS IN CAREER DEVELOPMENT

It is clear that appropriate career management should foster positive career development, alleviate burnout, reduce attrition, and promote productivity. Management functions in career development include disseminating career information and posting job openings. The manager should have a well-developed, planned system for career development for all employees; this system should include long-term coaching, the appropriate use of transfers, and how promotions are to be handled. These policies should be fair and communicated effectively to all employees.

With the integration of leadership, managers become more aware of how their own values shape personal career decisions. Additionally, the leader–manager shows genuine interest in the career development of all employees. Career planning is encouraged, and potential leaders are identified and developed. Leaders develop and share talent.

Effective managers recognize that in all career decisions, the employee must decide when he or she is ready to pursue promotions, return to school, or take on greater responsibility. Leaders are aware that every person perceives success in a different manner.

Although career development programs benefit all employees and the organization, there is an added bonus for the professional nurse. When professional nurses have the opportunity to experience a well-planned career development program, a greater viability for and increased commitment to the profession are often evident.

☀ Key Concepts

- There are many outcomes of a *career development program* that justify its implementation.
- Career job sequencing should assist the manager in career management.
- Career development programs consist of a set of personal responsibilities called *career planning* and a set of management responsibilities called *career management.*
- Employees often need to be encouraged to make more formalized long-term career plans.
- Designing *career paths* is an important part of organizational career management.
- Managers should plan specific interventions that promote growth and development in each of their subordinates.
- The *transfer,* when used appropriately, may be an effective way to provide career development.
- Policies regarding promotion should be in writing and communicated to all employees.
- Recruitment from within has been shown to have a positive effect on employee satisfaction.
- Recruitment from outside the organization allows for new ideas and prevents stagnation.
- To be successful, management development must be planned and supported by top-level management. This type of planned program is called *succession management.*
- If appropriate management attitudes and insight are goals of a management development program, social learning techniques need to be part of the teaching strategies used.
- *Long-term coaching* is a planned intervention on the part of the manager that results in the professional growth and development of subordinates.

More Learning Exercises and Applications

 Learning Exercise 11.6

Listing Policies Relating to Promotions
You have been appointed to a committee of staff nurses in your home health agency to assist in developing a set of policies regarding how future promotions are to be handled. Lately, there has been some unhappiness about how employees have been selected for promotions. Your committee is to focus on how shift and day charge nurses are to be selected.
Assignment: Develop a list of five to seven policies regarding such promotions. Be able to justify your promotion criteria and policies.

Learning Exercise 11.7

Preparing a Practice Résumé
The medical center where you have applied for a position has requested that you submit a résumé along with your application. Prepare a professional résumé using your actual experience and education. You may use any style and format you desire. The résumé will be critiqued on the basis of its professional appearance and appropriateness of included content.

Learning Exercise 11.8

Constructing a Management Development Plan
You are serving on an ad hoc committee to construct a management development program. Your organization has requested that the charge nurses work with staff development and plan a one-week training and education program that would be required of all new charge nurses before their appointment. Because the organization will be bearing the cost of the program (i.e., paying for the educators and employee time), you are required to select appropriate content and educational methods that will not exceed 40 hours, including actual orientation time by a charge nurse.
Assignment: Develop and write up such a plan and share it with the class. Your plan should depict hours, content, and educational methods.

Web Links

American Nurses Credentialing Center (ANCC)
http://www.nursingworld.org/ancc/
Provides a general overview of the ANCC as well as the more than 30 specialty and advanced practice areas of specialty certification/recertification offered.

Benner, J. (2000). How to Navigate Specialty Certification
http://www.springnet.com/certification/top.htm
Lists WEB sites and test locations/schedules for specialty certification examinations in nursing.

Career Mosaic's Health Opps
http://www.healthopps.com
Includes a healthcare jobs list, employer profiles and résumé postings.

Lenburg, C. L. (2000) ANA-COPA Model. Framework, Concepts and Methods of the Competency Outcomes and Performance Assessment
http://www.nursingworld.org
Suggests a cohesive conceptual framework that supports learning and assessment methods for nurses focused on practice competencies.

National Student Nurses Assoc. (NSNA). Planning Your Career
http://www.nsna.org
Includes resources for senior nursing students, new graduates, and registered nurses, with direct links to hospitals with positions for new graduates. Includes electronic articles on choosing the right first job, tips on getting the job you want, preparing for licensure as a registered nurse, specialty nursing, and others.

University of Sheffield Careers Service. Directions for Nurses and Midwives. Career Planning—Why Now?
http://www.shef.ac.uk/careers/students/nursing/planning.html
Includes job search strategies, the application process, interviewing, useful contacts, etc.

References

Chitty, K. K. (2001). *Professional nursing. Concepts & challenges* (3rd ed.). Philadelphia: W. B. Saunders.

Curran, C. R. (2003). Becoming the employer of choice. *Nursing Economic$, 21*(2), 57–58.

Johnstone, P. L. (2003). Nurse manager turnover in New South Wales during the 1990s. *Collegian, 10*(1), 8–16.

Kleinman, C. S. (2003). Leadership roles, competencies and education. *Journal of Nursing Administration,33*(9), 451–455.

Manchester, Inc. (2000). Executive coaching yields return on investment of almost six times its cost, says study. Available at: http://www.manchesterUS.com.

McNeese-Smith, D. K. (2000). Job stages of entry, mastery, and disengagement among nurses. *Journal of Nursing Administration, 30*(3), 140–147.

McPeck, P. (2001). Unlock your potential. *Nurseweek, 14*(16), 11–12.

Oermann, M. H. (2002). Developing a professional portfolio in nursing. *Orthopaedic Nursing, 21*(2), 73–79.

Savage, C. M. (2001). Executive coaching: Professional self-care for nursing. *Nursing Economic$, 19*(4), 178–182.

Smeltzer, C. H. (2002). Executive coaching: Succession planning. *Journal of Nursing Administration, 32*(12), 615–619.

Tuttas, C. (2002). Robbing Peter to pay Paul: Breaking the RN "recruitment cycle." *Journal of Nursing Care Quality. 16*(4), 39–45.

Bibliography

Allenbaugh, E. (2002). Six strategies to cultivate "bright eye" employees. *Patient Care Staff, 2*(12), 5–7.

Beaudin, C. L. (May 2001). Nursing professionals & career positioning in managed behavioral health care. *Journal of Psychosocial Nursing and Mental Health Services, 39*(5), 40–51.

Benner, J. (2001). How to navigate specialty certification. *Nursing 2001 Career Directory* (pp. 30–31). Springhouse, PA: Springhouse.

Chwedyk, P. (2002). Vital signs. Diversity leadership imitative aims to develop minority health care executives. *Minority Nurse, 11*(4), 8.

Curtin, L. (2002). Ethics in management. Reflections on integrity and career building. *Journal of Clinical Systems Management, 4*(9), 7.

Ingersoll, G. L, Olsan, T., Drew-Cates, J., Devinney, B. C., & Davies, J. (2002). Nurses' job satisfaction, organizational commitment, and career intent. *Journal of Nursing Administration, 32*(5), 253–263.

Maier, G. (2002). GN management. Career ladders: An important element in CAN retention. *Geriatric Nursing, 23*(40), 217–219.

Marshall, N. P. (2001). Career development. Networking is key to CFO career development. *Healthcare Financial Management, 55*(3), 70–71.

McVay, K. (2001). Making nursing an attractive career choice. *California Nurse, 97*(2), 3.

Robinson-Walker, C. (2002). The role of coaching in creating cultures of engagement. *Seminars for Nurse Managers, 10*(3), 150–156.

Shepherd, N. (2001). My profession, my choice. *Chart, 98*(3), 9.

Smeltzer, C. H. (2001). Executive coaching: Lack of power and influence. *Journal of Nursing Administration, 31*(7/8), 353–354.

CHAPTER

12

Organizational Structure

Society, community, family are all conserving institutions. They try to maintain stability, and to prevent, or at least to slow down, change. But the organization of the post-capitalist society of organizations is a destabilizer. Because its function is to put knowledge to work—on tools, processes, and products; on work; on knowledge itself—it must be organized for constant change.

—Peter Drucker

The preceding unit provided a background in planning, the first phase of the management process. Organizing follows planning as the second phase of the management process and is explored in this unit. In the organizing phase, relationships are defined, procedures are outlined, equipment is readied, and tasks are assigned. Organizing also involves establishing a formal structure that provides the best possible coordination or use of resources to accomplish unit objectives.

This chapter looks at how the structure of an organization facilitates or impedes communication, flexibility, and job satisfaction. Chapter 13 examines the role of authority and power in organizations and how power may be used to meet individual, unit, and organizational goals; Chapter 14 looks at how human resources can be organized to accomplish work.

Fayol (1949) suggested that an organization is formed when the number of workers is large enough to require a supervisor. Organizations are necessary because they accomplish more work than can be done by individual effort.

Organizational structure refers to the way in which a group is formed, its lines of communication, and its means for channeling authority and making decisions.

Because people spend most of their lives in social, personal, and professional organizations, they need to understand how the organizations are structured. *Organizational structure* refers to the way in which a group is formed, its lines of communication, and its means for channeling authority and making decisions.

Each organization has a *formal* and an *informal* organizational structure. The formal structure is generally highly planned and visible, whereas the informal structure is unplanned and often hidden. Formal structure, through departmentalization and work division, provides a framework for defining managerial authority, responsibility, and accountability. In a well-defined formal structure, roles and functions are defined and systematically arranged, different people have differing roles, and rank and hierarchy are evident.

Informal structure is generally social, with blurred or shifting lines of authority and accountability. People need to be aware that informal authority and lines of communication exist in every group, even when they are never formally acknowledged. The primary emphasis of this chapter, however, is the identification of components of organizational structure, the leadership roles and management functions associated with formal organizational structure, and the proper utilization of committees to accomplish organizational objectives (see **Display 12.1**).

ORGANIZATIONAL THEORY

Max Weber, a German social scientist, is known as the father of organizational theory. Generally acknowledged to have developed the most comprehensive classic formulation on the characteristics of *bureaucracy*, Weber wrote from the vantage point of a manager instead of that of a scholar. During the 1920s, Weber saw the growth of the large-scale organization and correctly predicted that this growth required a more formalized set of procedures for administrators. His statement on bureaucracy, published after his death, is still the most influential statement on the subject.

Weber postulated three "ideal types" of authority or reasons why people throughout history have obeyed their rulers. One of these, *legal-rational* authority, was based on a belief in the legitimacy of the pattern of normative rules and the rights of those

| Display 12.1 | Leadership Roles and Management Functions Associated with Organizational Structure |

Leadership Roles

1. Evaluates the organizational structure frequently to determine if management positions can be eliminated to reduce the chain of command.
2. Encourages and guides employees to follow the chain of command. Counsels employees who do not follow chain of command.
3. Supports personnel in advisory (staff) positions.
4. Models responsibility and accountability for subordinates.
5. Assists staff to see how their roles are congruent with and complement the organization's mission, vision, and goals.
6. Facilitates constructive informal group structure.
7. Encourages upward communication.
8. Fosters a consonant organizational culture between workgroups and subcultures through shared values and goals.
9. Promotes participatory decision making and shared governance to empower subordinates.
10. Uses committees to facilitate group goals, not to delay decisions.
11. Teaches group members how to avoid groupthink.

Management Functions

1. Continually identifies and analyzes stakeholder interests in the organization.
2. Is knowledgeable about the organization's internal structure, including personal and department authority and responsibilities within that structure.
3. Provides the staff with an accurate unit organizational chart and assists with interpretation.
4. When possible, maintains unity of command.
5. Clarifies unity of command when there is confusion.
6. Follows appropriate subordinate complaints upward through chain of command.
7. Establishes an appropriate span of control.
8. Is knowledgeable about the organization's culture.
9. Uses the informal organization to meet organizational goals.
10. Uses committee structure to increase the quality and quantity of work accomplished.
11. Works, as appropriate, to achieve a level of operational excellence appropriate to magnet status.

elevated to authority under such rules to issue commands. Obedience then was owed to the legally established impersonal set of rules, rather than to a personal ruler. It is this type of authority that is the basis for Weber's concept of bureaucracy.

Weber argued that the great virtue of bureaucracy—indeed, perhaps its defining characteristic—was that it was an institutional method for applying general rules to specific cases, thereby making the actions of management fair and predictable. Other characteristics of bureaucracies as identified by Weber include the following:

- A clear division of labor (i.e., all work must be divided into units that can be undertaken by individuals or groups of individuals competent to perform those tasks).

- A well-defined hierarchy of authority in which superiors are separated from subordinates; on the basis of this hierarchy, remuneration for work is dispensed, authority is recognized, privileges are allotted, and promotions are awarded.
- Impersonal rules and impersonality of interpersonal relationships. In other words, bureaucrats are not free to act in any way they please. Bureaucratic rules provide systematic control of superiors over subordinates, thus limiting the opportunities for arbitrary behavior and personal favoritism.
- A system of procedures for dealing with work situations (i.e., regular activities to get a job done) must exist.
- A system of rules covering the rights and duties of each position must be in place.
- Selection for employment and promotion based on technical competence.

Bureaucracy was the ideal tool to harness and routinize the energy and prolific production of the industrial revolution. Weber's work did not, however, consider the complexity of managing organizations in the 21st century. Weber wrote during an era when worker motivation was taken for granted, and his simplification of management and employee roles did not examine the bilateral relationships between employee and management prevalent in most organizations today.

Since Weber's research, management theorists have learned much about human behavior, and most organizations have modified their structures and created alternative organizational designs that reduce rigidity and impersonality. Current research also supports the thesis that changing an organization's structure in a manner that increases autonomy and work empowerment for nurses will also lead to more effective patient care (Miller, et al., 2001; Kramer & Schmalenberg, 2003). Yet, almost 100 years after Weber's findings, components of bureaucratic structure continue to be found in the design of most large organizations.

COMPONENTS OF ORGANIZATIONAL STRUCTURE

Weber also is credited with the development of the *organization chart* to depict an organization's structure. Because the organization chart (**Figure 12.1**) is a picture of an organization, the knowledgeable manager can derive much information from reading the chart. An organization chart can help identify roles and their expectations. By observing such elements as which departments report directly to the chief executive officer (CEO), the novice manager can make some inferences about the organization. For instance, having the top-level nursing manager reporting to an assistant executive officer rather than to the CEO might indicate the amount of value the organization places on nursing. Managers who understand an organization's structure and relationships will be able to expedite decisions and have a greater understanding of the organizational environment.

Relationships and Chain of Command

The organization chart defines formal relationships within the institution. Formal relationships, lines of communication, and authority are depicted on a chart by

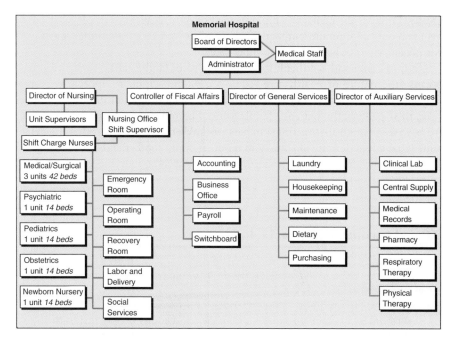

Figure 12.1 Sample organization chart.

unbroken (solid) lines. These line positions can be shown by solid horizontal or vertical lines. Solid horizontal lines represent communication between people with similar spheres of responsibility and power but different functions. Solid vertical lines between positions denote the official *chain of command,* the formal paths of communication and authority. Those having the greatest decision-making authority are located at the top; those with the least are at the bottom. The level of position on the chart also signifies status and power.

Dotted or broken lines on the organization chart represent *staff positions.* Because these positions are advisory, a staff member provides information and assistance to the manager but has limited organizational authority. Used to increase his or her sphere of influence, staff positions enable a manager to handle more activities and interactions than would otherwise be possible. These positions also provide for specialization that would be impossible for any one manager to achieve alone. Although staff positions can make line personnel more effective, organizations can function without them.

Advisory (staff) positions do not have inherent legitimate authority. Clinical specialists and in-service directors in staff positions often lack the authority that accompanies a line relationship. Accomplishing the role expectations in a staff position is therefore more difficult because typically little authority accompanies it. Because only line positions have authority for decision making, staff positions may result in an ineffective use of support services unless job descriptions and responsibilities for these positions are clearly spelled out.

Unity of command is indicated by the vertical solid line between positions on the organizational chart. This concept is best described as one person/one boss: employees have one manager to whom they report and to whom they are responsible. This greatly simplifies the manager–employee relationship because the employee needs to maintain only a minimum number of relationships and accept the influence of only one person as his or her immediate supervisor.

Unity of command is difficult to maintain in some large healthcare organizations because the nature of health care requires a multidisciplinary approach. Nurses frequently feel as though they have many bosses, including their immediate supervisor, their patient, the patient's family, central administration, and the physician. All have some input in directing a nurse's work. Weber was correct when he determined that a lack of unity of command results in some conflict and lost productivity. This is demonstrated frequently when healthcare workers become confused about unity of command.

Learning Exercise 12.1

Who's the Boss?
In groups or individually, analyze the following, and give an oral or written report.
1. Have you ever worked in an organization in which the lines of authority were unclear? Have you been a member of a social organization in which this happened? How did this interfere with the organization's functioning?
2. Do you believe the "one boss per person" rule is a good idea? Don't hospital clerical workers frequently have many bosses? If you have worked in a situation in which you had more than one boss, what was the result?

Span of Control

Span of control also can be determined from the organization chart. The number of people directly reporting to any one manager represents that manager's span of control and determines the number of interactions expected of him or her. Theorists are divided regarding the optimal span of control for any one manager. Quantitative formulas for determining the optimal span of control have been attempted; suggested ranges are from 3 to 50 employees. When determining an optimal span of control in an organization, the manager's abilities, the employees' maturity, task complexity, geographic location, and level in the organization at which the work occurs must all be considered. The number of people directly reporting to any one supervisor must be the number that maximizes productivity and worker satisfaction. Too many people reporting to a single manager delays decision making, whereas too few results in an inefficient, top-heavy organization.

Until the last decade, the principle of narrow spans of control at top levels of management, with slightly wider spans at other levels, was widely accepted. Now, with increased financial pressures on healthcare organizations to remain fiscally solvent and electronic communication technology advances, many have increased their spans of control and reduced the number of administrative levels in the organization.

Managerial Levels

In large organizations, several levels of managers often exist. *Top-level managers* look at the organization as a whole, coordinating internal and external influences, and generally make decisions with few guidelines or structures. Examples of top-level managers include the organization's chief operating officer (COO) or chief executive officer (CEO), and the highest-level nursing administrator. Current nomenclature for top-level nurse–managers varies; they might be called vice-president of nursing or patient care services, nurse administrator, director of nursing, chief nurse, assistant administrator of patient care services, or chief nurse officer (CNO).

Some top-level nurse–managers may be responsible for non-nursing departments. For example, a top-level nurse–manager might oversee the respiratory, physical, and occupational therapy departments in addition to all nursing departments. Likewise, the CEO might have various titles, such as president or director. It is necessary to remember only that the CEO is the organization's highest-ranking person and the top-level nurse–manager is its highest-ranking nurse.

Responsibilities common to top-level managers include determining the organizational philosophy, setting policy, and creating goals and priorities for resource allocation. Top-level managers have a greater need for leadership skills and are not as involved in routine daily operations as are lower-level managers.

Middle-level managers coordinate the efforts of lower levels of the hierarchy and are the conduit between lower and top-level managers. Middle-level managers carry out day-to-day operations but are still involved in some long-term planning and in establishing unit policies. Examples of middle-level managers include nursing supervisors, nurse–managers, head nurses, and unit managers. Currently, there are many health facility mergers and acquisitions, and reduced levels of administration are frequently apparent within these consolidated organizations. This often results in middle-level managers having increased responsibilities and role expansion. Consequently, many healthcare facilities have renamed middle-level managers using the title of "director" as a way to indicate new roles (Urden & Rogers, 2000). The old term director of nursing, still used in many small facilities to denote the CNO, is now used in many healthcare organizations to denote a middle-level manager. The proliferation of titles among healthcare administrators has made it imperative that individuals understand what roles and responsibilities go with each position.

First-level managers are concerned with their specific unit's work flow. They deal with immediate problems in the unit's daily operations, with organizational needs, and with personal needs of employees. The effectiveness of first-level managers tremendously affects the organization. First-level managers need good management skills. Because they work so closely with patients and healthcare teams, first-level managers also have an excellent opportunity to practice leadership roles that will greatly influence productivity and subordinates' satisfaction. Examples of first-level managers include primary care nurses, team leaders, case managers, and charge nurses. In many organizations, every registered nurse is considered a first-level manager. All nurses in every situation must manage themselves and those under their care. A composite look at top-, middle-, and first-level managers is shown in **Table 12.1.**

Table 12.1 Levels of Managers			
	Top Level	**Middle Level**	**First Level**
Examples	Chief nursing officer Chief executive officer Chief financial officer	Unit supervisor Department head Director	Charge nurse Team leader Primary nurse
Scope of responsibility	Look at organization as a whole as well as external influences	Focus is on integrating unit level day-to-day needs with organizational needs	Focus primarily on day-to-day needs at unit level
Primary planning focus	Strategic planning	Combination of long- and short-range planning	Short-range, operational planning
Communication flow	More often top down but receives subordinate feedback both directly and via middle-level managers	Upward and downward with great centrality	More often upward. Generally relies on middle-level managers to transmit communication to first-level managers

One of the leadership responsibilities of organizing is to periodically examine the number of people in the chain of command. Organizations frequently add levels until there are too many managers. Therefore, the nursing manager should carefully weigh the advantages and disadvantages of adding a management level. For example, does having a charge nurse on each shift aid or hinder decision making? Does having this position solve or create problems?

Centrality

Centrality refers to the location of a position on an organization chart where frequent and various types of communication occur.

Centrality is determined by organizational distance. Employees with relatively small organizational distance can receive more information than those who are more peripherally located. This is why the middle manager often has a broader view of the organization than other levels of management. A middle manager has a large degree of centrality because this manager receives information upward, downward, and horizontally.

Because all communication involves a sender and a receiver, messages may not be received clearly because of the sender's hierarchical position. Similarly, status and power often influence the receiver's ability to hear information accurately. An example of the effect of status on communication is found in the "principal syndrome."

Centrality refers to the location of a position on an organization chart where frequent and various types of communication occur.

Most people can recall panic, when they were school-aged, at being summoned to the principal's office. Thoughts of "what did I do?" travel through one's mind. Even adults find discomfort in communicating with certain people who hold high status. This may be fear or awe, but both interfere with clear communication. The difficulties with upward and downward communication are more fully discussed in Chapter 19.

Learning Exercise 12.2

Change Is Coming

This learning exercise refers to the organization chart in Figure 12.1. Because Memorial Hospital is expanding, the Board of Directors has made several changes that require modification of the organization chart. The directors have just announced the following changes:

- The name of the hospital has been changed to Memorial General Hospital and Medical Center.
- State approval has been granted for open-heart surgery.
- One of the existing medical-surgical units will be remodeled and will become two critical care units (one six-bed coronary and open-heart unit and one six-bed trauma and surgical unit).
- A part-time medical director will be responsible for medical care on each critical care unit.
- The hospital administrator's title has been changed to executive director.
- An associate hospital administrator has been hired.
- A new hospital-wide educational department has been created.
- The old pediatric unit will be remodeled into a seven-bed pediatric wing and a seven-bed rehabilitation unit.
- The nursing director's new title is vice-president of patient care services.

Assignment: If the hospital is viewed as a large, open system, it is possible to visualize areas where problems might occur. In particular, it is necessary to identify changes anticipated in the nursing department and how these changes will affect the organization as a whole. Depict all these changes on the old organization chart, delineating both staff and line positions. Give the rationale for your decisions. Why did you place the education department where you did? What was the reasoning in your division of authority? Where do you believe there might be potential conflict in the new organization chart? Why?

It is important, then, to be cognizant of how the formal structure affects overall relationships and communication. This is especially true because organizations change their structure frequently, resulting in new communication lines and reporting relationships. Unless one understands how to interpret a formal organization chart, confusion and anxiety will result when organizations are restructured.

Learning Exercise 12.3

Cultures and Hierarchies

Having been with the county health department for six months, you are very impressed with the physician who is the county health administrator. She seems to have a genuine concern for patient welfare. She has a tea for new employees each month to discuss the department's philosophy and her own management style. She says she has an open-door policy so employees are always welcome to visit her.

Since you have been assigned to the evening immunization clinic as charge nurse, you have become concerned with a persistent problem. The housekeeping staff often spends part of the evening sleeping on duty or socializing for long periods. You have reported your concerns to your health department supervisor twice. Last evening, you found the house-keeping staff having another get-together. This mainly upsets you because the clinic is chronically in need of cleaning. Sometimes the public bathrooms get so untidy that they embarrass you and your staff. You frequently remind the housekeepers to empty overflowing waste paper baskets. You believe this environment is demeaning to patients. This also upsets you because you and your staff work so hard all evening and rarely have a chance to sit down. You believe it is unfair to everyone that the housekeeping staff is not doing its share.

On your way to the parking lot this evening, the health administrator stops to chat and asks you how things are going. Should you tell her about the problem with the housekeeping staff? Is this an appropriate chain of command? Do you believe there is a dissonance between the housekeeping unit's culture and the nursing unit's culture? What should you do? List choices and alternatives. Decide what you should do and explain your rationale.

Note: Attempt to solve this problem before referring to a possible solution posted in the back of this book.

Is it ever appropriate to go outside the chain of command? Of course, there are isolated circumstances when the chain of command must be breached. However, those rare conditions usually involve a question of ethics. In most instances, those being bypassed in a chain of command should be forewarned. Remember that unity of command provides the organization with a workable system for procedural directives and orders, so that productivity is increased and conflict is minimized.

TYPES OF ORGANIZATION STRUCTURES

Traditionally, nursing departments have used one of the following structural patterns: bureaucratic, ad hoc, matrix, flat, or various combinations of these. The type of structure used in any healthcare facility affects communication patterns, relationships, and authority.

Line Structures

Bureaucratic organizational designs are commonly called line structures or *line organizations.* Those with staff authority may be referred to as *staff organizations.* Both of these types of organizational structures are found frequently in large healthcare facilities and usually resemble Weber's original design for effective organizations.

Because of most people's familiarity with these structures, there is little stress associated with orienting people to these organizations. In these structures, authority and responsibility are clearly defined, which leads to efficiency and simplicity of relationships. The organization chart in Figure 12.1 is a line-and-staff structure.

These formal designs have some disadvantages. They often produce monotony, alienate workers, and make adjusting rapidly to altered circumstances difficult. Another problem with line and line-and-staff structures is their adherence to chain of command communication, which restricts upward communication. Good leaders encourage upward communication to compensate for this disadvantage. However, when line positions are clearly defined, going outside the chain of command for upward communication is usually inappropriate.

Ad Hoc Design

The *ad hoc* design is a modification of the bureaucratic structure and is sometimes used on a temporary basis to facilitate completion of a project within a formal line organization. The ad hoc structure is a means of overcoming the inflexibility of line structure and serves as a way for professionals to handle the increasingly large amounts of available information. Ad hoc structures use a project team or task approach and are usually disbanded after a project is completed. This structure's disadvantages are decreased strength in the formal chain of command and decreased employee loyalty to the parent organization.

Matrix Structure

A *matrix* organization structure is designed to focus on both product and function. Function is described as all the tasks required to produce the product, and the product is the end result of the function. For example, good patient outcomes are the product and staff education and adequate staffing may be the functions necessary to produce the outcome.

The matrix organization structure has a formal vertical and horizontal chain of command. **Figure 12.2** depicts a matrix organizational structure and shows that the director of maternal childcare could report both to a vice president for maternal and women's services (product manager) and a vice president for nursing services (functional manager). Although there are less formal rules and fewer levels of the hierarchy, a matrix structure is not without disadvantages. For example, in this structure, decision making can be slow because of the necessity of information sharing, and it can produce confusion and frustration for workers because of its dual-authority hierarchical design. The primary advantage of centralizing expertise is frequently outweighed by the complexity of the design.

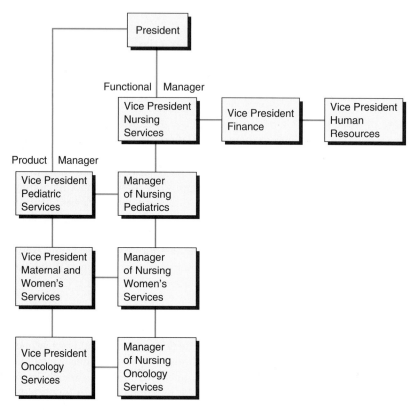

Figure 12.2 Matrix organizational structure.

Service Line Organization

Similar to the matrix design is *service line organization*, which can be used in some large institutions to address the shortcomings that are endemic to traditional large bureaucratic organizations. Service lines, sometimes called *care-centered organizations*, are smaller in scale than a large bureaucratic system. For example, in this organizational design the overall goals would be determined by the larger organization, but the service line would decide on the processes to be used to achieve the goals (Miller et al., 2001).

Flat Designs

Flat organizational designs are an effort to remove hierarchical layers by flattening the scalar chain and decentralizing the organization. There continues to be line authority, but because the organizational structure is flattened, more authority and decision making can occur where the work is being carried out. **Figure 12.3** shows

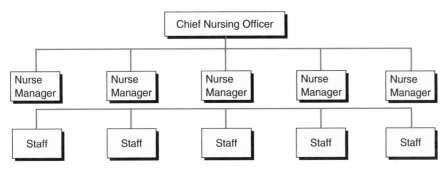

Figure 12.3 Flat organizational structure.

a flattened organizational structure. Many managers have difficulty letting go of centralized control, and even very flattened types of structure organizations often retain many characteristics of a bureaucracy.

DECISION MAKING WITHIN THE ORGANIZATIONAL HIERARCHY

The decision-making hierarchy, or pyramid, is often referred to as a *scalar chain*. By reviewing the organization chart in Figure 12.1, it is possible to determine where decisions are made within the management hierarchy. Although every manager has some decision-making authority, its type and level are determined by the manager's position on the chart.

In organizations with *centralized decision making,* a few managers at the top of the hierarchy make the decisions. *Decentralized decision making* diffuses decision making throughout the organization and allows problems to be solved by the lowest practical managerial level. Often this means that problems can be solved at the level at which they occur, which has the potential to improve quality care outcomes and increase organizational efficiency (Hagenstad, Weis, & Brophy, 2000; Krairiksh & Anthony, 2001). In general, the larger the organization, the greater the need to decentralize decision making.

Decision making needs to be decentralized in large organizations because the complex questions that must be answered can best be addressed by a variety of people with distinct areas of expertise. In addition, leaving such decisions in a large organization to a few managers burdens those managers tremendously and could result in devastating delays in decision making.

> In general, the larger the organization, the greater the need to decentralize decision making.

EXTERNAL STAKEHOLDERS

In addition to examining internal organizational structure, every organization should be viewed as being part of a greater community of stakeholders. Stakeholders are those entities in an organization's environment that play a role in the organization's health and performance, or that are affected by the organization (Borgatti, 2001). Examples of stakeholders for an acute care hospital might be the local School of Nursing, home health agencies, and managed care providers who contract with consumers in the area. Even the Chamber of Commerce in a city could be considered a stakeholder for a healthcare organization.

Stakeholders have interests in what the organization does, and may or may not have the power to influence the organization to protect their interests. Stakeholders' interests are varied, however, and their interests may coincide on some issues and not others. When stakeholders are unconnected, they have difficulty coordinating their efforts, and thus cannot control the organization. In contrast, when stakeholders are well connected, and the bonds among the stakeholders are closer than the bonds with the organization, stakeholders may side with each other against the organization, and be reluctant to act in ways that negatively affect other stakeholders (Borgatti, 2001).

Kerfoot (2002) suggests, however, that connected stakeholders can be a very positive thing and argues that the bottom line to success of any organization is the worth and value of the internal and external relationships that can be created. *Creating Communities of practice* (COP) (Wenger & Snyder, 2000) allows interested parties to come together to share their common vision and expertise and to create a plan for action. Astute leaders and managers then must always be cognizant of who their stakeholders are, what their connectedness is, and the opportunities for positive collaboration to achieve the organization's mission. A visual depiction of unconnected and connected stakeholders is shown in **Figure 12.4.**

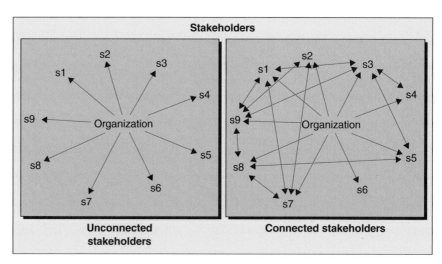

Figure 12.4 Unconnected stakeholders (left) work singly whereas connected stakeholders (right) can participate fully and share their vision and ideas.
(Source: Borgatti, S.P. [2001]. Organizational theory: Determinants of structure. Retrieved 11/21/03 from http://www.anlaytictech.com./mb021/orgtheory.htm)

LIMITATIONS OF ORGANIZATION CHARTS

Because organization charts show only formal relationships, what they can reveal about an institution is limited. The chart does not show the informal structure of the organization. Every institution has in place a dynamic informal structure that can be powerful and motivating. Knowledgeable leaders never underestimate its importance because the informal structure includes employees' interpersonal relationships, the formation of primary and secondary groups, and the identification of group leaders without formal authority.

The informal structure also has its own leaders. In addition, it also has its own communication channels, often referred to as the *grapevine*. These groups are important in organizations because they provide a feeling of belonging. They also have a great deal of power in an organization; they can either facilitate or sabotage planned change. Their ability to determine a unit's norms and acceptable behavior has a great deal to do with the socialization of new employees.

Informal leaders are frequently found among long-term employees or people in select gatekeeping positions, such as the CNO's secretary. Frequently the informal organization evolves from social activities or from relationships that develop outside the work environment.

Organization charts also are limited in their ability to depict each line position's degree of authority. Equating status with authority frequently causes confusion. The distance from the top of the organizational hierarchy usually determines the degree of status: the closer to the top, the higher the status. Status also is influenced by skill, education, specialization, level of responsibility, autonomy, and salary accorded a position. People frequently have status with little accompanying authority.

Because organizations are dynamic environments, an organization chart becomes obsolete very quickly. It also is possible that the organization chart may depict how things are supposed to be, when in reality the organization is still functioning under an old structure because employees have not yet accepted new lines of authority.

Another limitation of the organization chart is that although it defines authority, it does not define responsibility and accountability. The manager should understand the interrelationships and differences among these three terms.

Authority is defined as the official power to act. It is power given by the organization to direct the work of others. A manager may have the authority to hire, fire, or discipline others. Because the use of authority, power building, and political awareness are so important to functioning effectively in any structure, the next chapter discusses these organizational components in depth.

A *responsibility* is a duty or an assignment. It is the implementation of a job. For example, a responsibility common to many charge nurses is establishing the unit's daily patient care assignment. Managers should always be assigned responsibilities with concomitant authority. If authority is not commensurate to the responsibility, role confusion occurs for everyone involved. For example, supervisors may have the responsibility of maintaining high professional care standards among their staff. If the manager is not given the authority to discipline employees as needed, however, this responsibility is virtually impossible to implement.

> The informal structure also has its own leaders and its own communication channels, often referred to as the *grapevine*.

Display 12.2 **Advantages and Limitations of the Organization Chart**

Advantages
1. Maps lines of decision-making authority
2. Helps people understand their assignments and those of their coworkers
3. Reveals to managers and new personnel how they fit into the organization
4. Contributes to sound organizational structure
5. Shows formal lines of communication

Limitations
1. Shows only formal relationships
2. Does not indicate degree of authority
3. May show things as they are supposed to be or used to be rather than as they are
4. Possibility exists of confusing authority with status

Accountability is similar to responsibility but it is internalized. Thus to be accountable means that individuals agree to be morally responsible for the consequences of their actions. Thus, one individual cannot be accountable for another. Society holds us accountable for our assigned responsibilities, and people are expected to accept the consequences of their actions. A nurse who reports a medication error is being accountable for the responsibilities inherent in the position. **Display 12.2** discusses the advantages and limitations of an organizational chart.

ORGANIZATIONAL CULTURE

Organizational culture is a system of symbols and interactions unique to each organization. It is the ways of thinking, behaving, and believing that members of a unit have in common. It is the total of an organization's values, language, tradition, customs, and *sacred cows*—those few things present in an institution that are not open to discussion or change. For example, the hospital logo that had been designed by the original board of trustees is an item that may not be considered for updating or change.

Similarly, Waters (2004) defines organizational culture as "the source of motivated and coordinated activities within organizations, activities that serve as a foundation for practices and behaviors that endure because they're meaningful, have a history of working well, and are likely to continue working in the future" (p. 36). Both of these definitions impart a sense of the complexity and importance of organizational culture. It is the "operating system" of an organization and drives the organization and its actions (Waters).

Organizational culture is often confused with *organizational climate*—how employees perceive an organization. For example, an employee might perceive an organization as fair, friendly, and informal or as formal and very structured. The perception may be accurate or inaccurate, and people in the same organization may have different perceptions about the same organization.

The organization's climate and its culture may differ. Sleutel (2000), however, suggests that the phenomenon is the same, and it is only the perspective that is different. Although there are many differences between the constructs, there are also many similarities, and both areas deal with human behavior in organizations and how organizations influence group members (Sleutel, 2000).

Three types of organizational culture have been identified. Cooke and Lafferty (1989) call the first of these a *positive culture*. The positive culture is a constructive culture in which members are encouraged to interact with others and to approach tasks in proactive ways that will help them to meet their satisfaction needs. The constructive culture is based on achievement, self-actualization, encouragement of humanism, and affiliative norms.

In the other two cultures, *passive-aggressive* and *aggressive-defensive*, members interact in guarded and reactive ways and approach tasks in forceful ways to protect their status and security. These two cultures are based on approval, conventional, dependent, and avoidance norms and oppositional, power, competitive, and perfectionistic norms, respectively.

A constructive culture is one of the characteristics of a healthy organization and is set largely by leaders in the organization. The organization's culture provides the context for organizational behavior and, in turn, influences and sets the tone for employee behavior. However, culture is frequently modified with new leadership.

Although assessing unit culture is a management function, building a constructive culture, particularly if a negative culture is in place, requires the interpersonal and communication skills of a leader. "Healthcare organizations have lagged behind trends evident in corporate American that demonstrate how investments in organizational culture translate into high performance"(Wooten & Crane, 2003, p. 275). The leader must take an active role in creating the kind of organizational culture that will ensure success. The more entrenched the culture and pattern of actions, the more challenging the change process is for the leader. Indeed, Curran (2002) goes so far as to say that "culture eats strategy for lunch every time" (p. 267). In other words, culture is omnipotent and "if culture is the sum of our values, beliefs, rights and rituals, culture is reality" (p. 257). Given such entrenchment of culture, success in building a new culture often requires new leadership and/or assistance by the use of outside analysis.

Organizations, if large enough, also have many different and competing value systems that create subcultures. These subcultures shape perceptions, attitudes, and beliefs and influence how their members approach and execute their particular roles and responsibilities. Thus, these subcultures and members of their subcultures have their own perspectives and priorities (Mohr, Deatarick, Richmond, & Mahon, 2001). Baker, Beglinger, King, Salyards, and Thompson (2000) suggest that these subcultures can undermine the service delivery strategies of an organization, drain the energy of the managers who dare to take them on, and be remarkably resistant to change. A critical challenge then for the nurse leader–manager is to recognize these subcultures and to do whatever is necessary to create shared norms and priorities. "Defining a collective mission is a critical first step in creating the team efforts that drive collaborative and productive work and communication" (Wooten & Crane, 2003, p. 275).

If the unit culture is in harmony with the organizational culture and the nursing culture is in harmony with the other professional cultures, *consonance* is said to exist

(Fleeger, 1993). If the opposite is true, *incongruency* or *dissonance* occurs. Mohr, et al. (2001) states that incongruency between stated organizational values and behavior results in inflexibility due to the lack of a shared focus of attention to the organizational mission, a tendency to foster vicious or self-defeating circles, and tenuous emotional stability under conditions of stress. The characteristics of consonant and dissonant cultures are shown in **Table 12.2.**

Managers must be able to assess their unit's culture and choose management strategies that encourage consonance and discourage dissonance. Transforming negative work cultures is a difficult but not impossible task and requires the involvement and commitment of all parties (Baker et al., 2000). Such transformation requires both management assessment and leadership direction. Indeed, Wooten and Crane (2003) argue that nursing leaders should take on the responsibility of culture gatekeeper.

Much of an organization's culture is not available to staff in a retrievable source and must be related by others. For example, feelings about collective bargaining, nursing education levels, nursing autonomy, and nurse–physician relationships differ from one organization to another. These beliefs and values, however, are rarely written down or appear in a philosophy. Therefore, in addition to creating a constructive culture, a major leadership role is to assist subordinates in understanding the organization's culture. **Display 12.3** identifies questions leaders and followers should ask when assessing organizational culture.

Table 12.2 Characteristics of Consonant and Dissonant Cultures

Consonant Cultures	Dissonant Cultures
Collective spirit	Mismatch between professional and organizational goals
Golden rule norm	Stronger union affiliations than organizational
One supraordinate goal	Little staff representation on committees
Frequent staff–management interactions	Low staff participation in decision making
Clinical expertise valued	Do not have primary care models
Professional and organizational goals similar across work units	Competitive spirit
High cooperation between units	Them-versus-us norm
Primary care model promoting autonomy and independence	Low staff–management interactions
Formal and informal systems to address conflicts	Staff feel undervalued
Match between values and outcomes	Mismatch between values and outcomes
All nurses seen as members of same occupational group	Management seen as outside occupation; double standards for behaviors
All members seen as working toward same goal	Groups feel others not working toward common goal
Behavior norms same for everyone	Myths, stories, symbols not caring or positive

Display 12.3 Assessing the Organizational Culture

How does the organization view the physical environment?
1. Is the environment attractive?
2. Does it appear that there is adequate maintenance?
3. Are nursing stations crowded or noisy?
4. Is there an appropriate-size lobby? Are there quiet areas?
5. Is there sufficient seating for families in the dining room?
6. Are there enough conference rooms?

What is the organization's social environment?
1. Are many friendships maintained beyond the workplace?
2. Is there an annual picnic or holiday party that is well attended by the employees?
3. Do employees seem to generally like each other?
4. Do all shifts and all departments get along fairly well?
5. Are certain departments disliked or resented?
6. Are employees on a first-name basis with coworkers, doctors, charge nurses, and supervisors?

How supportive is the organization?
1. Is educational reimbursement available?
2. Are good, low-cost meals available to employees?
3. Are there adequate employee lounges?
4. Are funds available to send employees to workshops?
5. Are employees recognized for extra effort?
6. Does the organization help pay for the holiday party or other social functions?

What is the organizational power structure?
1. Who holds the most power in the organization?
2. Which departments are viewed as powerful? Which are viewed as powerless?
3. Who gets free meals? Who gets special parking places?
4. Who carries beepers? Who wears lab coats? Who has overhead pages?
5. Who has the biggest office?
6. Who is never called by his or her first name?

How does the organization view safety?
1. Is there a well-lighted parking place for employees arriving or departing when it is dark?
2. Is there an active and involved safety committee?
3. Are security guards needed?

What is the communicative environment?
1. Is upward communication usually written or verbal?
2. Is there much informal communication?
3. Is there an active grapevine? Is it reliable?
4. Where is important information exchanged? the parking lot? the doctors' surgical dressing room? the nurses' station? the coffee shop? in surgery or in the delivery room?

What are the organizational taboos? Who are the heroes?
1. Are there special rules and policies that can never be broken?
2. Are certain subjects or ideas forbidden?
3. Are there relationships that cannot be threatened?

SHARED GOVERNANCE: THE ORGANIZATIONAL DESIGN OF THE 21ST CENTURY?

Shared governance, one of the most innovative and idealistic of organization structures, was developed in the mid-1980s as an alternative to the traditional bureaucratic organizational structure. A flat type of organizational structure is often used to describe shared governance but differs somewhat, as shown in **Figure 12.5.** In shared governance, the organization's governance is shared among board members, nurses, physicians, and management. Thus, decision-making and communication channels are altered. Group structures, in the form of joint practice committees, are developed to assume the power and accountability for decision making, and professional communication takes on an egalitarian structure.

The stated aim of shared governance is the empowerment of people within the decision-making system. In healthcare organizations, this empowerment is directed at increasing nurses' authority and control over nursing practice. Shared governance thus gives nurses more control over their nursing practice by being an accountability-based governance system for professional workers.

Although *participatory management* lays the foundation for shared governance, they are not the same. Participatory management implies that others are allowed to participate in decision making over which someone has control. Thus, the act of "allowing" participation identifies the real and final authority for the participant.

There is no single model of shared governance, although all models emphasize the empowerment of staff nurses. Generally, issues related to nursing practice are the responsibility of nurses, not managers, and *nursing councils* are used to organize governance. These nursing councils, elected at the organization and unit levels,

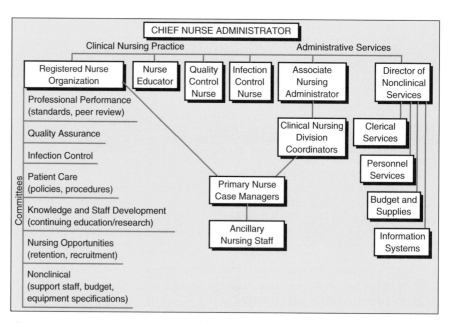

Figure 12.5 Shared governance model.

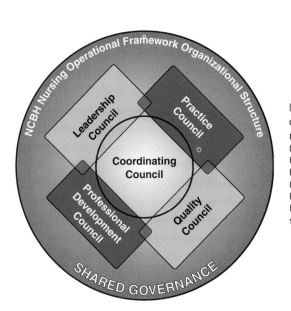

Figure 12.6 Sample nursing councils in a Shared Governance Model.
(Source: North Carolina Baptist Hospital, Wake Forest University Baptist Medical Center. (n.d.). Shared Governance. Retrieved 11/20/03 from http://www.wfubmc.edu/nursing/sharedgov.html.)

use a congressional format organized like a representative form of government, with a president and cabinet.

A sample operational framework of an organization using shared governance is shown in **Figure 12.6.** In this model from Wake Forest University, Baptist Medical Center, there are four Governance Councils and a Coordinating Council. The Governance Councils are Practice Council, Professional Development Council, Quality Council, and Leadership Council. The councils participate in decision making and coordination of the Department of Nursing and provide input through the Shared Governance process in all other areas where nursing care is delivered.

Black (2003) describes another shared governance model, called the *Professional Nurse Practice Model* (PNPM). This model was implemented at Central Iowa Health System, and involves staff nurses in making decisions about nursing practice via participation in a committee structure. Issues include nursing quality, nursing policy and procedure, nursing research, resource utilization, and professional growth. Some of the accomplishments of the PNPM over the past two years included the development of a model for evidence-based practice, a clinical advancement program that recognizes clinical excellence at the bedside, and nursing grand rounds. In addition, the staff nurse vacancy rate fell from 12% in 2000 to 4.3% by the end of 2002.

The number of healthcare organizations using shared governance models is increasing, and research supports that shared governance improves staff nurses' perceptions of their job and practice environment. Additionally, recent research comparing traditional and shared governance models in hospitals revealed that using a shared governance model results in a constructive hospital culture, nurse retention, work satisfaction, and positive patient outcomes (Stumpf, 2001).

However, a major impediment to the implementation of shared governance has been the reluctance of managers to change their roles. The nurse–manager's role

Research suggests that using a shared governance model results in a constructive hospital culture, nurse retention, work satisfaction, and positive patient outcomes.

becomes one of consulting, teaching, collaborating, and creating an environment with the structures and resources needed for the practice of nursing and shared decision making between nurses and the organization. This new role is foreign to many managers and difficult to accept. In addition, consensus decision making takes more time than autocratic decision making, and not all nurses want to share decisions and accountability. Although many positive outcomes have been attributed to implementation of shared governance, the expense of introducing and maintaining this model also must be considered. Shared governance requires a substantial and long-term commitment on the part of the workers and the organization.

ORGANIZATIONS AND MAGNET STATUS

During the early 1980s, the American Academy of Nursing (AAN) first began identifying hospitals that maintained well-qualified nurse executives in a decentralized environment, with organizational structures that emphasized open, participatory management (Upenieks, 2003). These *magnet* hospitals, as they came to be called, also offered autonomous, self-managing, self-governing climates that allowed nurses to fully practice their clinical expertise, flexible staffing, adequate staffing ratios and clinical career opportunities (Upenieks, 2003).

In 1994, some 12 years after the original magnet hospitals were identified, the American Nurses Association (ANA), through the American Nurses' Credentialing Center's (ANCC), established a "new" magnet hospital designation process that would allow hospitals to self-nominate under the "Magnet Nursing Services Recognition Program for Excellence in Nursing Services" (Havens, 2001).

Becoming a magnet hospital is not easy. First the hospital must create and promote a professional practice culture in all aspects of nursing care (Bumgarner & Beard, 2003). Then the hospital must apply to the ANCC, submit comprehensive documentation that demonstrates its compliance with standards in the ANA's *Scope and Standards for Nurse Administrators*, and undergo a multi-day onsite evaluation to verify the information in the documentation submitted and to assess the presence of the 14 "forces of magnetism" (see **Display 12.4**) within the organization (Joint Commission for the Accreditation of Hospitals, 2003). This process may take up to two years (Bumgarner & Beard, 2003). Magnet status is awarded for a four-year period, after which the organization must reapply.

The average RN vacancy rate at magnet hospitals is 8.19% and the average length of employment among RNs is 8.94 years (New Law, JCAHO Reports 2002), significantly better than non-magnet hospitals. RNs employed in magnet hospitals also experience better staffing, lower use of agency nurses, lower levels of burnout, and higher levels of job satisfaction. Patients fare better as well with improved outcomes, including lower morality rates (Spence-Laschinger, Almost, & Tuer-Hodes, 2003; Aiken, Havens, & Sloane, 2000; Havens, 2001).

As of October 15, 2003, there were 88 magnet-designated organizations (ANCC, 2003). The first ANCC magnet hospital, University of Washington, was designated in 1994 (New Law, 2002) and international certification began in 1999.

Display 12.4	The 14 Forces of Magnetism for Magnet Hospital Status

1. Quality of nursing leadership
2. Organizational structure
3. Management style
4. Personnel policies and programs
5. Professional models of care
6. Quality of care
7. Quality improvement
8. Consultation and resources
9. Autonomy
10. Community and the hospital
11. Nurses as teachers
12. Image of nursing
13. Interdisciplinary relationships
14. Professional development

Learning Exercise 12.4

Why Work for Them?

A list of current magnet hospitals and their contact information can be found at the American Nurses Credentialing Center website under the URL http://www.nursecredentialing.org/magnet/facilities.html.
Assignment: Select one of the current magnet hospitals and prepare a one-page written report about how that particular hospital demonstrates the excellence exemplified by magnet status. Speak to at least five of the "forces of magnetism." Would you want to work for this particular hospital?

COMMITTEE STRUCTURE IN AN ORGANIZATION

Managers also are responsible for designing and implementing appropriate committee structures. Poorly structured committees can be nonproductive for the organization and frustrating for committee members. However, there are many benefits to and justifications for well-structured committees. To compensate for some of the difficulty in organizational communication created by line and line-and-staff structures, committees are used widely to facilitate upward communication. The nature of formal organizations dictates a need for committees in assisting with management functions. Additionally, as organizations seek new ways to revamp old bureaucratic structures, committees may pave the road to increased staff participation in organization governance.

Committees may be advisory or may have a coordinating or informal function. Because committees communicate upward and downward and encourage the participation of interested or affected employees, they assist the organization in receiving

Display 12.5	Factors to Consider When Organizing Committees and Making Appointments

- The committee should be composed of people who want to contribute in terms of commitment, energy, and time.
- The members should have a variety of work experience and educational backgrounds. Composition should, however, ensure expertise sufficient to complete the task.
- Committees should have enough members to accomplish assigned tasks but not so many that discussion cannot occur. Six to eight members is usually ideal.
- The tasks and responsibilities, including reporting mechanisms, should be clearly outlined.
- Assignments should be given ahead of time, with clear expectations that assigned work will be discussed at the next meeting.
- All committees should have written agendas and effective committee chairs.

valuable feedback and important information. They generate ideas and creative thinking to solve operational problems or improve services and often improve the quality and quantity of work accomplished. Committees also can pool specific skills and expertise and help to reduce resistance to change.

However, all these positive benefits can be achieved only if committees are appropriately organized and led. If not properly used, the committee becomes a liability to the organizing process because it wastes energy, time, and money and can defer decisions and action. One of the leadership roles inherent in organizing work is to ensure that committees are not used to avoid or delay decisions but to facilitate organizational goals. **Display 12.5** lists factors to consider when organizing committees.

Responsibilities and Opportunities of Committee Work

Committees present the leader–manager with many opportunities and responsibilities. Managers need to be well grounded in group dynamics because meetings represent a major time commitment. Managers serve as members of committees and as leaders or chairpersons of committees.

Because committees make major decisions, managers should use the opportunities available at meetings to become more visible in the larger organization. The manager has a responsibility to select appropriate power strategies, such as coming to meetings well prepared, and to use skill in the group process to generate influence and gain power at meetings.

Another responsibility is to create an environment at unit committee meetings that leads to shared decision making. Encouraging an interaction free of status and power is important. Likewise, an appropriate seating arrangement, such as a circle, will increase motivation for committee members to speak up.

The responsible manager is also aware that staff from different cultures may have different needs in groups. When assigning members to committees, cultural diversity should always be a goal. In addition, because gender differences are increasingly being recognized as playing a role in problem solving, communication, and power, efforts should be made to include both men and women on committees.

The manager must not rely too heavily on committees or use them as a method to delay decision making. Numerous committee assignments exhaust staff, and committees then become poor tools for accomplishing work. An alternative that will decrease the time commitment for committee work is to make individual assignments and gather the entire committee only to report progress.

In the leadership role, an opportunity exists for important influence on committee and group effectiveness. A dynamic leader inspires people to put spirit into working for a shared goal. Leaders demonstrate their commitment to participatory management by how they work with committees. Leaders keep the committee on course. Committees may be chaired by an elected member of the group, appointed by the manager, or led by the department or unit manager. Informal leaders also may emerge from the group process.

It is important for the manager to be aware of the possibility for *groupthink* to occur in any group or committee structure. Groupthink occurs when group members fail to take adequate risks by disagreeing, being challenged, or assessing discussion carefully. If the manager is actively involved in the work group or on the committee, groupthink is less likely to occur. The leadership role includes teaching members to avoid groupthink by demonstrating critical thinking and being a role model who allows his or her own ideas to be challenged.

Organizational Effectiveness

There is no one "best" way to structure an organization. Variables as the size of the organization, the capability of its human resources, and the commitment level of its workers should always be considered. Regardless of what type of organizational structure is used, certain minimal requirements can be identified:

- The structure should be clearly defined so that employees know where they belong and where to go for assistance.
- The goal should be to build the fewest possible management levels and have the shortest possible chain of command. This eliminates friction, stress, and inertia.
- The unit staff need to be able to see where their tasks fit into common tasks of the organization.
- The organizational structure should enhance, not impede communication.
- The organizational structure should facilitate decision making that results in the greatest work performance.
- Staff should be organized in a manner that encourages informal groups to develop a sense of community and belonging.
- Nursing services should be organized to facilitate the development of future leaders.

Despite the known difficulties of bureaucracies, it has been difficult for some organizations to move away from the bureaucratic model. However, perhaps as a result of magnet hospital research demonstrating both improved patient outcomes and improved recruitment and retention of staff, there has been an increasing effort to redesign and restructure organizations to make them more flexible and decentralized. Still, progress toward these goals continues to be slow.

INTEGRATING LEADERSHIP ROLES AND MANAGEMENT FUNCTIONS ASSOCIATED WITH ORGANIZATIONAL STRUCTURE

Integrated leader–managers need to look at organizational structure as the road map that tells them how organizations operate. Without organizational structure, people would work in a chaotic environment. Structure becomes an important tool then to facilitate order and enhance productivity.

Astute leader–managers understand both the structure of the organization in which they work as well as external stakeholders. The integrated leader–manager, however, goes beyond personal understanding of the larger organizational design. The leader–manager takes responsibility for ensuring that subordinates also understand the overall organizational structure and the structure at the unit level. This can be done by being a resource and a role model to subordinates. The role modeling includes demonstrating accountability and the appropriate use of authority.

The effective manager recognizes the difficulties inherent in advisory positions and uses leadership skills to support staff in these positions. This is accomplished by granting sufficient authority to enable advisory staff to carry out the functions of their role.

Leadership requires that problems are pursued through appropriate channels, that upward communication is encouraged, and that unit structure is periodically evaluated to determine if it can be redesigned to enable increased lower-level decision making. The integrated leader–manager also facilitates constructive informal group structure. It is important for the manager to be knowledgeable about the organization's culture and subcultures. It is just as important for the leader to promote the development of a shared constructive culture with subordinates.

It is a management role to evaluate types of organizational structure and governance and to implement those that will have the most positive impact in the department. It is a leadership skill to role model the shared authority necessary to make newer models of organizational structure and governance possible.

When serving on committees, the opportunity should be used to gain influence to present the needs of patients and staff appropriately. The integrated leader–manager comes to meetings well prepared and contributes thoughtful comments and ideas. The leader's critical thinking and role-modeling behavior discourages groupthink among work groups or in committees.

Integrated leader–managers also refrain from judging and encourage all members of a committee to participate and contribute. An important management function is to see that appropriate works gets accomplished in committees, that they remain productive, and that they are not used to delay decision making. A leadership role is the involvement of staff in organizational decision making, either informally or through more formal models of organizational design, such as shared governance.

The integrated leader–manager understands the organization and recognizes what can be molded or shaped and what is constant. Thus, the interaction between the manager and the organization is dynamic.

※ Key Concepts

- Many modern healthcare organizations continue to be organized around a *line* or *line-and-staff* design and have many attributes of a bureaucracy; however, there is a movement toward less bureaucratic designs, such as ad hoc, matrix, or care-centered systems.
- A *bureaucracy*, as proposed by Max Weber, is characterized by a clear chain of command, rules and regulations, specialization of work, division of labor, and impersonality of relationships.
- An *organization chart* depicts formal relationships, channels of communication, and authority through *line* and *staff* positions, *scalar chains*, and *span of control*.
- *Unity of command* means that each person should have only one boss so there is less confusion and greater productivity.
- *Centrality* refers to the degree of communication a particular management position has.
- In *centralized decision making,* decisions are made by a few managers at the top of the hierarchy. In *decentralized decision making,* decision making is diffused throughout the organization, and problems are solved at the lowest practical managerial level.
- Organizational structure affects how people perceive their roles and the status given to them by other people in the organization.
- Organizational structure is effective when (1) the design is clearly communicated; (2) there are as few managers as possible to accomplish goals; (3) communication is facilitated; (4) decisions are made at the lowest possible level; (5) informal groups are encouraged; and (6) future leaders are developed.
- The sets of entities in an organization's environment that play a role in the organization's health and performance, or which are affected by the organization, are called *stakeholders.*
- *Authority, responsibility,* and *accountability* differ in terms of official sanctions, self-directedness, and moral integration.
- *Organizational culture* is the total of an organization's beliefs, history, taboos, formal and informal relationships, and communication patterns.
- Subunits of large organizations also have a culture. These subcultures may be *consonant* or *dissonant* with other professional cultures in the organization.
- Informal groups are present in every organization. They are often powerful, although they have no formal authority. Informal groups determine norms and assist members in the socialization process.
- *Shared governance* refers to an organizational design that empowers staff nurses by making them an integral part of patient care decision making and providing accountability and responsibility in nursing practice.

- *Magnet* hospital status is conferred by the American Nurses Credentialing Center on hospitals exemplifying well qualified nurse executives in a decentralized environment, with organizational structures that emphasize open, participatory management. Magnet hospitals demonstrate improved patient outcomes and higher staff nurse satisfaction than non-magnet hospitals.
- Too many committees in an organization is a sign of a poorly designed organizational structure.
- Committees should have an appropriate number of members, prepared agendas, clearly outlined tasks, and effective leadership if they are to be productive.
- *Groupthink* occurs when there is too much conformity to group norms.

More Learning Exercises and Applications

 Learning Exercise 12.5

Restructuring—*In Depth*

You are the staff coordinator at a home health agency. There are 22 registered nurses in your span of control. In a meeting today, John Dao, the chief nursing officer (CNO), tells you that your span of control needs adjustment to be effective. Therefore, the CNO has decided to decentralize the department. To accomplish this, he plans to designate three of your staff as shift coordinators. These shift coordinators will "schedule patient visits for all the staff on their shift and be accountable for the staff they supervise." The CNO believes this restructuring will give you more time for implementing a continuous quality improvement (CQI) program and promoting staff development.

Although you are glad to have the opportunity to begin these new projects, you are somewhat unclear about the role expectations of the new shift coordinators and how this will change your job description. Will these shift coordinators report to you? If so, will you have direct line authority or staff authority? Who should be responsible for evaluating the performance of the staff nurses now? Who will handle employee disciplinary problems? How involved should the shift coordinators be in strategic planning or determining next year's budget? What types of management training will be needed by the shift coordinators to prepare for their new role? Are you the most appropriate person to train them?

Assignment: There is great potential for conflict here. In small groups, make a list of 10 questions (not including the ones listed in the learning exercise) that you would want to ask the CNO at your next meeting to clarify role expectations. Discuss tools and skills you have learned in the preceding units that could make this role change less traumatic for all involved.

Learning Exercise 12.6

Problem Solving: Working Toward Shared Governance
You are the supervisor of a Surgical Services department in a non-union hospital. The staff on your unit have become increasingly frustrated with hospital policies regarding staffing ratios, on-call pay, and verbal medical orders, but feel they have limited opportunities for providing feedback to change the current system. You would like to explore the possibility of moving toward a shared governance model of decision making to resolve this issue and others like it, but are not quite sure where to start.
Assignment: Assume you are the supervisor in this case. Answer the following questions.
1. Who do I need to involve in this discussion and at what point?
2. How might I determine if the overarching organizational structure supports shared governance? How would I determine if external stakeholders would be impacted? How would I determine if organizational culture and subculture would support a shared governance model?
3. What types of Nursing Councils might be created to provide a framework for operation?
4. Who would be the members on these Nursing Councils?
5. What support mechanisms would need to be in place to ensure success of this project?
6. What would my role be as a supervisor in identifying and resolving employee concerns in a shared governance model?

Learning Exercise 12.7

Finding Direction
You are a new graduate working the 3 P.M. to 11 P.M. shift in a large metropolitan hospital on the pediatrics unit. You feel frustrated because you had many preceptors while you were being oriented and each told you slightly different variations of the unit routine. Additionally, the regular charge nurse has just been promoted and moved to another unit and the charge nurse position on your unit is being filled by two part-time nurses.

You feel inadequate for the job and do not know where to turn or to whom you should direct your questions. Assuming that your organization chart resembles the one in Figure 12.1, outline a plan of action that would be appropriate to take. Share your plan with a larger group.

Learning Exercise 12.8

Cultures and Countercultures
Review Display 12.2. Then select one of the following topics to discuss in small groups:
1. Identify key components of the professional nursing and medical cultures. Are the cultures of professional nursing and medicine consonant or dissonant? Give examples to support your position.
2. Identify key components of the registered nurse and licensed vocational nurse cultures. Are these two cultures consonant or dissonant? Do other members of the healthcare team (e.g., respiratory therapists, dietitians, occupational therapists, physical therapists) have a culture consonant with nursing? Give examples to support your position.
3. (For RN to BSN students) Have you found a difference between the culture of your baccalaureate nursing program and that of your ADN or diploma nursing program? If so, do you think this dissonance contributed to the failure of the 1985 American Nurses Association resolution to mandate the baccalaureate degree as the entry level to professional nursing practice?
4. Some clinicians have argued that nursing education is "carried out in an ivory tower, far removed from the real world of nursing practice." Do you believe there is dissonance between nursing education's culture and that of clinical practice? What are the key attributes of each of these cultures?

Learning Exercise 12.9

Thinking About Committee Work
As a writing exercise, choose one of the following to examine in depth:
1. What has contributed to the productivity of the committees on which you have served?
2. Have you ever served on a committee that made recommendations on which higher authority never acted? What was the effect on the group?

Learning Exercise 12.10

Participation and Productivity
You are a 3 to 11 charge nurse on a surgical unit. You have been selected
to chair the unit's safety committee. Each month, you have a short committee meeting with the other committee members. Your committee's
main responsibility is to report upward any safety issues that have been
identified. Lately, you have found an increase in needle-stick incidents,
and the committee has been addressing this problem.

The committee is made up of two nursing assistants, one unit clerk, two
staff RNs, and two LPNs. All shifts and staff cultures are represented. Lately,
you have found the meetings are not going well because one member of
the group, Mary, has begun to monopolize the meeting time. She is especially outspoken about the danger of HIV and seems more interested in
pointing blame regarding the needle sticks than in finding a solution to
the problem.

You have privately spoken to Mary about her frequent disruption of the
committee business; although she apologized, the behavior has continued. You feel some members of the committee becoming bored and rest-
less, and you believe the committee is making very little progress.
Assignment: Using your knowledge of committee structure and effectiveness, outline steps you would take to facilitate more group participation
and make the committee more productive. Be specific and explain exactly
what you would do at the next meeting to prevent Mary from taking over
the meeting.

 Web Links

American Nurses Credentialing Center:
http://www.nursingworld.org/ancc/magnet.html
*Accessed 11/20/03. Frequently asked questions about magnet hospital status as well as
current list of magnet hospitals.*

Organizational charts:
http://ftp.fcc.gov/fccorgchart.html
*Accessed 11/20/03. Site shows a typical government (Federal Communications Com-
mission) organization chart.*

Matrix Management in Changing Times:
http://www.nursingnetwork.com/matrix.htm
Accessed 11/20/03. An article by J. Klein on the use of the matrix organizational structure.

Max Weber, 1864-1920:
http://cepa.newschool.edu/het/profiles/weber.htm
*Accessed 11/20/03. Photo, biography, major works of sociologist and economist Max
Weber.*

References

Aiken, L. H., Havens, D. S. & Sloane, D. M. (2000). The Magnet Nursing Services Recognition program: A comparison of two groups of magnet hospitals. *American Journal of Nursing, 100* (3), 26–36.

American Nurses Credentialing Center. (2003). *Frequently asked questions.* Retrieved Nov. 20, 2003 from http://www.nursecredentialing.org/magnet/facilities.html.

Baker, C., Beglinger, J., King, S., Salyards, M., & Thompson, A. (2000). Transforming negative work cultures. *Journal of Nursing Administration, 30*(7/8), 357–363.

Bumgarner, S. D., & Beard, E. L. (2003). The magnet application: Pitfalls to avoid. *Journal of Nursing Administration, 33 (*11), 603–606.

Black, K. (2003). Recruitment & retention report. Innovative programs grab a thumbs up. *Nursing Management, 34* (6), 19–20, 22.

Borgatti, S. P. (Revised Oct. 8, 2001). *Organizational theory: Determinants of structure.* Retrieved 11/21/03 from http://www.analytictech.com/mb021/orgtheory.htm.

Cooke, R., & Lafferty, J. (1989). *Organizational culture inventory.* Plymouth, MI: Human Synergistics.

Curran, C. R. (2002). Editorial: Culture eats strategy for lunch every time. *Nursing Economics, 20* (6), 257.

Fayol, H. (1949). General and industrial management (C. Storrs, Trans.). London: Isaac Pittman and Sons.

Fleeger, M. E. (1993). Assessing organizational culture: A planning strategy. *Nursing Management, 24*(2), 39–41.

Hagenstad, R., Weis, C., & Brophy, K. (2000). Striking a balance with decentralized housekeeping. *Nursing Management, 31*(6), 39–43.

Havens, D. S. (2001). Comparing nursing infrastructure and outcomes: ANCC Magnet and non-magnet CNE's Report. *Nursing Economic$, 19* (6). 258–266.

Hill, V. L. (2004). Cultivate corporate culture and diversity. *Nursing Management, 35* (1), 36–37, 50.

Howell, J. N., Frederick, J., Olinger, B., Leftridge, D., Bell, T., Hess, R., & Clipp, E. C. (2001). Can nurses govern in a government agency? *Journal of Nursing Administration, 31* (4), 187–195.

Joint Commission for the Accreditation of Hospitals. (2003). Facts about American Nurses Credentialing Center Magnet Recognition program. Retrieved Nov. 20, 2003 from http://www.jcaho.com/news+room/press+kits/facts+about+magnet+hospitals.htm

Kerfoot, K. (2002). The leader as chief knowledge officer. *Nursing Economic$, 20* (1), 40, 43.

Krairiksh, M., & Anthony, M. K. (2001). Benefits and outcomes of staff nurses' participation in decision-making. *Journal of Nursing Administration, 31*(1), 16–23.

Kramer, M., & Schmalenberg, C. E. (2003). Magnet hospital nurses describe control over nursing practice. *Western Journal of Nursing Research, 25* (4), 434–452.

Miller, J., Galloway, M., Coughlin, C., & Brennan, E. (2001). Care-centered organizations. *Journal of Nursing Administration, 31*(2), 67–73.

Mohr, W. K., Deatrick, J., Richmond, T., & Mahon, M. M. (2001). A reflection on values in turbulent times. *Nursing Outlook, 49* (1), 30–36.

New law. JCAHO report recognizes success of Magnet status. (2002, September/October). *The American Nurse.* Retrieved 11/20/03 from http://nursingworld.org/tan/sepoct02/magnet.htm

Sleutel, M. R. (2000). Climate, culture, context, or work environment? *Journal of Nursing Administration, 30*(2), 53–58.

Spence-Laschinger, H. K., Almost, J., & Tuer-Hodes, D. (2003). Workplace empowerment and magnet hospital characteristics. *Journal of Nursing Administration, 33* (7/8), 410–422.

Stumpf, L. R. (2001). A comparison of governance types and patient satisfaction outcomes. *Journal of Nursing Administration, 31*(4), 196–202.

Upenieks, V. V. (2003). What's the attraction to magnet hospitals? *Nursing Management, 34* (2), 43–44.

Urden, L. D., & Rogers, S. (2000). Out in front: A new title reflects nurse managers; changing scope of accountabilities. *Nursing Management, 31*(7), 27–30.

Wake Forest University Baptist Medical Center. (n.d.). *Shared governance.* Retrieved 11/20/03 from http://www.wfubmc.edu/nursing/sharedgov.html

Waters, V. L. (2004). Cultivate corporate culture and diversity: Create and maintain a thriving environment in the midst of institutional change. *Nursing Management, 35*(1), 36–37, 50.

Wenger, E., & Snyder, W. (2000). Communities of practice: The new organizational frontier. *Harvard Business Review, 78*(1), 139–145.

Wooten, L. P., & Crane, P. (2003). Nurses as implementers of organizational culture. *Nursing Economic$, 21* (6), 275–279.

Bibliography

Aiken, L. H., & Patrician, P. (2000). Measuring organizational traits of hospitals: The revised nursing work index. *Nursing Research, 49*, 146–153.

Andrica, D. C. (2000). Working with a board. *Nursing Economic$, 18*(3), 167–168.

Burge, P., Nones-Cronin, S., Kramer, J., & Ober, J. (2003). Prepare to draw magnet recognition. *Nursing Management, 34* (11), 32–35.

Castleforte, M. R., & Milton, D. (2000). Rounding out the house supervisor role. *Nursing Management, 31*(11), 46.

Esler, R. O. & Nipp, D. A. (2001). Worker designed culture change. *Nursing Economic$, 19* (4), 161–163.

Gershon, R. R., Stone, P. W., Bakken, S., & Larson, E. (January 2004). Measurement of organizational culture and climate in healthcare. *Journal of Nursing Administration, 34* (1), 33–40.

Hospital's culture values employees. (2003). *OR Manager, 19* (4), 10.

How building a "just culture" helps an organization learn from errors. (2003). *OR Manager, 19* (5), 1, 14–15.

Ingersoll, G. I., Kirsch, J. C., Merk, S. E., & Lightfoot, J. (2000). Relationship of organizational culture and readiness for change to employee commitment to the organization. *Journal of Nursing Administration, 30*(1), 11–20.

Jones, J. M. (2003). Dual or dueling culture and commitment: The impact of a tri-hospital merger. *Journal of Nursing Administration, 33* (4), 235–242.

Jones-Schenk, J. (2001). How magnets attract nurses. *Nursing Management, 32*(1), 41–42.

Kennerly, S. (2000). Perceived worker autonomy: The foundation for shared governance. *Journal of Nursing Administration, 30*(12), 611–617.

Kramer, M., Schmalenberg, C. (2003). Magnet hospital staff nurses describe clinical autonomy. *Nursing Outlook, 51*(1), 13–19.

Neuheuser, P. C. (2002). Building a high-retention culture in healthcare: Fifteen ways to get good people to stay. *Journal of Nursing Administration, 32*(9), 470–478.

Perry-Wooten, L., & Crane, P. (2003). Nurses as implementers of organizational culture. *Nursing Economic$, 21*(6), 275–279.

Porter-O'Grady, T. (2001). Worker autonomy: The foundation of shared governance. *Journal of Nursing Administration, 31*(3), 100.

Porter-O'Grady, T. (2001). Is shared governance still relevant? *Journal of Nursing Administration, 31* (10), 468–473.

Porter-O'Grady, T. (2003). Researching shared governance: A futility of focus . . . "The value of collaborative governance/staff empowerment." *Journal of Nursing Administration, 33* (4), 251–252.

Salvage, J. (2003). It's time for nurses to file away the bureaucracy. *Nursing Times, 99*(4), 19.

Sim, J., Zadnik, M. G., & Radloff, A. (2003). University and workplace cultures: Their impact on the development of lifelong learners. *Radiography, 9*(2), 99–107.

Taylor, N.T. (2003). The magnetic pull. *Nursing Management, 34*(7), 48–56.

Upenieks, V. (2000). The relationship of nursing practice models and job satisfaction outcomes. *Journal of Nursing Administration, 30*(6), 330–335.

Understanding Organizational, Political, and Personal Power

. . . power is a positive concept, and several types of power are prerequisite for human development and self-expression.

—Sue Thomas Hegyvary

The previous chapter reviewed organizational structure and introduced status, authority, and responsibility at different levels of the organizational hierarchy. In Chapter 13, the organization is examined further, with emphasis on the management functions and leadership roles inherent in effective use of authority, establishment of a personal power base, empowerment of staff, and the impact of organizational politics on power.

The word *power* is derived from the Latin verb *potere* (to be able); thus, power may be appropriately defined as that which enables one to accomplish goals. Power can also be defined as the capacity to act or the strength and potency to accomplish something. Having power gives one the potential to change the attitudes and behaviors of individual people and groups.

Authority, or the right to command, accompanies any management position and is a source of legitimate power, although components of management, authority, and power are also necessary, to a degree, for successful leadership. The manager knowledgeable about the wise use of authority, power, and political strategy is more effective at meeting personal, unit, and organizational goals. Likewise, powerful leaders are able to build high morale because they delegate more and build with a team effort. Thus, their followers become part of the growth and excitement of the organization as their own status is enhanced. The leadership roles and management functions inherent in the use of authority and power are shown in **Display 13.1.**

Display 13.1 **Leadership Roles and Management Functions Associated with Organizational Politics, Power Acquisition, and Authority**

Leadership Roles
1. Creates a climate that promotes followership in response to authority.
2. Recognizes the dual pyramid of power that exists between the organization and its employees.
3. Uses a powerful persona to increase respect and decrease fear in subordinates.
4. Recognizes when it is appropriate to have authority questioned or to question authority.
5. Is personally comfortable with power in the political arena.
6. Empowers other nurses.
7. Assists staff in using appropriate political strategies.

Management Functions
1. Uses authority to ensure that organizational goals are met.
2. Uses political strategies that are complementary to the unit's and organization's functioning.
3. Builds a power base adequate for the assigned management role.
4. Maintains a small authority–power gap.
5. Is knowledgeable about the essence and appropriate use of power.
6. Maintains personal credibility with subordinates.
7. Serves as a role model of the empowered nurse.

UNDERSTANDING POWER

Power may be feared, worshipped, or mistrusted. It is frequently misunderstood. Our first experience with power usually occurs in the family unit. Power, in most ordinary uses of the term, appears to be more aligned with male than with female stereotypes (Ledet & Henley, 2000). Because children's roles are likened to later subordinate roles and the parental power position is similar to management, adult views of the management–subordinate relationship are influenced by how power was used in the family unit. A positive or negative familial power experience may greatly affect a person's ability to deal with power systems in adulthood. Sellers (1999) interviewed many of *Fortune* magazine's 50 most powerful women in America and found that many of them credited their powerful mothers in developing their potential for leading companies.

Gender and Power

Successful leaders are aware of their views on the use and abuse of power. Some women, in particular, may hold negative connotations of power and never learn to use power constructively. Women have traditionally demonstrated, at best, ambivalence toward the concept of power and until recently have openly eschewed the pursuit of power. This may have occurred because women as a whole have been socialized to view power differently than men do. For some women, power may be viewed as dominance versus submission; associated with personal qualities, not accomplishment; and dependent on personal or physical attributes, not skill. Many women may not believe they inherently possess power but instead must rely on others to acquire it. Rather than feeling capable of achieving and managing power, some women may feel that power manages them.

However, the historical view of women as less powerful than men appears to be changing. These changes are taking place within women, in women's view of other women holding power, in organizational hierarchies, and among both male subordinates and male colleagues (Fisher, 1999; Ledet & Henley, 2000).

Today gender differences regarding power are fading and the corporate world is beginning to look at new ways for leaders to obtain and handle power. Stahl (1999) maintains that nurse leaders in the 21st century will need to deal with organizational power and politics in a completely different way and will need to develop political strategies for team building and establishing trust. Political skill in developing consensus, inclusion, and involvement are also needed, skills that have often been linked to female characteristics (Carli, 1999; Fisher, 1999).

It is notable that these very attributes, which once closed corporate doors and created a glass ceiling, are now welcomed in the boardroom. These attributes are certainly not limited to women; many male leaders also possess these characteristics. However, despite significant gains, many women continue to remain unskilled in the art of the political process. While not all agree (Lips, 2000), many recent studies show that how others view men and women as being powerful has gradually changed over the last 10 years. At present it is difficult to say with certainty if the male or female is stereotypically viewed as the more powerful in organizations (Fisher, 1999; Ledet & Henley, 2000).

Learning Exercise 13.1

Is Power Different for Men and Women?
Research studies differ on how men and women view power and how others view men and women in positions of authority. Do you think there are gender differences in how people are viewed as being powerful? Discuss this in a group and then go to the library or use Internet sources to see if you can find recent studies that support your views.

Politics is the art of using legitimate power wisely. It requires clear decision making, assertiveness, accountability, and the willingness to express one's own views. It also requires being proactive rather than reactive and demands decisiveness. Women in power positions in today's healthcare settings are more likely to recognize their innate abilities that support the effective use of power.

In determining whether power is "good" or "bad," it may be helpful to look at its opposite: *powerlessness*. Most people agree that they dislike being powerless. Everyone needs some control in his or her life. Powerlessness tends to breed bossiness. Thus, the leader–manager who feels powerless often creates an ineffective, petty, dictatorial, and rule-minded management style. Individuals who feel powerless become bossy and rules-oriented. They may become oppressive leaders, punitive and rigid in decision making, or they withhold information from others, and become difficult to work with. Although the adage that power corrupts might be true for some, it may be more correct to say that powerlessness, not power, corrupts. Power is likely to bring more power in an ascending cycle, whereas powerlessness will only generate more powerlessness. Because the powerful have credibility to support their actions, they have greater capacity to get things accomplished and can enhance their base. As managers gain power, they are less coercive and rule-bound; thus, their peers and subordinates are more cooperative.

Apparently, then, power has a negative and a positive face. The negative face of power is the "I win, you lose" aspect of dominance versus submission. The positive face of power occurs when someone exerts influence on behalf of rather than over someone or something. Hegyvary (2003) maintains that several types of power are prerequisite for self-expression and human development. Power, therefore, is not good or evil; how it is used and for what purpose it is used determine if it is good or evil.

Types of Power

For leadership to be effective, some measure of power must often support it. This is true for the informal social group and the formal work group. French and Raven (1959) postulate that several bases, or sources, exist for the exercise of power: reward power, punishment or coercive power, legitimate power, expert power, and referent power.

Reward power is obtained by the ability to grant favors or reward others with whatever they value. The arsenal of rewards that a manager can dispense to get employees to work toward meeting organizational goals is very broad. Positive leadership through rewards tends to develop a great deal of loyalty and devotion toward leaders.

Punishment or *coercive power*, the opposite of reward power, is based on fear of punishment if the manager's expectations are not met. The manager may obtain compliance through threats (often implied) of transfer, layoff, demotion, or dismissal. The manager who shuns or ignores an employee is exercising power through punishment, as is the manager who berates or belittles an employee.

Legitimate power is position power. Authority also is called legitimate power. It is the power gained by a title or official position within an organization. Legitimate power has inherent in it the ability to create feelings of obligation or responsibility. As previously discussed, the socialization and culture of subordinate employees will influence to some degree how much power a manager has due to his or her position.

Expert power is gained through knowledge, expertise, or experience. Having critical knowledge allows a manager to gain power over others who need that knowledge. This type of power is limited to a specialized area. For example, someone with vast expertise in music would be powerful only in that area, not in another specialization. Fralic (2000) feels that Florence Nightingale was the first nurse to effectively use this expert power. When Nightingale used research to quantify the need for nurses in the Crimea (by showing that when nurses were present, fewer soldiers died), she was using her research to demonstrate expertise in the health needs of the wounded. Power derived from expert knowledge is fundamental for any profession (Hegyvary, 2003).

Referent power is power a person has because others identify with that leader or with what that leader symbolizes. Referent power also occurs when one gives another person feelings of personal acceptance or approval. It may be obtained through association with the powerful. People also may develop referent power because others perceive them as powerful. This perception could be based on personal charisma, the way the leader talks or acts, the organizations to which he or she belongs, or the people with whom he or she associates. People others accept as role models or leaders enjoy referent power. Physicians use referent power very effectively; society, as a whole, views physicians as powerful, and they carefully maintain this image.

Some theorists distinguish charismatic power from referent power. Willey (1990) states that charisma is a type of personal power, whereas referent power is gained only through association with powerful others.

Heineken and McCloskey (1985) add another type of power to the French and Raven power sources by identifying *informational power*. This source of power is obtained when people have information that others must have to accomplish their goals. Morrison (1988) refers to all these types of power as patriarchal in that they imply power over others. Morrison prefers a power defined as *feminist power* or *self-power*—the power a person gains over his or her own life—and maintains that this power is a personal power that comes from maturity, ego integration, security in relationships, and confidence in one's impulse. The various sources of power are summarized in **Table 13.1.**

Table 13.1 Sources of Power	
Type	**Source**
Referent	Association with others
Legitimate	Position
Coercive	Fear
Reward	Ability to grant favors
Expert	Knowledge and skill
Charismatic	Personal
Informational	The need for information
Self	Maturity, ego strength

THE AUTHORITY–POWER GAP

If authority is the right to command, then a logical question is, "Why do workers sometimes not follow orders?" The right to command does not ensure that employees will always follow orders. The gap that sometimes exists between a position of authority and subordinate response is called the *authority–power gap*. The term *manager power* may explain subordinates' response to the manager's authority. The more power subordinates perceive a manager to have, the smaller the gap between the right to expect certain things and the resulting fulfillment of those expectations by others.

The negative effect of a wide authority–power gap is that organizational chaos may develop. There would be little productivity if every order were questioned. The organization should rightfully expect that its goals would be accomplished. One of the core dynamics of civilization is that there will always be a few authority figures pushing the many for a certain standard of performance.

People in the United States are socialized very early to respond to authority figures. Children are conditioned to accept the directives of their parents, teachers, and community leaders. The traditional nurse–educator has been portrayed as an authoritarian who demands unconditional obedience. Educators who maintain a very narrow authority–power gap reinforce dependency and obedience by emphasizing the ultimate calamity—the death of the patient. Thus, nursing students may be socialized to be overly cautious and to hesitate when making independent nursing judgments.

Because of these types of early socialization, the gap between the manager's authority and the worker's response to that authority tends to be relatively small. In other countries, it may be larger or smaller, depending on how people are socialized to respond to authority. This authority dependence that begins with our parents and is later transferred to our employers may be an important resource to managers.

Although the authority–power gap continues to be small, it has grown in the last 20 years. Both the women's movement and the student unrest of the 1960s have contributed to the widening of the authority–power gap. This widening gap is evidenced when a 1970s college student asked her mother why she did not protest as a college student; the mother replied, "I didn't know we could."

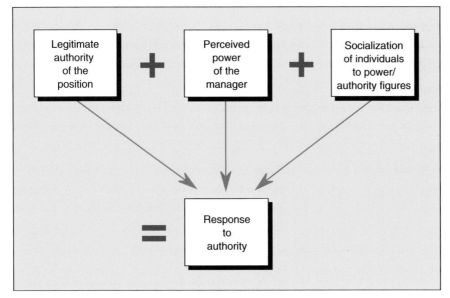

Figure 13.1 Interdependency of response to authority.

At times, however, authority should be questioned by either the leader or the subordinates. This is demonstrated in health care by the increased questioning of the authority of physicians—many of whom feel they have the authority to command— by nurses and consumers. **Figure 13.1** shows the dynamics of the relationships in organizational authority–power response.

Learning Exercise 13.2

Power and Authority
Think back to your childhood. Who did you feel was most powerful in your family? Why do you think that person was powerful? If you are using group work, how many in your group named powerful male figures; how many named powerful female figures?
  Did you grow up with a very narrow authority–power gap? Have your views regarding authority and power changed since you were a child? Do you believe children today have an authority–power gap similar to what you had as a child? Support your answers with examples.

Bridging the Authority–Power Gap

Sometimes subordinates feel badgered by very visible exercises of authority. Because overusing commands can stifle cooperation, naked commands should be used infrequently. Authority as a power tool should be used as a last resort.

A method to bridge the gap is for the leader to make a genuine effort to know and care about each subordinate as a unique individual. This is especially important because each person has a limited tolerance of authority, and subordinates are better able to tolerate authority if they believe the leader cares about them as people.

The manager needs to provide enough information about organizational and unit goals to subordinates so that they understand how their efforts and those of their manager are contributing to goal attainment. The manager will have bridged the authority–power gap if followers (1) perceive that the manager is doing a good job; (2) believe that the organization has their best interests in mind; and (3) do not feel controlled by authority.

Finally, the manager must be seen as credible for the authority–power gap not to widen. All managers begin their appointment with subordinates ready to believe them. This, again, is due to the socialization process that causes people to believe that those in power say what is true. However, the deference to authority will erode if managers handle employees carelessly, are dishonest, or seem incapable of carrying out their duties. When a manager loses credibility, the power inherent in his or her authority decreases.

Another dimension of credibility that influences the authority–power relationship is *future promising*. It is best to underpromise if promises must be made. Managers should never guarantee future rewards unless they have control of all possible variables. If managers revoke future rewards, they lose credibility in the eyes of their subordinates. However, managers should dispense present rewards to buy patronage, making the manager more believable and building greater power into his or her legitimate authority. A scenario that illustrates the difference in dispensing future and present awards follows.

An RN requests a day off to attend a wedding, and you are able to replace her. You use the power of your position to reward her and give her the day off. The RN is grateful to you, and this increases your power.

Another RN requests three months in advance to have every Thursday off in the summer to take a class. Although you promise this to her, on the first day of June three nurses resign, rendering you unable to fulfill your promise. This nurse is very upset, and you have lost much credibility and, therefore, power. It would have been wiser for you to say you could not grant her original request (underpromising) or to make it contingent on several factors. If the situation had remained the same and the nurses had not resigned, you could have granted the request. Less trust is lost between the manager and the subordinate when underpromising occurs than when a granted request is rescinded, as long as the subordinate believes the manager will make a genuine effort to meet his or her request.

> Empowerment is an interactive process that develops, builds, and increases power through cooperation, sharing, and working together.

Empowering Subordinates

The empowerment of staff is a hallmark of transformational leadership. To *empower* means to enable, develop, or allow.

Kreitner and Kinicki (1998) define *empowerment* as decentralization of power. Empowerment occurs when leaders communicate their vision, employees are given the opportunity to make the most of their talents, and learning, creativity, and exploration are encouraged. Empowerment plants seeds of leadership, collegiality, self-respect, and professionalism. Hegyvary (2003) maintains that nurses are empowered through nursing knowledge and research, which then frees staff from mechanistic thinking and encourages critical thinking, problem solving, and the application of knowledge to practice.

However, Fullam and associates (1998) maintain that empowerment is not an easy one-step process but a complex process that consists of three components. First, all practitioners must have professional traits, including responsibility for continuing education, participation in professional organizations, and political activism, and most importantly must have a sense of value about their work. Second, the nurse must work in an environment that encourages empowerment. Lastly, the process must include an effective leadership style. The leader–manager must be someone who nurtures the development of an empowered staff (Fullam, Lando, Johansen, Reyes, & Szaloczy, 1998).

> Empowerment requires professional traits, a supportive work environment, and effective leadership.

Leaders empower subordinates when they delegate assignments to provide learning opportunities and allow employees to share in the satisfaction derived from achievement. Empowerment is not the relinquishing of rightful power inherent in a position, nor is it a delegation of authority or its commensurate responsibility and accountability. Instead, the actions of empowered staff are freely chosen, owned, and committed to on behalf of the organization without any requests or requirements to do so. Empowerment creates and sustains a work environment that speaks to values that facilitate the employee's choice to invest in and own personal actions and behaviors resulting in positive contributions to the organization's mission (Fullam et al., 1998; Laschinger & Wong, 1999).

There are many barriers to creating an environment for empowerment in an organization. Seven barriers identified by Tebbitt (1993) are as follows:

- **Organizational beliefs about authority and status.** Empowerment is blocked if authority and power are viewed as the key motivational forces for achieving the organization's mission and strategic planning.
- **Controlling perceptions, needs, and attitudes.** If managers emphasize rules, regulations, mandated policies, and procedures, little room is left for employee participation and empowerment. The person who is unwilling to teach others and who does not want to see others succeed has been termed a queen bee and the activities and behaviors used to keep others from power, the *queen bee syndrome* (Spengler, 1976). The queen bee wants to be the main attraction and desires that subordinates remain powerless. Behaviors exhibited by nursing queen bees include identifying with others outside the profession (usually males who hold higher positions in the organization) and a disinterest in improving or changing the profession.
- **Organizational inertia.** Empowerment does not happen "naturally." It occurs only as a result of an organizational commitment of time, energy, and resources.
- **Personal and interdepartmental barriers.** Interdepartmental rivalries result in internal competition for resources. The more time managers must spend "defending their turf," the less organizational emphasis will be given to the empowerment process.

- **Employee number, mix, and skill.** Larger organizations with greater staff diversity face a greater challenge in developing focused yet flexible strategies to empower their work force. Not only are there gender differences in views of power but cultural differences as well.
- **A lack of ability and unwillingness of staff to assume responsibility and accountability for their attitudes and behaviors.** Clarity of job roles or job expectations encourages empowerment as staff understand what is expected of them and can identify areas for improvement.
- **Managerial incompetence.** The management skills required to empower staff are planning and goal setting, identifying and addressing problems, making decisions, defining priorities, implementing and managing change, forming interactive and self-directed teams, communicating, resolving conflict, fostering motivation, and building consensus. **Display 13.2** summarizes these barriers.

Learning Exercise 13.3

Cultural Diversity
Why do you think cultural diversity might be a challenge when empowering nurses? Do you agree with this or disagree? Think of ways that various cultures may view power and empowerment differently. If you know people from other cultures, ask them how powerful people or those in authority positions are viewed in their culture and compare that with your own culture.

Once organizational barriers have been eliminated, the leader–manager may develop strategies at the unit level to empower staff. The easiest strategy is to be a role model of an empowered nurse. Another strategy would be to assist staff in building their own personal power base. This can be accomplished by showing subordinates how their personal, knowledge, and referent power can be expanded. Empowerment also occurs when subordinates are involved in planning and implementing change; subordinates believe they have some input in what is about to happen to them and some control over the environment in which they will work in the future.

Display 13.2	Seven Impediments to Empowerment

- Authoritarianism
- Rigid control
- Inertia
- Internal competition
- Employee mix
- Lack of staff accountability
- Managerial incompetence

STRATEGIES FOR BUILDING A PERSONAL POWER BASE

Managers must build a personal power base to further organizational goals, fulfill the leadership role, carry out management functions, and meet personal goals. A beginning manager or even a newly graduated nurse can begin to build a power base in many ways. Habitual behaviors resulting from early lessons, passivity, and focusing on wrong targets can be replaced with new power-gaining behaviors. Marquis and Huston (1998) suggest some strategies for enhancing power:

Maintain Personal Energy

Power and energy go hand in hand. Effective leaders take sufficient time to unwind, reflect, rest, and have fun when they feel tired. Managers who do not take care of themselves begin to make mistakes in judgment that may result in terrible political consequences. Taking time for significant relationships and developing outside interests are important so that other resources are available for sustenance when political forces in the organization drain energy.

Present a Powerful Picture to Others

How people look, act, and talk influence whether others view them as powerful or powerless. The nurse who stands tall and is poised, assertive, articulate, and well groomed presents a picture of personal control and power. The manager who looks like a victim will undoubtedly become one.

Pay the Entry Fee

Newcomers who stand out and appear powerful are those who do more, work harder, and contribute to the organization. They are not clock watchers or "nine-to-fivers." They attend meetings and in-services, do committee work, and take their share of night shifts and weekend and holiday assignments without complaining. A power base is not achieved by slick, easy, or quick maneuvers but through hard work.

Determine the Powerful in the Organization

Understanding and working within the formal and informal power structures are necessary. People must be cognizant of their limitations and seek counsel appropriately. One should know the names and faces of those with both formal and informal power. The powerful people in the informal structure are often more difficult to identify than those in the formal. When working with powerful people, look for similarities and shared values and avoid focusing on differences.

Learn the Language and Symbols of the Organization

Each organization has its own culture and value system. New members must understand this culture and be socialized into the organization if they are to build a power base. Being unaware of institutional taboos and sacred cows often results in embarrassment for the newcomer.

Learn How to Use the Organization's Priorities

Every group has its own goals and priorities for achieving those goals. Those seeking to build a power base must be cognizant of organizational goals and use those priorities and goals to meet management needs. For example, a need for a new manager in a community health service might be to develop educational programs on chemotherapy because some of the new patient caseload includes this nursing function. If fiscal management is a high priority, the manager needs to show superiors how the cost of these educational programs will be offset by additional revenues. If public relations with physicians and patients are a priority, the manager would justify the same request in terms of additional services to patients and physicians.

Increase Professional Skills and Knowledge

Because employees are expected to perform their jobs well, one's performance must be extraordinary to enhance power. One method of being extraordinary is to increase professional skills and knowledge until reaching an expert level. Having knowledge and skill that others lack greatly augments a person's power base. Excellence that reflects knowledge and demonstrates skill enhances a nurse's credibility and determines how others view him or her.

Maintain a Broad Vision

Because people are assigned to a unit or department, they often develop a narrow view of the total organization. Power builders always look upward and outward. The successful manager recognizes not only how the individual unit fits within the larger organization, but also how the institution as a whole fits into the scheme of the total community. People without vision rarely become very powerful.

Use Experts and Seek Counsel

Newcomers should seek out role models. By looking to others for advice and counsel, people demonstrate that they are willing to be team players, that they are cautious and want expert opinion before proceeding, and that they are not rash newcomers who think they have all the answers. Aligning oneself with appropriate veterans in the organization is excellent for building power.

Be Flexible

Anyone wishing to acquire power should develop a reputation as someone who can compromise. The rigid, uncompromising newcomer is viewed as insensitive to the organization's needs.

Develop Visibility and a Voice in the Organization

Newcomers must become active in committees or groups that are recognized by the organization as having clout. When working in groups, the newcomer must not monopolize committee time. Novice leaders and managers must develop observational, listening, and verbal skills. Their spoken contributions to the committee should be valuable and articulated well.

Learn to Toot Your Own Horn

Accepting compliments is an art. One should be gracious but certainly not passive when praised for extraordinary effort. Additionally, people should let others know when some special professional recognition has been achieved. This should be done in a manner that is not bragging but reflects the self-respect of one who is talented and unique.

Maintain a Sense of Humor

Appropriate humor is very effective. The ability to laugh at oneself and not take oneself too seriously is a most important power builder.

Empower Others

Leaders need to empower others, and followers must empower their leaders. When nurses empower each other, they gain referent power. Individual nurses and the profession as a whole do not gain their share of power because they allow others to divide them and weaken their base (Huston & Marquis, 1988). Nurses can empower other nurses by sharing knowledge, maintaining cohesiveness, valuing the profession, and supporting each other. Power building political strategies are summarized in **Display 13.3.**

Display 13.3	Leadership Strategies: Developing Power and Political Savvy

Power-Building Strategies	Political Strategies
Maintain personal energy	Develop information acquisition skills
Present a powerful persona	Communicate astutely
Pay the entry fee	Become proactive
Determine the powerful	Assume authority
Learn the organizational culture	Network
Use organizational priorities	Expand personal resources
Increase skills and knowledge	Maintain maneuverability
Have a broad vision	Remain sensitive to people, timing, and situations
Use experts and seek counsel	Promote subordinates' identities
Be flexible	Meet organizational needs
Be visible and have a voice	Expand personal wellness
Toot your own horn	
Maintain a sense of humor	
Empower others	

Learning Exercise 13.4

Building Power As the New Nurse

You have been an RN for three years. Six months ago, you left your position as a day-charge nurse at one of the local hospitals to accept a position at the public health agency. You really miss your friends at the hospital and find most of the public health nurses older and aloof. However, you love working with your patients and have decided this is where you want to build a lifetime career. Although you believe you have some good ideas, you are aware that because you are new, you will probably not be able to act as change agent yet. Eventually, you would like to be promoted to agency supervisor and become a powerful force for stimulating growth within the agency. You decide that you can do a few things to build a power base. You spend a weekend plotting your political design.

Assignment: Make a power-building plan. Give six to ten specific examples of things you would do to build a power base in the new organization. Give rationales for each selection. (Do not merely select from the general lists in the text. Outline specific actions you would take.) It might be helpful to consider your own community and personal strengths when solving this learning exercise.

THE POLITICS OF POWER

Earlier in this chapter, politics was defined as the effective use of power or the art of using power. Although there continues to be a lack of empirical research to assist nurses within organizations to improve their power position (Sieloff, 2003), there are many strategies that are politically wise. For example, it is important for managers to understand politics within the context of their employing organization. After the employee has built a power base through hard work, increased personal power, and knowledge of the organization, developing skills in the politics of power is necessary. People often lose hard-earned power in an organization because they make political mistakes. Even seasoned leaders occasionally blunder in this arena.

It is useless to argue the ethics or value of politics in an organization because politics exists in every organization. Thus, nurses waste energy and remain powerless when they refuse to learn the art and skill of political maneuvers. Andrica (1999) states, "Though you may want to avoid office politics, sometimes you must become involved, whether it be for the good of yourself, the organization, or a peer. And it is not necessarily a negative thing. Office politics can prove positive and beneficial for those involved" (p. 156). Politics becomes divisive only whenever gossip, rumor, or unethical strategies occur.

Much attention is given to improving competence, but little time is spent in learning the intricacies of political behavior. The most important strategy is to learn to "read the environment" through observation, listening, reading, detachment, and analysis. Stahl (1999) maintains that the next millennium will see a change in organizational politics and that the new rules of engagement will be less about "who you know" and more about leadership with political savvy.

> Although power is a universally available resource that does not have a finite quality, it can be lost as well as gained.

Because power implies interdependence, nurses must not only understand the organizational structure in which they work, but also be able to function effectively within that structure, including dealing effectively with the institution's inherent politics. Only when managers understand power and politics will they be capable of recognizing limitations and potential for change. Being in touch with one's own power can be frightening. People may anticipate attacks from many fronts that will reduce their power. When these attacks occur, people who hold powerful positions may undermine themselves by regressing rather than progressing and by being reactive rather than proactive.

The following political strategies will help the novice manager negate the negative effects of organizational politics.

- **Become an expert handler of information and communication.** Beware that facts can be presented seductively and out of context. The manager must be cautious in accepting facts as presented because information is often changed to fit others' needs. Managers must become adept at the art of acquiring information and questioning others.

  Decisions should be delayed until adequate and accurate information has been gathered and reviewed. Managers who fail to do the necessary homework may make decisions with damaging political consequences. Additionally, managers must not allow themselves to be trapped into discussing something about which they know very little. The politically astute manager says, "I don't know" when inadequate information is available.

  This political astuteness in communication is often a difficult skill to master. Grave consequences can result from sharing the wrong information with the wrong people at the wrong time. Determining who should know, how much they should know, and when they should know requires great finesse.

  One of the most politically serious errors one can make is lying to others within the organization. Although withholding or refusing to divulge information are both good political strategies, lying is not. Lying destroys trust, and Fitzpatrick (2001) says leaders must never underestimate the power of trust.

- **Be a proactive decision maker.** Nurses have had such a long history of being reactive that they have had little time to learn how to be proactive. Although being reactive is better than being passive, being proactive means getting the job done better, faster, and more efficiently. The proactive leader prepares for the future instead of waiting for it to happen. He or she sees approaching change in the healthcare system and, instead of fighting those changes, prepares to meet them.

  One way the nurse can become proactive is by assuming authority. Part of power is the image of power; a powerful political strategy also involves image. Instead of asking, "May I?" leaders assume that they may. When people ask permission, they are really asking someone to take responsibility for them. If something is not expressly prohibited in the organization or in a job description, the powerful leader assumes that it may be done.

  Politically astute nurses have been known to create new positions or new roles within a position simply by gradually assuming that they could do things that no one else was doing. In other words, they saw a need in the organization and, instead of asking if they could do something, they started doing it. The organization, through default, allowed expansion of the role. People do need to be aware, however, that if they assume authority and something goes wrong, they will be held accountable, so this strategy is not without risk.

· **Expand personal resources.** Because organizations are dynamic and the future is impossible to predict, the proactive nurse prepares for the future by expanding personal resources. Personal resources include economic stability, higher education, and a broadened skill base. This is often called the political strategy of "having maneuverability"—that is, the person avoids having limited options. People who have "money in the bank and gas in the tank" have a political freedom of maneuverability that others do not.

People lose power if others within the organization know that they cannot afford to make a job change or do not have the necessary skills to do so. Those who become economically dependent on a position lose political clout. Likewise, the nurse who has not bothered to develop additional skills or seek further education loses the political strength that comes from having the option of being able to find quality employment elsewhere.

· **Develop political alliances and coalitions.** Nurses often can increase their power and influence by forming alliances with other groups. People can form alliances with peers, sponsors, or subordinates. The alliances may be from within their own group or from without.

One of the most effective methods of forming alliances is through networking. Managers can sharpen their political skills by becoming involved with peers outside the organization. In this manner, the manager is able to keep abreast of current happenings and to use others for advice and counsel. Although networking works among many groups, for the nurse–manager, few groups are as valuable as local and state nursing associations.

Networking—forming coalitions and alliances—also can be effective within the organization. This strategy is especially useful for some types of planned change. More power and political clout result from people working together rather than people acting alone. When a person is under political attack by others in the organization, group power is very useful.

· **Be sensitive to timing.** Successful leaders are sensitive to both the appropriateness and timing of their actions. The person who presents a request to attend an expensive nursing conference on the same afternoon that his or her supervisor just had extensive dental work is an example of someone with insensitivity to timing.

Besides being able to choose the right moment, the effective manager should develop skill in other areas of timing. One of these areas is to know when it is the appropriate time to do nothing. For example, in the case of a problem employee who is three months from retirement, time itself would resolve the situation.

The sensitive manager also learns when the time has come to stop requesting something, and that time should be before a superior has given a firm "no." Once this firm "no" has been reached, continuing to press the issue is politically unwise.

- **Promote subordinate identification.** There are many ways a manager can promote the identification of subordinates. A simple "thank you" for a fine job works especially well when spoken in front of someone else. By calling attention to the extra effort of your subordinates, you are saying in effect, "Look what a good job we are capable of doing." Sending subordinates sincere notes of appreciation is another way of praising and promoting. Rewarding the excellent employee's work is an effective political strategy.
- **View personal and unit goals in terms of the organization.** Even extraordinary and visible activities will not result in desired power unless those activities are used to meet organizational goals. Hard work for purely personal gain will become a political liability.

Frequently novice managers think only in terms of their needs and their problems rather than seeing the large picture. Additionally, people often look upward for solutions rather than attempting to find answers themselves. When problems are identified, it is more politically astute to take the problem

Learning Exercise 13.5

Turning Lemons into Lemonade

The following is based on a real event. The cast includes Sally Jones, the director of nursing; Jane Smith, the hospital administrator and CEO; and Bob Black, the assistant hospital administrator. Sally has been in her position at Memorial Hospital for two years. She has made many improvements in the nursing department and is generally respected by the hospital administrator, the nursing staff, and the physicians.

The present situation involves the newly hired Bob Black. Previously too small to have an assistant administrator, the hospital has grown, and this position was created. One of the departments assigned to Bob is the personnel and payroll department. Until now, nursing, which comprises 45% of all personnel, has done its own recruiting, interviewing, and selecting. Since Bob has been hired, he has shown obvious signs that he would like to increase his power and authority.

Now Bob has proposed that he hire an additional clerk who will do much of the personnel work for the nursing department, although nursing administration will be able to make the final selections in hiring. Bob proposes that his department should do the initial screening of applicants, seeking references, and so on.

Sally has grown increasingly frustrated in dealing with the encroachment of Bob. Having just received Bob's latest proposal, she has requested to meet with Jane Smith and Bob to discuss the plan.

Assignment: What danger, if any, is there for Sally Jones in Bob Black's proposal? Explain two political strategies you believe Sally could use in the upcoming meeting. Is it possible to facilitate a win–win solution to this conflict? If so, how? If there is not a win–win solution, how much can Sally win?

Note: Attempt to solve this case before reading the solution presented in the back of this book.

Learning Exercise 13.7

Friendships and Truth

You are a middle-level manager in a public health department. One of your closest friends, Janie, is a registered nurse under your span of control. Today, Janie calls and tells you that she injured her back yesterday during a home visit after she slipped on a wet front porch. She said that the homeowners were unaware that she fell and that no one witnessed the accident. She has just returned from visiting her doctor, who advises six weeks of bed rest. She requests that you initiate the paperwork for worker's compensation and disability, because she has no sick days left.

Shortly after your telephone conversation with Janie, you take a brief coffee break in the lounge. You overhear a conversation between Jon and Lacey, two additional staff members in your department. Jon says that he and Janie were water skiing last night, and she took a terrible fall and hurt her back. He planned to call her to see how she was feeling.

You initially feel hurt and betrayed by Janie because you believe she has lied to you. You want to call Janie and confront her. You plan to deny her request for worker's compensation and disability. You are angry that she has placed you in this position. You also are aware that proving Janie's injury is not work-related may be difficult.

Assignment: How should you proceed? What are the political ramifications if this incident is not handled properly? How should you use your power and authority when dealing with this problem?

Learning Exercise 13.8

Decision Making: Conflict and Dilemma

You are the director of a small Native American health clinic. Other than yourself and a part-time physician, your only professional staff are two RNs. The remaining staff members are Native Americans and have been trained by you.

Because nurse Bennett, a 26-year-old female BSN graduate, has had several years of experience working at a large southwestern community health agency, she is familiar with many of the patients' problems. She is hard working and extremely knowledgeable. Occasionally, her assertiveness is mistaken for bossiness among the Native American workers. However, everyone respects her judgment.

The other RN, nurse Mikiou, is a 34-year-old male Native American. He started as a medic in the Persian Gulf War and attended several career-ladder external degree programs until he was able to take the RN examination. He does not have a baccalaureate degree. His nursing knowledge is occasionally limited, and he tends to be very casual about performing his duties. However, he is competent and has never shown unsafe judgment. His humor and good nature often reduce tension in the clinic. The Native American population is very proud of him, and he has a special relationship with them. However, he is not a particularly good role model because his health habits leave much to be desired, and he is frequently absent from work.

Nurse Bennett has come to find nurse Mikiou intolerable. She believes she has tried working with him, but this is difficult because she doesn't respect him. As the director of the clinic, you have tried many ways to solve this problem. You feel especially fortunate to have nurse Bennett on your staff. It is difficult to find many nurses of her quality willing to come and live on a desolate Native American reservation. On the other hand, if the Native American health concept is really going to work, the Native Americans themselves must be educated and placed in the agencies so that one day they can run their own clinics. It is very difficult to find educated Native Americans who want to return to this reservation. Now you are faced with a management dilemma. Nurse Bennett has said either nurse Mikiou must go, or she will go. She has asked you to decide.

Assignment: List the factors bearing on this decision. What (if any) power issues are involved? Which choice will be the least damaging? Justify your decision.

Learning Exercise 13.9

Power Struggle

You are team leader on a medical unit of a small community hospital. Your shift is 3 PM to 11 PM. When leaving the report room, John, the day-shift team leader, tells you that Mrs. Jackson, a terminally ill patient with cancer, has decided to check herself out of the hospital "against medical advice." John states that he has already contacted Mrs. Jackson's doctor, who expressed his concern that the patient would have inadequate pain control at home and undependable family support. He believes she will die within a few days if she leaves the hospital. He did, however, leave orders for home prescriptions and a follow-up appointment.

You immediately go into Mrs. Jackson's room to assess the situation. She tells you that the doctor has told her that she will probably die within six weeks and that she wants to spend what time she has left at home with her little dog, who has been her constant companion for many years. In addition, she has many things "to put in order." She states that she is fully aware of her doctor's concerns and that she was already informed by the day-shift nurse that leaving "against medical advice" may result in the insurance company refusing to pay for her current hospitalization. She states that she will be leaving in 15 minutes when her ride home arrives.

When you go to the nurse's desk to get a copy of the home prescriptions and follow-up doctor's appointment for the patient, the ward clerk states, "The hospital policy says that patients who leave against medical advice have to contact the physician directly for prescriptions and an appointment, because they are not legally discharged. The hospital has no obligation to provide this service. She made the choice—now let her live with it." She refuses to give a copy of the orders to you and places the patient's chart in her lap. Short of physically removing the chart from the ward clerk's lap, it is clear that you have no immediate access to the orders.

You confront the charge nurse, who states that the hospital policy does give that responsibility to the patient. She is unsure what to do and has paged the unit director, who appears to be out of the hospital temporarily.

You are outraged. You believe the patient has the "right" to her prescriptions because the doctor ordered them, assuming she would receive them before she left. You also know that if the medications are not dispensed by the hospital, there is little likelihood that Mrs. Jackson will have the resources to have the prescriptions filled. Five minutes later, Mrs. Jackson appears at the nurse's station, accompanied by her friend. She states she is leaving and would like her discharge prescriptions.

Assignment: The power struggle in this scenario involves you, the unit clerk, the charge nurse, and organizational politics. Does the unit clerk in this scenario have informal or formal power? What alternatives for action do you have? What are the costs or consequences of each possible alternative? What action would you take?

Learning Exercise 13.10

When a Subordinate Goes Over Your Head

You are the day-shift charge nurse for the intensive care unit. One of your nurses, Carol, has just requested a week off to attend a conference. She is willing to use her accrued vacation time for this and to pay the expenses herself. The conference is in one month, and you are a little irritated with her for not coming to you sooner. Carol's request conflicts with a vacation that you have given another nurse. This nurse requested her vacation three months ago.

  You deny Carol's request, explaining that you will need her to work that week. Carol protests, stating that the educational conference will benefit the intensive care unit and repeating that she will bear the cost. You are firm but polite in your refusal. Later, Carol goes to the supervisor of the unit to request the time. Although the supervisor upholds your decision, you believe that Carol has gone over your head inappropriately in handling this matter. **Assignment:** How are you going to deal with Carol? Decide on your approach, and support it with political rationale.

Web Links

Maxi:
http://www.maximag.com/toc/toc.html
An on-line magazine that examines women's issues. Articles and interviews related to relationships, feminist politics, and glass ceilings.

Women Working 2000 and Beyond:
http://womenworking2000.com
Web site that springs from the television special, "Women Working 2000 and Beyond." Offers networking contacts, wisdom, and leadership.

Political Action Links for Nurses:
http://www.academic.scranton.edu/faculty/zalonm1/political.html
Links to workplace government organizations in health care, sponsored by the University of Scranton.

References

Andrica, D. C. (1999). Handling office politics. *Nursing Economic$*, 17(3), 156.

Baker, A. M., & Young, C. E. (1994). Transformational leadership: The feminist connection in postmodern organizations. *Holistic Nursing Practice, 9*(1), 16–25.

Carli, L. L. (1999). Gender, interpersonal power and social influence. *Journal of Social Issues, 55*(1), 81–100.

Fisher, H. E. (1999). *The First Sex: The Natural Talents of Women and How They Are Changing the World.* New York: Random House.

Fitzpatrick, M. A. (2001). Famous last words: Trust me! *Nursing Management, 32*(6), 6.

Fralic, M. F. (2000). What is leadership? *Journal of Nursing Administration, 30*(7/8), 340–341.

French, J., & Raven, B. (1959). The bases of social power. In D. Cartwright (Ed.). *Studies in social power.* Ann Arbor, MI: University of Michigan.

First- and middle-level managers generally have their greatest influence on the organizing phase of the management process at the unit or department level. It is here that managers organize how work is to be done, shape the organizational climate, and determine how patient care delivery is organized. It is the top-level manager, however, who is most likely to influence the philosophy and resources necessary for any selected care delivery system to be effective. Without a supporting philosophy and adequate resources, the most well-intentioned delivery system will fail.

The unit leader–manager determines how best to plan work activities so organizational goals are met effectively and efficiently. This involves using resources wisely and coordinating activities with other departments. How activities are organized can impede or facilitate communication, flexibility, and job satisfaction.

For organizing functions to be productive and facilitate meeting the organization's needs, the leader must know the organization and its members well. Activities will be unsuccessful if their design does not meet group needs. The roles and functions of the leader–manager in organizing groups for patient care are shown in **Display 14.1**.

MODES OF ORGANIZING PATIENT CARE

Choosing the most appropriate organizational mode to deliver patient care for each unit or organization depends on the skill and expertise of the staff, the availability of registered professional nurses, the economic resources of the organization, the acuity of the patients, and the complexity of the tasks to be completed.

The five most well known means of organizing nursing care for patient care delivery are (1) total patient care, (2) functional nursing, (3) team and modular nursing, (4) primary nursing, and (5) case management (see **Display 14.2**). Each of these basic types has undergone many modifications, often resulting in new terminology. For example, primary nursing has been called case method nursing in the past and is now frequently referred to as a professional practice model. Team nursing is sometimes called *partners in care* or *patient service partners* and case managers assume different titles, depending on the setting in which they provide care. When closely examined, many of the newer models of patient care delivery systems are merely recycled, modified, or retitled versions of older models. Indeed, it is sometimes difficult to find a delivery system true to its original version or one that does not have parts of others in its design. Although some of these care delivery systems were developed to organize care in hospitals, most can be adapted to other settings. Choosing the most appropriate organizational mode to deliver patient care for each unit or organization depends on the skill and expertise of the staff, the availability of registered professional nurses, the economic resources of the organization, the acuity of the patients, and the complexity of the tasks to be completed.

Total Patient Care Nursing or Case Method Nursing

Total patient care is the oldest mode of organizing patient care. In this method, nurses assume total responsibility during their time on duty for meeting all the needs of assigned patients. At the turn of the 19th century, total patient care was generally provided in the patient's home, and the nurse was responsible for cooking, house cleaning, and other activities specific to the patient and family, in addition to traditional nursing care (Nelson, 2000). It is important to note that most medical and nursing care for the

Display 14.1	**Leadership Roles and Management Functions Associated with Organizing Patient Care**

Leadership Roles

1. Periodically evaluates the effectiveness of the organizational structure for the delivery of patient care.
2. Determines if adequate resources and support exist before making any changes in the organization of patient care.
3. Examines the human element in work redesign and supports personnel during adjustment to change.
4. Inspires the work group toward a team effort.
5. Inspires subordinates to achieve higher levels of education, clinical expertise, competency, and experience in differentiated practice.
6. Ensures that chosen nursing care delivery models advance the practice of professional nursing.

Management Functions

1. Examines the unit philosophy to ensure it supports any change in patient care delivery system.
2. Selects a patient care delivery system most appropriate to the needs of the patients being served.
3. Uses scientific research and current literature to analyze proposed changes in nursing care delivery models.
4. Uses a patient care delivery system that maximizes human and physical resources as well as time.
5. Ensures that nonprofessional staff are appropriately trained and supervised in the provision of care.
6. Organizes work activities to attain organizational goals.
7. Groups activities in a manner that facilitates communication and coordination within and between departments.
8. Organizes work so that it is as cost-effective as possible.
9. Makes changes in work design to facilitate meeting organizational goals.
10. Clearly delineates criteria to be used for differentiated practice roles.

Display 14.2	**Common Patient Care Delivery Methods**

Total patient care
Functional nursing
Team and modular nursing
Primary nursing
Case management

wealthy and middle class during this time occurred in the home; hospitals at the time were used primarily by the poor and very acutely ill. Total patient care nursing is sometimes referred to as the *case method* of assignment because patients were assigned as cases, much like contemporary private-duty nursing is carried out.

During the Great Depression of the 1930s, people could no longer afford home care and began using hospitals for care that had been performed by private-duty nurses in the home. During that time, nurses and students were the caregivers in hospitals and in public health agencies. As hospitals grew during the 1930s and 1940s, providing total care continued as the primary means of organizing patient care. A structural diagram of this method is shown in **Figure 14.1.**

This method of assignment is still widely used in hospitals and home health agencies. This organizational structure provides nurses with high autonomy and responsibility. Assigning patients is simple and direct and does not require the planning that other methods of patient care delivery require. The lines of responsibility and accountability are clear. The patient theoretically receives holistic and unfragmented care during the nurse's time on duty.

Each nurse caring for the patient can, however, modify the care regimen. Therefore, if there are three shifts, the patient could receive three different approaches to care, often resulting in confusion for the patient. To maintain quality care, this method requires highly skilled personnel and thus may cost more than some other forms of patient care. This method's opponents argue that some tasks performed by the primary caregiver could be accomplished by someone with less training and therefore at a lower cost.

The greatest disadvantage of total patient care delivery occurs when the nurse is inadequately prepared to provide total care to the patient. In the early history of nursing, only RNs provided care; now a variety of nursing care personnel, many of who have no license and limited education, work with patients. During

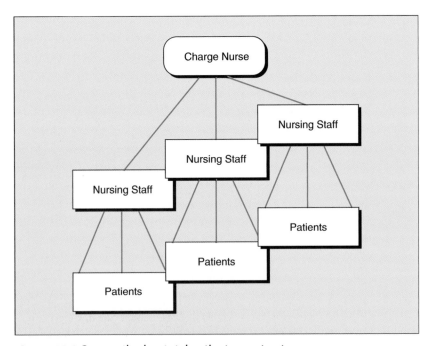

Figure 14.1 Case method or total patient care structure.

nursing shortages, many hospitals assign healthcare workers who are not RNs to provide most of the nursing care. Because the co-assigned RN may have a heavy patient load, little opportunity for supervision exists. This potentially could result in unsafe care.

Functional Nursing

The *functional method* of delivering nursing care evolved primarily as a result of World War II and the rapid construction of hospitals as a result of the Hill Burton Act. Because nurses were in great demand overseas and at home, a nursing shortage developed and ancillary personnel were needed to assist in patient care. These relatively unskilled workers were trained to do simple tasks and gained proficiency by repetition. Personnel were assigned to complete certain tasks rather than care for specific patients. Examples of functional nursing tasks were checking blood pressures, administering medication, changing linens, and bathing patients. Registered nurses became managers of care rather than direct care providers, and "care through others" became the phrase used to refer to this method of nursing care (Nelson, 2000, p. 156). Functional nursing structure is shown in **Figure 14.2.**

This form of organizing patient care was thought to be temporary as it was assumed that when the war ended, hospitals would not need ancillary workers. However, the baby boom and resulting population growth immediately following World War II left the country short of nurses. Thus, employment of personnel with various levels of skill and education proliferated as new categories of healthcare workers were created. Currently, most healthcare organizations have continued this practice of employing healthcare workers of many educational backgrounds and skill levels.

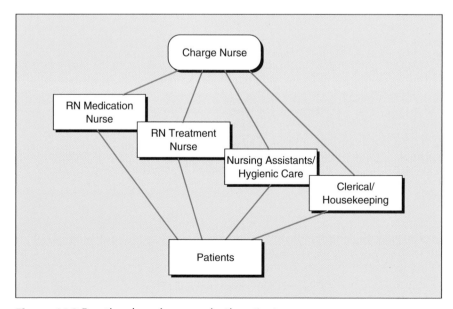

Figure 14.2 Functional nursing organization structure.

Most administrators consider functional nursing an economical means of providing care. This is true if quality care and holistic care are not regarded as essential. A major advantage of functional nursing is its efficiency; tasks are completed quickly, with little confusion regarding responsibilities. Functional nursing does allow care to be provided with a minimal number of registered nurses. In many areas, such as the operating room, the functional structure works well and is still very much in evidence. Long-term care facilities also frequently use a functional approach to nursing care.

During the past decade, the use of unlicensed assistive personnel (UAP) in healthcare organizations has increased. Many nurse administrators believe that assigning low-skill tasks to UAPs frees the professional nurse to perform more highly skilled duties and is therefore more economical; however, others argue that the time needed to supervise the UAP negates any time savings that might have occurred. Most modern administrators would undoubtedly deny that they are using functional nursing, yet the trend of assigning tasks to workers, rather than assigning workers to the professional nurse, resembles, at least in part, functional nursing.

Functional nursing may lead to fragmented care and the possibility of overlooking patient priority needs. Because some workers feel unchallenged and understimulated in their roles, functional nursing also may result in low job satisfaction. Nelson (2000) argues that functional nursing "mutes" the nursing process as nurses who are trained as clinicians become managers of patient care, and that keeping care patient-centered and individualized is jeopardized. In addition, functional nursing may not be cost-effective due to the need for many coordinators. Employees often focus only on their own efforts, with less interest in overall results.

Learning Exercise 14.1

Transitioning to Total Patient Care
Most nursing students begin their clinical training doing some form of functional nursing care and then advancing to total patient care for a small number of patients. Reflect back to your earliest clinical experiences as a student nurse. Which tasks were easiest for you to learn? How did you gain mastery of those tasks? Was task mastery a time consuming process for you? Was it difficult to make the transition to total patient care? If so, why? What skills were most difficult for you to learn in providing total patient care? Do you anticipate having to learn additional skills to feel comfortable in the role of total care provider as an RN? What higher level (non-functional) skills do you think will be the hardest to learn and be confident with?

Team and Modular Nursing

Team nursing was developed in the 1950s in an effort to decrease the problems associated with the functional organization of patient care. Many believed that despite a continued shortage of professional nursing staff, a patient care system had to be developed that reduced the fragmented care that accompanied functional nursing. Team nursing structure is shown in **Figure 14.3.**

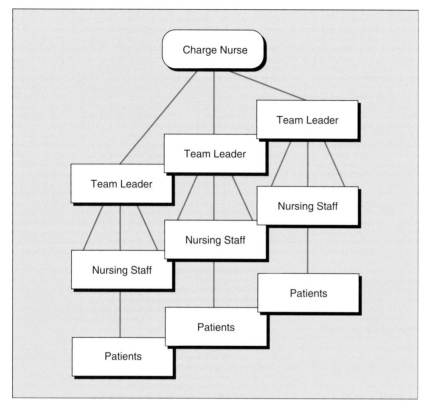

Figure 14.3 Team nursing organization structure.

In team nursing, ancillary personnel collaborate in providing care to a group of patients under the direction of a professional nurse. As the team leader, the nurse is responsible for knowing the condition and needs of all the patients assigned to the team and for planning individual care. The team leader's duties vary depending on the patient's needs and the workload. These duties may include assisting team members, giving direct personal care to patients, teaching, and coordinating patient activities.

Through extensive team communication, comprehensive care can be provided for patients despite a relatively high proportion of ancillary staff. This communication occurs informally between the team leader and the individual team members and formally through regular team planning conferences. A team should consist of not more than five people or it will revert to more functional lines of organization.

Team nursing is usually associated with democratic leadership. Group members are given as much autonomy as possible when performing assigned tasks, although the team shares responsibility and accountability collectively. The need for excellent communication and coordination skills makes implementing team nursing difficult and requires great self-discipline on the part of team members.

Team nursing allows members to contribute their own special expertise or skills. Team leaders, then, should use their knowledge about each member's abilities when making patient assignments. Recognizing the individual worth of all employees and giving team members autonomy result in high job satisfaction.

Disadvantages to team nursing are associated primarily with improper implementation rather than with the philosophy itself. Frequently, insufficient time is allowed for team care planning and communication. This can lead to blurred lines of responsibility, errors, and fragmented patient care. For team nursing to be effective, the leader must have good communication, organizational, management, and leadership skills and must be an excellent practitioner.

Team nursing, as originally designed, has undergone much modification in the last 30 years. Most team nursing was never practiced in its purest form but was instead a combination of team and functional structure. Recent attempts to refine and improve team nursing have resulted in the concept of *modular nursing*, which is a mini-team (two or three members) approach. Members of the modular nursing team are sometimes called *care pairs*. Keeping the team small and attempting to assign personnel to the same team as often as possible should allow the professional nurse more time for planning and coordinating team members. Additionally, a small team requires less communication, allowing members better use of their time for direct patient care activities.

Primary Nursing

Primary nursing, also known as *relationship-based nursing*, developed in the early 1970s, uses some of the concepts of total patient care and brings the registered nurse back to the bedside to provide clinical care. Indeed, Manthey (2001) suggests that primary nursing is the only type of patient care delivery that requires a one-to-one relationship between a nurse and a patient with responsibility for planning and managing care clearly established.

As originally designed, primary nursing requires a nursing staff comprised totally of RNs. The RN primary nurse assumes 24-hour responsibility for planning the care of one or more patients from admission or the start of treatment to discharge or the treatment's end. During work hours, the primary nurse provides total direct care for that patient. When the primary nurse is not on duty, associate nurses who follow the care plan established by the primary nurse provide care. Primary nursing structure is shown in **Figure 14.4.**

Although designed for use in hospitals, this structure lends itself well to home health nursing, hospice nursing, and other healthcare delivery enterprises. An integral responsibility of the primary nurse is to establish clear communication among the patient, the physician, the associate nurses, and other team members. Although the primary nurse establishes the care plan, feedback is sought from others in coordinating the patient's care. The combination of clear interdisciplinary group communication and consistent, direct patient care by relatively few nursing staff allows for holistic, high-quality patient care.

Although job satisfaction is high in primary nursing, this method is difficult to implement because of the degree of responsibility and autonomy required of the primary nurse. However, for these same reasons, once nurses develop skill in primary nursing care delivery, they feel challenged and rewarded.

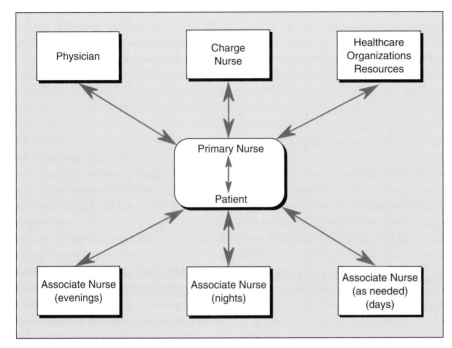

Figure 14.4 Primary nursing structure.

Disadvantages to this method, as in team nursing, lie primarily in improper implementation. An inadequately prepared or incompetent primary nurse may be incapable of coordinating a multidisciplinary team or identifying complex patient needs and condition changes. Many nurses may be uncomfortable in this role or initially lack the experience and skills necessary for the role. Although an all-RN nursing staff has not been proved to be more costly than other modes of nursing, it sometimes has been difficult to recruit and retain enough RNs, especially in times of nursing shortages. Currently, licensed vocational and practical nurses serve as associate nurses in some facilities, although the role of the primary nurse should be reserved for an experienced RN who has an appropriate scope of requisite skills for the role.

Case Management

Case management is the latest work design proposed to meet patient needs. Case management is defined by the Case Management Society of America (CMSA) as a collaborative process that assesses, plans, implements, coordinates, monitors, and evaluates options and services to meet an individual's health needs through communication and available resources to promote quality, cost-effective outcomes (Powell, 2000). The focus in case management is on individual patients, not populations of patients. Case managers handle each case individually, identifying the most cost-effective providers, treatments, and care settings for insured individuals (Finkleman, 2001).

Learning Exercise 14.2

Reorganizing to Accommodate a Change in Staffing Mix
You are the head nurse of an oncology unit. At present, the patient care delivery mode on the unit is total patient care. You have a staff composed of 60% RNs, 35% practical nurses (LPNs/LVNS), and 5% clerical staff. Your bed capacity is 28, but your average daily census is 24. An example of day-shift staffing follows:

- One charge nurse who notes orders, talks with physicians, organizes care, makes assignments, and acts as a resource person and problem solver
- Three RNs who provide total patient care, including administering all treatments and medications to their assigned patients, giving IV medications to the practical nurses' assigned patients, and acting as a clinical resource person for the practical nurses
- Two licensed practical nurses assigned to provide total patient care except for administering IV medications

  Your supervisor has just told all head nurses that because the hospital is having difficulty recruiting nurses, it has decided to hire nursing assistants. The nurses on your unit will have to assume more supervisory responsibilities and focus less on direct care. Your supervisor has asked you to reorganize the patient care management on your unit to best use the following day-shift staffing: three RNs, which will include the present charge nurse position; two practical nurses; and two nursing assistants. You may delete the past charge nurse position and divide charge responsibility among all three nurses or divide up the work any way you choose.

Assignment: Draw a new patient care organization diagram. Who would be most affected by the reorganization? Evaluate your rationale, both for the selection of your choice and the rejection of others. Explain how you would go about implementing this planned change.

> The focus in case management is on individual patients, not populations of patients.

While case management referrals often begin in the hospital inpatient setting, with length of stay and profit margin per confinement used as measures of efficiency, case management in the managed care era frequently extends to outpatient settings as well. Historically, however, the focus has been episodic or component-style orientation to the treatment of disease in inpatient settings and post acute care settings for insured individuals (Finkleman, 2001).

Acute care case management integrates utilization management and discharge planning functions and may be unit based, assigned by patient, disease based, or primary nurse case managed (Powell, 2000). Assignment by unit is most common, particularly in mid- to large-sized hospitals because patient units typically care for patients with like diagnoses (Smith, 2003). "The advantages of this model include additional work efficiency due to geographic proximity, but more importantly, the benefit of establishing solid working relationships with the nursing and ancillary staff working on the unit" (p. 238). In general, a case manager can handle a load of 25 patients (Smith).

The premise of inpatient case management is that hospitals are better off "managing the demand for care" than attempting to try to increase the "supply of resources" such as beds or personnel (Smith, 2003). Case managers do this by using *critical pathways* (see Chapter 10) and *multidisciplinary action plans (MAPs)* to plan patient care.

The care MAP is a combination of a *critical pathway* and a *nursing care plan*. In addition, the care MAP indicates times when nursing interventions should occur. All healthcare providers follow the care MAP to facilitate expected outcomes. If a patient deviates from the normal plan, a variance is indicated. A *variance* is anything that occurs to alter the patient's progress through the normal critical path. Benson et al. (2001) states that the true utility of clinical pathways is derived from information obtained through *variance tracking*—documenting when and why a patient's care varies from the clinical pathway.

Furlow (2003) suggests a different type of care MAP in her discussion of cycle time reduction. *Cycle time reduction* involves reviewing an existing process that provides a product or service, determining where there's wasted time or effort, and developing an improved, streamlined way to achieve the same results more efficiently.

Many other types of case management occur in outpatient settings, although only a few are discussed here. With *insurance case management* (also known as *third-party payor case management*), the case manager works as the insurer's liaison to resolve disputes between providers, patients, and the insurer regarding needed levels of care and authorizations for reimbursement. *Workers' compensation case management* is directed at preventing worker injuries, when possible, and managing such injuries when they occur (Powell, 2000). *Entrepreneurial case management* uses independent case management consultants who contract with patients, family members, physicians, or insurance companies. These individuals coordinate all aspects of care, in the home and in any level of care needed. *Hospice case managers* coordinate end of life care. Finally, *home health case managers* service the needs of the chronically ill in the home setting (Powell). This might include the coordination of wound care, infusion therapy services, physical therapy, speech therapy, occupational therapy, coordination of durable medical equipment, medication monitoring and skilled nursing services.

Because the role expectations and scope of knowledge required to be a case manager are extensive, some experts have argued that this role should be reserved for the advance practice nurse or registered nurse with advanced training (Huston, 2002), although this is not usually the case in the practice setting today. Smith (2003) argues that effective case managers should have three to five years of direct care experience, preferably within the specialty area in which they case manage. They should also be extremely bright, have well-developed interpersonal skills, be able to multitask, have a strong foundation in utilization review, and understand payer-patient specifics and hospital reimbursement mechanisms.

Learning Exercise 14.3

Developing a Case Management Plan

Jimmy Jansen is a 44-year-old man with type I diabetes mellitus. He was recently referred to your home health agency for case management follow-up at home. He is experiencing multiple complications from his diabetes including the recent onset of blindness and peripheral neuropathy. His left leg was amputated below the knee last year as a result of a gangrenous infection of his foot. He is unable to wear his prosthesis at present since he has a small ulcer at the stump site. His chart states that he has been only "intermittently compliant" with blood sugar testing or insulin administration in the past despite the visit of a community health nurse on a weekly basis the past year. His renal function has become progressively worse over the past six months and it is anticipated that he will need to begin hemodialysis soon.

His social history reveals that he recently separated from his wife and has no contact with an adult son who lives in another state. He has not worked for over 10 years and has no insurance other than Medicaid. The home he lives in is small and he says he hasn't been able to keep it up with his wife gone. No formal safety assessment of his home has been conducted. He also acknowledges that he's not eating right since he now must do his own cooking. He cannot drive and states "I don't know how I'm going to get to the clinic to have my blood cleaned by the kidney machine."

Assignment: Mr. Jansen has many problems that would likely benefit from case management intervention.

1. Make a list of five nursing diagnoses for Mr. Jansen that you would use to prioritize your interventions.
2. Then make a list of at least five goals you would like to accomplish in planning Mr. Jansen's care. Make sure these goals reflect realistic patient outcomes.
3. What referrals would you make? What interventions would you implement yourself? Would you involve other disciplines in his plan of care?
4. What is your plan for follow up and evaluation?

DISEASE MANAGEMENT AND CASE MANAGEMENT

One role increasingly assumed by case managers is coordinating *disease management* programs. Disease management (DM), also known as *population-based health care* and *continuous health improvement*, is a comprehensive, integrated approach to the care and reimbursement of high-cost, chronic illnesses. The goal of DM is to address such illnesses or conditions with maximum efficiency across treatment settings regardless of typical reimbursement patterns (Huston, 2002). Thus, a continuum of chronic illness care is established that includes early detection and early intervention. This prevents or reduces exacerbation of the disease, acute episodes (known as *cost drivers*), and the use of expensive resources such as hospital inpatient care, making prevention and proactive case management two important areas of emphasis (Huston). In addition, DM programs include comprehensive tracking of patient outcomes. Thus, the goals for disease management are focused on integrating components and improving long-term outcomes.

In DM programs, common high-cost, high-resource utilization diseases are identified and population groups are targeted for implementation. This is one of the most important differences between case management and disease management. In *population-based health care*, the focus is on "covered lives" or populations of patients, rather than on the individual patient (Huston, 2002). The goal in DM is to service the optimal number of covered lives required to reach operational and economic efficiency. Providing optimum, cost-effective care to individual patients is critical to the success of a DM program; however, the focus for planning, implementation, and evaluation is population based.

Other primary features of DM programs include the use of a multidisciplinary healthcare team, including specialists in the area, the selection of large population groups to reduce adverse selection, the use of standardized clinical guidelines–clinical pathways reflecting best practice research to guide provider practice, and the use of integrated data management systems to track patient progress across care settings and allow continuous and ongoing improvement of treatment algorithms (Reeder, 1999; Huston, 2002). Common features of DM programs are shown in **Display 14.3.**

One thing is clear; DM continues to grow as a means of organizing patient care. This is particularly true in the government sector where there was almost a complete absence of DM services in the traditional Medicare plan until early this decade (Huston, 2002). Beginning in 2000, Medicare embraced a new round of trial DM demonstration projects, many of which are now mainstream initiatives, in an effort to deliver better outcomes at better prices (Carroll, June 2000).

In addition, the National Committee for Quality Assurance (NCQA), the Department of Health and Human Services, the Joint Commission for the

> ➤ The goal of disease management is to address a high-cost, chronic illness or condition with maximum efficiency across treatment settings.

Display 14.3 | **Common Features of Disease Management Programs**

1. Provide a comprehensive, integrated approach to the care and reimbursement of common, high-cost, chronic illnesses.
2. Focus on prevention as well as early disease detection and intervention to avoid costly acute episodes, but provides comprehensive care and reimbursement.
3. Target population groups (population based) rather than individuals.
4. Employ a multidisciplinary healthcare team, including specialists.
5. Use standardized clinical guidelines–clinical pathways reflecting best practice research to guide providers.
6. Use integrated data management systems to track patient progress across care settings and allow continuous and ongoing improvement of treatment algorithms.
7. Frequently employ professional nurses in the role of case manager or program coordinator.

- How will a change in the patient care delivery system alter individual and group decision making? Who will be affected? Will autonomy decrease or increase?
- How will social interactions and interpersonal relationships change?
- Will employees view their unit of work differently? Will there be a change from a partial unit of work to a whole unit? (For example, total patient care would be a whole unit of work, whereas team nursing would be a partial unit.)
- Will the change require a wider or more restricted range of skills and abilities on the part of the caregiver?
- Will redesign change how employees receive feedback on their performance, either for self-evaluation or by others?
- Will communication patterns change?

DIFFERENTIATED NURSING PRACTICE

> The philosophy behind differentiated nursing practice is that registered nurses should work within the role structure and responsibilities that correspond best with their individual capabilities.

Differentiated nursing practice refers to "the sorting of the roles, functions, and work of registered nurses according to some identified criteria—usually education, experience, and competence—or some combination of these (Huber, 2000, p. 584). The philosophy behind differentiated nursing practice is that registered nurses should work within the role structure and responsibilities that correspond best with their individual capabilities.

Two basic models are used to differentiate practice (see **Display 14.4**). The older one, the *education model*, reflects the ADN, BSN, and MSN programs and includes three basic components of nursing: provision of care, communication, and management. The *competency model* is based partly on the eight American Nurses Association's Standards of Nursing and also reflects Benner's (1984) five levels of practice: novice, advanced beginner, competent, proficient, and expert. Brady et al. (2001) suggest, however, that the 21 Pew Health Professional Commission Competencies could serve as a useful tool to nurses and health system leaders as they attempt to adapt the current model of nursing practice to the demands and realities of the contemporary and continually evolving healthcare environment. Brady et al. argue that this framework would offer an approach to rationalizing both nursing education and practice, with the potential for improving the quality of care and reducing fragmentation, cost, and public confusion about a nurse's educational preparation and scope of practice.

Display 14.4	**Two Basic Differentiated Practice Models**
Type	**Type of Differentiation**
Education Model	Role differentiation based on type of educational preparation (ADN, BSN, and MSN)
Competency Model	Role differentiation based on individual nurse skill level, expertise, experience, etc.

The rationale for differentiated practice is to match patient needs with nursing competencies; facilitate the effective and efficient use of nursing resources; provide equitable compensation based on education, productivity, and expertise; increase nurse satisfaction; build loyalty; and increase the prestige of the nursing profession. It also recognizes the broad domain of professional nursing, the multiple roles and responsibilities that nurses assume, and the contribution of all nursing personnel as valuable and unique (Blais, Hayes, Kozier, & Erb, 2002). Differentiated nursing practice is still too new to determine whether it has met the intended goals. It is hoped that the effectiveness of this concept will be thoroughly demonstrated before it is widely embraced and, if it is proven to be effective, that it be implemented correctly so that its adaptation will be successful.

Learning Exercise 14.5

Differentiating Practice at the Unit Level

You are serving on a committee of nurse–managers and staff nurses to develop guidelines and job descriptions for a new pay structure based on differentiated nursing practice. Several members of the committee are resistant to change. Your committee is now looking at four clinical levels of registered nurses, with different salary ranges for each level. Some believe both education and expertise should be required for advancement from one level to the next, and others believe it should be based only on expertise.

So far, the committee has agreed that nurses who wish to advance to the next clinical level must (1) apply for an open position at that level, (2) be recommended by both their immediate supervisor and one other nurse of an advanced clinical level, and (3) possess the expertise and education necessary to fulfill the job functions. It is on number three that you are having difficulty. You cannot agree on the type (formal or certifications) and amount of education necessary for each level or on how you will document expertise.

Assignment: Write a proposal for differentiating practice at the unit level. Will you use education, years of experience, or skill level to differentiate your career ladder or will you use some combination of the three? What would you name each of the four levels of nursing? Will your minimum requirements for each level be fixed or will you allow for individual variations?

INTEGRATING LEADERSHIP ROLES AND MANAGEMENT FUNCTIONS IN ORGANIZING PATIENT CARE

Organizing is an important management function. The work must be organized so organizational goals are sustained. Activities must be grouped so resources, people, materials, and time are used fully. The integrated leader–manager understands that the organization and unit's nursing philosophy and the availability of resources greatly influence the type of patient care delivery system that should be chosen and the potential success of future work redesign.

The integrated leader–manager then is responsible for selecting and implementing a patient care delivery system that facilitates the accomplishment of unit goals. All members of the work group should be assisted with role clarification, especially when work is redesigned or new systems of patient care delivery are implemented. This team effort in work activity increases productivity and worker satisfaction. The emphasis is on seeking solutions to poor organization of work, rather than finding fault.

There is no one "best" mode for organizing patient care. Integrating leadership roles and management functions ensures that the type of patient care delivery model selected will provide quality care and staff satisfaction and that change in the mode of delivery will not be attempted without adequate resources, appropriate justification, and attention to how it will affect group cohesiveness. Historically, nursing has frequently adopted models of patient care delivery based on societal events (e.g., a nursing shortage, a proliferation of types of healthcare workers) rather than upon well-researched models with proven effectiveness that promote professional practice. The leadership role demands that the primary focus of patient care delivery be on promoting a professional model of practice that also reduces costs and improves patient outcomes.

☀ Key Concepts

- *Total patient care*, utilizing the case method of assignment, is the oldest form of patient care organization and is still widely used today.
- *Functional nursing* organization requires the completion of specific tasks by different nursing personnel.
- *Team or modular nursing* organization uses a leader who coordinates team members in the care of a group of patients.
- *Primary care nursing* is organized so the patient is at the center of the structure. One nurse has 24-hour responsibility for the nursing care plan.
- *Case management* is a collaborative process that assesses, plans, implements, coordinates, monitors, and evaluates options and services to meet an individual's health needs through communication and available resources to promote quality, cost-effective outcomes.
- While the focus historically for case management has been the individual patient, the case manager employed in a *disease management program* plans the care for populations or groups of patients with the same chronic illness.
- *Differentiated* nursing practice delineates different roles for nurses based on their skill, knowledge, educational level, and motivation.
- The *care MAP* (multidisciplinary action plan) is a combination of a critical path and a nursing care plan, except that it shows times when nursing interventions should occur as well as variances.
- Delivery systems may have elements of the various designs present in the system in use in any organization.

- Each unit's care delivery structure should (1) facilitate meeting the goals of the organization; (2) be cost-effective; (3) satisfy the patient; (4) provide role satisfaction to nurses; (5) allow implementation of the nursing process; and (6) provide for adequate communication among healthcare providers.
- When work is redesigned, it frequently has personal consequences for employees that must be considered. Social interactions, the degree of autonomy, the abilities and skills necessary, employee evaluation, and communication patterns are often affected by work redesign.

More Learning Exercises and Applications

 Learning Exercise 14.6

Creating a Plan to Reduce Resistance

You work in an intensive care unit where there is an RN staff. The unit works 12-hour shifts, and each nurse is assigned one or two patients, depending on the nursing needs of the patient. The unit has always used total patient care delivery assignments. Recently, your unit manager has informed the staff that all patients in the unit would be assigned a case manager in an effort to maximize the use of resources and to reduce length of stay in the unit. Many of the unit staff resent the case manager and believe this has reduced the RN's autonomy and control of patient care. They are resistant to the need to document variances to the care MAPs and are generally uncooperative, but not to the point that they are insubordinate.

Although you feel some loss of autonomy, you also think that the case manager has been effective in coordinating care to speed patient discharge. You believe that at present the atmosphere in the unit is very stressful. The unit manager and case manager have come to you and requested that you assist them in convincing the other staff to go along with this change.

Assignment: Using your knowledge of planned change and case management, outline a plan for reducing resistance.

 Learning Exercise 14.7

Types of Patient Care Delivery Models Used in Your Area

In a group, investigate the types of patient care delivery models used in your area. Do not limit your investigation to hospitals. One healthcare organization should be assigned to a group. If possible, conduct interviews with nurses from a variety of delivery systems. Share the report of your findings with your classmates. How many different models of patient care delivery did you find? What is the most widely used method in healthcare facilities in your area? Does this vary from models identified most frequently in current nursing literature?

Learning Exercise 14.8

Implementing a Managed Care System
You are the director of a home health agency that has recently come under a managed care system. In the past, only a physician's order was necessary for authorization from the Medicare system, but now approval must come from the managed care organization (MCO). In the past, public health certified nurses (all BSNs) have acted as case managers for their assigned caseload. Now the MCO case manager has taken over this role, creating much conflict among the staff. Additionally, there is pressure from your board to cut costs by using more less-skilled nonprofessionals for some of the home care. You realize that unless you do so, your agency will not survive.

You have visited other home health agencies and researched your options carefully. You have decided you must use some type of team approach.

Assignment: Develop a plan, objectives, and a time frame for implementation. In your plan, discuss who will be most affected by your changes. As a change agent, what will be your most important role?

Web Links

University of Colorado Health Sciences Center. Colorado Differentiated Practice Model.
http://www.uchsc.edu/ahec/cando/nursing/diffpractice97.htm
Examines history, purposes, goals, and implementation of Colorado Differentiated Practice Model for Nursing.

M. L. Birnbaum. Guidelines, Algorithms, Critical Pathways, Templates, and Evidence-based Medicine (Last modified June 2000)
http://pdm.medicine.wisc.edu/birnbaum6.htm
Differentiates between standardized guidelines, algorithms, critical pathways, and templates and urges critical analysis of all these components that form the standards of practice for evidence–based medicine.

Case Management Society of America
http://www.cmsa.org/
The professional society for case management professionals. This site includes society information, links to other case management sites, and other information about case management.

CNA's Position on Differentiated Practice/Competency-Based Role Differentiation in Nursing
http://www.calnurse.org/cna/np/np6101599.html
Examines the California Nurses Association's 1999 House of Delegates unanimous vote to reaffirm opposition to differentiated nursing practice.

References

A conversation with Bob Stone: How time and circumstance changed disease management. (2001, December). *Managed Care.* Available at: http://www.managedcaremag.com/archives/0112/0112.qna_stone.html. Accessed January 10, 2004.

Benner, P. (1984). *From novice to expert: Excellence and power in clinical nursing practice.* Menlo Park, CA: Addison-Wesley.

Benson, L. M., Bowes, J., Cheesebro, K., Stasa, C., Horst, T., Blyskal, S., et. al. (2001). Using variance tracking to improve outcomes and reduce costs. *Dimensions of Critical Care Nursing, 20*(2), 34–42.

Blais, K. K., Hayes, J. S., Kozier, B. & Erb, G. (2002). *Professional nursing practice: Concepts and perspectives* (4th ed.). Upper Saddle River, NJ: Prentice Hall Health.

Brady, M., Leuner, J. D., Bellack, J. P., Loquist, R. S., Cipriano, P. F, & O'Neil, E. H. (2001). A proposed framework for differentiating the 21 Pew competencies by level of nursing education. *Nursing and Health Care Perspectives, 22*(1), 30–35.

Carroll, J. (2000). DM vendors start to address costs created by comorbidities. *Managed Care.* Available at: http://www.managedcaremag.com/archives/0203/0203.dmconsolidate.html. Accessed January 10, 2004.

Carroll, J. (2000). DM and Medicare: A marriage made in heaven? *Managed Care.* Available at: http://www.managedcaremag.com/archives/0206/0206.medicare_dm.html. Accessed January 10, 2004.

DM program is first to be accredited by JCAHO . . . disease management. (2002). *Healthcare-Benchmarks, 9*(4), 46–47.

Finkelman, A. W. (2001). *Managed care: A nursing perspective.* Upper Saddle River, NJ: Prentice Hall.

Furlow, L. (2003). Cut the clutter with cycle time reduction. *Nursing Management, 34*(3), 42–44.

Huber, D. (2000). *Leadership and nursing care management* (2nd ed.). Philadelphia: W.B. Saunders.

Huston, C. (2002). The role of the case manager in a disease management program. *Lippincott's Case Management, 7*(6), 221–227.

Manthey, M. (2001). A core incremental staffing plan. *Journal of Nursing Administration, 31*(9), 424–425.

Nelson, J. W. (2000). Models of nursing care: A century of vacillation. *Journal of Nursing Administration, 30*(4), 156, 184.

Powell, S. K. (2000). *Case management: A practical guide to success in managed care* (2nd ed.). Philadelphia: Lippincott.

Reeder, L. (1999). Anatomy of a disease management program. *Nursing Management, 30*(4), 41–45.

Smith, A. P. (2003). Case management. Key to access, quality, and financial success. *Nursing Economic$, 21*(5), 237–240, 244.

Bibliography

Ackermann, R. J. (May 2001). Primary care. Nursing home practice: Strategies to manage most acute and chronic illnesses without hospitalization. *Geriatrics, 56*(5), 37, 40, 43–44.

Barkell, N. P. (2002). The relationship between nurse staffing models and patient outcomes: A descriptive study. *Outcomes Management, 6*(1), 27–33.

Burke, R. J. (2001). Surviving hospital restructuring. *Journal of Nursing Administration, 31*(4), 169–172.

Coughlin, C. (2000). Is now the time to design new care delivery models? *Journal of Nursing Administration, 30*(9), 403–404.

Drennan, V. (2001). An assessment of dual-role primary care nurses in the inner city. *British Journal of Community Nursing, 6*(7), 336–341.

Ebert, J. (2000). Utilizing the nursing "team model" to enhance the role of the case manager. *Lippincotts Case Management, 5*(5), 199–201.

Enhance care by making CM part of Medicare: Value of case managers "yet to be recognized." (2003*). Hospital Case Management, 11*(10), 157.

Gerrish, K., Ferguson, A., Kitching, N., & Mischenko, J. (2000). Developing primary care nursing: The contribution of nursing development units. *Journal of Community Nursing, 14*(6), 8, 10, 12.

Goode, D. (2001). Perceptions and experiences of primary nursing in an ICU: A combined methods approach. *Intensive Critical Care Nurse, 17*(5), 294–303.

Henderson, C. W. (2001, January 15). Study looks at case management intervention to improve access to care. *AIDS Weekly*, 10–12.

Horst, L., Werner, R. R., & Werner, C. L. (2000). Case management for children and families. *Journal of Child and Family Nursing, 3*(1), 5–15.

Ibbs, L. (2001). A team approach stretches RN's ability to care . . . "Kaiser outlines new nurse staffing ratios," July 30. *Nurseweek Calif, 14*(17), 2.

Kovner, C. (September 2001). The impact of staffing and the organization of work on patient outcomes and healthcare workers in healthcare organizations, *Joint Commission Journal on Quality Improvement, 27*(9), 458–468.

Make sure that you are culturally competent: CMs should prepare to treat a diverse population. (2003). *Hospital Case Management, 11*(10), 149–150.

Mancher, T. (May 2001). A better model by design—and it works. *Nursing Management, 32*(5), 45–47.

Makinen, A. (July 2003). Organization of nursing care and stressful work characteristics. *Journal of Advanced Nursing, 43*(2), 197–205.

Mueller, C. (2000). GN management: A framework for nurse staffing in long-term care facilities. *Geriatric Nursing, 21*(5), 262–267.

Pesut, D. (2002). Education. Differentiation: Practice versus services. *Journal of Professional Nursing, 18*(3), 118–119.

Potter, P. & Grant, E. (2004). Understanding RN and unlicensed assistive personnel working relationships in designing care delivery strategies. *Journal of Nursing Administration, 43*(1), 19–23.

Powell, S. (2000). *Advanced case management: Outcomes and beyond.* Philadelphia: Lippincott.

Rick, C. (2003). AONE's leadership exchange. Differentiated practice: Get beyond the fear factor. *Nursing Management, 34*(1), 11.

Ritter-Teitel, J. (2002). The impact of restructuring on professional nursing practice. *Journal of Nursing Administration, 32*(1), 31–41.

Ross, F. (2002). Mapping research in primary care nursing: Current activity and future priorities . . . including commentary by Pearson, P. *Nursing Research 7*(1), 46–59.

Schriefer, J. A., & Botter, M. L. (2001). Tools and systems for improved outcomes. Nurse case management skills required for care management. *Outcomes Management for Nursing Practice, 5*(2), 48–51.

Smith, A. P. (2003). Case management: Key to access, quality, and financial success. *Nursing Economic$, 21*(5), 237–240.

Strategies to build high performance nursing teams. (2003). *COR Clinical Excellence, 4* (1), 6–8.

CHAPTER

15

Preliminary Staffing Functions: Employee Recruitment, Selection, Placement, and Indoctrination

Recruitment and retention of staff is more than technique. It requires enthusiasm about nursing and caring for others.

—Louis Benson

After planning and organizing, *staffing* is the third phase of the management process. In staffing, the leader–manager recruits, selects, places, indoctrinates, and promotes personnel development to accomplish the goals of the organization. Healthcare managers have long been sensitive to the importance of physical resources (technology, space) and financial resources to the success of service delivery. During the last several decades, the value and potential for development of a third element, the human resource, has gained new recognition. The importance of viewing personnel as a critical resource is crucial to meet challenges faced in a rapidly changing healthcare environment with limited resources.

Staffing is an especially important phase of the management process in healthcare organizations because such organizations are usually labor intensive (i.e., many employees are required for an organization to accomplish its goals). Additionally, this large workforce must be composed of highly skilled, competent professionals. Ensuring the adequacy of skilled staff to accomplish organizational goals is an important management function. Unit 5 reviews the manager's responsibilities in executing the staffing functions of the management process.

The following are the sequential steps of staffing responsibilities, although each step has some interdependence with all staffing activities:

1. Determine the number and types of personnel needed to fulfill the philosophy, meet fiscal planning responsibilities, and carry out the chosen patient care delivery system selected by the organization.
2. Recruit, interview, select, and assign personnel based on established job description performance standards.
3. Use organizational resources for induction and orientation.
4. Ascertain that each employee is adequately socialized to organization values and unit norms.
5. Develop a program of staff education that will assist employees with meeting the goals of the organization.
6. Use creative and flexible scheduling based on patient care needs to increase productivity and retention.

This chapter examines national and regional trends for professional nurse staffing. It also addresses the preliminary staffing functions, namely determining present and future staffing needs and recruiting, interviewing, selecting, and placing personnel. It also includes two employee indoctrination functions: induction and orientation. The management functions and leadership roles inherent in these staffing responsibilities are shown in **Display 15.1**.

PLANNING FOR STAFFING AND RESPONDING TO SHORTAGES

Planning is a major leadership role in staffing and is often a neglected part of the staffing process. Because the success of many staffing decisions greatly depends on previous decisions made in the planning and organizing phases, one must consider staffing when making other plans. Consideration must be given to the type of patient care management used, the education and knowledge level of staff to be recruited,

| Display 15.1 | **Leadership Roles and Management Functions Associated with Preliminary Staffing Functions** |

Leadership Roles

1. Plans for future staffing needs proactively by being knowledgeable regarding current and historical staffing events.
2. Identifies and recruits talented people to the organization.
3. Seeks diversity in staffing, which reflects the diversity of the population being served.
4. Is self-aware regarding personal biases during the preemployment process.
5. Seeks to find the best possible fit between employee's unique talents and organizational staffing needs.
6. Periodically reviews induction and orientation programs to ascertain they are meeting unit needs.
7. Ensures that each new employee understands appropriate organizational policies.
8. Continually aspires to create a work environment that promotes retention and worker satisfaction.

Management Functions

1. Ensures that there is an adequate skilled workforce to meet the goals of the organization.
2. Shares responsibility for the recruitment of staff with organization recruiters.
3. Plans and structures appropriate interview activities.
4. Uses techniques that increase the validity and reliability of the interview process.
5. Applies knowledge of the legal requirements of interviewing and selection to ensure that the organization is not unfair in its hiring practices.
6. Develops established criteria for selection.
7. Uses knowledge of organizational needs and employee strengths to make placement decisions.
8. Interprets information in employee handbook and provides input for handbook revisions.
9. Participates actively in employee orientation.

budget constraints, the historical background of staffing needs and availability, and the diversity of the patient population to be served.

Accurately predicting staffing needs is a valuable management skill because it enables the manager to avoid staffing crises. Managers should know the source of their nursing pool, how many students are currently enrolled in local nursing schools, the usual length of employment of new hires, peak staff resignation periods, and times when patient census is highest. Analyzing historical patterns, using computers to sort personnel statistics, and keeping accurate unit records are examples of proactive planning.

The Value of Diversity

The manager should also be alert to the gender, culture, ethnicity, age, and language diversity in the communities the organization serves and should seek to recruit a staff that is both sensitive and responsive to that diversity. This requires seeking out and hiring staff who represent both the majority and minority cultures represented in the community. This valuing of diversity should become an integral part of the formal level of operations in the organization, with affirmative action committees monitoring the fairness of staffing policies and their implementation (Tappen, 2001). The importance of this goal cannot be understated. Traditionally, the nursing profession has been made up of approximately 90% white women, yet more than 40% of the population will reflect an ethnic or racial minority by 2020 (Frusti, Niesen, & Campion, 2003).

Impact of the Economy

The manager also should be aware of the role national and local economics play in planning for staffing. Historically, when the economy improves, nursing shortages occur. When the economy declines, nursing vacancy rates decline as well, since many unemployed nurses return to the workforce and part-time nurses return to full-time employment.

Third-party insurer reimbursement rates also impact staffing. As government and private insurer reimbursements declined in the 1990s, many healthcare organizations, hospitals in particular, began downsizing to achieve cost containment by eliminating registered nursing jobs or by replacing registered nursing positions with unlicensed assistive personnel. Even hospitals that did not downsize during this period often did little to recruit qualified registered nurses. This downsizing and short-sightedness regarding recruitment and retention contributed to the beginning of an acute shortage of registered nurses in many healthcare settings by the late 1990s.

Currently, the nursing shortage in this country is profound, exhibiting both demand and supply shortages. It is also widespread geographically and likely to worsen before it improves (Upenieks, 2003). The United States currently has just over 2.6 million registered nurses (RNs), and about 2.2 million of them are employed. One and one-half million nurses work full time (The Registered Nurse Population, 2000). The National Sample Survey of Registered Nurses projects that by the year 2005, approximately 2.6 million *full-time* registered nurses will be needed, a shortfall of 43% (The Registered Nurse Population).

Effects of Aging Workforce

Compounding the shortage is the fact that nurses are a graying population—even more so than the population at large. The average age of the working nurse today is 44 years (Buerhaus, Staiger, & Auerbach, 2000a), and the average retirement age for nurses is 49 years (The Registered Nurse Population, 2000). More than two thirds of registered nurses are age 40 and older, and less than 10% are under the age of 30 (Wakefield, 2001). By 2010, more than 40% of registered nurses will be over the age of 50 (Buerhaus et al., 2000a).

The shortage problem is complicated by the fact that simply recruiting *new* nurses to fill the void is not a viable solution. Recent data from the National League for Nursing indicates declines in enrollments in all types of entry-level nursing programs and a study by the American Association of Colleges of Nursing found that enrollments in entry-level baccalaureate programs decreased for six

There will likely be a vast exodus from the nursing workforce in the next two to ten years, at a time when 43% more nurses are needed.

consecutive years through 2002 (American Association of Colleges of Nursing, 2002; American Association of Colleges of Nursing, 1999). Some of this decline can be attributed to inadequate federal and state funding for nursing education; however, the popularity of nursing as a major field of study has declined as well. The most prominent factor seems to be the concurrent expansion of opportunities for capable young women to enter formerly male-dominated professions such as medicine, law, and business.

Only half as many women select nursing as a career today as compared with 25 years ago. This represents a drop of roughly 40% since 1973 in the percentage of college freshman who indicate that nursing is their top career choice (Staiger, Auerbach, & Buerhaus, 2000). In fact, a recent study reported that women graduating from high school in the 1990s were 35% less likely to become RNs than women who graduated in the 1970s (Buerhaus, Staiger, & Auerbach, 2000b).

To further confound the shortage and efforts to address it, the average age of nursing faculty members in this country is 50 (Buerhaus et al., 2000a), and the average age of professors in nursing programs is 52 (Buerhaus et al, 2000b). With less than 1% of nurses holding earned doctoral degrees and only 10% having master's degrees (Chitty, 2001), the educator pool is already small. In addition, the number of nurses with master's and doctoral degrees prepared for faculty roles has decreased dramatically over the past decade. Only 3.3% of students in master's programs in 1998 were enrolled in education tracks (Chitty, 2001). And the difficulty in recruiting a master's or doctorally prepared nurse to teach in academe is complicated by the fact that the service sector generally offers nurses with advanced degrees a much higher salary than academe offers (Huston, 2003).

Nursing in Community Settings

Another factor compounding the acute care shortage in acute care hospitals is the increasing number of nurses leaving the acute care hospital for employment in community health settings. Just over 18% of RNs are now employed in such settings (Wakefield, 2001). Although the majority of nurses continue to be employed in hospitals (59.1%), the average national hospital vacancy rate for registered nurses is between 12 and 15% (Case et al., 2002; Buerhaus, et al., 200b) and is expected to rise to 20% by the year 2020 (Buerhaus et al., 200b; Heinrich, 2001).

Besides shortages of nurses in acute care settings, the nursing workforce is poorly distributed geographically. As this decade began, the greatest concentration of employed nurses was in New England, with 1,075 RNs per 100,000 population. In contrast, the Pacific region had 596 RNs per 100,000 population (Wakefield, 2001). Although all states are affected by the current shortage, the situation in some states is especially dire. For example, California ranks second only to Nevada in the lowest proportion of working RNs per 100,000 population, yet newest figures suggest California will need at least 25,000 more registered nurses in the next five years than will be available (United States General Accounting Office, 2001) and 60,000 more by 2020 to maintain the current low levels (Case, Mowry, & Welebob, 2002). And out-of-state recruitment won't be the answer for California. Half of the RNs currently working in California already are educated in other states or countries (State of California, 1999).

All of these factors have led to a significant professional nursing shortage in the early 21st century. In February 2001, a forum entitled "Hard Numbers, Hard Choices: A Report on the Nation's Nursing Workforce" was held on Capitol Hill. Three members of Congress shared their views on the adverse consequences of insufficient numbers and distribution of nurses as well as a plan to begin addressing these problems (Wakefield, 2001). Wakefield goes on to say that clearly, the current and short-term future nursing workforce is insufficient to meet both the general healthcare demands of a growing U.S. population as well as demands from an increasingly graying society.

Acting to Resolve Staffing Shortages

Johnson (2000) states in regard to the current shortage: "We have spent lots of time denying, analyzing, and sometimes blaming as well. We have experienced 'analysis paralysis' despite the fact that the demand side of the profession grows higher while the supply side slides further into crisis. We must act collectively, collaboratively, and in concert with a whole host of stakeholders, including all members of the healthcare team, the community, and Congress as well"(p. 402).

Short-term solutions to the shortage have been attempted including the immigration of foreign nurses and increases in federal money for nursing education. The recent passage of legislation such as the Nurse Reinvestment Act encourages more students to choose nursing as a career and help students financially to complete their education. It also encourages graduate students to complete their studies and assume teaching positions in nursing schools.

In addition, many states have introduced or passed legislation designed to improve working conditions or attract more nurses. Four states have passed workforce study bills to study the nursing shortage, and two states have passed bills authorizing funding for nursing education (Williams, 2001). Long-term planning and aggressive intervention, however, will be needed for some time at the national and regional level to ensure that an adequate, highly qualified nursing workforce will be available in the future to meet the healthcare needs of the citizens of this country.

RECRUITMENT

Recruitment is the process of actively seeking out or attracting applicants for existing positions. Although at any given time an organization may have an adequate supply of RNs to meet demand, historical data support the idea that recruitment should be an ongoing process. Nevidjon and Erickson (2001) suggest that the retention of nurses begins with how much the organization does or does not value the staff. "Rhetoric notwithstanding, most healthcare executives view staff as an expense and in times of financial constraint, as is currently the state, watch the personnel budget line very closely. Instead of viewing staff as an expense, managers should view staff as an asset on the balance sheet that will drive different decisions about the work environment" (p. 7).

Learning Exercise 15.1

Choosing Your Place in the Workforce

You are a baccalaureate nursing student who will graduate in three months. You are aware that there are multiple vacancies at almost every acute care hospital in the area as well as more limited openings in home health, public health, community health, tele-health, and case management. The local community hospital is offering a significant sign-on bonus for new graduates who are willing to sign a two-year contract. This would be helpful in paying off school loans you have accrued. You really enjoyed, however, the autonomy and patient interaction you experienced in your public health practicum as part of school and the Monday to Friday work schedule of the public health nurses appeals to you, since you have small children. The salary, however, would be significantly lower than if you worked in an acute care setting. Moreover, the orientation period at the public health facility is fairly short. Finally, you have always had an interest in pediatric oncology, a specialty not available to you, unless you relocate to a regional medical center. No sign-on bonus is available at the medical center; however, there are more opportunities for advancement and professional development there. Your spouse is willing to make this move if this is what you really want.

Assignment:

1. Determine how you will move forward in making a decision about where you will seek employment.
2. Make a list of 10 factors you need to consider in weighting conflicting wants, needs, and obligations.
3. What evaluation criteria can you generate to look at both the process you used to make your decision as well as the decision itself?

In complex organizations, work must be accomplished by groups of people; wise managers, therefore, try to surround themselves with people of ability, motivation, and promise. Unfortunately, some managers feel threatened by bright and talented people and surround themselves with mediocrity. The organization's ability to meet its goals and objectives is directly related to the quality of its employees. Excellent employees reflect well on the manager because they prevent stagnation and increase productivity within the organization. A leadership role in staffing includes identifying, recruiting, and hiring gifted people.

> The organization's ability to meet its goals and objectives is directly related to the quality of its employees.

The Nurse Recruiter

The manager may be greatly or minimally involved with recruiting, interviewing, and selecting personnel depending on (1) the size of the institution; (2) the existence of a separate personnel department; (3) the presence of a nurse recruiter within the organization; and (4) the use of centralized or decentralized nursing management. Howell (1999) states that in the era of downsizing or "rightsizing," nurse recruiters have become an endangered species: "The onus to interview and choose candidates is on managers and directors, who often have little or no interviewing experience" (p. 25).

Generally speaking, the more decentralized nursing management and the less complex the personnel department, the greater the involvement of the lower-level manager in selecting personnel for individual units or departments. When deciding whether to hire a nurse recruiter or decentralize the responsibility for recruitment, the organization needs to weigh benefits against costs. Costs include more than financial considerations. For example, an additional cost to an organization employing a nurse recruiter might be the eventual loss of interest by managers in the recruiting process. The organization loses if managers relegate their collective and individual responsibilities to the nurse recruiter.

When organizations use nurse recruiters, a collaborative relationship must exist between managers and recruiters. Managers must be aware of recruitment constraints, and the recruiter must be aware of individual department needs and culture. Both parties must understand the organization's philosophy, benefit programs, salary scale, and other factors that influence employee retention.

Recruitment and Retention

Recruiting adequate numbers of nurses is less difficult if the organization is located in a progressive community with several schools of nursing and if the organization has a good reputation for quality patient care and fair employment practices. It will likely be much more difficult to recruit nurses to rural areas that historically have experienced less appropriation of healthcare professionals per capita than urban areas.

Because most recruiting methods are expensive, healthcare organizations often seek less costly means of recruitment. One of the best ways to maintain an adequate employee pool is by word of mouth, the recommendation of the organization's own satisfied and happy staff. Recruitment, however, is not the key to adequate staffing in the long term. *Retention* is, and it only occurs when the organization is able to create a work environment that makes staff want to stay. Some turnover, however, is normal and in fact, desirable. *Turnover* infuses the organization with fresh ideas. It also reduces the probability of "groupthink," in which all the people in the organization share similar thought processes, values, and goals. However, excessive or unnecessary turnover reduces the ability of the organization to produce its end-product and is expensive. The HSM Group (2002) reported that the nurse turnover rate in 2000 was 21.3%. In fact, 33% of nurses who are younger than age 30 plan to leave their nursing position within a year (Hopkins, 2001).

The average hidden and total cost of turnover in 2000 was estimated to be $64,000 for an ICU nurse and $42,000 for a medical–surgical nurse (The Advisory Board, 2000). Atencio, Cohen, and Gorenberg (2003) suggest the cost is actually up to twice a nurse's annual salary, or $92,422 for a medical–surgical nurse. The costs of replacing a specialty nurse then could be as high as $145,000 (Atencio, et al.). Such costs generally include human resource expenses for advertising and interviewing; recruitment fees such as sign-on bonuses, increased use of traveling nurses, overtime, and temporary replacements for the lost worker; lost productivity; and the costs of training time to bring the new employee up to desired efficiency.

It is critical, then, that the manager recognize the link between retention and recruitment. Some healthcare organizations find it necessary to do external recruitment, partly because of their lack of attention to retention. Atencio et al. (2003) state that the literature clearly supports that the social climate of the workplace is the primary initiator of a nurse's intent to stay or leave and that this social climate may reflect either work frustration or work excitement. Research by Strachota, Normandin, O'Brien, Clary, and Krukow (2003) concurs, citing work hours (having to work the majority of holidays, every other weekend, nights with no possibility of changing to day shift, and lack of scheduling flexibility) as the number one reason nurses leave their position. The middle level manager has the greatest impact in addressing these concerns and creating a positive social climate.

In addition, the closer the fit between what the nurse is seeking in employment and what the organization can offer, the greater the chance that the nurse will be retained. Often those recruiting during a nursing shortage inadvertently misrepresent the organization. At times, this behavior borders on unethical conduct but most often occurs because of the recruiter's overzealousness.

 Learning Exercise 15.2

Examining Recruitment Advertisements
Select one of the following:
1. In small groups, examine several nursing journals that carry job advertisements. Select three ads that particularly appeal to you. What do these advertisements say, or what makes them stand out? Are similar key words used in all three ads? What bonuses or incentives are being offered to attract qualified professional nurses?
2. Select a healthcare agency in your area. Write an advertisement or recruitment poster that accurately depicts the agency and the community. Compare your completed advertisement or recruitment flyer with those created by others in your group.

THE INITIAL CONTACT

Many prospective employees will make their first contact with an organization through the Human Resources Department or the recruiter. Generally, these employees are directed to complete an application and set up an appointment for an interview. Research by Kalisch (2003) suggests, however, that this process is often fraught with problems and that many (25%) potential employees never receive a response to letters or end up in an extensive and frustrating "telephone tag" (83%). In 21 of the 122 hospitals in Kalisch's study, the applications or resumes provided by the applicant were lost either temporarily or permanently. Interview wait times ranged from 1 to 90 minutes and interview length ranged from 5 to 95 minutes.

Only two applicants were offered coffee or refreshments of any kind and 32% reported reluctance or refusal to set up an appointment for an interview by the human resources secretary. Clearly, this conveys a lack of valuing of the potential employee and most healthcare institutions cannot afford this neglect of common courtesy in an era of nursing shortages.

INTERVIEWING

An *interview* may be defined as a verbal interaction between individuals for a particular purpose. Although other tools, such as testing and reference checks, may be used, the interview is frequently accepted as the foundation for selecting people for positions. The purposes or goals of the selection interview are threefold: (1) the interviewer seeks to obtain enough information to determine the applicant's suitability for the available position; (2) the applicant obtains adequate information to make an intelligent decision about accepting the job, should it be offered; and (3) the interviewer seeks to conduct the interview in such a manner that, regardless of the interview's result, the applicant will continue to have respect for and goodwill toward the organization.

Interviews may be unstructured or structured. The *unstructured* interview requires little planning because the goals for hiring may be unclear, questions are not prepared in advance, and often the interviewer does more talking than the applicant. The *structured* interview requires greater planning time because questions must be developed in advance that address the specific job requirements, information must be offered about the skills and qualities being sought, examples of the applicant's experience must be received, and the willingness or motivation of the applicant to do the job must be determined. The interviewer who uses a structured format would ask the same essential questions of all applicants.

Limitations of Interviews

> In reality, interviews generally require an interviewer to use judgments, biases, and values to make decisions based on a short interaction with an applicant in an unnatural situation.

The major defect of the interview is its subjectivity. Most interviewers feel confident that they can overcome this subjectivity and view the interview as a reliable selection tool whereas most interviews still have an element of subjectivity. The applicant, trying to create a favorable impression, also may be unduly influenced by the interviewer's personality.

Research findings regarding the validity and reliability of interviews have been inconsistent. However, the following findings are generally accepted:

- The same interviewer will consistently rate the interviewee the same. Therefore, the *intra-rater reliability* is said to be high.
- If two different interviewers conduct unstructured interviews of the same applicant, their ratings will not be consistent. Therefore, the inter-rater reliability is extremely low in unstructured interviews.
- *Inter-rater reliability* is satisfactory if the interview is structured and the same format is used by both interviewers.

- Even if the interview has *reliability* (i.e., it measures the same thing consistently), it still may not be valid. *Validity* occurs when the interview measures what it is supposed to measure, which, in this case is the potential for productivity as an employee. Structured interviews have greater validity than unstructured interviews. Thus, the structured interview was found to be a much better predictor of job performance and overall effectiveness than the unstructured interview.
- High interview assessments are not related to subsequent high-level job performance.
- Validity increases when there is a team approach to the interview.
- The attitudes and biases of interviewers greatly influence how candidates are rated. Although steps can be taken to reduce subjectivity, it cannot be eliminated entirely.
- The interviewer is more influenced by unfavorable than by favorable information. Negative information is weighed more heavily than positive information about the applicant.
- Interviewers tend to make up their minds about hiring applicants very early in the job interview. Decisions are often formed in the first few minutes of the interview.
- In unstructured interviews, the interviewer tends to do most of the talking, whereas in structured interviews, the interviewer does only about 50% of the talking. The goal should be to have the interviewee do 90% of the talking (Howell, 1999).

Regardless of the defects inherent in interviewing, the method remains a widely used and accepted way of selecting from among many applicants to fill a limited number of positions. By knowing the limitations of interviews and using findings from current research, interviewers should be able to conduct interviews so they will have an increased predictive value.

Overcoming Interview Limitations

Interview research has helped managers develop strategies for overcoming many of interviewing's inherent limitations. The following guidelines will assist the manager in developing an interview process that results in increased reliability and validity.

Use a Team Approach

Having more than one person interview the job applicant reduces individual bias. Staff involvement in hiring can be viewed on a continuum from no involvement to a team approach, using unit staff for the hiring decisions. When hiring a manager, using a staff nurse as part of the interview team is effective, especially if the staff nurse is mature enough to represent the interests and needs of the unit rather than his or her own self-interests.

Involving staff on hiring committees or panels to interview job applicants can involve a significant commitment of employee time and thus expense on the part of the organization. This expense may be justified if attrition rates are particularly high or if prior hiring outcomes have not been satisfactory to the organization. Any organization that has a high attrition rate should look very carefully at its selection process.

Develop a Structured Interview Format for Each Job Classification

Because each job has different position requirements, interviews must be structured to fit the position. The same structured interview should be used for all employees applying for the same job classification. A well-developed structured interview uses open-ended questions and provides ample opportunity for the interviewee to talk. The structured interview is advantageous because it allows the interviewer to be consistent and prevents the interview from becoming sidetracked. **Display 15.2** is an example of a structured interview.

Display 15.2 Sample Structured Interview

Motivation
Why did you apply for employment with this company?
Physical
Do you have any physical limitations that would prohibit you from accomplishing the job?
How many days have you been absent from work during the last year of employment?
Education
What was your grade point average in nursing school?
What were your extracurricular activities, offices held, awards conferred?
For verification purposes, are your school records listed under the name on your
    application form?
Professional
In what states are you licensed to practice?
Do you have your license with you?
What certifications do you hold?
What professional organizations do you currently participate in that would be of value
    in the job for which you are applying?
Military Experience
What are your current military obligations?
Which military assignments do you think have prepared you for this position?
Present Employer
How did you secure your present position?
What is your current job title? What was your title when you began your present position?
What supervisory responsibilities do you currently have?
How would you describe your immediate supervisor?
What are some examples of success at your present job?
How do you get along with your present employer?
How do you get along with your present colleagues?
What do you like most about your present job?
What do you like least about your present job?
May we contact your present employer?
Why do you want to change jobs?
For verification purposes only, is your name the same as it was while employed with your
    current employer?

Display 15.2	**Sample Structured Interview**

Previous Position(s)
Ask similar questions about recent past employment. Depending on the timespan and type of other positions held, the interviewer does not usually review employment history that took place beyond the position just previous to the current one.

Specific Questions for RNs
What do you like most about nursing?
What do you like least about nursing?
What is your philosophy of nursing?

Personal Characteristics
Which personal characteristics are your greatest assets?
Which personal characteristics cause you the most difficulty?

Professional Goals
What are your career goals?
Where do you see yourself 10 years from now?

Contributions to Organization
What can you offer this company?

Questions from Interviewee
What questions do you have about the organization?
What questions do you have about the position?
What other questions do you have?

Evaluation
Evaluation should be objective and relate to the applicant's qualifications for the specific position.

Use Scenarios to Determine Decision-making Ability

In addition to obtaining answers to a particular set of questions, the interview also should be used to determine the applicant's decision-making ability. This can be accomplished by designing scenarios that require problem-solving and decision-making skills. The same set of scenarios should be used with each category of employee. For example, a set could be developed for new graduates, critical care nurses, unit secretaries, and practical nurses. Patient care situations, as shown in **Display 15.3,** require clinical judgment and are very useful for this purpose.

Conduct Multiple Interviews

Candidates should be interviewed more than once on separate days. This prevents applicants from being accepted or rejected merely because they were having a good or bad day. Regardless of the number of interviews held, the person should be interviewed until all the interviewers' questions have been answered, and they feel confident they have enough information to make the right decision.

Provide Training in Effective Interviewing Techniques

Training should focus on communication skills and advice on planning, conducting, and controlling the interview. It is unfair to expect a manager to make appropriate hiring decisions if he or she has never had adequate training in interview techniques. Unskilled interviewers often let subjective rather than objective data affect their

Display 15.3	**Sample Interview Questions Using Case Situations**

Each recent graduate applying for a position at Country Hospital will be asked to respond to the following:

Case 1
You are working on the evening shift of a surgical unit. Mr. Jones returned from the postanesthesia care unit following a cholecystectomy two hours ago. While in the recovery room, he received 10 mg of morphine sulfate intravenously for incisional pain. Thirty minutes ago, he complained of mild incisional pain but then drifted off to sleep. He is now awake and complaining of moderate to severe incisional pain. His orders include the following pain relief order: morphine sulfate 8–10 mg, IV push every three hours for pain. It has been 2½ hours since Mr. Jones' last pain medication. What would you do?

Case 2
One of the practical nurses on your team seems especially tired today. She later tells you that her new baby kept her up all night. When you ask her about the noon finger-stick blood glucose level on Mrs. White (82 years old), she looks at you blankly and then says quickly that it was 150. Later, when you are in Mrs. White's room, she tells you that she doesn't remember anyone checking her blood glucose level at noon. What do you do?

hiring evaluation. In addition, unskilled interviewers may ask questions that could be viewed as discriminatory or that are illegal.

Planning, Conducting, and Controlling the Interview

Planning the interview in advance is vital to its subsequent success as a selection tool. If other interviewers are to be present, they should be available at the appointed time. The plan also should include adequate time for the interview. Before the interview, all interviewers should review the application, noting questions concerning information supplied by the applicant. Although it takes considerable practice, consistently using a planned sequence in the interview format will eventually yield a relaxed and spontaneous process. The following is a suggested interview format:

1. Introduce yourself and greet applicant.
2. Make a brief statement about the company and the available positions.
3. Ascertain the position for which the person is applying.
4. Discuss the information on the application, and seek clarification or amplification as necessary.
5. Discuss employee qualifications, and proceed with the structured interview format.
6. If applicant appears qualified, discuss the company and the position further.
7. Explain the subsequent procedures for hiring, such as employment physicals and hiring date. If the applicant is not hired at this time, discuss how and when he or she will be notified of the interview results.
8. Terminate the interview.

Remember that the interviewer should have control of the interview and set the tone. Try to create and maintain a comfortable environment throughout the interview. If the manager has opened well and the applicant is at ease, the interview will usually proceed smoothly. During the meeting, the manager should pause frequently to allow the applicant to ask questions. The format should always encourage and include ample time for questions from the applicant. Often interviewers are able to infer much about applicants by the types of questions they ask.

Moving the conversation along, covering questions on a structured interview guide, and keeping the interview pertinent but friendly becomes easier with experience. Methods that help reach the goals of the interview follow:

- Ask only job-related questions.
- Use open-ended questions that require more than a "yes" or "no" answer.
- Pause a few seconds after the applicant has seemingly finished before asking the next question. This gives the applicant a chance to talk further.
- Return to topics later in the interview on which the applicant offered little information initially.
- Ask only one question at a time.
- Restate part of the applicant's answer if you need elaboration.
- Ask questions clearly, but do not verbally or nonverbally indicate the correct answer. Otherwise, by watching the interviewer's eyes and observing other body language, the astute applicant may learn which answers are desired.
- Always appear interested in what the applicant has to say. The applicant should never be interrupted, nor should the interviewer's words ever imply criticism of or impatience with the applicant.
- Language should be used that is appropriate for the applicant. Terminology or language that makes applicants feel the interviewer is either talking down to them or talking over their heads is inappropriate.

A written record should be kept of all interviews. Notetaking ensures accuracy and serves as a written record to recall the applicant. Keep notetaking or use of a checklist, however, to a minimum so that you do not create an uncomfortable climate.

As the interview draws to a close, the interviewer should make sure that all questions have been answered and that all pertinent information has been obtained. Usually applicants are not offered a job at the end of a first interview unless they are clearly qualified and the labor market is such that another applicant would be difficult to find. In most cases, interviewers need to analyze their impressions of the applicant, compare these perceptions with members of the selection team, and incorporate those impressions with other available data about the applicant. Frequently, the interviewer needs to consult with others in the organization before a job offer can be made. It is important, however, to let applicants know if they are being seriously considered for the position and how soon they can expect to hear a final outcome.

When the applicant is obviously not qualified, the interviewer needs to be extremely tactful. The interviewer should not give false hope but should advise the person as soon as possible that he or she does not have the proper qualifications for the position. Such applicants should believe they have been treated fairly. The interviewer should, however, maintain records of the exact reasons for rejection in case of later discrimination charges.

Evaluation of the Interview

Interviewers should plan post-interview time to evaluate the applicant's interview performance. Interview notes are often taken in shorthand and may be difficult to read later. To avoid this problem, notes should be reviewed as soon as possible and necessary points clarified or amplified. Using a form to record the interview evaluation is a good idea. The final question on the interview report form is a recommendation for or against hiring. In answering this question, two aspects must carry the most weight:

1. **The requirements for the job.** Regardless of how interesting or friendly people are, unless they have the basic skills for the job, they will not be successful at meeting the expectations of the position. Likewise, those overqualified for a position will usually be unhappy in the job.
2. **Personal bias.** Because completely eliminating the personal biases inherent in the interview is impossible, it is important for the interviewer to examine any negative feelings that occurred during the interview. Often the interviewer discovers that the negative feelings have no relation to the criteria necessary for success in the position. Leadership requires that individual bias is minimized in personnel decisions.

Legal Aspects of Interviewing

The organization must ascertain that the application form does not contain questions that violate various employment acts. Likewise, managers must avoid unlawful inquiries during the interview. Inquiries cannot be made regarding age, marital status, children, race, sexual preference, financial or credit status, national origin, or religion. In addition to federal legislation, many states have specific laws pertaining to information that can be obtained during the process. For example, some states prohibit asking about a woman's ability to reproduce or her attitudes toward family planning. **Table 15.1** lists subjects that are most frequently part of the interview process or applicant form, with examples of acceptable and unacceptable inquiries.

Managers who maintain interview records and receive applicants with an open and unbiased attitude have little to fear regarding charges of discrimination. Remember, the third goal of the interview process is that each applicant should feel good about the organization when the interview concludes. Regardless of the interview's outcome, each applicant and each interviewer should remember the experience as a positive one. It is a leadership responsibility to see that this goal is accomplished.

Tips for the Interviewee

Just as there are things the interviewer should do to prepare and conduct the interview, there are things interviewees should do to increase the likelihood that the interview will be a mutually satisfying and enlightening experience (**Display 15.4**).

Table 15.1 Acceptable and Unacceptable Interview Inquiries

Subject	Acceptable Inquiries	Unacceptable Inquiries
Name	If applicant has worked for the company under a different name. If school records are under another name. If applicant has another name.	Inquiries about name that would indicate lineage, national origin, marital, or criminal status.
Marital and family status	Whether applicant can meet specified work schedules or has commitments that may hinder attendance requirements. Inquiries as to anticipated stay in the position.	Any question about applicant's marital status or number or age of children. Information about child care arrangements. Any questions concerning pregnancy.
Address or residence	Place of residence and length resided in city or state.	Former addresses, names or relationships of people with whom applicant resides, or if owns or rents home.
Age	If over 18 or statement that hire is subject to age requirement. Can ask if applicant is between 18 and 70.	Inquiry of specific age or date of birth.
Birthplace	Can ask for proof of U.S. citizenship.	Birthplace of applicant or spouse or any relative.
Religion	No inquiries allowed.	
Race or color	Can be requested for affirmative action but not as employment criteria.	All questions about race are prohibited.
Character	Inquiry into actual convictions that relate to fitness to perform job.	Questions relating to arrests or conviction of a crime.
Relatives	Relatives employed in company. Names and addresses of parents if applicant is a minor.	Questions about who applicant lives with or number of dependents.
Notice in case of emergency	Name and address of a *person* to be notified.	Name and address of a *relative* to be notified.
Organizations	Professional organizations.	Requesting a list of all memberships.
References	Professional or character reference.	Religious references.

continued

Table 15.1 Acceptable and Unacceptable Interview Inquiries

Subject	Acceptable Inquiries	Unacceptable Inquiries
Physical condition	All applicants can be asked if they are able to carry out the physical demands of the job.	Employers must be prepared to justify any mental or physical requirements. Specific questions regarding handicaps are forbidden.
Photographs	Statement that a photograph may be required *after* employment.	Requirement that a photograph be taken before interview or hiring.
National origin	If necessary to perform job, languages applicant speaks, read, or writes.	Inquiries about birthplace, native language, ancestry, date of arrival in United States, or native language.
Education	Academic, vocational, or professional education. Schools attended. Ability to read, speak, and write foreign languages.	Inquiries into racial or religious affiliation of a school. Inquiry into dates of schooling.
Sex	Inquiry or restriction of employment is only for bona fide occupational qualification, which is interpreted very narrowly by the courts.	Cannot ask sex on application. Sex cannot be used as a factor for hiring decisions.
Credit rating	No inquiries.	Questions about car or home ownership also are prohibited.
Other	Notice may be given that misstatements or omissions of facts may be cause for dismissal.	

The interviewee must also prepare in advance for the interview. Obtaining copies of the philosophy and organization chart of the organization to which you are applying should give you some insight as to the organization's priorities and should help you identify appropriate questions you may want to ask the interviewer. Speaking to individuals who already work at the organization should also be helpful in determining whether the organization philosophy is actually implemented in practice.

Schedule an appointment for the interview. Do not allow yourself to be drawn into an impromptu interview when you are dropping off an application or seeking information from the human resource department. You will want to be professionally dressed and will likely need time to reflect and prepare for the interview.

Practice responses to potential interview questions in advance. It is very difficult to spontaneously answer questions about your personal philosophy of nursing, your individual strengths and weaknesses, and your career goals if you have not given

Display 15.4   Interviewing Tips for Applicants

1. Prepare in advance for the interview.
2. Obtain copies of the philosophy and organization chart of the organization to which you are applying to determine if the organization philosophy is implemented in practice.
3. Schedule an appointment for the interview.
4. Dress professionally and conservatively.
5. Practice responses to potential interview questions in advance.
6. Arrive early on the day of the interview.
7. Greet the interviewer formally and do not sit down before he or she does, unless given permission to do so.
8. Shake the interviewer's hand upon entering the room and smile.
9. During the interview, sit quietly, be attentive, and take notes only if absolutely necessary.
10. Do not chew gum, fidget, slouch, or play with your hair, keys, or writing pen.
11. Ask appropriate questions about the organization or the specific job for which you are applying.
12. Avoid a "what can you do for me?" approach and focus instead on whether your unique talents and interests are a fit with the organization.
13. Answer interview questions as honestly and confidently as possible.
14. Shake the interviewer's hand at the close of the interview and thank him or her for his or her time.
15. Send a brief, typed thank-you note to the interviewer within 24 hours of the interview.

Learning Exercise 15.3

Assessing Personal Bias in Interviewing

You are a new evening charge nurse on a medical floor in an acute care hospital. This is your first management position. You graduated 18 months ago from the local university with a bachelor's degree in nursing. Your immediate supervisor has asked you to interview two applicants who will be graduating from nursing school in three months. Your supervisor believes that they both are qualified. Because the available position is on your shift, she wants you to make the final hiring decision.

Both applicants seem equally qualified in academic standing and work experience. Last evening, you interviewed Lisa and were very impressed. Tonight, you interviewed John. During the meeting, you kept thinking that you knew John from somewhere but couldn't recall where. The interview went well, however, and you were equally impressed with John.

After John left, you suddenly remembered that one of your classmates used to date him, and he had attended some of your class parties. You recall that, on several occasions, he appeared to abuse alcohol. This recollection bothers you, and you are not sure what to do. You know that tomorrow your supervisor wants to inform the applicants of your decision. **Assignment:** Decide what you are going to do. Support your decision with appropriate rationale. Explain how you would determine which applicant to hire. How great a role did your personal values play in your decision?

them advance thought. On the day of the interview, arrive about 10 minutes early to allow time for you to collect your thoughts and be mentally ready. Anticipate some nervousness (this is perfectly normal). Greet the interviewer formally (not by first name) and do not sit down before the interviewer does, unless given permission to do so. Be sure to shake the interviewer's hand upon entering the room and to smile. Smiling will reduce both your anxiety and that of the interviewer. Remember that many interviewers make up their mind early in the interview process, so first impressions count a lot.

During the interview, sit quietly, be attentive, and take notes only if absolutely necessary. Do not chew gum, fidget, slouch, or play with your hair, keys, or writing pen. Dress conservatively and make sure you are neatly groomed. Ask appropriate questions about the organization or the specific job for which you are applying. Questions about wages, benefits, and advancement opportunities should likely come later in the interview. Avoid a "what can you do for me?" approach and focus instead on whether your unique talents and interests are a fit with the organization. Answer interview questions as honestly and confidently as possible. Avoid rambling and never lie. If you do not know the answer to a question, say so. Also, if you need a few moments to reflect on a complex question before answering, state that as well.

At the close of the interview, shake the interviewer's hand and thank him or her for taking time to talk with you. It is always appropriate to clarify at that point when hiring decisions will be made and how you will be notified about the interview's outcome. You may want to send a brief thank-you note to the interviewer as well. If you do send a follow up thank-you note, be sure to type it and send it within 24 hours of the interview (Hawke, 2003). Thank the interviewer once again and reinforce that you want the job and can do it (Hawke).

SELECTION

After applicants have been recruited, have completed their applications, and have been interviewed, the next step in the preemployment staffing process is *selection*. Selection is the process of choosing from among applicants the best-qualified individual or individuals for a particular job or position. The selection process involves verifying the applicant's qualifications, checking his or her work history, and deciding if a good match exists between the applicant's qualifications and the organization's expectations. Can the applicant contribute to the organization in some unique way? Are the goals of the applicant and the institution compatible? Determining whether a "fit" exists between an employee and an organization is not easy. Furlow (2000) suggests that job profiling should be used as an adjunct to the regular hiring process. A *job profile* is an analysis of the criteria that define top performers in a specific job, thus allowing the organization to prescreen applicants for the "fit" to the job.

Employee diversity should also be considered in making selection decisions. Having a staff that is diverse in terms of gender, age, culture, ethnicity, and language is helpful in meeting the needs of an increasingly diverse patient population. In addition, having a diverse staff enhances the morale and productivity of the minority groups within the organization and enriches the entire organization, bringing new perspectives to the thinking and problem solving that occur daily, as well as providing more complex and creative solutions (Tappen, 2001).

Educational and Credential Requirements

Consideration should be given to educational requirements and credentials for each job category as long as a relationship exists between these requirements and success on the job. If requirements for a position are too rigid, the job may remain unfilled for some time. Additionally, people who might be able to complete educational or credential requirements for a position are sometimes denied the opportunity to compete for the job. Therefore, many organizations have a list of preferred criteria for a position and a second list of minimal criteria. Frequently, organizations will accept substitution criteria in lieu of preferred criteria. For example, a position might require a bachelor's degree, but a master's degree is preferred. However, five years of nursing experience could be substituted for the master's degree.

It is very important to check the academic and professional credentials of all job applicants. In a competitive job market, candidates may succumb to the pressure of telling "white lies" about their qualifications.

Reference Checks

All applications should be examined to see if they are complete and to ascertain that the applicant is qualified for the position. At this point, references are requested and employment history is verified. Usually the personnel department carries out some of these functions. Excellent references do not necessarily guarantee excellent job performance; however, poor references may help to prevent a bad hiring decision. Whenever possible, references should be checked and work experience and credentials should be verified before the interview. Some managers prefer to interview first so time is not wasted processing the application if the interview results in a decision not to hire. Although this is a personal choice, positions should never be offered until information on the application has been verified and references have been checked.

Occasionally, reference calls will reveal unsolicited information about the applicant. Information obtained by any method may not be used to reject an applicant unless a justifiable reason for disqualification exists. For example, if the applicant volunteers information about his or her driving record or if this information is discovered by other means, it cannot be used to reject a potential employee unless the position requires driving.

Preemployment Testing

Preemployment testing is used only when such testing is directly related to the ability to perform a specific job. Although testing is not a stand-alone selection tool, it can, when coupled with excellent interviewing and reference checking, provide additional information about a candidate to make the best selection.

Lawsuits resulting from allegedly improper implementation and interpretation of preemployment testing, have made employers shy away from preemployment testing. Some major corporations, but few healthcare organizations, still use testing as a selection tool. Some healthcare organizations, however, do use post-employment testing to determine learning needs or skill deficiencies.

Physical Examination

A medical examination is generally a requirement for hiring. This examination determines if the applicant can meet the requirements for a specific job and provides a record of the physical condition of the applicant at the time of hire. The physical examination also may be used to identify applicants who will potentially have unfavorable attendance records or may file excessive future claims against the organization's health insurance.

Only those selected for hire can be required to have a physical examination, which is nearly always conducted at the employer's expense. If the physical examination reveals information that disqualifies the applicant, he or she is not hired. Most employers make job offers contingent on meeting certain health or physical requirements.

Making the Selection

When processing applications and determining the most appropriate person to fit the job, the manager must be sure that the same standards are used to evaluate all candidates. Final selection should be based on established criteria, not on value judgments and personal preferences.

Frequently, managers fill positions with internal applicants. These positions might be entry level or management. These applicants are interviewed in the same manner as newcomers to the organization; however, some organizations give special consideration and preference to their own employees. Every organization should have guidelines and policies regarding how transfers and promotions are to be handled. Transfers and promotions were discussed more fully in Chapter 11.

Finalizing the Selection

Once a final selection has been made, the manager is responsible for the following closure of the preemployment process:

1. Follow up with applicants as soon as possible, thanking them for their applications and informing them when they can expect to be notified about a decision.
2. Candidates not offered a position should receive a timely written notice of their elimination. Whenever appropriate, applicants not being hired should be given reasons why they were not hired (e.g., insufficient education or work experience), whether their application will be held for possible later employment, or if they should reapply in the future.
3. Applicants offered a position should be informed in writing of the benefits, salary, and placement. This avoids misunderstandings later regarding what employees think they were promised by the nurse recruiter or the interviewer.

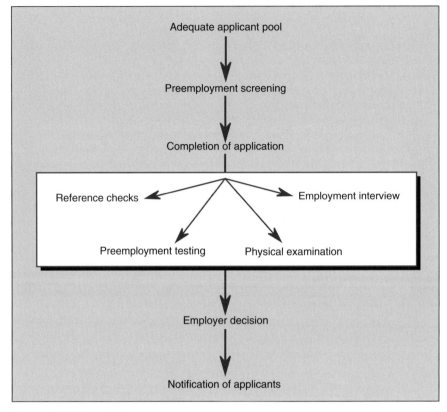

Figure 15.1 The selection process.

4. Applicants who accept job offers should be informed as to preemployment procedures, such as physical examinations, and supplied with the date to report to work.
5. Applicants who are offered positions should be requested to confirm in writing their intention to accept the position.

Because selection involves a process of reduction (i.e., diminishing the number of candidates for a particular position), the person making the final selection has a great deal of responsibility. These decisions have far-reaching consequences, both for the organization and for the people involved. For these reasons, the selection process should be as objective as possible. The selection process is shown in **Figure 15.1.**

PLACEMENT

The astute leader is able to assign a new employee to a position within his or her sphere of authority where the employee will have a reasonable chance for success. Nursing units and departments develop subcultures that have their own norms, values, and methods of accomplishing work. It is possible for one person to fit in

Learning Exercise 15.4

Creating Additional Interview Criteria
You are a home health nurse with a large caseload of low-income, inner-city families. Because of your spouse's job transfer, you have just resigned from your position of three years to take a similar position in another public health district.

Your agency supervisor has asked that you assist her with interviewing and selecting your replacement. Five applicants meet the minimum criteria. They each have at least two years of acute care experience, a baccalaureate nursing degree, and a state public health credential.

Because you know the job requirements better than anyone, your supervisor has asked that you develop additional criteria and a set of questions to ask each applicant.

Assignment:
1. Use a decision grid (see Figure 2.3) to develop additional criteria. Weight the criteria so the applicants will have a final score.
2. Develop an interview guide of six appropriate questions to ask the applicants.

well with an established group, whereas another equally qualified person would never become part of that group.

Additionally, many positions within a unit or department require different skills. For example, in a hospital, decision-making skills might be more important on a shift where leadership is less strong; communication skills might be the most highly desired skill on a shift where there is a great deal of interaction among a variety of nursing personnel.

Frequently, newcomers suffer feelings of failure because of inappropriate placement within the organization. This can be as true for the newly hired experienced employee as for the novice nurse. Appropriate placement is as important to the organization's functioning as it is to the new employee's success. Faulty placement can result in reduced organizational efficiency, increased attrition, threats to organizational integrity, and frustration of personal and professional ambitions.

Conversely, proper placement fosters personal growth, provides a motivating climate for the employee, maximizes productivity, and increases the probability that organizational goals will be met. Managers who are able to match employee strengths to job requirements facilitate unit functioning, accomplish organizational goals, and meet employee needs.

INDOCTRINATION

Indoctrination, as a management function, refers to the planned, guided adjustment of an employee to the organization and the work environment. Although the words "induction" and "orientation" are frequently used to describe this function, the indoctrination process includes three separate phases: induction, orientation, and socialization. Because socialization is part of the staff development and team-building process, it will be covered in the next chapter.

Indoctrination denotes a much broader approach to the process of employment adjustment than either induction or orientation. It seeks to (1) establish favorable employee attitudes toward the organization, unit, and department; (2) provide the necessary information and education for success in the position; and (3) instill a feeling of belonging and acceptance. Effective indoctrination programs result in higher productivity, fewer rule violations, less attrition, and greater employee satisfaction. The employee indoctrination process begins as soon as a person has been selected for a position and continues until the employee has been socialized to the norms and values of the work group. See **Display 15.5** for employee indoctrination content. Effective indoctrination programs assist employees in having a successful employment tenure.

Display 15.5 Employee Indoctrination Content

1. Company history, mission, and philosophy
2. Company service and service area
3. Organizational structure, including department heads, with an explanation of the functions of the various departments
4. Employee responsibilities to the company
5. Organizational responsibilities to the employee
6. Payroll information, including how increases in pay are earned and when they are given (Progressive or unionized companies publish pay scales for all employees.)
7. Rules of conduct
8. Tour of the company and of the assigned department
9. Work schedules, staffing and scheduling policies
10. When applicable, a discussion of the collective bargaining agreement
11. Benefit plans, including life insurance, health insurance, pension, and unemployment
12. Safety and fire programs
13. Staff development programs, including in-service, and continuing education for relicensure
14. Promotion and transfer policies
15. Employee appraisal system
16. Workload assignments
17. Introduction to paperwork/forms used in the organization
18. Review of selection in policies and procedures
19. Specific legal requirements, such as maintaining a current license, reporting of accidents, and so forth
20. Introduction to fellow employees
21. Establishment of a feeling of belonging and acceptance, showing genuine interest in the new employee

Note: Much of this content could be provided in an employee handbook, and the fire and safety regulations could be handled by a media presentation. *Appropriate* use of videotapes or film strips can be very useful in the design of a good orientation program. All indoctrination programs should be monitored to see if they are achieving their goals. Most programs need to be revised at least annually.

Induction

Induction, the first phase of indoctrination, takes place after the employee has been selected but before performing the job role. The induction process includes all activities that educate the new employee about the organization and employment and personnel policies and procedures.

Induction activities are often performed during the placement and preemployment functions of staffing or may be included with orientation activities. However, induction and orientation are often separate entities, and new employees suffer if content from either program is omitted. The most important factor is to provide the employee with adequate information.

Employee handbooks, an important part of induction, are usually developed by the personnel department. Managers, however, should know what information the employee handbooks contain and should have input into their development. Most employee handbooks contain a form that must be signed by the employee, verifying that he or she has received and read it. The signed form is then placed in the employee's personnel file.

The handbook is important because employees cannot assimilate all the induction information at one time, so they need a reference for later. However, providing an employee with a personnel handbook is not sufficient for real understanding. The information must be followed with discussion by various people during the employment process, such as the personnel manager and staff development personnel during orientation. The most important link in promoting real understanding of personnel polices is the first-level manager.

Orientation

Induction provides the employee with general information about the organization, whereas *orientation* activities are more specific for the position. A sample two-week orientation schedule is shown in **Display 15.6.** Organizations may use a wide variety of orientation programs. For example, a first-day orientation could be conducted by the hospital's personnel department, which could include a tour of the hospital and all of the induction items listed in Display 15.5. The next phase of the orientation program could take place in the staff development department, where aspects of concern to all employees, such as fire safety, accident prevention, and health promotion, would be presented. The third phase would be the individual orientation for each department. At this point, specific departments, such as dietary, pharmacy, and nursing, would each be responsible for developing their own programs. A sample distribution of responsibilities for orientation activities is shown in **Display 15.7.**

Because induction and orientation involve many different people from a variety of departments, they must be carefully coordinated and planned to achieve preset goals. The overall goals of induction and orientation include helping employees by providing them with information that will smooth their transition into the new work setting. The purpose of the orientation process is to make the employee feel a part of the team. This will reduce burnout and help new employees more quickly become independent in their new roles.

Display 15.6	Sample Two-Week Orientation Schedule for Experienced Nurses

Week One
Day 1, Monday:

8:00 AM–10:00 AM	Welcome by personnel department; employee handbooks distributed and discussed
10:00 AM–10:30 AM	Coffee and fruit served; welcome by staff development department
10:30 AM–12:00 PM	General orientation by staff development
12:00 PM–12:30 PM	Tour of the organization
12:30 PM–1:30 PM	Lunch
1:30 PM–3:00 PM	Fire and safety films; body mechanics demonstration
3:00 PM–4:00 PM	Afternoon tea and introduction to each unit supervisor

Day 2, Tuesday:

8:00 AM–10:00 AM	Report to individual units Time with unit supervisor; introduction to assigned preceptor
10:00 AM–10:30 AM	Coffee with preceptor
10:30 AM–12:00 PM	General orientation of policies and procedures
12:00 PM–12:30 PM	Lunch
12:30 PM–4:30 PM	CPR recertification
Day 3, Wednesday:	Assigned all day to unit with preceptor
Day 4, Thursday:	Assigned all day to unit with preceptor
Day 5, Friday:	Morning with preceptor, afternoon with supervisor and staff development for wrap-up

Week Two

Monday to Wednesday:	Work with preceptor on shift and unit assigned, gradually assuming greater responsibilities
Thursday:	Assign 80% of normal assignment with assistance and supervision from preceptor
Friday:	Carry normal workload. Have at least a 30-minute meeting with immediate supervisor to discuss progress

It is important to look at productivity and retention as the orientation program is planned, structured, and evaluated. Organizations should periodically assess their induction and orientation program in light of organizational goals; programs that are not meeting organizational goals should be restructured. For example, if employees consistently have questions about the benefit program, this part of the induction process should be evaluated.

Too often, various people having partial responsibility for induction and orientation "pass the buck" regarding failure of or weaknesses in the program. It is the joint responsibility of the personnel department, the staff development department, and each nursing service unit to work together to provide an indoctrination program that meets the needs of employees and the organization.

Display 15.7 **Responsibilities for Orientation**

1. *Personnel Department:* Performs salary and payroll functions, insurance forms, physical exams, income withholding forms, tour of the organization, employee responsibilities to the organization and vice versa, additional labor–management relationships, and benefit plan.
2. *Staff Development Department:* Hands out and reviews employee handbook; discusses organizational philosophy and mission; reviews history of the organization; shows media presentation of various departments and how they function (if a media presentation is not available, introduces various department heads and shares how departments function); discusses organizational structure, fire and safety programs, CPR certification and verifications; discusses available educational and training programs, reviews selected policies and procedures including medication, treatment, and charting policies.
3. *The Individual Unit:* Tour of the department, introductions, review of specific unit policies that differ in any way from general policies, review of unit scheduling and staffing policies and procedures, work assignments, promotion and transfer policies, and establishment of a feeling of belonging, acceptance, and socialization.

For some time, managers in healthcare organizations, especially hospitals, did not fulfill their proper role in the orientation of new employees. Managers assumed that between the personnel and staff development, or in-service, departments, the new employee would become completely oriented. This often frustrated new employees because although they received an overview of the organization, they received little orientation to the specific unit. Because each unit has many idiosyncrasies, the new employee was left feeling inadequate and incompetent. The latest trend in orientation is for the nursing unit to take a greater responsibility for individualizing orientation.

The unit manager must play a key role in the orientation of the new employee. An adequate orientation program minimizes the likelihood of rule violations, grievances, and misunderstandings; fosters feelings of belonging and acceptance; and promotes enthusiasm and morale.

INTEGRATING LEADERSHIP ROLES AND MANAGEMENT FUNCTIONS IN PRELIMINARY STAFFING RESPONSIBILITIES

Productivity is directly related to the quality of an organization's personnel. Active recruitment allows institutions to bring in the most qualified personnel for a position. After those applicants have been recruited, managers, using specified criteria, have a critical responsibility to see that the best applicant is hired. To ensure that all applicants are evaluated using the same standards and that personal bias is minimized, the manager must be skilled in interviewing and other selection processes.

Learning Exercise 15.5

How Would You Strengthen This Orientation Process?
As a new head nurse, one of your goals is to reduce attrition. You plan to do this by increasing retention, thus reducing costs for orienting new employees. In addition, you believe the increased retention will provide you with a more stable staff.

In studying your notes from exit interviews, it appears that new employees seldom develop a loyalty to the unit but instead use the unit to gain experience for other positions. You believe one difficulty with socializing new employees might be your unit's orientation program. The agency allows two weeks of orientation time (80 hours) when the new employee is not counted in the nursing care hours. These are referred to as nonproductive hours and are charged to the education department. Your unit has the following two-week schedule for new employees:

Week One

| Monday, Tuesday | 9 AM to 5 PM | Classroom |
| Wednesday, Thursday, Friday | 7 AM to 11 AM | Assigned to work with someone on the unit |

Week Two

| Monday, Tuesday | 7 AM to 3:30 PM | Assigned to unit with an employee |
| Wednesday, Thursday, Friday | | Assigned to shift they will be working for orientation to shift |

Following this two-week orientation, the new employee is expected to function at 75% productivity for two or three weeks and then perform at full productivity. The exception to this is the new graduate (RN) orientation. These employees spend one extra week on 7 AM to 3 PM and one extra week assigned to their particular shift before being counted as staff.

Your nursing administrator has stated that you may alter the orientation program in any way you wish as long as you do not increase the nonproductive time and you ensure that the employee receives information necessary to meet legal requirements and to function safely.
Assignment: Is there any way for you to strengthen the new employee orientation to your unit? Outline your plans (if any), and state the rationale for your decision.

Leadership roles in preliminary staffing functions include planning for future staffing needs and keeping abreast of changes in the healthcare field. Leadership also is necessary in the interview process to ensure that all applicants are treated fairly and that the interview terminates with applicants having positive attitudes about the organization. Because leaders are fully aware of nuances, strengths, and weaknesses within their sphere of authority, they are able to assign newcomers to areas that offer the greatest potential for success.

The integration of leadership roles and management functions in the organization ensures good public relations within the community because applicants know that they will be treated fairly. The pool of applicants will be sufficient because future needs are planned for proactively. The leader–manager uses the selection and placement process as a means to increase productivity and retention, accomplish the goals of the organization, and meet the needs of new employees.

The integrated leader–manager knows that a well-planned and implemented induction and orientation program is a wise investment of organizational resources. It provides the opportunity to mold a team effort and infuse employees with enthusiasm for the organization. New employees' impressions of an organization during this period will stay with them a long time. If the impressions are positive, they will be remembered in the difficult times that will ultimately occur during any long tenure of employment.

☼ Key Concepts

- The first step in the staffing process is to determine the type and number of personnel needed.
- A number of factors have contributed to a severe nursing shortage, particularly in acute care hospitals, in the early 21st century. These factors include a nationwide downsizing of hospitals in the 1990s, the transition of employed nurses from acute care hospitals to outpatient settings, a geographically maldistributed workforce, the aging of the nursing workforce, accelerating innovations in treatment and diagnostic technology, and a significant decline in nursing school enrollments.
- Successfully *recruiting* an adequate workforce depends on many variables, including financial resources, an adequate nursing pool, competitive salaries, the organization's reputation, the location's desirability, and the status of the national and local economy.
- Effective recruiting methods include advertisements, career days, literature, and the informal use of members of the organization as examples of satisfied employees.
- Despite their limitations, interviews are widely used as a method of selecting which employees to hire.
- The interview should meet the goals of the applicant and the manager.
- Managers must be skilled in planning, conducting, and controlling interviews.
- Due to numerous federal acts that protect the rights of job seekers, managers must be cognizant of the legal constraints on interviews.
- *Selection* should be based on the requirements necessary for the job; these criteria should be developed before beginning the selection process.
- Managers should seek to proactively recruit and hire staff that represent age, gender, cultural, ethnic, and language diversity in response to the rapidly increasing diversity of the communities they serve.

- Managers should place new employees on units, departments, and shifts where they have the best chance of succeeding.
- *Indoctrination* consists of induction, orientation, and socialization of employees.
- A well-prepared and executed orientation program educates the new employee about the desired behaviors and expected goals of the organization and actively involves the new employee's immediate supervisor.

More Learning Exercises and Applications

 Learning Exercise 15.6

Ethical Issues in Hiring

You are the head nurse of an intensive care unit and are interviewing Sam, a prospective charge nurse for your evening shift. Sam is currently the head nurse at Memorial Hospital, which is the other local hospital and your organization's primary competitor. He is leaving Memorial Hospital for personal reasons.

Sam, well qualified for the position, has strong management and clinical skills. Your evening shift needs a strong manager with the excellent clinical skills that Sam also has. You feel fortunate that Sam is applying for the position.

Just before the close of the interview, however, Sam shuts the door, lowers his voice secretively, and tells you that he has vital information regarding Memorial's plans to expand and reorganize its critical care unit. He states that he will share this information with you if you hire him.

Assignment: How should you respond to Sam? Should you hire him? Identify the major issues in this situation. Support your hiring decision with rationale from this chapter and other readings.

Learning Exercise 15.7

Making a Hiring Selection and Assessing Its Impact

You are the head nurse of a surgical unit, a position you have held for six years. You are comfortable with your role and know your staff well. Recently, the day charge nurse resigned. Two of your staff, Nancy and Sally, have applied for the position.

Nancy, an older nurse, has been with the organization for eight years but has been assigned to your department for only five years. She has 12 years' experience in acute care nursing. She performs her job competently and has good interpersonal relationships with the other staff and with patients and physicians. Although her motivation level is adequate for her current job, she has neither demonstrated much creativity or initiative in helping the surgical unit establish a reputation for excellence nor demonstrated specific skills in predicting or planning for the future.

Sally, a nurse in her mid-30s, has been with the organization and the unit for three years. She has been a positive driving force behind many of the changes that have occurred. She is an excellent clinician and highly respected by physicians and staff. The older staff, however, appear to resent her because they feel she attempted too much change before "paying her dues."

Both nurses have baccalaureate degrees and meet all the position qualifications for the job. Both nurses can be expected to work at least another five years in the new position. There is no precedent for your decision.

You must make a selection. If you do not use seniority as a primary selection criterion, many of the long-term employees may resent both Sally and you, and they may become demotivated. You are aware that Nancy is limited in her futuristic thinking and that the unit may not grow and develop under her leadership as it could under Sally's.

Assignment: Identify how your own values will affect your decision. Rank your selection criteria, and make a decision about what you will do. Determine the personal, interpersonal, and organizational impact of your decision.

Learning Exercise 15.8

Which Two Grads Would You Choose—and Why?

You are the supervisor of a critical care surgical unit. For the past several years, you have been experimenting with placing four newly graduated nurses directly into the unit, two from each spring and fall graduating class. These nurses are from the local BSN program. You consult closely with the nursing faculty and their former employers before making a selection.

Overall, this experiment has worked well. Only two new graduates were unable to develop into critical care nurses. Both of these nurses later transferred back into the unit after two years in a less intensive medical–surgical area.

Because of the new graduates' motivation and enthusiasm, they have complemented your experienced critical care staff nicely. You believe your success with this program has been due to your well-planned and structured four-month orientation and education program, careful selection, and appropriate shift placement.

This spring, you have narrowed the selection down to four acceptable and well-qualified candidates. You plan to place one on the 3 PM to 11 PM shift and one on the 11 PM to 7 AM shift. You sit in your office and review the culture of each shift and your notes on the four candidates. You have the following information:

3 PM to 11 PM shift: A very assertive, all-female staff; 85% RNs and 15% practical nurses. This is your most clinically competent group. They are highly respected by everyone, and although the physicians often have confrontations with them, the physicians also tell you frequently how good they are. The nurses are known as a group that lacks humor and does not welcome newcomers. However, once the new employee earns their trust, they are very supportive. They are intolerant of anyone not living up to their exceptionally high standards. Your two unsuccessful new graduate placements were assigned to this shift.

11 PM to 7 AM shift: A very cohesive and supportive group. Although overall these nurses are competent, this shift has some of your more clinically weak staff. However, it also is the shift that rates the highest with families and patients. They are caring and compassionate. Every new graduate you have placed on this shift has been successful. Thirty percent of the nurses on this shift are men. The group tends to be very close and has a number of outside social activities.

Your four applicants consist of the following:

John: A 30-year-old married man without children. He has had a great deal of emergency room experience as a medical emergency technician. He appears somewhat aloof. His definite career goals are two years in critical care, three years in emergency room, and then flight crew. Instructors praise his independent judgment but believe he was somewhat of a loner in school. Former employers have rated him as an independent thinker and very capable.

Sally: A 22-year-old unmarried woman. She is at the top of her class clinically and academically. She has not had much work experience until the last two years as a summer nursing intern at a medical center, where her performance appraisal was very good. Instructors believe she lacks some maturity and interpersonal skills but praise her clinical judgment. She does not want to work in a regular medical–surgical unit. She believes she can adapt to critical care.

Joan: A mature, divorced 38-year-old woman. She has no children. She has had a great deal of health-related work experience in counseling and has had limited clinical work experience (only nursing school). Former employers praise her attention to detail and her general competence. Instructors praise her interpersonal skills, maturity, and intelligence. She is quite willing to work elsewhere if not selected. She has a long-term commitment to nursing.

Mary: A dynamic, 28-year-old married mother of two. She was previously a practical nurse and returned to school to get her degree. She did not do as well academically due to working and family commitments. Former employers and instructors speak of her energy, organization, and interpersonal skills. She appears to have fewer independent decision-making skills than the others do. She previously worked in a critical care unit.

Assignment: Select the two new graduates, and place them on the appropriate shift. Support your decisions with rationale.

 Web Links

American Health Information Management Association (AHIMA)
http://library.ahima.org/xpedio/groups/public/documents/ahima/pub_bok1_015763.html
Statement on the Health Information Management Workforce. Approved by AHIMA Board of Directors—July 18, 2002. The American Health Information Management Association is an organization of more than 41,000 specially educated professionals dedicated to accurate and timely information regarding healthcare workforce supply.

Career Mosaic's Health Opps
www.healthopps.com
This site includes a healthcare jobs list, employer profiles, and résumé posting. Resumes can be reviewed. The site also offers a healthcare recruiter connection for human resources professionals, including a section on market trends.

Interviewing Tips
http://www.careercc.com/interv3.shtml
This site includes general interviewing tips, questions the interviewer might ask applicants, and questions the applicant should consider asking the interviewer.

Monster Career Center—Interview Tips (2003)
http://content.monster.com/jobinfo/interview/
Includes a practice virtual interview, questions to ask the interviewer, and an interview planner.

HRSA- Bureau of Health Professions. National Sample Survey of Registered Nurses (July 2002)
http://bhpr.hrsa.gov/healthworkforce/reports/rnproject/
The nation's most extensive and comprehensive source of statistics on nurses with current licenses to practice in the United States, whether they are employed in nursing or not.

References

Advisory Board Company (2000). *Enfranchising nursing in cost reform.* Washington, D.C.: Author.

American Association of Colleges of Nursing. (1999). *1998–1999 Enrollment and graduations in baccalaureate and graduate programs in nursing.* Washington, D.C.: American Association of Colleges of Nursing.

American Association of Colleges of Nursing. (2002, Februrary 17). *Nursing school enrollments fall as demand for RNs continues to climb.* Washington, D.C.: AACN.

Atencio, B. L., Cohen, J., & Gorenberg, B. (2003). Nurse retention: Is it worth it? *Nursing Economic$, 21*(6), 262–268.

Buerhaus, P., Staiger, D., & Auerbach, I. (2000a). Policy responses to an aging registered nurse workforce. *Nursing Economic$, 18*(6), 278–284, 303.

Buerhaus, P. I., Staiger, D. O., & Auerbach, D. I. (2000b). Implications of an aging registered nurse workforce. *Journal of the American Medical Association (JAMA), 283*(22), 2948–2954.

Case, J., Mowry, M., & Welebob, E. (2002, June). *First Consulting Group. The nursing shortage: Can technology help?* Oakland, CA: California Healthcare Foundation.

Chitty, K. K. (2001). *Professional nursing. Concepts and challenges* (3rd ed., p. 59). Philadelphia: Saunders.

Frusti, D. K., Niesen, K. M., & Campion, J. K. (2003). Creating a culturally competent organization. *Journal of Nursing Administration, 33*(1), 31–38.

Furlow, L. (2000). Job profiling: Building a winning team using behavioral assessments. *Journal of Nursing Administration, 30*(3), 107–111.

Hawke, M. (2003, Fall). Ten killer interview tips. *Nursing Spectrum Career Fitness Guide for Students.* 24–25.

Heinrich, J. (2001, July). GAO report to health subcommittee on health. GAO-01-944 Nursing workforce: Emerging nurse shortages due to multiple factors (pp. i–15). Washington, D. C.: United States General Accounting Office.

Hopkins, M. E. (2001). Critical condition. *Nurse Week, 2,* 15–18.

Howell, S. B. (1999). It's a match. *Nursing Management, 30*(2), 25–30.

HSM Group, Ltd., The (2002). Acute care hospital survey of RN vacancy turnover rates in 2000. *Journal of Nursing Administration, 32*(9) 437–439.

Huston, C. (2003). Quality health care in an era of diminished resources: Challenges and opportunities. *Journal of Nursing Care Quality, 18*(4), 295–301.

Johnson, J. (2000). The nursing shortage. A difficult conversation. *Journal of Nursing Administration, 30*(9), 401–402.

Kalisch, B. J. (2003). Recruiting nurses. The problem is the process. *Journal of Nursing Administration, 33*(9), 408–477.

Nevidjon, B., & Erickson, J. I. (2001). The nursing shortage: Solutions for the short and long term. *Online Journal of Issues in Nursing.* Available at: *http://www.nursing world.org/ojin/topic14/tpc14_4.htm.* Accessed July 4, 2001.

Staiger, D. O., Auerbach, D. I., & Buerhaus, P. I. (2000). Expanding career opportunities for women and the declining interest in nursing as a career. *Nursing Economic$, 18*(5), 230–236.

State of California, Department of Consumer Affairs, Board of Registered Nursing. (BRN) (1999). *Unpublished license data.*

Strachota, E., Normandin, P., O'Brien, N., Clary, M., & Krukow, B. (2003). Reasons registered nurses leave or change employment status. *Journal of Nursing Administration, 33*(2), 111–117.

Tappen, R. M. (2001). Nursing leadership and management: Concepts and practices. (4th ed.). Philadelphia: F. A. Davis Co.

Registered nurse population, (the) *(march 2000).* Available at *http://bhpr.hrsa.gov/healthworkforce/reports/rnsurvey/rnss1.htm* Retrieved November 7, 2004. Also see 'Office of the Profession: The nursing shortage. Available at: *http://www.op.nysed.gov/nurseshortage.htm.*

United States General Accounting Office. (2001, July). *Nursing workforce. Emerging nurse shortages due to multiple factors.* GAO-01-944. p. 2.

Upenieks, V. (2003). Recruitment and retention strategies: A magnet hospital prevention program. *Nursing Economic$, 21*(1), 7–13, 23.

Wakefield, M. K. (2001). Hard numbers, hard choices: Seeking solutions to the nursing shortage. *Nursing Economic$, 19*(2), 80–82.

Williams, S. (2001). Common cause: State and federal measures to address shortage find bipartisan support. *NurseWeek, 14*(15), 10–11.

Bibliography

American Association of Colleges of Nursing (AACN). (2001). *Enrollment and graduations in baccalaureate and graduate programs in nursing.* Washington, D.C.: AACN.

Andrica, D. C. (2000). Answering tough questions on interview. *Nursing Economic$, 18*(1), 45–46.

Boyce, V. J. (2002). Nursing shortage. Everything old is new again. *Policy, Politics, & Nursing Practice, 3*(2), 177–183.

Bozell, J. (2001). In the driver's seat. *Nursing 2001 Career Directory,* 44.

Brewer, C., & Tassone Kovner, C. (2001). Is there another nursing shortage? What the data tell us. *Nursing Outlook, 49*(1), 20–26.

Cardillo, D. (2003, Fall). The right approach for the right interview. *Nursing Spectrum Career Fitness Guide for Students.* 14–15.

Cardillo, D. (2003, Fall). Juggling job offers. *Nursing Spectrum Career Fitness Guide for Students.* 30–31.

Cline, D., Reilly, C., & Moore, J. F. (2003). What's behind RN turnover? *Nursing Management, 34*(10), 50–53.

DeMarco, R. F., Horowitz, J. A., & McLeod, D. (2000). A call to intraprofessional alliances. *Nursing Outlook, 48*(4), 172–178.

Greipp, M.E. (2003). Salary compression. Its effect on nurse recruitment and retention. *Journal of Nursing Administration, 33*(6), 321–330.

Jeffries, E. (2002). Creating a great place to work. Strategies for retaining top talent. *Journal of Nursing Administration, 32*(6), 303–305.

Kerfoot, K. (2000). The leader as a retention specialist. *Nursing Economic$, 18*(4), 216–218.

Kubar, P. A., Miller, D., & Spear, B. T. (2004). The meaningful retention strategy inventory. *Journal of Nursing Administration, 34*(1), 10–18.

Murray, M. K. (2002). The nursing shortage. Past, present and future. *Journal of Nursing Administration, 32*(2), 79–84.

Nierenberg, R. J. (2003). The use of a strategic interviewing technique to select the nurse manager. *Journal of Nursing Administration, 33*(10), 500–505.

Pinkerton, S. E. (2002). A system approach to retention and recruitment. *Nursing Economic$, 20*(6), 296, 299.

Purnell, M. J., Horner, D., Gonzalez, J., & Westman, N. (2001). The nursing shortage. *Journal of Nursing Administration, 31*(4), 179–186.

Rambur, B., Palumbo, M.V., McIntosh, B., & Mongeon, J. (2003). A statewide analysis of RN's intention to leave their position. *Nursing Outlook, 51*(4), 182–188.

Roark, D. C. (2001). Against the odds: Defining and overcoming the nursing shortage. *Nursing 2001 Career Directory*, 14.

Rudy, S., & Sions, J. (2003). Floating. Managing a recruitment and retention issue. *Journal of Nursing Administration, 33*(4), 196–198.

Wagner, C. M., & Huber, D. (2003). Catastrophe and nursing turnover. *Journal of Nursing Administration, 33*(9), 486–492.

Wittmann-Price, R., & Kuplen, C. (2003). A recruitment and retention program that works. *Nursing Economic$, 21*(1), 35–38.

Meeting Staff Socialization and Educational Needs for Team Building

Environments rich in continuing education ripen staff development, morale and retention.

—Diane Postlen-Slattery and Kathryn Foley

Socialization is the process by which a person acquires the technical skills of his or her society, the knowledge of the kinds of behavior that are understood and acceptable in that society, and the attitudes and values that make conformity with social rules personally meaningful, even gratifying (Hyperdictionary, 2003). Socialization has also been called *enculturation*.

Socialization differs from orientation in that it involves little structured information. Rather, socialization is a sharing of the values and attitudes of the organization by the use of role models, myths, and legends. During the socialization phase of indoctrination, the leader introduces employees to unit values and culture and uses the socialization process to mold a fit between new staff members and the unit. Socialization into the organization is critical for the novice professional, and adequate socialization of all employees, has been shown to reduce attrition and increase satisfaction (Cable & Parsons, 2001; Apker, Zabava, Ford, & Fox, 2003). During this phase of indoctrination, employees are instilled with high morale and enthusiasm for the organization, which is primarily a leadership role.

The unit leader–manager bears the greatest responsibility for meeting staff socialization needs. Once staff are selected, inducted, and oriented, the manager must see that they are appropriately socialized in order to build a cohesive and effective team. Orientation alone is usually inadequate to ensure that new employees are properly socialized into the organization.

The leader–manager also has a responsibility for training and maintaining a competent staff, but this responsibility is shared with other members of the organization. Because new equipment, procedures, and knowledge are constantly being introduced, the leader must develop skills in assessing staff learning needs. Educational needs of staff are partially dependent on the staffing mix and position responsibilities that were developed during the organizing and planning phases of management. For example, the more experienced and educated the staff, the less educational and training needs they will have.

This chapter examines the responsibilities of the manager in socializing, educating, and training employees. The delineation between education and training is made as well as the differences between role models, preceptors, and mentors. The needs of the adult learner are explored and the concept of coaching as a staff development tool is introduced. Finally, the need to build a cohesive team from a culturally diverse workforce, through appropriate socialization and education strategies, is explored. The leadership roles and management functions in using socialization and education inherent for team building are shown in **Display 16.1.**

SOCIALIZATION AND RESOCIALIZATION

There is no one theory of socialization. Among sociologists, the phenomenon of socialization has generally focused on *role theory*—that is, the behaviors that accompany each role are learned socially and by instruction, observation, and trial and error. Much has been written about the importance of socializing new members into their professional roles (Kramer, 1974; Lindeman, 2000; Tanner, 2000).

Display 16.1	Leadership Roles and Management Functions Associated with Meeting Staff Socialization and Educational Needs

Leadership Roles

1. Clarifies department norms and values to all new employees.
2. Infuses a team spirit among employees.
3. Serves as a role model to all employees and a mentor to select employees.
4. Encourages mentorship between senior staff and junior employees.
5. Observes carefully for signs of knowledge or skill deficit in new employees and intervenes appropriately.
6. Assists employees in developing personal strategies to cope with role transition.
7. Applies adult learning principles when helping employees learn new skills or information.
8. Coaches employees spontaneously regarding knowledge and skill deficits.
9. Is sensitive to the unique socialization and education needs of a culturally and ethnically diverse staff.
10. Continually assesses the learning deficits of the staff and creatively minimizes these deficits.

Management Functions

1. Is aware of and clarifies organizational and unit goals for all employees.
2. Clarifies role expectations for all employees.
3. Uses positive and negative sanctions appropriately to socialize new employees.
4. Carefully selects preceptors and encourages role modeling of the senior staff.
5. Provides methods of meeting the special orientation needs of new graduates, international nurses, and experienced nurses changing roles.
6. Works with the education department to delineate shared and individual responsibility for staff development.
7. Ensures that there are adequate resources for staff development and makes appropriate decisions regarding resource allocation during periods of fiscal restraint.
8. Assumes responsibility for quality and fiscal control of staff development activities.
9. Ensures that all staff are competent for roles assigned.
10. Provides input in formulating staff development policies.

The first *socialization* to the nursing role occurs during nursing school, and continues after graduation. Because nurse administrators and nursing faculty have been found to hold different values and both of these groups assist in socializing the new nurse, there is potential for the new nurse to develop conflict and frustration (Lindeman, 2000). (Socialization of the new graduate nurse is discussed in greater depth later in this chapter). However, less research exists on the unique resocialization needs of nurses as they change roles throughout their professional careers.

Resocialization occurs when individuals are forced to learn new values, skills, attitudes, and social rules as a result of changes in the type of work they do, the scope of responsibility they hold, or in the work setting itself. Individuals who frequently need resocialization include new graduates leaving nursing school and entering the work world, experienced nurses who change work settings, either within the same organization or in a new organization, and nurses who undertake new roles. Some employees adapt easily to resocialization, but most experience some stress with role change. Organizations can plan in advance to ease the stress of resocialization by the conscious use of appropriate interventions.

CLARIFYING ROLE EXPECTATIONS THROUGH ROLE MODELS, PRECEPTORS, AND MENTORS

Role expectations can be clarified by using role models, preceptors, and mentors. Although all three clarify roles through social interaction and educational processes, each has a different focus and uses different mechanisms. All have an appropriate place in employee socialization and resocialization.

A *role model* is defined as someone worthy of imitation (Hyperdictionary, 2003). Role models in nursing are experienced, competent employees. The relationship between the new employee and the role model is a passive one (i.e., employees see that role models are skilled and attempt to emulate them, but the role model does not actively seek this emulation). One of the exciting aspects of role models is their cumulative effect. The greater the number of excellent role models available for new employees to emulate, the greater the possibilities for new employees to perform well.

The educational process in role modeling is passive, but the preceptor role is active and purposeful. The assumption that a one-on-one relationship increases learning is the basis for the use of preceptors. A *preceptor* is an experienced nurse who provides knowledge and emotional support, as well as a clarification of role expectations, on a one-to-one basis. An effective preceptor can role model and adjust teaching to each learner as needed.

Occasionally, the fit between a preceptor and preceptee is not good. This risk is lower if preceptors willingly seek out this responsibility and if they have attended educational courses outlining preceptor duties and responsibilities. In addition, preceptors need to have an adequate knowledge of adult learning theory (Currie, Vierke, & Greer, 2000). Organizations that use preceptors to help new employees clarify their roles and improve their skill level should be careful not to overuse preceptors to the point that that they become tired or demotivated. In addition, workload assignments for the preceptor should be decreased whenever possible so that adequate time can be devoted to helping the preceptee problem solve and learn. Incentive pay for preceptors reinforces that the organization values this role.

Mentors take on an even greater role in using education as a means for role clarification. Lee (2000) describes *mentoring* as a distinctive interactive relationship between two individuals, occurring most commonly in a professional setting. Some individuals use the term preceptor and mentor interchangeably. While a preceptor takes on some of the roles of a mentor, they are not the same. For example, preceptors are usually assigned, but true mentors freely choose who they will mentor. The mentor makes a conscious decision to assist the protégé in attaining expert status and in furthering his or her career development. Preceptors have a relatively short

Learning Exercise 16.1

Criteria for Preceptorship
You have been selected to represent your unit on a committee to design a preceptor program for the nursing department. One of the committee's first goals is to develop criteria for the selection of preceptors.
Assignment: In groups, select a minimum of five and a maximum of eight criteria that would be appropriate for selecting preceptors on your unit. Would you have minimum education or experience requirements? What personality or behavioral traits would you seek? Which of the criteria that you identified are measurable?

> Not every nurse will be fortunate enough to have a mentor to facilitate each new career role. Most nurses will be lucky if they have one or two mentors throughout their careers.

relationship with the person they have been assigned, but the relationship between the mentor and mentee is longer and more intense.

Hurst et al. (2002) maintains that there are four phases in mentoring relationships. The first phase, *initiation*, occurs when the relationship is established. The second phase, *cultivation*, is characterized by coaching, protection, and sponsorship as well as counseling, acceptance, and the creation of a sense of competence. During this phase, the relationship develops through established meeting times to share and evaluate progress (Pinkerton, 2003). The third phase is *separation* and the fourth is *redefinition* in which the relationship takes on a new form or ends. Separation and redefinition are often difficult as the mentor and mentee may share different perceptions about whether it is time to separate and what their new relationship should be. Separation and redefinition are critical, however, as mentees should outgrow the need for such intense coaching if the mentor has done a good job of cultivation. Covan (2000) maintains that the mentoring process is part of the interactional work that is essential for socialization and career development.

Mentors serve a particularly useful role in acclimating nurses to management roles. Those lucky enough to find a mentor as they move into roles with increased responsibilities and status will find that resocialization will be smoother. A mentor, as no other, is able to instill the values and attitudes that accompany each role. This is because mentors lead by example. A mentor's strong moral and ethical fiber encourages mentees to think critically and take a stand on ethical dilemmas in the workplace (Shaffer, Tallarica, & Walsh, 2000). Becoming a mentor requires committing to a personal relationship. It also requires teaching skills and a genuine interest and belief in the capabilities of others (Shaffer et al., 2000). The roles of the mentor are shown in **Display 16.2.**

Byrne and Keefe (2002) suggest that mentoring activities can and should be incorporated into all stages of education and professional development. Projects over short periods, multiple sources of mentors across careers, and mutually beneficial peer relationships all provide infusions of mentoring techniques requiring limited resources (Byrne & Keefe).

Display 16.2 Roles of the Mentor

1. *Model:* Someone you admire or want to emulate.
2. *Envisioner:* Someone who can see and communicate a meaning of professional nursing and its potential.
3. *Energizer:* Someone whose dynamism stimulates you to take action.
4. *Investor:* Someone who invests his or her time and energy into your personal and professional growth.
5. *Supporter:* Someone who offers you emotional support and builds self-confidence.
6. *Standard prodder:* Someone who refuses to accept less than standards of excellence.
7. *Teacher–coach:* Someone who teaches you interpersonal, technical, or political skills essential for advancement.
8. *Feedback giver:* Someone who gives honest positive and negative feedback for growth.
9. *Eye opener:* Someone who broadens your perspective and gives you new ways of viewing situations.
10. *Door opener:* Someone who, by virtue of his or her position, can provide you with new opportunities or experiences.
11. *Idea bouncer:* Someone who will listen and discuss your ideas.
12. *Problem solver:* Someone who can help you examine problems and identify possible solutions.
13. *Career counselor:* Someone who helps you to make short- and long-term career plans.
14. *Challenger:* Someone who encourages you to investigate issues more critically or in greater detail.

Adapted from Darling, L. A. (1984). What do nurses want in a mentor? *Journal of Nursing Administration, 14*(29), 42–44.

ASSISTANCE IN MEETING ROLE DEMANDS

When meeting role demands, people generally need assistance in two areas: the specific skills and knowledge requirements for the role, and the values and attitudes that accompany any given role. To assist the employee in meeting the demands of the job, the manager needs to determine what those needs are. This requires more than just asking employees about their knowledge deficits or giving employees a skills checklist or test; it requires careful observation by the manager and preceptor so deficiencies are identified and corrected before they handicap the employee's socialization. Careful observation is a leadership role. When such deficiencies are not corrected early, other employees often create a climate of nonacceptance that prevents assimilation of the new employee.

The second area in which employees often need assistance is in meeting value and attitude requirements for their roles. Values and attitudes may be a source of conflict as nurses learn new roles. However, organizations can assist new employees in meeting this requirement of socialization. Useful strategies are providing role models; providing a safe climate for new employees to ventilate their frustration with value conflicts; clarifying differing role expectations that are held by physicians, patients, and other staff; and assisting new employees in developing strategies to cope with and resolve value and attitude conflicts (Tanner, 2000).

OVERCOMING MOTIVATIONAL DEFICIENCIES

Although *sanctions* occur at many levels during the socialization process, they are rarely carried out on a systematic and planned basis. Yet, most employees learn what behavior is rewarded in an organization.

If difficulties in socialization or resocialization occur because of motivational deficiencies, a planned program should occur to correct the deficiencies using positive and negative sanctions.

For example, new employees determine quickly if getting off duty on time or excellent patient care receives reward sanctions. Cable and Parsons (2001) found that informal types of socialization had more effect than formal tactics on the perceived fit of a new individual within an organization. Effective leadership requires a conscious awareness of how unit values and behavior norms affect employee socialization.

Positive Sanctions

Positive sanctions can be used as an interactional or educational process of socialization. If deliberately planned, they become educational. However, sanctions given informally through the group process, or reference group, use the social interaction process. The reference group sets norms of behavior and then applies sanctions to ensure that new members adopt the group norms before acceptance into the group. These informal sanctions offer an extremely powerful tool for socialization and resocialization in the workplace. Managers should become aware of what role behavior they reward and what new employee behavior senior staff is rewarding.

Negative Sanctions

Negative sanctions, like rewards, provide cues that enable people to evaluate their performance consciously and to modify behavior when needed. For positive or negative sanctions to be effective, they must result in the role learner internalizing the values of the organization.

Negative sanctions are often applied in very subtle and covert ways. Making fun of a new graduate's awkwardness with certain skills or belittling a new employee's desire to use nursing care plans is a very effective negative sanction that may be used by group members to mold individual behavior to group norms. The manager should know what the group norms are and be observant of sanctions used by the group to make newcomers conform, and take appropriate intervention if group norms are not part of the organizational culture.

This is not to say that negative sanctions should never be used. New employees should be told when their behavior is not an acceptable part of their role. However, the sanctions used should be constructive and not destructive.

Learning Exercise 16.2

Great Influences
Who or what has been the greatest influence on your socialization to the nursing role? Were positive or negative sanctions used? Write a short essay (three or four paragraphs) describing this socialization. If appropriate, share this in a group.

EMPLOYEES WITH UNIQUE SOCIALIZATION NEEDS

The previous discussion has focused on the problems that frequently occur in role adaptation for all new employees. However, some employees have unique problems in socializing to new roles. These include the new nurse, the international nurse, the minority student, employees with role status change, and the experienced nurse in role transition. Managers providing appropriate socialization assistance for these groups increase the chance of a positive employment outcome.

The New Nurse

One group with unique socialization needs is the new nursing graduate. Kramer (1974) described special fears and difficulties in adapting to the work setting that are common to new graduate nurses and named this fear *reality shock* because it occurs as a result of conflict between a new graduate's expectations of the nursing role and the reality of the actual role in the work setting.

Schmalenberg and Kramer (1979) built on this original work in their assertion that there are four phases of role transition from student nurse to staff nurse: *the honeymoon* phase, followed by the *shock*, *recovery*, and *resolution* phases. As long as the novice nurse is sincerely welcomed into the workplace, the new nurse has little difficulty in the honeymoon phase. During the second phase of reality shock, however, there is often great personal conflict as the nurse discovers that many nursing school values are not prized in the workplace. The organization and the manager then must take sufficient action during the recovery and resolution phases if the new graduate is to be successfully socialized.

Research by Duchscher (2001) also attests to the unique socialization needs of the new graduate. Duchscher's qualitative research study found that new graduates experience an enormous amount of frustration during the initial several months of their introduction to clinical nursing practice and that much of this frustration originates from issues that conflict with one another. "There was a desire to deliver quality nursing care, but participants had neither the knowledge, focus, time, nor energy to do so" (p. 427). New graduates also reported a fear of physicians, self-absorption, a traumatic transition from academe to the reality of nursing practice and an "unwelcoming wagon" where colleagues viewed them with criticism rather than acceptance (p. 427).

Managers can use several mechanisms to ease the role transition of new graduates. *Anticipatory socialization* carried out in educational settings will help prepare new nurses for their professional role. However, managers should not assume that such anticipatory socialization has occurred. Instead, they should build opportunities for sharing and clarifying values and attitudes about the nursing role into orientation programs. Use of the group process is an excellent mechanism to promote the sharing that provides support for new graduates and assists them in recovering from reality shock.

Additionally, managers should be alert for signs and symptoms of the shock phase of role transition; they should intervene by listening to new graduates and helping them cope in the real world. Managers must recognize the intensity of new nurses' practice experience, encourage them to have a balanced life, foster a work environment that has zero tolerance for disrespect, and strive to create work relationship models that promote interdependency of physicians and nursing staff (Duchscher, 2001).

Managers should also ensure that some of the new nurse's values are supported and encouraged so that work and academic values can blend. New professionals need to understand the universal nature of role transition and know it is not limited to nurses. Providing a class on role transition also may assist new graduates in socialization.

To combat reality shock, some hospitals have developed prolonged orientation periods for new graduates that last from six weeks to six months. This extended orientation, or *internship,* contrasts sharply with the routine two-week orientation that is normal for most other employees. During this time, graduate nurses are usually assigned to work with a preceptor and gradually takes on a patient assignment equal to that of the preceptor. Some internship programs also include a mentor to sponsor the new graduate into the nursing profession, as well as debriefing and self-care sessions for discussion about difficulties encountered during the internship as well as strategies to deal with those difficulties (Beecroft, Kunzman, & Krozek, 2001). Some hospitals have discontinued internship programs due to their expense; however, Beecroft, et al. (2001) argue that the resultant lower turnover levels more than offset the expense.

> It is important to remember that no one is immune to a loss of idealism and commitment in response to stress in the workplace.

Many of the potential hazards of internship (and preceptorship) programs can be overcome by (1) carefully selecting the preceptors, (2) selecting only preceptors who have a strong desire to be role models, (3) preparing preceptors for their role by giving formal classes in adult learning and other social–learning concepts, and (4) having either experienced staff development or supervisory personnel monitor the preceptor and new graduate closely to ensure that the relationship continues to be beneficial and growth producing for both.

Learning Exercise 16.3

Investigating Reality Shock
Talk with at least four nursing graduates who have been working as nurses for anywhere from three months to three years. Make sure at least two of them are recent graduates and two of them have been working at least 18 months. Ask them about their socialization to nursing after graduation. Did any of them experience reality shock? How long did it last? Did they recover from the shock? If so, how? Share your findings with other members of your group.

International Nurses

One solution to the current nursing shortage has been the active recruitment of nurses from overseas. Ryan (2003) suggests that socialization to the professional nursing role is one of four basic needs that must be addressed if foreign nurses are to adapt successfully to American workplaces. Ryan suggests that initially, foreign nurses must be introduced to American jargon and variations in nursing practice delivery. Then many must be supported through a period of cultural, professional, and psychological dissonance that is associated with anxiety, homesickness, and isolation. Finally, these nurses must be integrated within the institution so that they develop a sense of community life on the nursing unit.

Bola, Driggers, Dunlap, and Ebersole (2003) state that international nurses also frequently experience culture shock regarding nonverbal communication that may interfere with their assimilation. "Patients or staff with limited cultural competence may interpret nonverbal communication, such as eye contact or smiling, as disrespectful" (Bola et al., p. 41).

Ryan (2003) suggests that using a *cultural diversity enhancement group* (CDEG) and a "buddy program" may assist in socializing these international nurses. The CDEG includes staff nurses and management personnel from varied ethnic backgrounds who agree to buddy with the international nurses to make them feel welcomed in the organizational culture and to assist them regarding basic services, places, or necessary items they need to know about or have. Bola et al. (2003) concur, suggesting that without a support system, international nurses may question their ability to solve problems and function successfully since the values and behaviors helpful in solving problems in their home country may not be helpful in the United States.

Culturally and Ethnically Diverse Student Nurses

Another strategy for addressing the current nursing shortage has been to attract groups to nursing who might otherwise not choose it as a career; especially ethnic minorities (Harrigan, Gollin, & Casken, 2003). Federal, state, and private initiatives over the past 25 years have been directed at increasing minority representation in nursing with only limited success. Part of the difficulty in retaining such students is that they have unique socialization needs. Harrigan et al. (2003) suggest that minority students often need socialization to the role of higher education as well as to the idea that nursing is not menial labor.

Minority nursing students also experience many of the same issues already discussed for international nurses including differences in language and cultural values. It is important to remember that non-native speakers of English may be reticent to participate in the small group activities that are often a part of nursing school. This reticence may be attributable to insecurity about their English proficiency or a general lack of familiarity with group process. They may also be reluctant to speak out or offer opinions if they have been educated in a traditional hierarchical system in which the instructor or manager is regarded with unquestioned authority. Encouraging participation by drawing reticent members into discussions through requests for their views may be helpful in gaining their involvement.

In addition, using role models and preceptors representing the different ethnic minorities is appropriate both for recruiting and retaining minority students in nursing. The environment at the school of nursing must also be one that not only accepts cultural and ethnic diversity but actively encourages and values it. Finally, ongoing coaching and guidance throughout the nursing program may be needed for minority students to overcome these obstacles and succeed (Harrigan et al., 2003).

Employees with Role Status Change

Probably no other aspect of an employee's work life has as great an influence on productivity and retention as the quality of supervision exhibited by the immediate manager. Unfortunately, the orientation of new managers is often neglected by organizations. A qualitative study undertaken by Sullivan, Bretschneider, and McCausland (2003) found that many new managers perceived themselves as lacking basic and introductory managerial skills related to communication, conflict resolution, role transitioning, scheduling, budgeting and payroll management, performance evaluation, and staff counseling. This lack of skills may result in management errors.

Additionally, many restructured hospital organizational designs have created different and expanded roles for existing managers without ensuring that managers are adequately prepared for these new roles. Indeed, Kleinman (2003) argues that nurse managers are often less well prepared to manage the business activities than the clinical activities and that organizations must develop strategies to help nurse–managers develop the business knowledge and skills essential for the role.

There is a growing recognition that good managers do not emerge from the workforce without a great deal of conscious planning on the part of the organization. A management development program should be ongoing and individuals should receive some management development instruction before their appointment to a management position.

When an individual is filling a position where the previous manager is still available for orientation, the orientation period should be relatively short. The previous manager usually spends no longer than one week working directly with the new manager, especially when the new manager is familiar with the organization. A short orientation by the outgoing manager allows the newly appointed manager to gain control of the unit quickly and establish his or her own management style. If the new manager has been recruited from outside the organization, the orientation period may need to be extended.

Frequently, a new manager will be appointed to a vacant or newly established position. In either case, no one will be readily available to orient the new manager. In such cases, the new manager's immediate superior appoints someone to assist the new manager in learning the role. This could be a manager from another unit, the manager's supervisor, or someone from the unit who is familiar with the manager's duties and roles.

A new manager's orientation does not cease after the short introduction to the various tasks. Every new manager needs guidance, direction, and continued orientation and development during the first year in this new role. This direction comes from several sources in the organization:

- **The new manager's immediate superior.** This could be the unit supervisor if the new manager is a charge nurse, or it could be the chief nursing executive if the new manager is a unit supervisor. The immediate superior should have regularly scheduled sessions with the new manager to continue the ongoing orientation process.

- **A group of the new manager's peers.** There should be a management group in the organization with which the new manager can consult. The new manager should be encouraged to use the group as a resource.
- **A mentor.** If someone in the organization decides to mentor the new manager, it will undoubtedly benefit the organization. Although mentors cannot be assigned, the organization can encourage experienced managers to seek out individuals to mentor.

Clinical nurses who have recently assumed management roles often experience guilt when they decrease their involvement with direct patient care. When employees and physicians see a nurse–manager assuming the role of caregiver, they often make disparaging remarks such as, "Oh, you're working as a real nurse today." This tends to reinforce the nurse's value conflict in the new role.

Nurses moving into positions of increased responsibility also experience role stress created by role ambiguity and role overload. *Role ambiguity* describes the stress that occurs when job expectations are unclear. *Role overload* occurs when the demands of the role are excessive. Role overload is a major source of stress for nurse–managers. In addition, as nurses move into positions with increased status, their job descriptions tend to become increasingly vague. Therefore, clarifying job roles becomes an important tool in the resocialization process.

The Experienced Nurse in a New Position

For many reasons, nurses make frequent career moves. Experienced nurses often make lateral transfers within the same organization. Others take new positions that are quite different from their previous role; these new positions may be in their present organization or with a new one. Specific orientation needs arise for these nurses:

- **Transition from expert to novice.** This is a very difficult role transition. Many nurses transfer or change jobs because they no longer find their present job challenging. However, this results in the necessity of assuming a learning role in their new environment. The employee assigned to orient the nurse in role transition should be aware of the difficulties this nurse will experience. Transferred employees' lack of knowledge in the new area should never be belittled; whenever possible, the special expertise they bring from their former work area should be acknowledged and utilized.
- **Transition from familiar to the unfamiliar.** In the old surroundings, the employee knew everyone and where everything was located. In the new position, the employee will not only be learning new job skills, but will also be in an unfamiliar environment.

The managers of departments that receive frequent transfers should prepare a special orientation for experienced nurses transferring to the department. In addition to providing necessary staff development content, these orientation programs should focus on efforts to promote the self-esteem of these nurses as they learn the skills necessary for their new role. The special socialization needs of these new employees are often overlooked; these people need special attention that many organizations neglect.

> Organizations often fail to address socialization problems that occur in job, position, or status change.

Transitioning into a new job would result in less role strain if programs were designed to facilitate role modification and role expansion. For example, when a nurse moves from a medical floor to labor and delivery, the nurse does not know the group norms, is unsure of expected values and behaviors, and goes from being an expert to being a novice. All of these create a great deal of *role strain*. This same type of role stress occurs when experienced nurses move from one organization to another or from an inpatient setting to a community setting. Nurses often feel powerless during role transitions, which may culminate in anger and frustration as they seek to become socialized to a different role.

Assisting the Experienced Nurse in Role Transition

Programs designed to assist the nurse with the role transition of position change should do more than just provide an orientation to the new position; they also should address specific values and behaviors necessary for the new roles. The values and attitudes expected in a hospice nursing role may be very different than those expected of a trauma nurse. Managers should not assume that the experienced nurse is aware of the new role's expected attitudes. Excellent companies have leaders who take responsibility for shaping the values of new employees. By instilling and clarifying organizational values, managers are able to create a homogeneous staff who function as a team.

Employees adopting new values often experience role strain because they may need to give up a former value. Managers need to support employees during this value resocialization. Members of the reference group often use negative sanctions. For example, saying things like, "Well, we don't believe in doing that here" can make new, experienced employees feel as though the values held in other nursing roles were bad or wrong. Therefore, the manager should make efforts to see that formerly held values are not belittled.

STAFF DEVELOPMENT

The staff's knowledge level and capabilities are a major factor in determining the number of staff required to carry out unit goals. The better trained and more competent the staff, the fewer staff required. Staff development then is a cost-effective method of increasing productivity.

Education and training are two components of staff development that occur after an employee's indoctrination. Early staff development emphasized orientation and in-service training. In the last 20 years, however, other forms of education have become common in healthcare organizations. Management development, certification classes, and continuing education courses to meet relicensure requirements are now a part of many staff development programs. Because these forms of education are also a part of career planning they were discussed further in Chapter 11.

Training Versus Education

Managers have a greater responsibility for seeing that staff are properly trained than they do for meeting educational needs. *Training* may be defined as an organized method of ensuring that people have knowledge and skills for a specific purpose and that they have acquired the necessary knowledge to perform the duties of the job. The knowledge may require increased affective, motor, or cognitive skills. It is expected that acquiring new skills will increase productivity or create a better product.

Education is more formal and broader in scope than training. Whereas training has an immediate use, education is designed to develop the person in a broader sense. Recognizing educational needs and encouraging educational pursuits are roles and responsibilities of the leader. Managers may appropriately be requested to teach classes or courses; however, unless they have specific expertise, managers would not normally be responsible for an employee's formal education.

Responsibilities of the Education Department

Most education departments on the organization chart are depicted as having staff or advisory authority rather than line authority. Difficulties inherent in staff positions were discussed in Chapter 12. Because staff positions do not have line authority, education personnel generally have little or no authority over those for whom they are providing educational programs. Likewise, the unit manager has no authority over personnel in the education department.

Because of the ambiguity of overlapping roles and difficulties inherent in line and staff positions, educating and training employees may be neglected. If staff development activities are to be successful, it is necessary to delineate and communicate the authority and responsibility for all components of education and training.

Other difficulties arising from the shared responsibility among managers, personnel department staff, and educators for the indoctrination, education, and training of personnel are a frequent lack of cost-effectiveness evaluation and little accountability for the quality and outcomes of the educational activities.

The following suggestions can help overcome the difficulties inherent in a staff development system in which there is shared authority:

- The nursing department must ensure that all parties involved in the indoctrination, education, and training of nursing staff understand and carry out their responsibilities in that process.
- If the nursing department is not directly responsible for the staff development department (in large institutions, a non-nursing administrator may have authority for this department), there must be input from the nursing department in formulating staff development policies and delineating duties.
- An advisory committee should be formed with representatives from top-, middle-, and first-level management; staff development; and the human resource department. Representatives from all classifications of employees receiving training or education should be part of this committee.
- Accountability for various parts of the staff development program must be clearly communicated.
- Some method of determining the cost and benefits of various programs should be used.

Theories of Learning

Because all levels of management have a responsibility to improve employee performance through teaching, they must be familiar with learning theories. Understanding teaching–learning theories allows managers to structure training and use teaching techniques to change employee behavior and improve competence, which is the goal for all staff development.

Adult Learning Theory

> By understanding the assets adults bring to the classroom and the obstacles that might interfere with their learning, trainers and educators are able to create an effective learning environment.

Many managers attempt to teach adults using pedagogical or child learning strategies, the same method used in school. This type of teaching is usually ineffective for mature learners because adults have special needs. Knowles (1970) developed the concept of *androgogy*, or adult learning, to separate adult learner strategies from *pedagogy*, or child learning. **Display 16.3** summarizes the basic differences between the two learners. Adult learners are mature, self-directed people who have learned a great deal from life experiences and are focused toward solving problems that exist in their immediate environments.

Adult learning theory has contributed a great deal to the manner in which adults are taught.

Display 16.4 depicts the obstacles and assets to adult learning, and **Display 16.5** shows how the child and adult learning environments should differ. Knowles' studies have the following implications for trainers and educators:

- A climate of openness and respect will assist in the identification of what the adult learner wants and needs to learn.
- Adults enjoy taking part in and planning their learning experiences.
- Adults should be involved in the evaluation of their progress.
- Experiential techniques work best with adults.
- Mistakes are opportunities for adult learning.
- If the value of the adult's experience is rejected, the adult will feel rejected.

Display 16.3	Characteristics of Pedagogy and Androgogy

Pedagogy
Learner is dependent.
Learner needs external rewards and punishment.
Learner's experience is unimportant or limited.
Subject-centered.
Teacher-directed.

Androgogy
Learner is self-directed.
Learner is internally motivated.
Learner's experiences are valued and varied.
Task- or problem-centered.
Self-directed.

Display 16.4 **Obstacles and Assets to Adult Learning**

Obstacles to Learning
Institutional barriers
Time
Self-confidence
Situational obstacles
Family reaction
Special individual obstacles

Assets for Learning
High self-motivation
Self-directed
A proven learner
Knowledge experience reservoir
Special individual assets

Display 16.5 **Learning Environment of Pedagogy and Androgogy**

Pedagogy
The climate is authoritative.
Competition is encouraged.
Teacher sets goals.
Decisions are made by teacher.
Teacher lectures.
Teacher evaluates.

Androgogy
The climate is relaxed and informal.
Collaboration is encouraged.
Teacher and class set goals.
Decisions are made by teacher and students.
Students process activities and inquire about projects.
Teacher, self, and peers evaluate.

- Adults' readiness to learn is greatest when they recognize that there is a need to know (such as in response to a problem).
- Adults need the opportunity to apply what they have learned very quickly after the learning.
- Assessment of need is imperative in adult learning.

Social Learning Theory
Social learning theory builds on reinforcement theory as part of the motivation to learn and has many of the same components as the theories of socialization discussed in

previous chapters. Bandura (1977) suggests that people learn most behavior by direct experience and observation, and behaviors are retained or not retained based on positive and negative rewards.

Social learning theory involves four separate processes. First, people learn as a result of the direct experience of the effects of their actions. Second, knowledge is frequently obtained through vicarious experiences, such as by observing someone else's actions. Third, people learn by judgments voiced by others, especially when vicarious experience is limited. Fourth, people evaluate the soundness of the new information by reasoning through inductive and deductive logic. Social learning theory also acknowledges that anticipation of reinforcement influences what is observed and what goes unnoticed (Bandura, 1977). **Figure 16.1** depicts the social learning theory process.

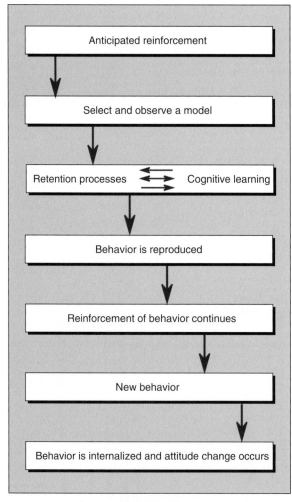

Figure 16.1 The social learning theory process.

The soundness of social learning theory is demonstrated by the effectiveness of role models, preceptors, and mentors. Because the cognitive process is very much a part of social learning, observational learning will be more effective if the learner is informed in advance of the benefits of adopting a role model's behavior.

Other Learning Theories

The following learning concepts may also be helpful to the leader–manager in meeting the learning needs of staff:

- **Readiness to learn.** This refers to the maturational and experiential factors in the learner's background that influence learning and is not the same as motivation to learn. *Maturation* means that the learner has received the prerequisites for the next stage of learning. The prerequisites could be behaviors or prior learning. *Experiential factors* are skills previously acquired that are necessary for the next stage of learning.
- **Motivation to learn.** If learners are informed in advance about the benefits of learning specific content and adopting new behaviors, they are more likely to be motivated to attend the training sessions and learn. Telling employees why and how specific educational or training programs will benefit them personally is a vital management function in staff development.
- **Reinforcement.** Because a learner's first attempts are often unsuccessful, a preceptor is essential. Good preceptors can reinforce desired behavior. Once the behavior or skill is learned, it needs continual reinforcement until it becomes internalized.
- **Task learning.** The learning of complex tasks is facilitated when tasks are broken into parts, beginning with the simplest and continuing to the most difficult. It is necessary, however, to combine *part learning* with *whole learning*. When learning motor skills, *spaced practice* is more effective than *massed practice*.
- **Transfer of learning.** The goal of training is to transfer new learning to the work setting. For this to occur, there should first be as much similarity between the training context and the job as possible. Second, adequate practice is mandatory, and *overlearning* (learning repeated to the degree that it is difficult to forget) is recommended. Third, the training should include a variety of different situations so that the knowledge is generalized. Fourth, whenever possible, important features or steps in a process should be identified. Finally, the learner must understand the basic principles underlying the tasks and how a variety of situations will modify how the task is accomplished. Learning in the classroom will not be transferred without adequate practice in a simulated or real situation and without an adequate understanding of underlying principles.
- **Span of memory.** The effectiveness of staff development activities depends to some extent on the ability of the participants to retain information. Effective strategies include the chance for repeated rehearsal, grouping items to be learned (three or four items for oral presentations and four to six visually), having the material presented in a well-organized manner, and *chunking*.
- **Chunking.** This occurs when two independent items of information are presented and then grouped together into one unit. While the mind can

remember only a limited number of chunks of data, experienced nurses can include more data in the chunks than novice nurses.

· **Knowledge of results.** Research has demonstrated that people learn faster when they are informed of their progress. The knowledge of results must be automatic, immediate, and meaningful to the task at hand. People need to experience a feeling of progress, and they need to know how they are doing when measured against expected outcomes.

Assessing Staff Development Needs

Although managers may not be involved in implementing all educational programs, they are responsible for identifying learning needs. Staff development activities are normally carried out for one of three reasons: to establish competence, to meet new learning needs, and to satisfy interests the staff may have in learning in specific areas. If educational resources are scarce, staff desires for specific educational programs may need to be sacrificed to fulfill competency and new learning needs. Because managers and staff may identify learning needs differently, an educational needs assessment should be carried out before developing programs.

Many staff development activities are generated to ensure that workers at each level are competent to perform the duties assigned to the position. *Competence* is defined as having the abilities to meet the requirements for a particular role. Healthcare organizations use many resources to determine competency. State board licensure, national certification, and performance review are some of the methods used to satisfy competency requirements. Other methods are self-administered checklists, record audits, and peer evaluation. Many of these methods are explained in Unit 7. It is important for staff development purposes to remember that in the case of deficient competencies, some staff development activity must be implemented to correct the deficiencies.

Another learning need that frequently affects healthcare organizations is the need to meet new technological and scientific challenges. Medical technology and science are developing rapidly, resulting in the need to learn new skills and procedures and acquire the knowledge necessary to operate complex equipment. Much of a manager's educational resources will be used to meet these new learning needs.

Some organizations implement training programs because they are faddish and have been advertised and marketed well. Educational programs are expensive, however, and should not be undertaken unless a demonstrated need exists. Educational resources should be able to be justified. In addition to developing rationale for education programs, the use of an assessment plan will be helpful in meeting learner needs. The following plan outlines the sequence that should be used in developing an educational program:

1. Identify the desired knowledge or skills the staff should have.
2. Identify the present level of knowledge or skill.
3. Determine the deficit of desired knowledge and skills.

4. Identify the resources available to meet needs.
5. Make maximum use of available resources.
6. Evaluate and test outcomes after use of resources.

Evaluation of Staff Development Activities

Because staff development includes participation and involvement from many departments, it is very difficult to control this important function effectively. *Control*, the evaluation phase of the management process, becomes extremely difficult when accountability is shared. It is very easy for the personnel department, middle-level managers, and the education department to "pass the buck" among one another for accountability regarding staff development activities.

Currently, in most organizations responsibility for staff development is decentralized and includes the nurse–manager. This has occurred as a result of fiscal concerns, the awareness of the need to socialize new employees at the unit level, and recognition of the relationship between employee competence and productivity. It is generally accepted that the ultimate responsibility for staff training and education rests with the manager, although the manager does not personally provide all aspects of staff development.

Some difficulties associated with decentralized staff development include the conflict created by role ambiguity whenever two people share responsibility. Role ambiguity is sometimes reduced when staff development personnel and managers delineate the difference between training and education.

Evaluation of staff development consists of more than merely having class participants fill out an evaluation form at the end of the class session, signing an employee handbook form, or assigning a preceptor for each new employee. Evaluation of the three components of staff development (indoctrination, training, and education) should include the following four criteria:

- **Learner's reaction.** How did the learner perceive the orientation, the class, the training, or the preceptor?
- **Behavior change.** What behavior change occurred as a result of the learning? Was the learning transferred? Testing someone at the end of a training or educational program does not confirm that the learning changed behavior. There needs to be some method of follow-up to observe if behavior change occurred.
- **Organizational impact.** Although it is often difficult to measure how staff development activities affect the organization, efforts should be made to measure this criterion. Examples of measurements are assessing quality of care, medication errors, accidents, quality of clinical judgment, turnover, and productivity.
- **Cost-effectiveness.** All staff development activities should be quantified in some manner. This is perhaps the most neglected aspect of accountability in staff development. All staff development activities should be evaluated for quality control, impact on the institution, and cost-effectiveness. This is true regardless of whether the education and training activities are carried out by the manager, the preceptor, the personnel department, or the education department.

Learning Exercise 16.4

Designing a Teaching Plan

You have been working in a home health agency for three years. During that time, the acuity of your caseload has increased dramatically, and you find that teaching home health aides has become more difficult as the equipment they need to use has become more complex. The home health aides seem motivated to learn, but you believe that part of the difficulty lies with how you are presenting the material. Many of them have a limited knowledge of nursing procedures.

One of your clients is Mr. Jones, who has no family. His insurance company has approved a visit from a home health aide every other day to bathe him and help him ambulate with a walker. Because of his chronic severe respiratory disease, he must be ambulated with oxygen but does not need it when resting.

Today, you have scheduled a session with Mr. Jones' home health aide for a demonstration and return demonstration on how to connect and disconnect the oxygen and how to use the walker. The aide is very competent in basic hygiene skills but has not always used good body mechanics when providing patient care, and she seems intimidated by new equipment.

Assignment: Using your knowledge of the learning theories presented in this chapter, construct a teaching plan for this aide. Support your plan with appropriate rationale.

Coaching as a Teaching Strategy

Coaching as a means to develop and train employees is a teaching strategy rather than a learning theory. Coaching is one of the most important tools for empowering subordinates, changing behavior, and developing a cohesive team. It is perhaps the most difficult role for a manager to master. Coaching is one person helping the other to reach an optimum level of performance. The emphasis is always on assisting the employee to recognize greater options, to clarify statements, and to grow. Fitzpatrick (2001) says that successful nurse leaders are good coaches who support new nurses and new hires by building safety nets to ensure their prosperity.

Coaching may be long term or short term. *Short-term coaching* is effective as a teaching tool, for assisting with socialization, and for dealing with short-term problems. *Long-term coaching* as a tool for career management and in dealing with disciplinary problems is different and is discussed in other chapters.

Short-term coaching frequently involves spontaneous teaching opportunities. Learning Exercise 16.5 is an example of how a manager can use short-term coaching to guide an employee in a new role.

Meeting the Educational Needs of a Culturally Diverse Staff

In the 21st century, nurse–leaders should expect to work with a more diverse workforce. In discussing the management of a diverse workforce, Seago (2000) states

Learning Exercise 16.5

Paul's Complaint

Paul is the charge nurse on a surgical floor from 3 pm to 11 pm. One day, he comes to work a few minutes early, as he occasionally does, so he can chat with his supervisor, Mary, before taking patient reports. Usually Mary is in her office around this time. Paul enjoys talking over some of his work-related management problems with her because he is fairly new in the charge nurse role, having been appointed three months ago. Today, he asks Mary if she can spare a minute to discuss a personnel problem.

Paul: Sally is becoming a real problem to me. She is taking long break times and has not followed through on several medication order changes lately.
Mary: What do you mean by "long breaks" and not following through?
Paul: In the last two months, she has taken an extra 15 minutes for dinner three nights a week and has missed changes in medication orders eight times.
Mary: Have you spoken to Sally?
Paul: Yes, and she said she had been an RN on this floor for four years, and no one had ever criticized her before. I checked her personnel record, and there is no mention of those particular problems, but her performance appraisals have only been mediocre.
Mary: What do you recommend doing about Sally?
Paul: I could tell her that I won't tolerate her extended dinner breaks and her poor work performance.
Mary: What are you prepared to do if her performance does not improve?
Paul: I could give her a written warning notice and eventually fire her if her work remains below standard.
Mary: Well, that is one option. What are some other options available to you? Do you think Sally really understands your expectations? Do you feel she might resent you?
Paul: I suppose I ought to sit down with Sally and explain exactly what my expectations are. Since my appointment to charge nurse, I've talked with all the new nurses as they have come on shift, but I just assumed the old-timers knew what was expected on this unit. I've been a little anxious about my new role; I never thought about her resenting my position.
Mary: I think that is a good first option. Maybe Sally interpreted your not talking with her, as you did all the new nurses, as a rejection. After you have another talk with her, let me know how things are going.

Analysis: The supervisor has coached Paul toward a more appropriate option as a first choice in solving this problem. Although Mary's choice of questions and guidance assisted Paul, she never "took over" or directed Paul, but instead let him find his own better solution. As a result of this conversation, Paul had a series of individual meetings with all his staff and shared with them his expectations. He also enlisted their assistance in his efforts to have the shift run smoothly. Although he began to see an improvement in Sally's performance, he realized she was a marginal employee who would need a great deal of coaching. He reported back to Mary and outlined his plans for improving Sally's performance further. Mary reinforced his handling of the problem by complimenting Paul.

that, although it has become a cliché of the current era, it is much easier to talk about than actually do. Her suggestions for creating an organization that celebrates a diverse workforce, rather than merely tolerating it, require well-planned learning activities. There should also be sufficient opportunity for small group so that personnel can begin recognizing their own biases and prejudices. This type of learning activity is especially important as more unlicensed assistive personnel (UAP) are added to the staff. Education to support cultural diversity should be part of the staff development of RNs and UAP to facilitate their learning to work together in teams.

Heterogeneity of staff in a teaching–learning setting may add strength or create difficulty. Factors, such as gender, age, English language proficiency, and culture, may affect success and cooperative learning of groups. Although meeting the educational needs of a heterogeneous staff may be more time consuming and beset with communication problems, the educational needs must be met. The ability of all nurses to work well with a culturally diverse staff is essential. Managers should respect cultural diversity and recognize the desirability of having nurses from numerous cultures on their staff.

Education staff should be aware that learners with diverse learning styles and cultural backgrounds may perceive both the classroom and instruction differently than learners who have never experienced a culture different from that of the mainstream United States. Whether in a classroom or at the bedside teaching, there are

Learning Exercise 16.6

Cultural Considerations in Teaching
You are the evening charge nurse for a large surgical unit. Recently, your long-time and extremely capable unit clerk retired, and the manager of the unit replaced the clerk with 23-year-old Nan, who does not have a healthcare background and is a recent immigrant. She speaks English with an accent but can be easily understood. She appears highly intelligent, but shy and unassertive.

Nan received a two-week unit clerk orientation that consisted of actual classroom time and working directly with the retiring clerk. She has been functioning on her own for two weeks, and you realize that her orientation has not been sufficient. Last evening after her tenth mistake, you became rather sharp with her, and she broke down in tears.

You are very frustrated by this situation. Your unit is very busy in the evening with returning surgeries and surgeons making rounds and leaving a multitude of orders. On the other hand, you believe that Nan has great potential. You realize there is much to learn in this job and, for a person without a healthcare background, learning the terminology, physicians' names, and unit routine is difficult. You spend the morning devising a training plan for Nan.

Assignment: Using your knowledge of learning theories, explain your teaching plan, and support your plan with appropriate rationale. How might Nan's lack of an American education and socialization influence her learning?

several things staff development personnel can do to facilitate the learning process, such as giving the learner plenty of time to respond to questions and restating information that is not understood.

Managers should also consider older nurses' learning styles and preceptor needs. Older nurses learn differently than new graduates do and respond well to sharing anecdotal case histories. LaDuke (2001) maintains that pairing an older nurse with a much younger one could result in conflict and mutual disrespect and result in less-effective learning during a critical time in the older nurse's socialization to the facility.

Building Team Unity Through Staff Development

The new momentum in organizations is toward encouraging a team effort through team building and providing a continual supportive learning environment. Healthcare science and technology change so rapidly that without adequate teaching–learning skills and educational services, organizations will get left behind. Likewise, it has become obvious in the new millennium that teams, rather than individuals, function more efficiently. Fitzpatrick (2001) thinks that a leader who is a good coach, and who can inspire others to join and remain with the team, ignites the team spirit.

INTEGRATING LEADERSHIP AND MANAGEMENT IN TEAM BUILDING VIA SOCIALIZATION AND EDUCATION

Socialization, a critical component of indoctrinating the employee into the organization, is a complex process directed at the acquisition of appropriate attitudes, cognition, emotions, values, motivations, skills, knowledge, and social patterns necessary to cope with the social and professional environment. Socialization differs from and has a greater impact than either induction or orientation on subsequent productivity and retention. It can also help to build loyalty and team spirit. This is the time to instill the employee with pride in the organization and the unit. This type of affective learning becomes the foundation for subsequent increased satisfaction and motivation.

The integrated leader–manager supports employees during difficult role transitions. Mentoring and role modeling are encouraged, and role expectations are clarified. The manager recognizes that employees who are not supported and socialized to the organization will not develop the loyalty necessary in the competitive marketplace. Leaders understand that creating a positive work environment where there is interdisciplinary respect will assist employees in their role transitions.

The integrated leader–manager knows that a well-planned and well-implemented indoctrination program is a wise investment of organizational resources. It provides the opportunity to mold a team effort and infuse employees with enthusiasm for the organization. There is perhaps no other part of management that has as great an influence on reducing burnout as successful indoctrination. New employees' impressions of an organization during their adjustment period stay with them a long time.

The manager recognizes the ultimate responsibility for staff development and uses appropriate teaching theories to assist with teaching and training staff. There is a shared responsibility for assessing educational needs, educational quality, and fiscal accountability of all staff development activities.

The leader uses knowledge of androgogy in dealing with all employees, is able to coach spontaneously and effectively, and seeks opportunities to be personally involved with teaching, training, and staff development. By integrating the leadership role with the management functions of staff development, the manager is able to collaborate with education personnel and others so the learning needs of unit employees are met.

The manager ensures that resources for staff development are used wisely. A focus of staff development should be keeping staff updated with new knowledge and ascertaining that all personnel remain competent to perform their roles. The integrated leader–manager is the role model of a good teacher, using teaching–learning theory to empower staff.

The integrated leader–manager is also one who encourages continuous learning from all individuals in the organization and is a role model of the life-long learner. He or she understands that by building and supporting a knowledgeable team, the collective knowledge generated will be greater than any single individual's contribution.

✳ Key Concepts

- The socialization of people into roles occurs with all professions and is a normal sociological process.
- *Socialization* and *resocialization* are often neglected areas of the indoctrination process.
- The terms *role model, preceptor,* and *mentor* are not synonymous, and all play an important role in assisting with the socialization of employees.
- New graduates, international nurses, minority student nurses, new managers, and experienced nurses in new roles have unique socialization needs.
- Difficulties with resocialization usually center around unclear role expectations *(role ambiguity)*, an inability to meet job demands, or deficiencies in motivation. *Role strain* and *role overload* contribute to the problem.
- *Training* and *education* are important parts of staff development.
- Managers and education department staff have a shared responsibility for the education and training of staff.
- Theories of learning and principles of teaching must be considered if staff development activities are to be successful.
- *Social learning* theory suggests that people learn most behavior by direct experience and observation.
- People from different cultures and age groups may have different socialization and learning needs.
- All staff development activities should be evaluated for quality control and fiscal accountability.
- The leader is a role model of the life-long learner.

More Learning Exercises and Applications

Learning Exercise 16.7

Accepting Additional Responsibility

You are an experienced staff nurse on an inpatient specialty unit. Today, a local nursing school instructor approaches you and asks if you would be willing to become a preceptor for a nursing student as part of his 10 week leadership-management clinical rotation. The instructor relays that there would be no instructor on site and that the student has had only minimum acute care clinical skills exposure. The student would have to work very closely with you on a 1:1 basis. The school of nursing can offer no pay for this role but the instructor states she would be happy to write a thank-you letter for your personnel file and that she would be available anytime to address questions that might arise.

The unit does not reduce workload for preceptors although credit for service is given on the annual performance review. The unit supervisor states that the choice is yours but warns that you may also be called upon to assist with the orientation of a nurse who will transfer to the unit in six weeks time.

You have mixed feelings about whether to accept this role. Although you enjoy having students on the unit as well being in the teaching role, you are unsure if you can do both your normal, heavy workload as well as give the students the time they will undoubtedly need to learn. You do feel a "need to give back to your profession" and personally believe that nurses need to be more supportive of each other, but are significantly concerned about role overload.

Assignment: Decide if you will accept this role. Would you place any constraints upon the instructor, the student, or your supervisor as a condition of accepting the role? What were the strongest driving forces for your decision? What were the greatest restraining forces? What evaluation criteria would you develop to assess whether your final decision was a good one?

Learning Exercise 16.8

Addressing Resocialization Issues

You are one of the care coordinators for a home health agency. One of your duties is to orient new employees to the agency. Recently, the chief nursing executive hired Brian, an experienced acute care nurse, to be one of your team members. Brian seemed eager and enthusiastic. He confided in you that he was tired of acute care and wanted to be more involved with long-term patient and family caseloads.

During Brian's orientation, you became aware that his clinical skills were excellent, but his therapeutic communication skills were inferior to the rest of your staff. You discussed this with Brian and explained how important communication is in gaining the trust of agency patients and that trust is necessary if the needs of the patients and the goals of the agency are to be met. You referred Brian to some literature that you believed might be helpful to him.

After a three-week orientation program, Brian began working unsupervised. It is now four weeks later. Recently, you received a complaint from one of the other nurses and one from a patient regarding Brian's poor communication skills. Brian seems frustrated and has not gained acceptance from the other nurses in your work group. You suspect that some of the nurses resent Brian's superior clinical skills, whereas others believe he does not understand his new role and are becoming impatient with him. You are genuinely concerned that Brian does not seem to be fitting in.

Assignment: Could this problem have been prevented? Decide what you should do now. Outline a plan to resocialize Brian into his new role and make him feel a valued part of the staff.

Learning Exercise 16.9

Effective Interpersonal Problem Solving

You have been working at Memorial Hospital for three months and have begun to feel fairly confident in your new role. However, one of the older nurses working on your shift constantly belittles your nursing education. Whenever you request assistance in problem solving or in learning a new skill, she says, "Didn't they teach you anything in nursing school?" Your charge nurse has given you a satisfactory three-month evaluation, but you are becoming increasingly defensive regarding the comments of the other nurse.

Assignment: Explain how you plan to evaluate the accuracy of the older nurse's comments. Might you be contributing to the problem? How will you cope with this situation? Would you involve others? What efforts can you make to improve your relationship with this coworker?

Learning Exercise 16.10

Changing Learning Needs

Learning needs and the maturity of those in a class often influence course content and teaching methods. Look back at how your learning needs and maturity level have changed since you were a beginning nursing student. When viewed as a whole, were you and the other beginning nursing students child or adult learners? Compare Knowles' pedagogy and androgogy characteristics to determine this.

Are pedagogical teaching strategies appropriate for beginning nursing students? If so, when does the nursing student make a transition from child to adult learner? What teaching modes do you believe would be most conducive to learning for a beginning nursing student? Would this change as students progressed through the nursing program? Support your beliefs with rationale.

Web Links

Multicultural Pavilion
http://curry.edschool.virginia.edu/go/multicultural
Provides instructional resources for those creating a multicultural curriculum, along with a discussion board dealing with diversity.

Peer Resources
http://peer.ca/mentor.html (last updated Jan. 2, 2004)
Information on mentoring resources/publications, mentor programs between students and people of diverse ages and backgrounds, mentor profiles.

National Mentoring Partnership
http://www.mentoring.org//become_a_mentor/become_a_mentor.adp?Entry=home
An organization that promotes, advocates, and is a resource for mentors and mentoring initiatives nationwide. Includes information on becoming a mentor, basics of mentoring, and mentoring stories.

Role Guidelines for Preceptors
http://www.acnp.utoronto.ca/npdiploma/Role%20Guidelines520for%preceptors.htm
The University of Toronto faculty of nursing has created this website with guidelines for preceptors as well as learners

Free Learning Games and Tips for Staff Development Educators
http://www.nurselearn.com/free_game_&_tips.htm
Includes word games, word searches, and crossword puzzles for use as staff development pretests or posttests with a classroom presentation, self-study program, poster presentation, etc.

References

Apker, J., Zabava Ford, W. S., & Fox. D. H. (2003). Predicting nurses' organizational and professional identification: The effect of nursing roles, professional autonomy, and supportive communication. *Nursing Economic$, 21*(5), 226–232.

Bandura, A. (1977). *Social learning theory.* Englewood Cliffs, NJ: Prentice-Hall.

Beecroft, P. C., Kunzman, L., & Krozek, C. (2001). RN internship. Outcomes of a one-year pilot program. *Journal of Nursing Administration, 31*(12), 575–582.

Bola, T.V., Driggers, K., Dunlap, C., & Ebersole, M. (2003). Foreign-educated nurses. Strangers in a strange land. *Nursing Management, 34*(7), 39–42.

Byrne, M. W., & Keefe, M. R. (2002). Building research competence in nursing through mentoring. *Journal of Nursing Scholarship, 34*(4), 391–396.

Cable, D. M., & Parsons, C. K. (2001). Socialization tactics and person–organization fit. *Personnel Psychology, 54*(1), 1–24.

Covan, E. K. (2000). Revisiting the relationship between elder modelers and their protégés. *Sociological Perspectives, 43*(1), S7–21.

Currie, D. L., Vierke, J., & Greer, K. (2000). Making a nurse intern program pay off. *Nursing Management, 31*(6), 12–13.

Darling, L. A. (1984). What do nurses want in a mentor? *Journal of Nursing Administration, 14*(29), 42–44.

Duchscher, J. E. B. (2001). Out in the real world. Newly graduated nurses in acute care speak out. *Journal of Nursing Administration, 31*(9), 426–439.

Fitzpatrick, M. A. (2001). Coaching champions. *Nursing Management, 32*(3), 7, 39–45.

Harrigan, R. C. Gollin, L. X., & Casken, J. (2003). Barriers to increasing native Hawaiian, Samoan, and Filipino nursing students: Perceptions of students and their families. *Nursing Outlook, 51*(1), 25–30.

Hurst, S., Koplin-Baucum, S., Wilkins, B., Merkel, D., Lujan, L., Helmich, C., Henry, C., & Mosesman, A. (2002). Mentoring program. Phoenix, AZ: Good Samaritan Regional Medical Center.

Hyperdictionary. (2003). Available at http://hyperdictionary.com/dictionary. Retrieved January 2, 2004.

Kleinman, C. S. (2003). Leadership roles, competencies, and education. How prepared are our nurse managers? *Journal of Nursing Administration, 33*(9), 451–455.

Knowles, M. (1970). *The modern practice of adult education: Androgogy versus pedagogy.* New York: Association Press.

Kramer, M. (1974). *Reality shock: Why nurses leave nursing.* St. Louis, MO: C. V. Mosby.

LaDuke, S. D. (2001). Shades of gray. *Nursing Management, 32*(4), 42–43.

Lee, L. A. (2000). Buzzwords with a basis. Motivation, mentoring, empowerment. *Nursing Management, 31*(10), 25–27.

Lindeman, C. A. (2000). Nursing's socialization of nurses. *Creative Nursing, 6*(4), 3–5.

Pinkerton, S. E. (2003). Mentoring new graduates. *Nursing Economic$, 21*(4), 202–203.

Postlen-Slattery, D. & Foley, K. (2003). The fruits of lifelong learning. *Nursing Management, 34*(2), 35–37.

Ryan, M. (2003). A buddy program for international nurses. *Journal of Nursing Administration, 33*(6), 350–352.

Schaffer, B., Tallarica, B., & Walsh, J. (2000). Win-win mentoring. *Nursing Management, 31*(1), 32–34.

Schmalenberg, C., & Kramer, M. (1979). *Coping with reality shock.* Wakefield, MA: Nursing Resources.

Seago, J. A. (2000). Registered nurses, unlicensed assistive personnel, and organizational culture in hospitals. *Journal of Nursing Administration, 30*(5), 278–286.

Sullivan, J., Bretschneider, J., & McCausland, M. P. (2003). Designing a leadership development program for nurse managers. *Journal of Nursing Administration, 33*(10), 544–549.

Tanner, C. (2000). Socializing students on the complexities of nursing practice. *Creative Nursing, 6*(4), 8–12.

Bibliography

Broome, M. E. (2003). Mentoring: To everything a season. *Nursing Outlook, 51*(6), 249–250.

Eifried, S. J. (2003). Bearing witness to suffering: The lived experience of nursing students. *Journal of Nursing Education, 42*(2), 59–67.

Findlay, P., & McKinlay, A. (2000). In search of perfect people: Teamwork and team players in the Scottish spirits industry. *Human Relations*, 53(12), 1549–1475.

Girard, N. G. (2003). Lifelong learning. *American Operating Room Nurse's Journal (AORN), 78*(3), 365–366.

Goggin, M. (2000). I'm behind you! The manager as coach. *Nursing Economic$, 18*(3), 160–162.

Gooden, M. B., & Porter, C. P. (2001). Rethinking the relationship between nursing and diversity. *American Journal of Nursing, 101*(1), 63–65.

Grindel, C. G. (2003). Mentoring managers. *Nephrology Nursing Journal, 30*(5), 517–522.

Jackson, M. (2001). A preceptor incentive program. *American Journal of Nursing, 101*(6), 24–27.

Koskinen, L. (May 2003). Charactersistics (sic) of intercultural mentoring—A mentor perspective. *Nurse Educator Today, 23*(4), 278–285.

Liebowitz, B. (2003). Leadership and management. Coaching managers. *Healthcare Financial Management, 57*(4), 108–10, 112.

Lockerwood-Rayermann, S. (2003). Preceptor leadership style and the nursing practicum. *Journal of Professional Nursing, 19*(1), 32–37.

Mamchur, C. J. (2003). Preceptorship and interpersonal conflict: A multidisciplinary study. *Journal of Advanced Nursing, 43*(2), 188–196.

McBee, P. (July 2003). When a bonus isn't enough: How one hospital used a unit-specific orientation survival guide to recruit and retain RNs. *Nursing, 33*(7), 32cc1–2.

Newhouse, R., & Dang, D. (2001). Measuring role changes for nurses. *Journal of Nursing Administration, 31*(4), 173–175.

Oermann, M. H. (2001). One-minute mentor. *Nursing Management, 32*(4), 12–14.

Olson, R. K., Nelson, M., Stuart, C., Young, L., Kleinsasser, A., Schroedermeier, R., & Newstrom, P. (2001). Nursing student residency program. *Journal of Nursing Administration, 31*(1), 40–48.

Pontius, C. (2001). Meant to be a mentor. *Nursing Management, 32*(5), 35–36.

Smeltzer, C. H. (December 2002). Executive coaching. Succession planning. *Journal of Nursing Administration, 32*(12), 615.

Tanner, A. (2002). Professional staff education. Quantifying costs and outcomes. *Journal of Nursing Administration, 32*(2), 91–97.

Staffing Needs and Scheduling Policies

Accurate definition and quantification of the work of nursing is critical to the identification of appropriate nursing resource requirements.

—Graf, Millar, Feilteau, Coakley, and Erickson, 2003

In addition to selecting, developing, and socializing staff, the manager must ascertain that adequate numbers and an appropriate mix of personnel are available to meet daily unit needs and organizational goals. Because staffing patterns and scheduling policies directly affect the daily lives of all personnel, it is important that they be administered fairly as well as economically.

This chapter examines different methods for determining staffing needs, communicating staffing plans, and developing and communicating scheduling policies. Unit fiscal responsibility is discussed, with sample formulas and instructions for calculating daily staffing needs.

The manager's responsibility for adequate and well-communicated staffing and scheduling policies is stressed. The need for periodic re-evaluation of staffing philosophy in order to meet stated care delivery outcomes is discussed. There is a focus on the leadership responsibility for developing trust through fair staffing and scheduling procedures. Recent legislation regarding mandatory staffing requirements is also discussed, including the manager's role for ensuring that the organization is able to facilitate the changes required by law. The leadership roles and management functions inherent in staffing and scheduling are shown in **Display 17.1**.

Display 17.1 **Leadership Roles and Management Functions Associated with Staffing and Scheduling**

Leadership Roles
1. Identifies creative and flexible staffing methods to meet the needs of patients, staff, and the organization.
2. Is knowledgeable regarding contemporary methods of scheduling and staffing.
3. Assumes a responsibility toward staffing that builds trust and encourages a team approach.
4. Periodically examines the unit standard of productivity to determine if changes are needed.
5. Is alert to extraneous factors that have an impact on staffing.
6. Is ethically accountable to patients and employees for adequate and safe staffing.
7. Plans for staffing shortages so patient care goals will be met.
8. Assesses if and how workforce intergenerational values impact staffing needs and responds accordingly.

Management Functions
1. Provides adequate staffing to meet patient care needs according to the philosophy of the organization.
2. Uses organizational goals and patient classification tools to minimize understaffing and overstaffing as patient census and acuity fluctuate.
3. Schedules staff in a fiscally responsible manner.
4. Develops fair and uniform scheduling policies and communicates these clearly to all staff.
5. Ascertains that scheduling policies are not in violation of local and national labor laws, organizational policies, or union contracts.
6. Assumes accountability for quality and fiscal control of staffing.
7. Evaluates scheduling and staffing procedures and policies on a regular basis.

UNIT MANAGER'S RESPONSIBILITIES IN MEETING STAFFING NEEDS

The requirement for night, evening, weekend, and holiday work that is frequently necessary in healthcare organizations is stressful and frustrating for some nurses. Inflexible scheduling is a major contributor to job dissatisfaction and turnover on the part of nurses (Shullanberger, 2000). Managers should do whatever they can to see that employees feel they have some control over scheduling, shift options, and staffing policies.

Although many organizations now use staffing clerks and computers to assist with staffing, the overall responsibility for scheduling continues to be an important function of first- and middle-level managers. Each organization has different expectations regarding the unit manager's responsibility in long-range human resource planning and in short-range planning for daily staffing.

Some organizations decentralize staffing by having unit managers make scheduling decisions. Other organizations use *centralized staffing*, where staffing decisions are made by personnel in a central office or staffing center. Such centers may or may not be staffed by registered nurses, although someone in authority would be a nurse even when a staffing clerk carries out the day-to-day activity.

In organizations with *decentralized staffing*, the unit manager is often responsible for covering all scheduled staff absences, reducing staff during periods of decreased patient census or acuity, adding staff during periods of high patient census or acuity, preparing monthly unit schedules, and preparing holiday and vacation schedules. Budreau, Balakrishnan, Titler, and Hafner (1999) state that nursing management is highly decentralized in most hospitals, with considerable variation found in staffing among patient care units. This means that many nurse–managers have some control over factors that affect cost on their specific units.

Advantages of decentralized staffing are that the unit manager understands the needs of the unit and staff intimately, which leads to the increased likelihood that sound staffing decisions will be made. Additionally, the staff feels more in control of their work environment because they are able to take personal scheduling requests directly to their immediate supervisor. Also, decentralized scheduling and staffing leads to increased autonomy and flexibility, thus, decreasing nurse attrition.

Decentralized staffing, however, carries the risk that employees will be treated unequally or inconsistently. Additionally, the unit manager may be viewed as granting rewards or punishments through the staffing schedule. Decentralized staffing also is time consuming for the manager and often promotes more "special pleading" than centralized staffing. However, undoubtedly the major difficulty with decentralized staffing is ensuring high-quality staffing decisions throughout the organization (Budreau et al., 1999).

In centralized staffing, the manager's role is limited to making minor adjustments and providing input. For example, the manager would communicate special staffing needs and assist with obtaining staff coverage for illness and sudden changes in patient census. Therefore, the manager in centralized staffing continues to have ultimate responsibility for seeing that adequate personnel are available to meet the needs of the organization.

Centralized staffing is fairer to all employees because policies tend to be employed more consistently and impartially. In addition, centralized staffing frees the middle-level manager to complete other management functions. Centralized staffing also allows for the most efficient (cost effective) use of resources since the more units that can be considered together, the easier it is to deal with variations in patient census and staffing needs (Wing, 2001).

Centralized staffing, however, does not provide as much flexibility for the worker, nor can it account as well for a worker's desires or special needs. Additionally, managers may be less responsive to personnel budget control if they have limited responsibility in scheduling and staffing matters.

Regardless of whether the organization has centralized or decentralized staffing, all unit managers should understand scheduling options and procedures and accept fiscal responsibility for staffing.

Managers must also be cognizant of the need to have an ethnically and culturally diverse staff to meet the needs of an increasingly diverse patient population. Indeed, national standards for providing culturally and linguistically appropriate services (CLAS) in health care were released by the Department of Health and Human Services Office of Minority Health in 2000 (Xu, 2001). Of the 14 standards put forth, several directly address the need for cultural and linguistic diversity in staffing. For example, Standard 4 requires that healthcare organizations offer language assistance services, including bilingual staff and interpreter services, at no cost to clients with limited English proficiency. Standard 6 assures the competency of this language assistance by interpreters and bilingual staff and Standard 5 requires that all verbal offers and written notices regarding patient's access to these services be available to patients in their preferred languages. Managers then must clearly understand the unique cultural and linguistic needs represented in their patient population and try to address these needs through an appropriately diverse staff. Indeed, Malloch, Davenport, and Hatler (2003) suggest that the importance of providing culturally competent caregivers cannot be overstated since health care congruent with cultural beliefs and values is essential for optimal outcomes.

> *It is important to remember that centralized and decentralized staffing are not synonymous with centralized and decentralized management decision making. For example, a manager can work in an organization that has centralized staffing but decentralized organizational decision making.*

Moreover, as the current healthcare system is evaluated, nurse–managers must be cognizant of new recommendations and legislation affecting staffing. There has been movement in at least fifteen states to impose mandatory staffing requirements (Spetz, 2001), and one state (California) has already enacted legislation requiring mandatory staffing rates that affect hospitals and long-term care facilities. Under Assembly Bill 394, passed in 1999 and crafted by the California Nurses Association, all hospitals in California had to comply with the minimum staffing ratios shown in **Display 17.2,** by January 1, 2004 (California Nurses Association, 2003a). These ratios, developed by the California Department of Health Services, represent the maximum number of patients an RN can be assigned to care for, under any circumstance. Similar bills have failed in Virginia, New Jersey, Hawaii, and Missouri (Hopkins, 2000).

Proponents of legislated minimum staffing ratios say that ratios are needed because many hospitals' current staffing levels are so low that both RNs and their patients are negatively affected (Kovner, 2000). In addition, numerous articles have appeared in the media attesting to grossly inadequate staffing in hospitals and

Display 17.2	Minimum Staffing Ratios for Hospitals in California Effective January 2004

Unit	Nurse-Patient Ratio
Critical Care/ICU	1:2
Neonatal ICU	1:2
Operating Room	1:1
Labor & Delivery	1:2
Ante partum	1:4
Post-partum couplets	1:4
Post-partum women only	1:6
Pediatrics	1:4
Step-down (Initial)	1:4
Step-down (in 2008)	1:3
Medical/Surgical (Initial)	1:6
Medical/Surgical (deferred from 2005 to 2008)	1:5
Oncology (Initial)	1:5
Oncology (in 2008)	1:4
Psychiatry	1:6
Emergency Room	1:4

Source: California Nurses Association (2003b). RN alert. Final ratios approved. CNA wins protection for RNs. Available at: http://www.calnurse.org/finalrat/finratrn7103.pdf. Retrieved November 28, 2003.

nursing homes, and professional nursing organizations such as the American Nurse's Association have expressed concern about the effect poor staffing has on both nurses' health and safety and on patient outcomes (Kovner). Adequate staffing then is needed to assure that care provided is at least safe, and hopefully more. Proponents of state regulation of RN to patient ratios suggest that such ratios protect the most basic elements of the public health we take for granted and argue that the government must take on this responsibility to ensure that safe health care is provided to all Americans (Kovner).

Hopkins (2000) suggests, however, that there are three arguments against staffing ratios. First, the current nursing shortage will make it difficult to fill the slots when the ratios appear. Second, the ratios may merely serve as a Band-Aid to the greater problems of quality of care. And finally, numbers alone do not ensure improved patient care since not all registered nurses have equivalent clinical experience and skill levels. Other critics have argued that staffing may actually decline with ratios since they might be used as the ceiling or as ironclad criteria if institutions are not willing to make adjustments for patient acuity or RN skill level. Vessey, Andres, Fountain, and Wheeler (2002) also suggest that mandatory staffing ratios create significant opportunity costs that may restrict employers and payors from responding to market forces; subsequently they may not be able to take advantage of improved technological support or respond to changes in patient acuity.

The bottom line, however, is that minimum staffing ratios would not have been proposed in the first place had staffing abuses and the resultant declines in the quality of patient care not occurred in the past. The implementation and subsequent evaluation of mandatory staffing ratios in California, beginning in 2004, should provide greater insight to the ongoing debate about the need for mandatory staffing ratios.

Learning Exercise 17.1

Comparing Staffing Ratios
California has often served as a bellwether for national healthcare trends and, surely the rest of the nation will be monitoring the implementation of minimum staffing ratios and assessing outcomes (Kovner, 2000).
Assignment: Compare the current staffing ratios used at the facility in which you work or do clinical practicums with those shown in Display 17. 2. How do they compare? Is there an effort to legislate minimum staffing ratios in the state in which you live? Who or what would you anticipate to be the greatest barrier to implementation of staffing ratios in your state?

Staffing and Scheduling Options

It is beyond the scope of this book to discuss all the creative staffing and scheduling options available and thus only a few are discussed here. Some of the more frequently used creative staffing and scheduling options include:

- 10- or 12-hour shifts
- Premium pay for weekend work
- Part-time staffing pool for weekend shifts and holidays
- Cyclical staffing, which allows long-term knowledge of future work schedules because a set staffing pattern is repeated every few weeks. **Figure 17.1** shows a master staffing pattern that repeats every four weeks.
- Job sharing
- Allowing nurses to exchange hours of work among themselves
- Flextime
- Use of supplemental staffing from outside registries and float pools
- Staff self-scheduling

There are advantages and disadvantages to each type of scheduling. Because extending the workday with 10- or 12-hour shifts may require overtime pay, the resultant nurse satisfaction must be weighed against the increased costs. Additionally, extending the length of shifts may result in increased judgment errors as nurses become fatigued. For this reason, many organizations limit the number of consecutive 10- or 12-hour days a nurse can work or the number of hours that can be worked in a given day.

Position	Name	Week I							Week II							Week III							Week IV						
		S	M	T	W	T	F	S	S	M	T	W	T	F	S	S	M	T	W	T	F	S	S	M	T	W	T	F	S
Full time	RN 1				X		X		X					X					X		X		X					X	
Full time	RN 2	X				X						X		X		X					X					X			X
Full time	RN 3		X				X		X			X					X				X		X				X		
Full time	RN 4	X			X							X		X		X			X								X		X
Full time	RN 5				X		X		X					X					X		X		X					X	
Full time	RN 6	X			X					X					X	X			X					X				X	
Full time	RN 7		X				X		X			X					X				X		X			X			
Full time	RN 8	X				X						X		X		X			X					X					X
Part time 8 hrs/wk	RN 9	On													On	On													On
Part time 8 hrs/wk	RN 10							On	On													On	On						
Part time 8 hrs/wk	RN 11	On													On	On													On
Part time 8 hrs/wk	RN 12							On	On													On	On						
Total RNs on duty each day		6	7	7	6	6	6	6	6	7	7	6	6	6	6	6	7	7	6	6	6	6	6	7	6	7	6	6	6

Elements: Every other weekend off   Number of split days off each period: 2   X: Scheduled day off
Maximum days worked: 4   Operates in multiples of 4, 8, 12...
Minimum days worked: 2   Schedule repeats itself every 4 weeks

Figure 17.1 Four-week cycle master time sheet.

 Learning Exercise 17.2

Choosing 8- or 12-Hour Shifts
You are the manager of an intensive care unit. Many of the nurses have approached you requesting 12-hour shifts. Other nurses have approached you stating that they will transfer out of the unit if 12-hour shifts are implemented. You are exploring the feasibility and cost-effectiveness of using both 8-hour and 12-hour shifts so that staff could select which type of scheduling they wanted.
Assignment: Would this create a scheduling nightmare? Will you limit the number of 12-hour shifts staff could work in a week? Would you pay overtime for the last four hours of the 12-hour shift? Would you allow staff to choose freely between 8- and 12-hour shifts? What other problems may result from mixing 8- and 12-hour shifts?

Another increasingly common staffing and scheduling alternative is the use of supplemental nursing staff such as *agency nurses* or *travel nurses*. These nurses are usually directly employed by an external nursing broker and work for premium pay (often two to three times that of a regularly employed staff nurse), without benefits. While such staff provide scheduling relief, especially in response to unanticipated increases in census or patient acuity, their continuous use is expensive and can result in poor continuity of nursing care.

Some hospitals have created their own internal supplemental staff by hiring *per-diem* employees and creating *float pools*. Per-diem staff generally have the flexibility to choose if and when they want to work. In exchange for this flexibility, they receive a higher rate of pay, but usually no benefits. Float pools are generally composed of employees who agree to cross train on multiple units so that they can work additional hours during periods of high census or worker shortages. Wing (2001) argues, however, that float pools are adequate for filling intermittent staffing holes but, like agency or registry staff, are not an answer to the ongoing need to alter staffing according to census. In addition, they result in a lack of staff continuity.

Some organizations have made an effort to meet the needs of a diverse workforce by using flextime and self-scheduling. *Flextime* is a system that allows employees to select the time schedules that best meet their personal needs while still meeting work responsibilities. In the past, most flextime has been possible only for nurses in roles that did not require continuous coverage. However, staff nurses recently have been able to take part in a flextime system through prescheduled shift start times. Variable start times may be longer or shorter than the normal 8-hour workday. When a hospital uses flextime, units have employees coming and leaving the unit at many different times. Although flextime staffing creates greater employee choices, it may be difficult for the manager to coordinate and could easily result in overstaffing or understaffing.

Developed in the 1960s, *self-scheduling* allows nurses in a unit to work together to construct their own schedules rather than have schedules created by management. With self-scheduling, employees typically are given four to six week schedule worksheets to fill out several weeks in advance of when the schedule is to begin. These employees typically have one to two weeks to fill in the blanks on the schedule, following whatever guidelines or requirements are set by management (i.e., number of weekend shifts that must be worked, maximum number of consecutive shifts) (Hung, 2002). The nurse–manager then reviews the worksheet to make sure all guidelines or requirements have been met.

Although self-scheduling offers nurses greater control over their work environment, it is not easy to implement. Success depends on the leadership skills of the manager to support the staff and demonstrate patience and perseverance throughout the implementation.

In a review of self-scheduling research, Shullanberger (2000) found that self-scheduling provides greater worker participation in decision making but requires greater worker involvement and management flexibility to be successful. Self-scheduling also saves management time, improves morale and professionalism, and reduces personnel turnover (Hung, 2002). Those nurses most satisfied with self-scheduling were those who shared responsibility for adequate staffing and those who had developed good negotiating skills.

Obviously, all scheduling and staffing patterns, from traditional to creative, have shortcomings. Therefore, any changes in current policies should be evaluated carefully as they are implemented. Because all scheduling and staffing patterns have a heavy impact on employees personal lives, productivity, and budgets, it is wise to have a six-month trial of new staffing and scheduling changes, with an evaluation at the end of that time to determine the impact on financial costs, retention, productivity, risk management, and employee and patient satisfaction.

> Self-scheduling provides greater worker participation in decision making but requires greater worker involvement and management flexibility to be successful.

Learning Exercise 17.3

Self-Scheduling Holiday Dilemma

You graduated last year from your nursing program and were excited to obtain the job you wanted most. The unit where you work has a very progressive supervisor who believes in empowering the nursing staff.

Approximately six months ago, after considerable instruction, the unit began self-scheduling. You have enjoyed the freedom and control this has given you over your work hours. There have been some minor difficulties among staff, and occasionally the unit was slightly overstaffed or understaffed, but overall the self-scheduling has seemed to work well.

Today (September 15), you come to work on the 3 PM to 11 PM shift after two days off and see that the schedule for the upcoming Thanksgiving and Christmas holiday period has been posted, and many of the staff have already scheduled their days on and their days off. When you take a close look, it appears that no one has signed up to work Christmas Eve, Thanksgiving Day, or Christmas Day. You are very concerned because self-scheduling includes responsibility for adequate coverage. There are still a few nurses, including yourself, who have not added their days to the schedule, but even if all the remaining nurses worked all three holidays, it would provide only scant coverage.

Assignment: What leadership role (if any) should you take in solving this dilemma? Should you ignore the problem and schedule yourself for only one holiday and let your supervisor deal with the issue? Remember, you are a new nurse, both in experience and on this unit. List the options for decision making available to you and, using rationale to support your decision, plan a course of action.

WORKLOAD MEASUREMENT TOOLS

Requirements for staffing are based on whatever standard unit of measurement for productivity is used in a given unit. A formula for calculating nursing care hours per patient day (NCH/PPD) is reviewed in **Figure 17.2.** This is the simplest formula in use and continues to be used widely. In this formula, all nursing and ancillary staff are treated equally for determining hours of nursing care and no differentiation is made for differing acuity levels of patients. These two factors alone may result in an incomplete or even inaccurate picture of nursing care needs. Jennings, Loan, DePaul, Brosch, and Hildreth (2001) concur, suggesting that the use of NCH/PPD as a workload measurement tool may be too restrictive, since it may not represent the reality of today's inpatient care setting, where staffing fluctuates not only among shifts, but within shifts.

At the national level, the use of a PCS is a condition for participation in Medicare and is required by the Joint Commission for certification.

$$\text{NCH/PPD} = \frac{\text{Nursing Hours Worked in 24 Hours}}{\text{Patient Census}}$$

Figure 17.2 Standard formula for calculating nursing care hours (NCH) per patient-day (PPD).

As a result, *patient classification systems* (PCS), also known as *workload management*, or *patient acuity tools*, were developed in the 1960s. *PCSs* group patients according to specific characteristics that measure acuity of illness in an effort to determine both the number and mix of the staff needed to adequately care for those patients. Because other variables within the system have an impact on nursing care hours, it is usually not possible to transfer a patient classification system from one facility to another. Instead, each basic classification system must be modified to fit a specific institution.

Seago (2002) suggests that most PCSs can be classified as either the *critical indicator* or *criterion* type or the *summative task* type. The critical indicator PCS uses broad indicators such as bathing, diet, intravenous fluids and medications, and positioning to categorize patient care activities. The summative task type requires the nurse to note the frequency of occurrence of specific activities, treatments, and procedures for each patient. For example, a summative task type PCS might ask the nurse whether a patient required nursing time for teaching, elimination, or hygiene. Both types of PCSs are generally filled out prior to each shift although the summative task type typically has more items to fill out than the critical incident or criterion type (Agency for Healthcare Research and Quality).

Once an appropriate PCS is adopted, hours of nursing care must be assigned for each patient classification. Although an appropriate number of hours of care for each classification is generally suggested by companies marketing patient classification systems, each institution is unique and must determine to what degree that classification system must be adapted for them. White (2003) suggests that each patient population is different and that each unit must examine clinical profiles of patients, average length of stay, and practitioner specialty in defining their patient population. In addition, staff competency, core staff versus visiting staff, and skill mix must be considered (White, 2003).

Federal and state regulations mandating the use of a PCS to determine staffing levels have increased since the 1990s. At the national level, use of a PCS is a condition for participation in Medicare and is required by the Joint Commission for certification (O'Bryan, Krueger, & Lusk, 2002). In California, objective staffing systems, driven by patient acuity or need, are mandated by Title 22 (O'Bryan, et. al., 2002; Seago, 2002).

Any patient classification system has many variables, and all systems have their faults. It is a mistake for managers to think that patient classification systems will solve all staffing problems. Although such systems provide a better definition of problems, it is up to people in the organization to make judgments and use the information obtained by the system appropriately to solve staffing problems. A sample classification system is illustrated in **Table 17.1.**

Table 17.1 Patient Care Classification Using Four Levels of Nursing Care Intensity

Area of Care	Category 1	Category 2	Category 3	Category 4
Eating	Feeds self or needs little food	Needs some help in preparing; may need encouragement	Cannot feed self but is able to chew and swallow	Cannot feed self and may have difficulty swallowing
Grooming	Almost entirely self-sufficient	Needs some help in bathing, oral hygiene, hair combing, and so forth	Unable to do much for self	Completely dependent
Excretion	Up and to bathroom alone or almost alone	Needs some help in getting up to bathroom or using urinal	In bed, needs bedpan or urinal placed; may be able to partially turn or lift self	Completely dependent
Comfort	Self-sufficient	Needs some help with adjusting position or bed (e.g., tubes, IVs)	Cannot turn without help, get drink, adjust position of extremities, and so forth	Completely dependent
General health	Good—in for diagnostic procedure, simple treatment, or surgical procedure (D & C, biopsy, minor fracture)	Mild symptoms—more than one mild illness, mild debility, mild emotional reaction, mild incontinence (not more than once per shift)	Acute symptoms—severe emotional reaction to illness or surgery, more than one acute illness, medical or surgical problem, severe or frequent incontinence	Critically ill—may have severe emotional reaction

Table 17.1 Patient Care Classification Using Four Levels of Nursing Care Intensity

Area of Care	Category 1	Category 2	Category 3	Category 4
Treatments	Simple— supervised ambulation, dangle, simple dressing, test procedure preparation not requiring medication, reinforcement of surgical dressing, x-pad, vital signs once per shift	Any category 1 treatment more than once per shift, Foley catheter care, I & O; bladder irrigations, sitz bath, compresses, test procedures requiring medications of follow-ups, simple enema for evacuation, vital signs every four hours	Any treatment more than twice per shift, medicated IVs, complicated dressings, sterile procedures, care of tracheotomy, Harris flush, suctioning, tube feeding, vital signs more than every four hours	Any elaborate or delicate procedure requiring two nurses, vital signs more often than every two hours
Medications	Simple, routine, not needing preevaluation or post-evaluation; medications no more than once per shift	Diabetic, cardiac, hypotensive, hypertensive, diuretic, anticoagulant medications, prn medications, more than once per shift, medications needing preevaluation or postevaluation	Unusual amount of category 2 medications; control of refractory diabetics (need to be monitored more than every four hours)	More intensive category 3 medications; IVs with frequent, close observation and regulation

continued

Table 17.1 Patient Care Classification Using Four Levels of Nursing Care Intensity

Area of Care	Category 1	Category 2	Category 3	Category 4
Teaching and emotional support	Routine follow-up teaching; patients with no unusual or adverse emotional reactions	Initial teaching of care of ostomies; new diabetics; tubes that will be in place for periods of time; conditions requiring major change in eating, living, or excretory practices; patients with mild adverse reactions to their illness (e.g., depression, overly demanding)	More intensive category 2 items; teaching of apprehensive or mildly resistive patients; care of moderately upset or apprehensive patients; confused or disoriented patients	Teaching of resistive patients, care and support of patients with severe emotional reaction

The middle-level manager must be alert to internal or external forces affecting unit needs that may not be reflected in the organization's patient care classification system. Examples of such forces could be a sudden increase in nursing or medical students using the unit, a lower skill level of new graduates, or cultural and language difficulties of recently hired foreign nurses. The organization's classification system may prove to be inaccurate, or the hours allotted for each category or classification of patient may be inadequate. This does not imply that unit managers should not be held accountable for the standard unit of measurement, but rather they must be cognizant of justifiable reasons for variations.

Some futurists have suggested that eventually *workload measurement* systems may replace acuity-based staffing systems. Workload measurement is a relatively new technique that evaluates work performance as well as necessary resource levels (Walsh, 2003). Thus, it goes beyond patient diagnosis or acuity level, and examines the specific number of care hours needed to meet a given population's care needs. Thus, workload measurement systems capture census data, care hours, patient acuity, and patient activities. This tool, while more complicated, holds great promise for better predicting the nursing resources needed to staff hospitals effectively.

Regardless of the workload measurement tool used (NCH/PPD, PCS, workload measurement system, etc), the units of workload measurement that are used need to be reviewed periodically and adjusted as necessary. This is both a leadership role and a management responsibility.

Learning Exercise 17.4

Calculating Staffing Needs

You use a PCS to assist you with your daily staffing needs. The following are the hours of nursing care needed for each acuity level patient per shift:

	Category I Acuity Level	Category II Acuity Level	Category III Acuity Level	Category IV Acuity Level
NCHPPD needed for day shift	2.3	2.9	3.4	4.6
NCHPPD needed for P.M. shift	2.0	2.3	2.8	3.4
NCHPPD needed for night shift	0.5	1.0	2.0	2.8

When you came on duty this morning, you had the following patients:

1 patient in category I acuity level
2 patients in category II acuity level
3 patients in category III acuity level
1 patient in category IV acuity level

Note that you must be overstaffed or understaffed by more than one half of the hours a person is working to reduce or add staff. For example, for nurses working 8-hour shifts, the staffing must be over or under more than four hours to delete or add staff.

Assignment: Calculate your staffing needs for the day shift. You have on duty one RN and one LVN/LPN working 8-hour shifts and a ward clerk for four hours. Are you understaffed or overstaffed?

If you had the same number of patients, but the acuity levels were the following, would your staffing needs be the same?

2 patients in category I acuity level
3 patients in category II acuity level
2 patients in category III acuity level
0 patients in category IV acuity level

THE RELATIONSHIP BETWEEN NURSING CARE HOURS, STAFFING MIX, AND QUALITY OF CARE

It is difficult to pick up a nursing journal today that does not have at least one article that speaks to the relationship between nursing care hours, staffing mix, and quality of care. This has occurred in response to the "restructuring" and "reengineering" boom that occurred in many acute care hospitals in the 1990s. Restructuring and reengineering was done to reduce costs, increase efficiency, decrease waste and duplication, and reshape the way care was delivered (Urden & Walston, 2001).

Given that health care is labor intensive, cost cutting under restructuring and reengineering often included staffing models that reduced RN representation in the staffing mix and increased the use of unlicensed assistive personnel (UAP). This fairly rapid and dramatic shift in both registered nurse care hours and staffing mix provided fertile ground for comparative studies that examined the relationship between nursing care hours, staffing mix, and patient outcomes.

Although early research on nursing care hours, staffing mix, and patient outcomes lacked standardization in terms of tools used and measures examined, nationwide attention shifted to this issue and a plethora of better funded and more rigorous scientific study followed. A current review of the literature consistently and overwhelmingly demonstrates that as RN hours decrease in NCHPPD, adverse patient outcomes increase, including increased medication errors and patient falls and decreased patient satisfaction with pain management (Kovner, Jones, & Gergen, 2000; Sovie & Jawad, 2001; Agency for Healthcare Research and Quality, 2001; Clarke, 2003; Potter, Barr, McSweeney & Sledge, 2003; Huston, 2001).

Unit managers must understand the effect that major restructuring and redesign have on their staffing and scheduling policies as well. As new practice models are introduced, there must be a simultaneous examination of the existing staff mix and patient care assessments to ensure that appropriate changes are made in staffing and scheduling policies.

For example, decreasing licensed staff, increasing numbers of unlicensed assistive staff, and developing new practice models have a tremendous impact on patient care assignment methods. Past practices of relying on part-time staff, responding to staff preferences for work, and providing a variety of shift lengths and shift rotations may no longer be enough. Administrative practices also have saved money in the past by sending people home when there was low census; they have also floated them to other areas to cover other unit needs, not scheduled staff for consecutive shifts because of staff preferences, and had scheduling polices that were unreasonably accommodating. Lastly, patient assignments in the past were often made without attention to patient continuity and assigned by numbers rather than workload. Some of these past practices have benefited staff, and some have been for the benefit of the organization, but few of them have benefited the patient. Indeed, assigning a different nurse to care for a patient each day of an already reduced length of stay may contribute to negative patient outcomes.

Therefore, there must be an honest appraisal of current staffing, scheduling, and assignment policies simultaneously as organizations are restructured and new practice models are engineered. Changing these policies often has far-reaching consequences, but in order for new models of care to be successfully implemented this must be done. For example, if primary nursing is to be effective, then nurses must work a number of successive days with a client to ensure there is time to formulate and evaluate a plan of care. In this example, floating policies and requests for days off may need to be changed or modified to fit the philosophy of primary nursing care delivery.

Shullanberger (2000) states that having an adequate number of knowledgeable, trained nurses is imperative to attaining desired patient outcomes. Ascertaining an appropriate skill mix depends on the patient care setting, acuity of patients, and other factors. There is no national standard to determine whether staffing decisions are suitable for a given setting. Additionally, many of the tools and methods used to determine staffing have been unreliable and invalid, either in their development or their application (Shullanberger, 2000). However, some formulas developed recently

A current review of the literature consistently and overwhelmingly demonstrates that patient outcomes improve as RN hours increase in NCH/PPD.

allow for adjustment for variations in the skill mix of staff. These formulas are still relatively new but may be a better tool to use when making staffing decisions (Budreau et al., 1999). In addition, Manthey (2001) describes several factors that will drive additional new staffing plans in the coming decade. These factors, which she calls "Work Force 2000," include the increased importation of foreign nurses who must be safely incorporated into the care delivery system, ongoing fiscal restraints that result in the need for lean staffing, and plentiful, attractive career options for nurses outside the hospital.

GENERATIONAL CONSIDERATIONS FOR STAFFING

Some researchers suggest that the different generations represented in nursing today have different value systems, which may impact staffing (**Display 17.3**). Hill (2004) describes the "*veteran generation*" as those nurses born between 1925 and 1942. Having lived through several international military conflicts (World War II, the Korean War, and Vietnam), they're often risk adverse regarding personal finances, respectful of authority, supportive of hierarchy, and disciplined (Hill). Therefore, these nurses may be less likely to question staffing assignments and may work best in a more structured patient care delivery system.

McNeese-Smith and Crook (2003) posit that the *boom generation* (born between 1943 and 1960) and the *silent generation* (born between 1925 and 1942) have more traditional work values and ethics; however, the boomers are more materialistic and are willing to work long hours at their jobs. Hill (2004) points out, however, that many nurses in the boomer age group have been taught from a young age to think as individuals and to express themselves creatively. These nurses then may be best suited for staffing assignments that require flexibility, independent thinking, and creativity.

Generation Xers (born between 1961 and 1981), in contrast, may lack the interest in lifetime employment at one place that prior generations have valued; instead, this generation values the more flexible part-time and 12-hour shift options (McNeese-Smith & Crook, 2003). Hill (2004) argues this is because

Display 17.3	Generational Work Groups	
Generation	**Year of Birth**
Silent Generation or Veteran Generation	1925 to 1942
Baby Boomer or Boom	1943 to early 1960s
Generation X	Early 1960s to 1980
Generation Y	Late 1970s to 1986

Source: Adapted from Hill, K. S. (2004). Defy the decades with multigenerational teams. *Nursing Management, 35*(1), 32–35; McNeese-Smith, D.K., & Crook, M. (2003). Nursing values and a changing nurse workforce: Values, age, and job stages. *Journal of Nursing Administration, 33*(5), 260–270; Martin, C. A. (April 2003). Transcend generational timelines. *Nursing Management, 34*(4), 25–26, 28.

and accuracy in any system, the longer the time required to make staffing computations. Perhaps the greatest danger in staffing by acuity is that many organizations are unable to supply the extra staff when the system shows unit understaffing. However, the same organization may use the acuity-based staffing system to justify reducing staff on an overstaffed unit. Therefore, a staffing classification system can be demotivating if used inconsistently or incorrectly.

Employees have the right to expect a reasonable workload. Managers must ensure that adequate staffing exists to meet the needs of staff and patients. Managers who constantly expect employees to work extra shifts, stay overtime, and carry unreasonable patient assignments are not being ethically accountable.

Effective managers, however, do not focus totally on numbers of personnel, but look at all components of productivity; they examine nursing duties, job descriptions, patient care organization, staffing mix, and staff competencies. Such managers also use every opportunity to build a productive and cohesive team.

Uncomplaining nursing staff have often put forth superhuman efforts during periods of short staffing simply because they believed in their supervisor and in the organization. However, just as often the opposite has occurred: Units that were only moderately understaffed spent an inordinate amount of time and wasted energy complaining about their plight. The difference between the two examples has much to do with trust that such conditions are the exception, not the norm; that real solutions and not Band-Aid approaches to problem solving will be used to plan for the future; that management will work just as hard as the staff in meeting patient needs; and that the organization's overriding philosophy is based on patient interest and not financial gain.

Developing Staffing and Scheduling Policies

Nurses will be more satisfied in the workplace if staffing and scheduling policies and procedures are clearly communicated to all employees. Written policies provide a means for greater consistency and fairness. Personnel policies represent the standard of action that is communicated in advance so that employees are not caught unaware regarding personnel matters. In addition to being standardized, personnel policies should be written in a manner that allows some flexibility. A leadership challenge for the manager is to develop policies that focus on outcomes rather than constraints or rules that limit responsiveness to individual employee needs.

Scheduling and staffing policies should be reviewed and updated periodically. When formulating policies, management must examine its own philosophy and consider prevailing community practices. Unit-level managers will seldom have complete responsibility for formulating organizational personnel policies but should have some input as policies are reviewed. There are, however, nursing department and unit personnel policies that supervisors develop and implement.

The policies in **Display 17.4** should be formalized by the manager and communicated to all personnel. To ensure that unit-level staffing policies do not conflict with higher-level policies, there should be adequate input from the staff and they should be developed in collaboration with personnel and nursing departments. For example, some states have labor laws that prohibit 12-hour shifts. Other states

Display 17.4 Unit Checklist of Employee Staffing Policies

1. The person responsible for the staffing schedule and the authority of that individual if it is other than the employee's immediate supervisor
2. Type and length of staffing cycle used
3. Rotation policies, if shift rotation is used
4. Fixed shift transfer policies, if fixed shifts are used
5. Time and location of schedule posting
6. When shift begins and ends
7. Day of week schedule begins
8. Weekend off policy
9. Tardiness policy
10. Low census procedures
11. Policy for trading days off
12. Procedures for days-off requests
13. Absenteeism policies
14. Policy regarding rotating to other units
15. Procedures for vacation time requests
16. Procedures for holiday time requests
17. Procedures for resolving conflicts regarding requests for days off, holidays, or requested time off
18. Emergency request policies
19. Policies and procedures regarding requesting transfer to other units

allow workers to sign away their rights to overtime pay for shifts greater than 8 or 12 hours. Additionally, in organizations with union contracts, many staffing and scheduling policies are incorporated into the union contract. In such cases, staffing changes might need to be negotiated at the time of contract renewal.

INTEGRATING LEADERSHIP ROLES AND MANAGEMENT FUNCTIONS IN STAFFING

The manager is responsible for providing adequate staffing to meet patient care needs. Attention must be paid to fluctuations in patient census and workload units to ensure that understaffing or overstaffing is minimized and to ensure fiscal accountability to the organization. The prudent manager involves employees when developing unit staffing and scheduling policies and ascertains that adopted policies are not in violation of organizational policies, union contracts, or labor laws.

When leadership roles are integrated with management functions, creative staffing and scheduling options can occur. Knowing that staff needs are in part related to work design, the prudent leader–manager looks for ways to redesign work to reduce staffing needs.

The leader keeps abreast of changes in community and national trends and uses contemporary methods of staffing and scheduling. The leader also assumes an ethical accountability to patients and employees for adequate and appropriate staffing.

Unit policies are reviewed and revised on a timely basis. Additionally, the leader is alert for factors that affect the standard of productivity and negotiates changes in the standard when appropriate.

The effective leader–manager knows that establishing trust helps build the team spirit needed to deal with temporary staff shortages. The leader also looks for innovative methods to overcome staffing difficulties.

✳ Key Concepts

- The manager has both a fiscal and ethical duty to plan for adequate staffing to meet patient care needs.
- Innovative and creative methods of staffing and scheduling should be explored to avoid understaffing and overstaffing as patient census and acuity fluctuate.
- Staffing and scheduling policies must not violate labor laws, state laws, or union contracts.
- Workload measurement tools include NCH/PPD, PCS, and workload measurement systems. All workload measurement tools should be periodically reviewed to determine if they are a valid and reliable tool for measure staffing needs in a given organization.
- Mandatory overtime should be a last resort and not standard operating procedure because an institution does not have enough staff.
- Research clearly shows that as RN representation in the skill mix increases, patient outcomes improve and adverse incidents decline.
- Fair and uniform staffing and scheduling policies and procedures must be written and communicated to all staff.
- Existing staffing policies must be examined periodically to determine if they still meet the needs of the staff and the organization.

More Learning Exercises and Applications

Learning Exercise 17.5

Implementing a New Nursing Care Delivery Model
You are serving on an ad-hoc committee to examine ways to improve the continuity of patient assignments because your unit is thinking about switching from total patient care to a primary nursing care delivery model. The committee is having a difficult time formulating policies because you currently have a great number of nurses who work part-time, two days on and two days off. Additionally, your unit has a census that goes up and down unexpectedly, resulting in nurses being floated out of the unit often. The committee is committed to providing continuity of care in the new patient care delivery system.
Assignment: Develop some scheduling and staffing policies that have the probability of increasing continuity of assignment and will not result in a financial liability to the unit. How will these policies be fairly executed, and do they have the potential to cause staff to leave the unit?

Learning Exercise 17.6

Making Sound Staffing Decisions

You are the staffing coordinator for a small community hospital. It is now 12:30 P.M. and your staffing plan for the 3–11 P.M. shift must be completed no later than 1 P.M. (The union contract stipulates that any "call offs" that must be done for low census must be done at least two hours before the shift begins, or employees receive a minimum of four hours of pay.) You do, however, have the prerogative to call off staff for only half a shift (four hours). If they are needed for the last half of the shift (7–11 P.M.), you must notify them by 5 P.M. tonight. A local outside registry is available for supplemental staff; however, their cost is two and a half times that of your regular staff, so you must use this resource sparingly. Mandatory overtime is also used, but only as a last resort.

The current hospital census is 52 patients although the emergency department is very busy and has four possible patient admits. There are also two patients with confirmed discharge orders and three additional potential discharges on the 3–11 P.M. shift. All units have just submitted their PCS calculations for the 3–11 P.M. shift

You have five units to staff: the ICU, pediatrics, obstetrics (includes labor, delivery and post-partum), medical, and surgical departments. The ICU department must be staffed with a minimum of a 1:2 nurse–patient ratio. The pediatric unit is generally staffed at a 1:4 nurse–patient ratio and the medical and surgical departments at a 1:6 ratio. In obstetrics, a 1:2 ratio is used for labor and delivery and a 1:6 ratio is used in post-partum.

On reviewing the staffing you note the following:

ICU

Census = 6. Unit capacity = 8. The PCS shows a current patient acuity level requiring 3.2 staff. One of the potential admits in the ER is a patient who would need cardiac monitoring. One patient, however, will likely be transferred to the medical floor on 3–11 P.M. shift. Four RNs are assigned for the 3–11 p.m. shift.

Pediatrics

Census = 8. Unit capacity = 10. The PCS shows a current acuity level requiring 2.4 staff. There are two RNs and one CNA assigned for the 3–11 P.M. shift. There are no anticipated discharges or transfers.

Obstetrics

Census = 6. Unit capacity = 8. Three women are in active labor and three women are in the post-partum unit with their babies. Two RNs are assigned to the Obstetrics department for the 3–11 p.m shift. There are no in-house staff on 3–11 P.M. shift that have been cross trained for this unit.

Medical Floor

Census = 19. Unit capacity = 24. The PCS shows a current acuity level requiring 4.4 staff. There are two RNs, one LVN, and two CNA assigned for the 3–11 P.M. shift. Three of the potential emergency department admits would come to this floor. Two of the potential patient discharges are on this unit.

Surgical Floor
Census = 13. Unit capacity = 18. The PCS shows a current acuity level requiring 3.6 staff. Because of sick calls, you have only one RN and two CNAs assigned for the 3–11 P.M. shift. Both confirmed patient discharges as well as one of the potential discharges are from this unit.
Assignment: Answer the following questions.
1. Which units are overstaffed and which are understaffed?
2. Of those units that are overstaffed, what will you do with the unneeded staff?
3. How will you staff units that are understaffed? Were outside registry or mandatory overtime used?
4. Did staffing mix and PCS acuity levels factor into your decisions?
5. What safeguards can you build into the staffing plan for unanticipated admissions or changes in patient acuity during the shift?

 Learning Exercise 17.7

Reviewing Pros and Cons of Staffing Solutions
You are serving on a committee to help resolve a chronic problem with short staffing on your unit, a pediatric intensive care unit. Volunteer overtime, cross-training with the regular nonintensive care pediatric unit, and closed-unit staffing have been suggested as possible solutions.
Assignment: Make a list of the pros and cons of each of these suggestions to bring back to the committee for review. Share your list with group members.

Learning Exercise 17.8

Choosing a Delivery Care Model and Staffing Pattern

You have been hired as the unit supervisor of the new Rehabilitation Unit at Memorial Hospital. Memorial Hospital decentralizes the responsibility for staffing, but you must adhere to the following constraints:

1. All staff must be licensed staff.
2. The ratio of LVNs/LPNs to RNs is one to one.
3. An RN must always be on duty.
4. Your budgeted NCH/PPD is 8.2.
5. You are not counted into the NCH/PPD, but ward clerks are counted.
6. Your unit capacity is seven, and you anticipate a daily average census of six.
7. You may use any mode of patient care organization.

   Your patients will be chronic, not acute, but will be admitted for an active 2- to 12-week rehabilitation program. The emphasis will be in returning the patient home with adequate ability to perform activities of daily living. Many other disciplines, including occupational and physical therapy, will be part of the rehabilitation team. A waiting list for the beds is anticipated because this service is needed in your community. You anticipate that the majority of your patients will have had cerebrovascular accidents, spinal cord injuries, other problems with neurological deficits, and amputations.

   You have hired four full-time RNs and two part-time RNs. The part-time RNs would like to have at least two days of work in a two-week pay period; in return for this work guarantee, they have agreed to cover for most sick days and vacations and some holidays for your regular RN full-time staff.

   You also have hired three full-time LVNs/LPNs and two part-time LVNs/LPNs. However, the part-time LVNs/LPNs would like to work at least three days per week. You have decided not to hire a ward clerk but to use the pediatric ward clerk four hours each day to assist with various duties. Therefore, you need to calculate the ward clerk's four hours each day into the total hours worked.

   You have researched various types of patient care delivery models (see Chapter 14) and staffing patterns. Your newly hired staff is willing to experiment with any type of patient care delivery model and staffing pattern that you select.

Assignment: Determine what patient care delivery model and staffing pattern you will use. Explain why and how you made the choice you did. Next, show a 24-hour and 7-day staffing pattern. Were you able to create a schedule that adhered to the given constraints? Was this a time-consuming process?

Web Links

California Nurses Association Position Statement on RN Staffing Ratio
http://www.calnurse.org/12202/posrnlvn202.html
Argues in support of CA AB 394 and differentiates between scope of practice of RNs and LVNs in staffing ratios.

American Nurses Association (2002). Background Information and Legislative Maps. Nurse Staffing Plans and Ratios
http://www.nursingworld.org/GOVA/STATE/2004/staffing.pdf
Addresses need for nurse staffing ratios.

American Medical Directors Association
http://www.amda.com/library/governance/resolutions/h02.htm
Resolution and position statements on direct care staffing in nursing homes.

National Academies Press
http://www.nap.edu/books/0309053986/html/241.html
Information regarding the congressionally mandated study of the adequacy of nurse staffing in hospitals and nursing facilities by the Institute of Medicine, entitled. Nursing Staff in Hospitals and Nursing Homes: Is It Adequate? (1996).

References

Agency for Healthcare Research and Quality. (2001). *Nurse staffing. Models of care delivery and interventions.* (AHRQ Publication No. 01-EO58). Rockville, MD: Seago, J.

Aiken, L. H., Clarke, S. P., & Sloane, D. M. (2000). Hospital restructuring. Does it adversely affect care and outcomes? *Journal of Nursing Administration, 30*(10), 457–465.

Budreau, G., Balakrishnan, R., Titler, M., & Hafner, M. J. (1999). Caregiver-patient ratio: Capturing census and staffing variability. *Nursing Economic$, 17*(6), 317–325.

Calarco, M. M. (2001). Given the nursing shortage, is mandatory overtime a necessary evil? *Nursing Leadership Forum, 6*(2), 33–35.

California Nurses Association (2003a). *RN staffing ratios: It's the law.* Available at: http://www.calnurse.org/102103/safestaffqa.html. Retrieved November 26, 2003.

California Nurses Association. (2003b). RN alert. Final ratios approved. CNA wins protection for RNs. Available at: http://www.calnurse.org/finalrat/finratrn7103.pdf. Retrieved November 28, 2003.

Clarke, S. P. (2003). Balancing staffing and safety. *Nursing Management, 34*(6), 44–48.

Graf, C. M., Millar, S., Feilteau, C., Coakley, P. J., & Erickson, J. I. (2003). Patients' needs for nursing care. *Journal of Nursing Administration, 33*(2), 76–81.

Hill, K. S. (2004). Defy the decades with multigenerational teams. *Nursing Management, 35*(1), 32–35.

Hopkins, M. E. (2000). *Tip of the iceberg. Amid a sea of hot button issues, staffing ratios rise to the surface.* Nurseweek. Available at: http://www.nurseweek.com/news/features/00-10/wages.asp. Retrieved November 26, 2003.

Hung, R. (2002). A note on nurse self-scheduling. *Nursing Economic$, 20*(1), 37–39.

Huston, C. (2001). Contemporary staffing mix changes: Impact on post-operative pain management. *Pain Management Nursing, 2*(2), 65–72.

Huston, C. (2002). The role of the case manager in a disease management program. *Lippincott's Case Management.* Baltimore, MD: Lippincott.

Jennings, B. M., Loan, L. A., DePaul, D., Brosch, L. & Hildreth, P. (2001). Lessons learned while collecting ANA indicator data. *Journal of Nursing Administration, 31*(1), 121–129.

Kovner, C. T. (2000). State regulation of RN-to-patient ratios. *American Journal of Nursing, 100*(11), 61–63.

Kovner, C. T., Jones, C. B., & Gergen, P. J. (2000). Nurse staffing in acute care hospitals, 1990–1969. *Policy, Politics, & Nursing Practice, 1*(3), 194–204.

Malloch, K., Davenport, S. & Hatler, C. (2003). Nursing workforce management. Using benchmarking for planning and outcomes monitoring. *Journal of Nursing Administration, 33*(10), 538–543.

Manthey, M. (September 2001). A core incremental staffing plan. *Journal of Nursing Administration, 31*(9), 424–425.

Martin, C. A. (April 2003). Transcend generational timelines. *Nursing Management, 34*(4), 25–26, 28.

McNeese-Smith, D. K., & Crook, M. (2003). Nursing values and a changing nurse workforce: Values, age, and job stages. *Journal of Nursing Administration, 33*(5), 260–270.

Mee, C. L. (2001). Dear colleague. Mandatory madness. *Nursing 2001 31*(9), 6.

O'Bryan, L. O., Krueger, J., & Lusk, R. (2002). Rework the workload. *Nursing Management, 33*(3), 38–40.

Potter, P., Barr, N., McSweeney, M., & Sledge, J. (2003). Identifying nurse staffing and patient outcome relationships: A guide for change in care delivery. *Nursing Economic$, 21*(4), 158–166.

Seago, J. (2002). A comparison of two patient classification instruments in an acute care hospital. *Journal of Nursing Administration, 32*(5), 243–249.

Shullanberger, G. (2000). Nurse staffing decisions: An integrative review of the literature. *Nursing Economic$, 18*(3), 124–136.

Sovie, M. D. & Jawad, A. F. (2001). Hospital restructuring and its impact on outcomes. *Journal of Nursing Administration, 31*(12), 588–600.

Spetz, J. (2001). What should we expect from California's minimum nurse staffing legislation? *Journal of Nursing Administration, 31*(3), 132–140.

Urden, L. D., & Walston, S. L. (2001). Outcomes of hospital restructuring and reengineering. How is success or failure being measured? *Journal of Nursing Administration, 31*(4), 203–209.

Vernarec, E. (2000). Just say "no" to mandatory overtime? *RN, 63,*(12) 69–70, 72, 74.

Vessey, J. A., Andres, S., Fountain, M., & Wheeler, A. (2002). Rx for the nursing crisis? The economic impact of mandatory RN staffing to patient ratios. *Policy, Politics & Nursing Practice, 3*(3), 220–227.

Walsh, E. (2003). Get real with workload measurement. *Nursing Management, 34*(2), 38–42.

White, K. (2003). Effective staffing as a guardian of care. *Nursing Management, 34*(7), 20–24.

Wing, K. T. (2001). When flex comes to shove: Staffing and hospital census. *Nursing Management, 32*(1), 43–46.

Xu, Y. (2001). National standards for providing culturally and linguistically appropriate health care: Policy Implications for Nursing. *Nursing Economic$, 19*(5), 240–241.

Bibliography

Austin, S. (2000). Staffing: Knowing your liability. *Nursing Management, 311*(7), 19–20.

Blakeman Hodge, M., Asch, S. M., Olson, V. A., Kravitz, R. L. & Sauve, M. J. (2002). Developing indicators of nursing quality to evaluate nurse staffing ratios. *Journal of Nursing Administration, 32*(6), 338–345.

Buerhaus, P. I., & Needleman, J. (2000). Policy implications of research on nurse staffing and quality of patient care. *Policy, Politics & Nursing Practice, 1*(1), 5–16.

Charles, J. (2002). Ethical considerations. Mandatory overtime: Conflicts of conscience. *JONA's Healthcare Law, Ethics, and Regulation, 4*(1), 10–12.

DeWolf Bosek, M. S. (2001). Spotlight on . . . Mandatory overtime: Professional duty, harms, and justice. *JONA's Healthcare Law, Ethics, and Regulation. 3*(4), 99–102.

Gonzales-Torre, P. L., Adenso-Diaz, B., & Sanchez-Molero, O. (2002). Capacity planning in hospital nursing: A model for minimum staff calculation. *Nursing Economic$, 20*(1), 28–36.

Kany, K. (2001). Mandatory overtime. *American Journal of Nursing, 101*(5), 67–71.

Kaufman, S. (2000). Desperate strategies for last-minute staffing. *Nursing Management, 31*(1), 35.

Klitch, B. A. (2000). Staffing strategies for survey success. *Nursing Homes Long-Term Care Management, 49*(3), 12–17.

Kovner, C. T., & Harrington, C. (2000) Quality of care linked to nurse staffing levels. *American Journal of Nursing, 100*(9), 54.

Mark, B. A. (2002). What explains nurses' perceptions of staffing adequacy? *Journal of Nursing Administration, 32*(5), 234–242.

Mason, D. J. (2003). How many patients are too many? Legislating staffing ratios is good for nursing. *American Journal of Nursing, 103*(11), 7.

Maxwell. M. (2004). HR help for religious holiday scheduling, behavior issues, and turnover. *Nursing Economic$, 22*(1), 39–40.

McConnell, E. A. (2000). Staffing and scheduling at your fingertips. *Nursing Management, 31*(3), 52–54.

McGillis, L., Doran, D., & Pink, G. H. (2004). Nurse staffing models, nursing hours, and patient safety outcomes. *Journal of Nursing Administration, 34*(1), 41–45.

McKinnon, C. (2002). You can do it too in 2002. Registry reduction. *Journal of Nursing Administration, 32*(10), 498–500.

McVay, K., & DeMoro, D. (2002). Point/counterpoint. Regulated staffing ratios: Not "if" but "how." *Nursing Leadership Forum, 6*(4), 92, 95–99.

Pinkerton, S. E., & Rivers, R. (2001). Factors influencing staffing needs. *Nursing Economic$, 19*(5), 236–237, 208.

Price, C. (2000). A national uprising. *American Journal of Nursing, 100*(12), 75–77.

Wendling, L. A. (2003). Clocking care hours with workload measurement tools. *Nursing Management, 34*(8), 34–39.

CHAPTER

18

Creating a Motivating Climate

How we feel about and enjoy our work is crucial to how we perceive the quality of our lives.

—Jo Manion

This unit reviews the fourth phase of the management process: *directing*. This phase also may be referred to as *coordinating* or *activating*. Regardless of the nomenclature, this is the "doing" phase of management, requiring the leadership and management skills necessary to accomplish the goals of the organization. Managers direct the work of their subordinates during this phase. Components of the directing phase discussed in this textbook include creating a motivating climate, establishing organizational communication, managing conflict, facilitating collaboration, negotiating, and the impact of collective bargaining and employment laws on management.

In planning and organizing, managers attempt to establish an environment that is conducive to getting work done. In directing, the manager sets those plans into action. This chapter focuses on creating a motivating climate as a critical element in meeting employee and organizational goals.

The amount and quality of work accomplished by managers directly reflect their motivation and that of their subordinates. Why are some managers or employees more motivated than others? How do demotivated managers affect their subordinates? What can the manager do to help the employee who is demotivated? The motivational problems frequently encountered by the manager are complex. To respond to demotivated staff, managers need an understanding of the relationship between motivation and behavior.

Motivation may be defined as the force within the individual that influences or directs behavior. Because motivation comes from within the person, managers cannot directly motivate subordinates. The humanistic manager can, however, create an environment that maximizes the development of human potential. Management support, collegial influence, and the interaction of personalities in the work group can have a synergistic effect on motivation. The leader–manager must identify those components and strengthen them in maximizing motivation at the unit level.

All human beings have needs that motivate them. The leader focuses on the needs and wants of individual workers and uses motivational strategies appropriate for each person and situation.

> The leader also is the role model, listener, supporter, and encourager for demotivated employees.

Lee (2000) states that, "motivation, mentoring, and empowerment aren't just management jargon: they should be resources you use every day" (p. 25). Leaders should apply techniques, skills, and knowledge of motivational theory to help nurses achieve what they want out of work. At the same time, these individual goals should complement the goals of the organization. The manager bears primary responsibility for meeting organizational goals, such as reaching acceptable levels of productivity and quality.

The leader–manager, then, must create a work environment in which both organizational and individual needs can be met. Adequate tension must be created to maintain productivity while encouraging subordinates' job satisfaction. Thus, while the worker is achieving personal goals, organizational goals are being met. The leadership roles and management functions inherent in creating such an environment are included in **Display 18.1**.

This chapter examines motivational theories that have guided organizational efforts and resource distribution for the last 80 years. Special attention is given to the concepts of intrinsic versus extrinsic motivation and organizational motivation versus self-motivation.

Display 18.1 Leadership Roles and Management Functions Associated with Creating a Motivating Work Climate

Leadership Roles

1. Recognizes each worker as a unique individual who is motivated by different things.
2. Identifies the individual and collective value system of the unit, and implements a reward system that is consistent with those values.
3. Listens attentively to individual and collective work values and attitudes to identify unmet needs that can cause dissatisfaction.
4. Encourages workers to "stretch" themselves in an effort to promote self-growth and self-actualization.
5. Maintains a positive and enthusiastic image as a role model to subordinates in the clinical setting.
6. Encourages mentoring, sponsorship, and coaching with subordinates.
7. Devotes time and energy to create an environment that is supportive and encouraging to the discouraged individual.
8. Develops a unit philosophy that recognizes the unique worth of each employee and promotes reward systems that make each employee feel like a winner.
9. Demonstrates through actions and words a belief in subordinates that they desire to meet organizational goals.
10. Is self-aware regarding own enthusiasm for work and takes steps to remotivate self as necessary.

Management Functions

1. Uses legitimate authority to provide formal reward systems.
2. Uses positive feedback to reward the individual employee.
3. Develops unit goals that integrate organizational and subordinate needs.
4. Maintains a unit environment that eliminates or reduces job dissatisfiers.
5. Promotes a unit environment that focuses on employee motivators.
6. Creates the tension necessary to maintain productivity while encouraging subordinate job satisfaction.
7. Clearly communicates expectations to subordinates.
8. Demonstrates and communicates sincere respect, concern, trust, and a sense of belonging to subordinates.
9. Assigns work duties commensurate with employee abilities and past performance to foster a sense of accomplishment in subordinates.
10. Identifies achievement, affiliation, or power needs of subordinates, and develops appropriate motivational strategies to meet those needs.

INTRINSIC VERSUS EXTRINSIC MOTIVATION

Motivation is the action people take to satisfy unmet needs. It is the willingness to put effort into achieving a goal or reward to decrease the tension caused by the need. *Intrinsic motivation* comes from within the person, driving him or her to be productive. To be intrinsically motivated at work, the worker must value job performance and productivity.

The *intrinsic motivation to achieve is directly related to a person's level of aspiration. Extrinsic motivation* is motivation enhanced by the job environment or external rewards.

The intrinsic motivation to achieve is directly related to a person's level of aspiration. Parents and peers play major roles in shaping a person's values about what he or she wants to do and be. Parents who set high but attainable expectations for their children, and who constantly encourage them in a nonauthoritative environment, tend to impart strong achievement drives in their children. Cultural background also has an impact on intrinsic motivation; some cultures value career mobility, job success, and recognition more than others.

Extrinsic motivation is motivation enhanced by the job environment or external rewards. The reward occurs after the work has been completed. Although all people are intrinsically motivated to some degree, it is unrealistic for the organization to assume that all workers have adequate levels of intrinsic motivation to meet organizational goals. Thus, the organization must provide a climate that stimulates both extrinsic and intrinsic drives.

 Learning Exercise 18.1

Thinking about Motivation
Think back to when you were a child. What rewards did your parents use to promote good behavior? Was your behavior more intrinsically or extrinsically motivated? Were strong achievement drives encouraged and supported by your family? If you have children, what rewards do you use? Are they the same rewards your parents used? Why or why not?

Because motivation is so complex, the leader faces tremendous challenges in accurately identifying individual and collective motivators.

Because people have constant needs and wants, people are always motivated to some extent. In addition, because all human beings are unique and have different needs, they are motivated differently. The difference in motivation can be explained in part by our large- and small-group cultures. For example, because American culture values material goods and possessions more highly than many other cultures, rewards in this country are frequently tied to these values.

Organizations also have cultures and values. Motivators vary between organizations and even between units in organizations. Even in similar or nearly identical work environments, large variations in individual and group motivation often exist. Much research has been undertaken by behavioral, psychological, and social scientists to develop theories and concepts of motivation. Economists and engineers have focused on extrinsic fiscal rewards to improve performance and productivity, whereas human relations scientists have stressed intrinsic needs for recognition, self-esteem, and self-actualization. To better understand the current view that both extrinsic and intrinsic rewards are necessary for high productivity and worker satisfaction, one needs to look at how motivational theory has evolved over time.

MOTIVATIONAL THEORY

Chapter 2 introduced traditional management philosophy that emphasizes paternalism, worker subordination, and bureaucracy as a means to predictable but moderate productivity. In this philosophy, high productivity means greater monetary incentives for the worker, and workers are viewed as being motivated primarily by economic factors. This traditional management philosophy is still in use today. Many factory and assembly line production jobs and jobs that use production incentive pay are based on these principles.

The shift from traditional management philosophy to a greater focus on the human element and worker satisfaction as factors in productivity began during the human relations era (1930–1970). The best-known human motivation studies in this era were the Hawthorne studies conducted by Elton Mayo (1953).

Maslow

Continued focus on human motivation did not occur until Abraham Maslow's work in the 1950s. Most nurses are familiar with Maslow's hierarchy of needs and theory of human motivation. Maslow (1970) believed that people are motivated to satisfy certain needs, ranging from basic survival to complex psychological needs, and that people seek a higher need only when the lower needs have been predominantly met. Maslow's hierarchy of needs is depicted in **Figure 18.1.**

Although Maslow's work helps explain personal motivation, his early work, unfortunately, was not applied to motivation in the workplace. His later work, however, offers much insight into motivation and worker dissatisfaction. Because of Maslow's work, managers began to realize that people are complex beings, not solely economic animals, and that they have many needs motivating them at any one time. It also became clear that motivation is internalized and that if productivity is to increase, management must help employees meet lower-level needs. This shifting focus on what motivates employees has tremendously affected how organizations value workers today.

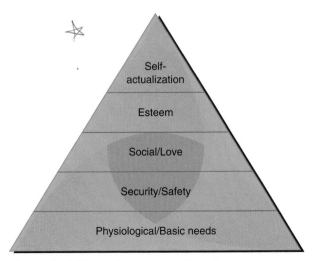

Figure 18.1 Maslow's hierarchy of needs.

Skinner

B. F. Skinner was another theorist in this era who contributed to the understanding of motivation, dissatisfaction, and productivity. Skinner's (1953) research on *operant conditioning* and *behavior modification* demonstrated that people could be conditioned to behave in a certain way based on a consistent reward or punishment system. Behavior that is rewarded will be repeated, and behavior that is punished or goes unrewarded is extinguished. Skinner's work continues to be reflected today in the way many managers view and use discipline and rewards in the work setting.

Herzberg

Frederick Herzberg (1977) believed that employees can be motivated by the work itself and that there is an internal or personal need to meet organizational goals. He believed that separating personal motivators from job dissatisfiers was possible. This distinction between *hygiene* or *maintenance factors* and *motivator factors* was called the Motivation–Hygiene theory or Two Factor theory. **Display 18.2** lists motivator and hygiene factors identified by Herzberg.

Herzberg maintained that motivators or job satisfiers are present in work itself; they give people the desire to work and to do that work well. Hygiene or maintenance factors keep employees from being dissatisfied or demotivated but do not act as real motivators. It is important to remember that the opposite of dissatisfaction may not be satisfaction. When hygiene factors are met, there is a lack of dissatisfaction, not an existence of satisfaction. Likewise, the absence of motivators does not necessarily cause dissatisfaction.

For example, salary is a hygiene factor. Although it does not motivate in itself, when used in conjunction with other motivators, such as recognition or advancement, it can be a powerful motivator. If, however, salary is deficient, employee dissatisfaction can result. Some argue that money can truly be a motivator, as evidenced by people who work insufferable hours at jobs they truly do not enjoy. Some theorists would argue that money in this case might be taking the place of some other unconscious need.

Display 18.2 **Herzberg's Motivators and Hygiene Factors**	
Motivators	**Hygiene Factors**
Achievement	Salary
Recognition	Supervision
Work	Job security
Responsibility	Positive working conditions
Advancement	Personal life
Possibility for growth	Interpersonal relationships and peers
	Company policy
	Status

Some people in Herzberg's studies, however, did report job satisfaction solely from hygiene or maintenance factors. Herzberg asserts that these people are only temporarily satisfied when hygiene factors are improved, show little interest in the kind and quality of their work, experience little satisfaction from accomplishments, and tend to show chronic dissatisfaction with other hygiene factors, such as salary, status, and job security.

Herzberg's work suggests that although the organization must build on hygiene or maintenance factors, the motivating climate must actively include the employee. The worker must be given greater responsibilities, challenges, and recognition for work well done. The reward system must meet both motivation and hygiene needs, and the emphasis given by the manager should vary with the situation and employee involved. Although hygiene factors in themselves do not motivate, they are needed to create an environment that encourages the worker to move on to higher-level needs. Hygiene factors also combat employee dissatisfaction and are useful in recruiting an adequate personnel pool. Vaughn's (2003) study showed that among the numerous retention factors suggested by Herzberg's Two Factor theory, nurses most desired a sense of recognition and achievement.

Vroom

Victor Vroom (1964), another motivational theorist in the human relations era, developed an expectancy model, which looks at motivation in terms of the person's *valence*, or preferences based on social values. In contrast to *operant conditioning*, which focuses on observable behaviors, the expectancy model says that a person's expectations about his or her environment or a certain event will influence behavior. In other words, people look at all actions as having a cause and effect; the effect may be immediate or delayed, but a reward inherent in the behavior exists to motivate risk taking. In Vroom's expectancy model (**Figure 18.2**), people make conscious

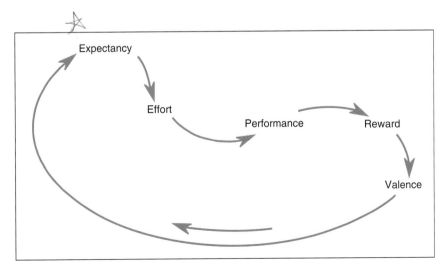

Figure 18.2 Vroom's expectancy model.

decisions in anticipation of reward; in operant conditioning, people react in a stimulus–response mode. Managers using the expectancy model must become personally involved with their employees to understand better the employees' values, reward systems, strengths, and willingness to take risks.

McClelland

> The challenge is to energize people to enjoy the beauty of pushing themselves beyond what they thought they could do.

David McClelland (1971) has examined what motives guide a person to action. McClelland states that people are motivated by three basic needs: achievement, affiliation, and power. *Achievement-oriented* people actively focus on improving what is; they transform ideas into action, judiciously and wisely, taking risks when necessary. In contrast, *affiliation-oriented* people focus their energies on families and friends; their overt productivity is less because they view their contribution to society in a different light than those who are achievement oriented. Research has shown that women generally have greater affiliation needs than men and that nurses generally have high affiliation needs. *Power-oriented* people are motivated by the power that can be gained as a result of a specific action. They want to command attention, get recognition, and control others. McClelland theorizes that managers can identify achievement, affiliation, or power needs of their employees and develop appropriate motivational strategies to meet those needs. Learning Exercise 18.2 is a self-evaluation tool that can be used to assess individual achievement, affiliation, and power needs.

Learning Exercise 18.2

Identifying Goals and Motivation
List six goals you hope to accomplish in the next five years. Identify which goals are most related to achievement needs, affiliation needs, and power needs. Remember that most people are motivated in part by all three needs, and no one motivational need is better than the others. However, each person must recognize and understand which basic needs motivate him or her most.

Gellerman

Saul Gellerman (1968), another humanistic motivational theorist, has identified several methods to motivate people positively. One such method, *stretching*, involves assigning tasks that are more difficult than what the person is used to doing. Stretching should not, however, be a routine or daily activity. Kerfoot (2001) stated, "Just as an Olympic coach teaches, trains, inspires, and creates a culture and discipline to achieve extraordinary outcomes, the successful leader also helps people achieve outcomes they didn't think were possible" (p. 125). Kerfoot goes on to say that "raising the bar" is a consistent part of excellence in leadership.

Another method, *participation*, entails actively drawing employees into decisions affecting their work. Gellerman strongly believed that motivation problems usually stem from the way the organization manages and not from the staff's unwillingness to work hard. According to Gellerman, most managers "overmanage"—they make the employee's job too narrow and fail to give the employee any decision-making power. Indeed, Friedrich (2001) asserts that decision-making input, autonomy, and independence are critical elements to nurses for staying motivated in the work environment.

McGregor

Douglas McGregor (1960) examined the importance of a manager's assumptions about workers on the intrinsic motivation of the workers. These assumptions, which McGregor labeled *Theory X* and *Theory Y* (depicted in **Display 18.3**), led to the realization in management science that how the manager views, and thus treats, the worker will have an impact on how well the organization functions.

McGregor did not consider Theory X and Theory Y as opposite points on the spectrum, but rather as two points on a continuum extending through all perspectives of people. McGregor believed that people should not be artificially classified as always having Theory X or Theory Y assumptions about others; instead, most people fall on some point on the continuum. Likewise, McGregor did not promote either Theory X or Theory Y as being the one superior management style, although many managers have interpreted Theory Y as being the ultimate management model. No one style is effective in all situations, at all times, and with all people. McGregor, without making value judgments, simply stated that in any situation, the manager's assumptions about people, whether grounded in fact or not, affect motivation and productivity.

The work of all these theorists has added greatly to the understanding of what motivates people in and out of the work setting. Research has revealed that motivation is extremely complex and that there is tremendous variation in what motivates different people. Therefore, managers must understand what can be done at the unit level to create a climate that allows the worker to grow, increases motivation and productivity, and eliminates dissatisfiers that drain energy and cause frustration.

Display 18.3 McGregor's Theory X and Theory Y	
Theory X Employees	**Theory Y Employees**
Avoid work if possible	Like and enjoy work
Dislike work	Are self-directed
Must be directed	Seek responsibility
Have little ambition	Are imaginative and creative
Avoid responsibility	Have underutilized intellectual capacity
Need threats to be motivated	Need only general supervision
Need close supervision	Are encouraged to participate in
Are motivated by rewards and punishment	problem solving

Learning Exercise 18.3

Crossword Puzzle: A Review of Motivational Theory

ACROSS

1. Maslow's _____ of needs.
3. One of the three basic motivators identified by McClelland.
5. Theorist who stated that one's assumptions about human nature influence his or her managerial behavior.
7. Factor that keeps the worker from being dissatisfied but is not a true motivator.
8. Developed the expectancy theory.
9. Described operant conditioning.

DOWN

2. Theorist who encouraged managers to "stretch" employees.
4. Manager who believes workers are inherently lazy, need total direction, and are externally motivated.
6. These studies were completed by Elton Mayo and suggested that individuals respond to the fact that they are being studied.

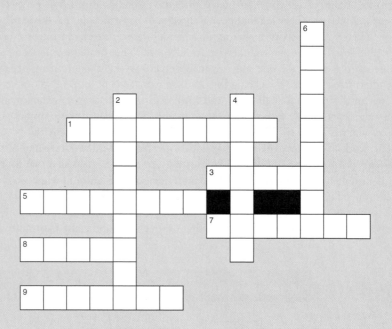

Note: Puzzle solution may be found in the appendix.

CREATING A MOTIVATING CLIMATE

Because the organization has such an impact on extrinsic motivation, it is important to examine organizational climates or attitudes that directly influence worker morale and motivation. For example, organizations frequently overtly or covertly reinforce the image that each employee is expendable and that individual recognition is in some way detrimental to the employee and his or her productivity within the organization. Just the opposite is true. "Employees are an organization's most valuable asset" (Andrica, 2000, p. 307), and people who have a strong self-concept and perceive themselves as winners are willing to take risks and increase their productivity to achieve greater recognition. Friedrich (2001) states that nurses who feel that their contributions are noticed experience satisfaction, and nurses who experience satisfaction stay where they are, contributing to an organization's retention.

Some organizations, on the other hand, erroneously believe that if a small reward results in desired behavior, then a larger reward will result in even more of the desired behavior. Thus, an employee's motivation should increase proportionately with the amount of the incentive or reward. This simply is not true. There appears to be a perceived threshold beyond which increasing the incentive results in no additional meaning or weight. Organizations must be cognizant of the need to offer incentives at a level where employees value them. This requires that the organization and its managers understand employees' collective values and devise a reward system that is consistent with that value system.

Managers also must be cognizant of an employee's individual values and attempt to reward each worker accordingly. Levin (2001) stated, "Each employee's commitment to the organization reflects the degree to which it can fulfill his/her tangible and intangible needs"(p. 18). Therefore, the manager must assess individual employee values and needs as well as organization values and then use his or her authority to bring these values together. The ability to recognize each worker as a unique person who is motivated differently and then to act upon those differences is a leadership skill.

In a study by Prothero, Marshall, Fosbinder, and Hendrix (2000) of RNs working in two hospitals in the United States, the values of sense of accomplishment, equality, and being imaginative, helpful, self-controlled, and obedient were significantly associated with total work satisfaction. A sense of accomplishment, equality, comfortable life, pleasure and being imaginative, helpful, self-controlled, and courageous were associated with satisfaction with the task requirements of the job. The study concluded that managerial consideration of nurses' personal values might be a critical factor in increasing employee work satisfaction.

In addition to the climate created by the organization's beliefs and attitudes, the unit supervisor or unit manager also has a tremendous impact on motivation at the unit level. Friedrich (2001) states that "the manner in which a first-line manager communicates with employees affects staff attitude toward the organization, for he or she usually has more influence over employees than any other level of manager" (p. 28).

Clearly, then, the interpersonal relationship between an employee and his or her supervisor is critical to the employee's motivation level. Kerfoot (2001) states, "As leaders, it is often easy to get lost in the goals of our units and organizations. We often forget that the only way to achieve our goals is through the people who work with us" (p. 125). Therefore, although managers cannot directly motivate employees, they can create a climate that demonstrates positive regard for their employees, encourages open communication, recognizes achievement, and encourages growth and productivity.

Learning Exercise 18.4

The Strongest Motivator
Identify the greatest motivator in your life at this time. Has it always been the strongest motivator? Could you list the strongest motivator for the significant others in your life? If so, have you ever used this awareness to motivate those people to do something specific?

One of the most powerful, yet frequently overlooked or underused, motivators the manager can use to create a motivating climate is *positive reinforcement*. Peters and Waterman (1982) have identified the following simple approaches for an effective reward–feedback system that uses positive reinforcement:

- Positive reinforcement must be specific or relevant to a particular performance. The manager should praise an employee for a specific task accomplished or goal met. This praise should not be general. For example, saying, "Your nursing care is good" has less meaning and reward than, "The communication skills you showed today as an advocate for Mr. Jones were excellent. I think you made a significant difference in his care."
- Positive reinforcement must occur as close to the event as possible.
- Reward–feedback system must be achievable. All performance goals must be attainable, and both large and small achievements should be recognized or rewarded in some way.
- Rewards should be unpredictable and intermittent. If rewards are given routinely, they tend to lose their value.

Making rewards unpredictable and intermittent is an approach that is open to several interpretations. If Peters and Waterman are advocating inconsistency when granting rewards, the authors disagree because there must be consistency in how and when rewards are given. When rewards lack consistency, there is greater risk that the reward itself will become a source of competition and thereby lower morale. An attitude prevails that "there are a limited number of awards, and an award received by anyone else limits the chances of my getting one; thus, I cannot support recognition for my peers." Likewise, rewarding one person's behavior and not another's who has accomplished a similar task at a similar level promotes jealousy and can demotivate.

If, however, Peters and Waterman mean that rewards and praise should be spontaneous and not relegated to predictable events, such as routine annual performance reviews or recognition dinners, then the authors agree. Rewards and praise should be given whenever possible and whenever they are deserved.

If positive reinforcement and rewards are to be used as motivational strategies, then rewards must represent a genuine accomplishment on the part of the person and should be somewhat individual in nature. For example, many managers erroneously consider annual merit pay increases as rewards that motivate employees.

Most employees, however, recognize annual merit pay increases as a universal "given"; thus, this reward has little meaning and little power to motivate. Managers should promote excellence within achievable goals and reward performance in a way that is valued by their staff. These are the cardinal elements for a successful motivation–reward system for the organization.

It is important to remember that all nurse–managers can enhance the work of their subordinates by providing them with more opportunities to experience the challenges that make their jobs exciting. Through shared governance, empowerment, and participative management, managers can have a direct impact on motivation at the unit level.

Finding Joy at Work: A Shared Responsibility

For many in today's healthcare organizations, some of the joy has gone from work, but it is possible to rekindle joy and to find both staff nurses and leaders who find true joy in their work. Manion (2003) says that positive mood is directly linked to many different performance-related behaviors, including enhanced creativity, greater helping behavior, integrative thinking, inductive reasoning, more efficient decision making, greater cooperation, and the use of more successful negotiation strategies. Manion elaborates by saying joyful people positively effect relationships and make the workplace more appealing.

How is joy found in work? In Manion's (2003) study, most of the participants felt that joy was an individual thing. However, her findings strongly suggested that the organization played a role in setting a climate for joy in work to occur; the creation of a positive work environment, hiring and retaining good people, adequate benefits and compensation, providing adequate resources, and living up to its mission were identified as contributing factors.

Pathways to Joy

Manion (2003) found that there were several personal pathways (see **Display 18.4**) that individual's used to find joy in their work. These pathways, summarized below, closely match Herzberg's and Maslow's theories of motivation.

- **Connections Pathway.** This pathway is based on relationships. This was the primary source of joy for all participants in the study. This relationship connection occurred with colleagues, patients, and families. Caring for, talking with, relating to, and helping others exemplified this pathway to joy.

Display 18.4	Pathways to Joy

Personal pathway via connections
Love of work pathway via the work itself
Achievement pathway via goal accomplishment and attainment
Recognition pathway via acknowledgement of good work by others

- **Love of Work Pathway.** This is the pathway that is based on the joy found in ones work itself. There was a strong connection and identification with the work that resulted in excitement and enthusiasm that brought joy to the participants.
- **Achievement Pathway.** Achievement, accomplishments, and positive work outcomes brought joy to some participants in the study. There was a sense of pride for a job well done, or for being a successful change agent. Personal assessment of achievement was also more important than external rewards for achievement.
- **Recognition Pathway.** Recognition and appreciation also brought people joy in their work. The recognition could be attained through a patient's gratitude, patient's families appreciation, or though praise or thanks from colleagues, or the organization.

STRATEGIES FOR CREATING A MOTIVATING CLIMATE

In addition to providing a climate that promotes joy in people's work, the leader–manager can do many other things that create an environment that is motivating. Sometimes fostering a subordinate's motivation is as simple as establishing a supportive and encouraging environment. The cost of this strategy is only the manager's time and energy. The strategies outlined in **Display 18.5** should be used consistently to create a motivating climate.

Display 18.5	**Strategies to Create a Motivating Climate**

1. Have clear expectations for workers, and communicate these expectations effectively.
2. Be fair and consistent when dealing with all employees.
3. Be a firm decision maker using an appropriate decision-making style.
4. Develop the concept of teamwork. Develop group goals and projects that will build a team spirit.
5. Integrate the staff's needs and wants with the organization's interests and purpose.
6. Know the uniqueness of each employee. Let each know that you understand his or her uniqueness.
7. Remove traditional blocks between the employee and the work to be done.
8. Provide experiences that challenge or "stretch" the employee and allow opportunities for growth.
9. When appropriate, request participation and input from all subordinates in decision making.
10. Whenever possible, give subordinates recognition and credit.
11. Be certain that employees understand the reason behind decisions and actions.
12. Reward desirable behavior; be consistent in how you handle undesirable behavior.
13. Let employees exercise individual judgment as much as possible.
14. Create a trustful and helping relationship with employees.
15. Let employees exercise as much control as possible over their work environment.
16. Be a role model for employees.

Learning Exercise 18.5

Write a Detailed Plan to Motivate—Quickly!

You are the manager of a medical unit in a community hospital. The hospital has faced extreme budget cuts during the last five years as a result in decreased reimbursement. Your unit used to be a place that nurses wanted to work and you rarely had openings for long, even though it was necessary for the hospital to contain costs and shorten nursing care hours per patient day. However recently there has been a severe nursing shortage in your community and it seems to have accelerated worker dissatisfaction in your staff.

In the last week, five of the unit nurses, all excellent long-time employees, have stopped by your office either in tears, anger, or frustration and had various comments, including: "Working here is no longer fun," "I used to love my job," "I am tired of working with incompetent people," and "I am sick to death of calling for supplies that should be stocked on the floor."

You know that there will not be more funding in the near future, but you feel that perhaps there are things you could do to make the situation better for your staff.

Assignment: In examining the strategies for creating a motivating climate and the atmosphere that supports finding joy in work, decide what you as an individual unit manager can do to provide a more positive work environment. Don't just take things from the list in Display 18.5, but write a detailed plan that is feasible, and one you could begin implementing fairly quickly, that would have the potential to turn this situation around.

PROFESSIONAL SUPPORT SYSTEMS FOR THE MANAGER

Managers also can create a motivating climate by being a positive and enthusiastic role model in the clinical setting. Managers who frequently project unhappiness to subordinates contribute greatly to low unit morale. A burned-out, tired manager will develop a lethargic and demotivated staff. Therefore, managers must constantly monitor their own motivational level and do whatever is necessary to restore their motivation to be a role model to staff.

> The attitude and energy level of managers directly affect the attitude and productivity of their employees.

Managers must be internally motivated before they can motivate others. It is imperative that discouraged managers acknowledge their own feelings and seek assistance accordingly. Managers are responsible to themselves and to subordinates to remain motivated to do the best job possible.

Nursing is a stressful profession, and managers must practice health-seeking behaviors and find social supports when confronted with stress or else risk burnout as a result. *Burnout* is defined as "a syndrome of emotional exhaustion, depersonalization, and reduced personal accomplishment which happens as a result of the chronic emotional strain of working extensively with other human beings, particularly when they are troubled" (Schwab, 1996, p. 172). Kalliath and Morris (2002) found that the degree of job satisfaction was the greatest predictor of burnout.

Garrett and McDaniel's (2001) research suggests that environmental uncertainty is positively associated with burnout in nurses and that social climate in a workplace is negatively associated with burnout. Thus, they conclude that social networks are important during times of change and uncertainty in the work environment; in other words, a supportive workplace can protect against burnout.

Burnout and other forms of work-related stress are related to negative organizational outcomes such as illness, absenteeism, turnover, performance deterioration, decreased productivity, and job dissatisfaction. These outcomes cost the organization and impede quality of care.

Perhaps the most important strategy for avoiding burnout and maintaining a high motivation level is *self-care*. Ellis (2000) defines self-care as caring for yourself physically, mentally, and spiritually to maximize your potential. Self-care gives the manager personal insight, which increases his or her self-esteem and self-efficacy.

For self-care, the manager should seek time off on a regular basis to meet personal needs, have recreation, form relationships outside the work setting, and have fun. Friends and colleagues are essential for emotional support, guidance, and renewal. A proper diet and exercise are important to maintain physical health as well as emotional health. Finally, the manager must be able to separate his or her work life and personal life; the manager should remember that there is life outside of work, and that time should be relished and protected. Ellis (2000) suggests that writing a self-care contract is one way to put a commitment for self-care into motion. Ultimately, the decision to practice self-care rests with each and every nurse.

INTEGRATING LEADERSHIP ROLES AND MANAGEMENT FUNCTIONS IN MOTIVATING

Most human behavior is motivated by a goal the person wants to achieve. Identifying employee goals and fostering their attainment allow the leader to motivate employees to reach personal and organizational goals. The motivational strategy the leader uses should vary with the situation and the employee involved; it may be formal or informal. It also may be extrinsic, although because of a limited formal power base, the leader generally focuses on the intrinsic aspects of motivation.

The leader also must be a listener, supporter, or encourager to the discouraged employee. Perhaps the most important role the leader has in working with the demotivated employee, however, is that of role model. "When we feel strong physically, mentally, spiritually, and emotionally, we have the energy to create the passion that drives excellence. When we don't, we aren't able to renew and recover the energy necessary to perform at our desired level" (Kerfoot, 2001, p. 126). Leaders who maintain a positive attitude and high energy levels directly and profoundly affect the attitude and productivity of their followers.

When creating a motivating climate, the manager uses formal authority to reduce dissatisfiers at the unit level and to implement a reward system that reflects individual and collective value systems. This reward system may be formalized, or it may be as informal as praise. Managers, by virtue of their position, have the ability to motivate subordinates by "stretching" them intermittently with increasing responsibility and assignments they are capable of achieving. The manager's role, then, is to create the tension necessary to maintain productivity while encouraging subordinates' job satisfaction. Therefore, the success of the motivational strategy is measured by the increased productivity and benefit to the organization and by the growth in the person, which motivates him or her to accomplish again.

☀ Key Concepts

- Because human beings have constant needs and wants, they are always motivated to some extent. However, human beings are motivated differently.
- Managers cannot intrinsically motivate people because motivation comes from within the person. The humanistic manager can, however, create an environment in which the development of human potential can be maximized.
- Maslow stated that people are motivated to satisfy certain needs, ranging from basic survival to complex psychological needs, and that people seek a higher need only when the lower needs have been predominantly met.
- Skinner's research on *operant conditioning* and behavior modification demonstrates that people can be conditioned to behave in a certain way based on a consistent reward or punishment system.
- Herzberg maintained that *motivators*, or *job satisfiers*, are present in the work itself and encourage people to want to work and to do that work well. *Hygiene* or *maintenance factors* keep the worker from being dissatisfied or demotivated but do not act as true motivators for the worker.
- Vroom's *expectancy model* says that people's expectations about their environment or a certain event will influence their behavior.
- McClelland's studies state that all people are motivated by three basic needs: *achievement*, *affiliation*, and *power*.
- Gellerman states that most managers in organizations *overmanage*, making the responsibilities too narrow and failing to give employees any decision-making power or to stretch them often enough.
- Douglas McGregor shows the importance of a manager's assumptions about workers on the intrinsic motivation of the worker.
- There appears to be a perceived threshold beyond which increasing reward incentives results in no additional meaning or weight in terms of productivity.
- *Positive reinforcement* is one of the most powerful motivators the manager can use and is frequently overlooked or underused.
- The supervisor's or manager's personal motivation is an important factor affecting staff's commitment to duties and morale.
- Managers should network with a professional support system for positive reinforcement, information, and guidance in their professional development.
- The success of a motivational strategy is measured by the increased productivity and benefit to the organization and by the growth in the person, which motivates him or her to accomplish again.

More Learning Exercises and Applications

Learning Exercise 18.6

Create a Plan to Remotivate a New Employee

You are a county public health coordinator. You have grown concerned about the behavior of one of the new RNs assigned to work in the agency. This new nurse, Sally Brown, is a recent graduate of a local BSN program. Sally came to work for the agency immediately after her graduation six months ago. For the first few months, Sally appeared to be extremely hard working, knowledgeable, well liked, and highly motivated. Recently, though, several small incidents happened to Sally. The medical director of the agency became very angry with her over a minor medication error she had made; Sally was already feeling badly about the careless error. After this episode, a different patient's husband began disliking Sally for no discernible reason; he then refused to allow Sally to come into their home to care for his wife. Then two weeks ago, a diabetic patient died fairly suddenly from renal failure, and although no one was to blame, Sally apparently believed that if she had been more observant and skilled in assessment, she would have picked up the subtle changes in the patient's condition sooner.

Although you have been supportive of Sally, you recognize that she is in danger of becoming demotivated. Her once-flawless appearance now borders on being unkempt; she is frequently absent from work; and her once-pleasant personality has been exchanged for withdrawal from her coworkers.

Assignment: Using your knowledge of new role identification, assimilation, and motivational theory, develop a plan to assist this young nurse. What can you do to provide a climate that will remotivate her and decrease her job dissatisfaction? Explain what you think is happening to this nurse and the rationale behind your plan. Your plan should be realistic in terms of the time and energy you have to spend on one employee. Be sure to identify the responsibilities of the employee as well.

Learning Exercise 18.7

A Nursing Officer's Dilemma

You are the chief nursing officer of County Hospital. Dr. Jones, a cardiologist, has approached you about having an ICU/CCU nurse make rounds with him each morning on all the patients in the hospital with a cardiac-related diagnosis. He believes this will probably represent a 90-minute commitment of nursing time daily. He is vague about the nurse's exact role or purpose, but you believe there is great potential for better and more consistent patient education and care planning.

Beth, one of your finest ICU/CCU nurses, agrees to assist Dr. Jones. Beth has always wanted to have an expanded role in teaching. However, because of personal constraints, she has been unable to relocate to a larger city where there are more opportunities for teaching. You warn Beth that it might be some time before this role develops into an autonomous position, but she is eager to assist Dr. Jones. The other ICU/CCU staff agree to cover Beth's patients while she is gone, although it is obviously an extension of an already full patient load.

After three weeks of making rounds with Dr. Jones, Beth comes to your office. She tearfully reports that rounds frequently take two to three hours and that making rounds with Dr. Jones amounts to little more than "carrying his charts, picking up his pages, and being a personal handmaiden." She has assertively stated her feelings to him and has attempted to demonstrate to Dr. Jones how their allegiance could result in improved patient care. She states that she has not been allowed any input into patient decisions and is frequently reminded of "her position" and his ability to have her removed from her job if she does not like being told what to do. She is demoralized and demotivated. In addition, she believes that her peers resent having to cover her workload because it is obvious that her role is superficial at best.

You ask Beth if she wants you to assign another nurse to work with Dr. Jones, and she says that she would really like to make it work but does not know what action to take that would improve the situation.

You call Dr. Jones, and he agrees to meet with you at your office when he completes rounds the following morning. At this visit, Dr. Jones confirms Beth's description of her role but justifies his desire for the role to continue by saying, "I bring $10 million of business to this hospital every year in cardiology procedures. The least you can do is provide the nursing assistance I am asking for. If you are unable to meet this small request, I will be forced to consider taking my practice to a competitive hospital." However, after further discussion, he does agree that eventually he would consider a slightly more expanded role for the nurse after he learns to trust her.

Assignment: Do you meet Dr. Jones' request? Does it make any difference whether Beth is the nurse, or can it be someone else? Does the revenue Dr. Jones generates supersede the value of professional nursing practice? Should you try to talk Beth into continuing the position for a while longer? While trying to reach a goal, people must sometimes endure a difficult path, but at what point does the means not justify the end? Be realistic about what you would do in this situation. What do you perceive to be the greatest obstacles in implementing your decision?

Learning Exercise 18.8

To Work or Not to Work?
You are a nurse in a long-term care facility. The facility barely meets minimum licensing standards for professional nursing staffing. Although agency recruiters have been actively seeking to hire more licensed staff, pay at the facility for professional staff is less than at local acute care hospitals and the patient–nurse ratio is significantly higher. There appears to be little chance of improving the RN staffing mix in your agency in the near future. The nursing administrator is extremely supportive of the staff's efforts but can do little to ease the current workload for licensed staff, other than to turn away patients or close the agency. As a result, all the nurses on the unit have been working at least 48 hours per week during the last six months; many have been working several double shifts and putting in many overtime hours each pay period.

Morale is deteriorating, and the staff has begun to complain. Most of the licensed staff are feeling burned out and demotivated. Many have started refusing to work extra shifts or do overtime. You feel a responsibility to the patients, community, and organization and have continued to work the extra hours but are exhausted.

Today is your first evening off in six days. At 2 P.M., the phone rings, and you suspect it is the agency calling you to come in to work. You delay answering while you decide what to do. The answering machine turns on, and you hear your administrator's voice. She says that they are desperate. Two new patients were admitted during the day, and the facility is full. She says she appreciates all the hours you've been working but needs you once again, although she is unable to give you tomorrow off in compensation. You feel conflicting loyalties to the unit, patients, supervisor, and yourself.

Assignment: Decide what you will do. Will you agree to work? Will you return the administrator's telephone call, or pretend you are not home? When do your loyalties to your patients and the organization end and your loyalties to yourself begin? Is the administrator taking advantage of you? Are the other staff being irresponsible? What values have played a part in your decision making?

Learning Exercise 18.9

Remotivating Oneself

You are a school nurse and have worked in the same school for two years. Before that time, you were a staff nurse at a local hospital working in pediatrics and later for a physician. You have been an RN for six years.

When you began your job, it was exciting. You believed you were really making a difference in children's lives. You started several good health promotion programs and worked hard upgrading your health aides' education and training.

Several months ago, funding for the school was drastically cut, and several of your favorite programs were eliminated. You have been very depressed about this and lately have been short-tempered at work. Today, one of your best health aides gave you her two-week notice and said, "This isn't a good place to work anymore." You realize that many of the aides and several of the schoolteachers have picked up your negative attitude.

There is much you still love about your job, and you are not sure if the budget problems are temporary or long term. You go home early today and contemplate what to do.

Assignment: Should you stay in this job or leave? If you stay, how can you get remotivated? Can you remotivate yourself if the budget cuts are long term? Make a plan about what to do.

Learning Exercise 18.10

Downsizing Panic and Anxiety

As the result of rising costs and shrinking reimbursement, many hospitals downsized their staffs in an effort to shrink costs. Because the hospital where you are the chief nursing administrator is faced with mandatory staffing ratios, it is impossible to cut further staff nurse positions and meet requirements for state licensing.

Therefore, the CEO of the hospital has mandated that management positions be reduced by 30% throughout the hospital. The CEO has decided that department heads can reduce management positions by any method they choose as long as it is done in six months. Job duties are to be reassigned among the remaining managers.

This affects you significantly, as nursing has more managers than any other department. It does not appear that attrition, or turnover, rates in the next months will be adequate to eliminate the need for some reassignments, demotions, or termination of your group of 17 managers. This includes both house supervisors and unit managers.

The news travels rapidly through the hospital grapevine. Semi-hysteria prevails, with many managers consulting you regarding whether their position is in jeopardy and what they can to do to increase the likelihood of their retention. Morale is rapidly plummeting, and relationships are becoming increasingly competitive rather than cooperative.

Assignment: Determine how you will handle this situation. What strategies might you implement to reduce the immediate anxiety level? What advice can you give to staff who may face either a layoff or a demotion? Is it possible to preserve the morale of your mangers in an uncertain situation such as this?

Web Links

Understanding Human Motivation
http://www.utoledo.edu/~ddavis/maslow.htm
Provides a synopsis about the work of Abraham Maslow.

Landmark Education—Motivation
http://www.landmarkeducation.com
The Landmark Forum is a collaborative seminar focused on motivation.

Motivation Theory—The Theorists and Their Theories
http://www.accel-team.com/motivation/theory_01.html *and*
http://www.accel-team.com/motivation/theory_02.html
Reviews the work of theorists Simon, McGregor, Maslow, Herzberg, Argyris, Likert, Luthans, Vroom, Mayo, and McClelland.

Theories About the Need for Achievement
http://mentalhelp.net/psyhelp/chap4/chap4j.htm
A psychological self-help site dedicated to the achievement needs to succeed and excel.

Strategies for Life
http://www.yourbestyear.com
Offers proven methods for setting and achieving your goals for the coming year.

References

Andrica, D. C. (2000). Employee satisfaction. *Nursing Economic$, 18*(6), 307.

Ellis, L. L. (2000). Have you and your staff signed self-care contracts? *Nursing Management, 31*(3), 47–48.

Friedrich, B. (2001). Staying power: First-line managers keep nurses satisfied with their jobs. *Nursing Management, 32*(7), 26–28.

Garrett, D. K., & McDaniel, A. M. (2001). A new look at nurse burnout. *Journal of Nursing Administration, 31*(2), 91–96.

Gellerman, S. W. (1968). *Management by motivation.* American Management Association.

Herzberg, F. (1977). One more time: How do you motivate employees? In L. Carroll, R. Paine, & A. Miner (Eds.), *The management process* (2nd ed.). New York: Macmillan.

Kalliath, T. & Morris, R. (2002). Job satisfaction among nurses: A predictor of burnout levels. *Journal of Nursing Administration, 32*(12), 648–654.

Kerfoot, K. (2001). The art of raising the bar. *Nursing Economic$, 19*(3), 125–128.

Lee, L. A. (2000). Buzzwords with a basis. *Nursing Management, 31*(10), 25–27.

Levin, P. M. (2001). The loyal treatment. *Nursing Management, 32*(1), 17–20.

Manion, J. (2003). Joy at work! Creating a positive workplace. *Journal of Nursing Administration, 33*(12), 652–659.

Maslow, A. (1970). *Motivation and personality* (2nd ed.). New York: Harper & Row.

Mayo, E. (1953). *The human problems of an industrialized civilization.* New York: Macmillan.

McClelland, D. C. (1971). *Assessing human motivation.* Morristown, NJ: General Learning Press.

McGregor, D. (1960). *The human side of enterprise.* New York: McGraw-Hill.

Peters, T., & Waterman, R. H. (1982). *In search of excellence.* New York: Harper & Row.

Prothero, M. M., Marshall, E. S., Fosbinder, D. M., & Hendrix, L. J. (2000). Personal values and work satisfaction. Registered nurses working in hospitals. *Image-Journal of Nursing Scholarship, 32*(1), 81–82.

Schwab, L. (1996). Individual hardiness and staff satisfaction. *Nursing Economic$, 14*(3), 171–173.

Skinner, B. F. (1953). *Science and human behavior.* New York: Free Press.

Vroom, V. (1964). *Work and motivation.* New York: John Wiley and Sons.

Vaughn, G. R. M. (2003). Motivators get creative. *Nursing Management, 34*(4), 12–14.

Bibliography

Asselin, M. E. (2003). Motivating LPNs. *Nursing Management, 34*(8), 40–45.

Cohen, S. (2003). Manager's fast track. Motivation: Your key IC ingredient. *Nursing Management, 34*(6), 10.

Fletcher, C. E. (2001). Hospital RN's job satisfactions and dissatisfactions. *Journal of Nursing Administration, 31*(6), 324–331.

Goggin, M. (2000). I'm behind you! The manager as coach. *Nursing Economic$, 18*(3), 160–161.

How motivated are you? (2001). *Training, 38*(3), 32–33.

Fenner, K. (2003). Workforce management. Thriving during a nursing crisis: Part III: Adding the contributions of individual staff nurses. *Journal of Clinical Systems Management, 5*(5), 14–15.

Joshua-Amadi, M. (2003). A study in motivation: Recruitment and retention in the NHS. *Nursing Management, London, 9*(9), 14–19.

Kerfoot, K. (2000). Leadership: Creating a shared destiny. *Nursing Economic$, 18*(5), 263–264.

Laschinger, H. K. S., Finegan, J., & Shamian, J. (2001). Promoting nurses' health: Effect of empowerment on job strain and work satisfaction. *Nursing Economic$, 19*(2), 42–52.

Mahoney, J. (2000). The importance of job satisfaction in retaining nurses. *Home Healthcare Nurse Manager, 4*(1), 28–30.

McGirr, M., & Bakker, D. A. (2000). Shaping positive work environments for nurses: The contributions of nurses at various organizational levels. *Canadian Journal of Nursing Leadership, 13*(1), 7–14.

Prencipe, L. W. (2001). Reenergize the disengaged worker. *InfoWorld, 23*(16), 95–99.

Schrage, M. (2001). Actually, I'd rather have that favor than a raise. *Fortune, 143*(8), 412.

Organizational, Interpersonal, and Group Communication

Organizations cannot operate effectively without effective communication.

—Euan Henderson

Although some functions of management, such as planning, organizing, and controlling, can be reasonably isolated, communication forms the core of management activities and cuts across all phases of the management process. Organizational communication is a management function; it must be systematic, have continuity, and be fully integrated into the organizational structure, encouraging an exchange of views and ideas. In addition, communication involves language, which is culturally bound and influenced, further adding to its complexity (Brice, 2000). Developing expertise in all aspects of communication is critical to managerial success.

Because the majority of managerial communication time is spent speaking and listening, it is clear that in a leadership role, one must have excellent interpersonal communication skills. These are perhaps the most critical leadership skills. The nurse–leader communicates with clients, colleagues, superiors, and subordinates. In addition, because nursing practice tends to be group-oriented, interpersonal communication among group members is necessary for continuity and productivity. The leader is responsible for developing a cohesive team to meet organizational goals. To do this, the leader must articulate issues and concerns so workers will not become confused about priorities. The ability to communicate effectively often determines success as a leader–manager.

Leadership skills and management functions inherent in organizational, interpersonal, and group communication are listed in **Display 19.1.** This chapter examines both organizational and interpersonal communication. Barriers to communication in large organizations and managerial strategies to overcome those difficulties are presented. Channels and modes of communication are compared, and guidelines are given for managerial selection of the optimum channel or mode. In addition, assertiveness, nonverbal behavior, and active listening as interpersonal communication factors are discussed. The chapter concludes with a discussion of how technology is altering communication in healthcare settings and the ever-increasing challenge of maintaining confidentiality in a system where so many people have access to so much information.

THE COMMUNICATION PROCESS

Chitty (2001) defines *communication* as the complex exchange of thoughts, ideas, or information on at least two levels: verbal and nonverbal. Thus, communication begins the moment two or more people become aware of each other's presence. What happens, however, when the thoughts, ideas, and information exchanged do not have the same meaning for both the sender and the receiver of the message? What if the verbal and nonverbal messages are not congruent? Does communication occur if an idea is transmitted but not translated into action?

Because communication is so complex, many models exist to explain how organizations and individuals communicate. Basic elements common to most models are shown in **Figure 19.1.** In all communication, there is at least one sender, one

Display 19.1 Leadership Roles and Management Functions Associated with Organizational, Interpersonal, and Group Communication

Leadership Roles

1. Understands and appropriately uses the informal communication network in the organization.
2. Communicates clearly and precisely in language others will understand.
3. Is sensitive to the internal and external climate of the sender or receiver and uses that awareness in interpreting messages.
4. Appropriately observes and interprets the verbal and nonverbal communication of followers.
5. Role-models assertive communication and active listening.
6. Demonstrates congruency in verbal and nonverbal communication.
7. Recognizes status, power, and authority as barriers to manager–subordinate communication. Uses communication strategies to overcome those barriers.
8. Maximizes group functioning by keeping group members on course, encouraging the shy, controlling the garrulous, and protecting the weak.
9. Seeks a balance between technological communication options and the need for human touch, caring, and one-on-one, face- to-face interaction.

Management Functions

1. Understands and appropriately uses the organization's formal communication network.
2. Determines the appropriate communication mode or combination of modes for optimal distribution of information in the organizational hierarchy.
3. Prepares written communications that are clear and uses language that is appropriate for the message and the receiver.
4. Consults with other departments or disciplines in coordinating overlapping roles and group efforts.
5. Differentiates between "information" and "communication" and appropriately assesses the need for subordinates to have both.
6. Prioritizes and protects client and subordinate confidentiality.
7. Ensures that staff and self are trained to appropriately and fully utilize technological communication tools.
8. Uses knowledge of group dynamics for goal attainment and maximizing organizational communication.

receiver, and one message. There also is a mode or medium through which the message is sent, such as verbal, written, or nonverbal.

An internal and an external climate also exist in communication. The *internal climate* includes the values, feelings, temperament, and stress levels of the sender and the receiver. Weather conditions, temperature, timing, and the organizational climate itself are parts of the *external climate*. The external climate also includes status, power, and authority as barriers to manager–subordinate communication.

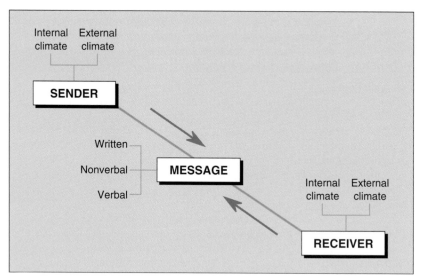

Figure 19.1 The communication process.

Both the sender and the receiver must be sensitive to the internal and external climate, because the perception of the message is altered greatly depending on the climate that existed at the time the message was sent or received. For example, an insecure manager who is called to meet with superiors during a period of stringent layoffs will probably view the message with more trepidation than a manager who is secure in his or her role.

Because each person is different and thus makes decisions and perceives differently, assessing external climate is usually easier than internal climate. In assessing internal climate, remember that the human mind perceives only what it expects to perceive. The unexpected is generally ignored or misunderstood. In other words, receivers cannot communicate if the message is incompatible with their expectations. Therefore, effective communication requires the sender to determine what receivers see and hear.

> Effective communication requires the sender to determine what receivers see and hear.

VARIABLES AFFECTING ORGANIZATIONAL COMMUNICATION

Formal organizational structure has an impact on communication. People at lower levels of the organizational hierarchy are at risk for inadequate communication from higher levels. This occurs because of the number of levels communication must filter through in large organizations. As the number of employees increases (particularly more than 1,000 employees), the quantity of communication generally increases; however, employees may perceive it as increasingly closed.

In addition, in large organizations, it is impossible for individual managers to communicate personally with each person or group involved in organizational decision making. Anthony and Preuss (2002) state that within hospitals there are multiple complex systems with rules, contingencies, exceptions, and multiple intermember communications, all of which make effective communication difficult. Jackson (1984) identified the following characteristics of large organizations make communication particularly problematic:

- Spatial distance within an organization can be a barrier to communication.
- Different subgroups or subcultures within the organization have their own value systems and identities. Members within that subgroup form an allegiance to their own members. This results in different translations of messages from management, depending on the significance of the message to the things the subgroup values and is striving to accomplish.
- People are structured into different systems of relationships in organizations. A work structure exists in which certain people are expected to complete tasks with other people. An authority structure exists when some workers are in charge of supervising others. A status structure determines which people have rights and privileges. A prestige structure allows some people to expect deferential treatment from others. The friendship structure encourages interpersonal trust. All of these systems influence who should communicate with whom and in what manner.
- Organizations are in a constant state of flux. Relationships (subgroups or subcultures) and geographical locations constantly change. It is difficult to communicate decisions to all the people who are affected by them because of this constant state of change.

Gender is also a significant factor in organizational communication since men and women communicate and use language differently. Indeed, Rudan's (2003) study of gender differences in team building showed that leadership style was an extension of communication style. He found that when conducting business meetings, the males were "all business" while the females discussed other personal and social issues with team members. Men also frequently held "meetings before the meeting" where things were agreed upon prior to the meeting, and women were not present at these small meetings.

Complicating the picture further is the historical need in the healthcare industry for a predominantly male medical profession to closely communicate with a predominantly female nursing profession. Chitty (2001) states that during female-dominated nursing school experiences, most nurses are encouraged to view physicians as teammates and to collaborate with them whenever possible. Male-dominated medical schools, however, tend to instill in their graduates a hierarchical model of teamwork with the physician at the top of the hierarchy. The combination of difference in use of language and perceived difference in status often results in patterns of male dominance and female deference in communication.

In addition, the majority of healthcare administrators continue to be male. Therefore, male physicians and male administrators may feel little incentive to seek a collaborative approach in communication that female nurses often desire. These differences in gender and in power and status continue to affect tremendously the types and quality of organizational and unit-level communication.

> Gender is a significant factor in organizational communication because men and women communicate and use language differently.

Learning Exercise 19.1

Large Organization Communication
Have you ever been employed in a large organization? Was the communication within that organization clear and timely? What or who was your primary source of information? Were you a part of a subgroup or subculture? If so, how did that affect communication?

ORGANIZATIONAL COMMUNICATION STRATEGIES

Although organizational communication is complex, the following strategies can increase the likelihood of clear and complete communication:

- Managers must assess organizational communication. Who communicates with whom in the organization? Is the communication timely? Does communication within the formal organization concur with formal lines of authority? Are there conflicts or disagreements about communication? What modes of communication are used?
- Managers must understand the organization's structure and recognize who will be affected by decisions that are made. Both formal and informal communication networks need to be considered. *Formal communication networks* follow the formal line of authority in the organization's hierarchy. *Informal communication networks* occur between people at the same or different levels of the organizational hierarchy but do not represent formal lines of authority or responsibility. For example, an informal communication network might occur between a hospital's CEO and her daughter, who is a clerk on a medical wing. Although there may be a significant exchange of information about unit or organizational functioning, this communication network would not be apparent on the organization chart. It is imperative, then, that managers be very careful of what they say and to whom until they have a good understanding of the formal and informal communication networks.
- Communication is not a one-way channel. If other departments or disciplines will be affected by a message, the manager must consult with those areas for feedback before the communication occurs.
- The communication must be clear, simple, and precise. The manager (sender) is responsible for ensuring the message is understood.
- Managers should seek feedback regarding whether their communication was accurately received. One way to do this is to ask the receiver to repeat the communication or instructions. In addition, the sender should continue follow-up communication in an effort to determine if the communication is being acted upon.
- Multiple communication methods should be used when possible if a message is important. Using a variety of communication methods in combination increases the likelihood that everyone in the organization who needs to hear the message will.

- Managers should not overwhelm subordinates with unnecessary information. Although information and communication are different, they are interdependent. *Information* is formal, impersonal, and unaffected by emotions, values, expectations, and perceptions. *Communication*, on the other hand, involves perception and feeling. It does not depend on information and may represent shared experiences. In contrast to information sharing, superiors must continually communicate with subordinates.

For example, most staff need little information about ordering procedures or organizational supply vendors as long as supplies are adequate and appropriate to meet unit needs. If, however, a vendor is temporarily unable to meet unit supply needs, the use of supplies by staff becomes an issue requiring close communication between managers and subordinates. The manager must communicate with the staff about which supplies will be inadequately stocked and for how long. In addition, the manager may choose to discuss this inadequacy of resources with the staff to identify alternative solutions.

CHANNELS OF COMMUNICATION

Because large organizations are so complex, communication channels used by the manager may be upward, downward, horizontal, diagonal, or through the "grapevine." In *upward communication*, the manager is a subordinate to higher management. Needs and wants are communicated upward to the next level in the hierarchy. Those at this higher level make decisions for a greater segment of the organization than the lower-level manager.

In *downward communication*, the manager relays information to subordinates. This is a traditional form of communication in organizations and helps coordinate activities in various levels of the hierarchy.

In *horizontal communication*, managers interact with others on the same hierarchical level as themselves who are managing different segments of the organization. The need for horizontal communication increases as departmental interdependence increases.

In *diagonal communication*, the manager interacts with personnel and managers of other departments and groups, such as physicians, who are not on the same level of the organizational hierarchy. Although these people have no formal authority over the manager, this communication is vital to the organization's functioning. Diagonal communication tends to be less formal than other types of communication.

The most informal communication network is often called the *grapevine*. Grapevine communication flows haphazardly between people at all hierarchical levels and usually involves three or four people at a time. Grapevine communication is subject to error and distortion because of the speed at which it passes and because the sender has little formal accountability for the message. Ribeiro and Blakeley (1998) suggest this distortion occurs because transmitters using grapevine communication often do one of the following: (1) elaborate on the original story but convey its original intent, (2) distort the message either deliberately or unintentionally, or (3) start a contradictory message because they disagree with the original message received. Given the frequency of grapevine communication in all organizations, all managers must attempt to better understand how the grapevine works in their own organization as well as who is contributing to it.

Learning Exercise 19.2

When and How Will You Tell?
Assume that you are the project director of a small, family planning clinic. You have just received word that your federal and state funding has been slashed and that the clinic will probably close in three months. Although an additional funding source may be found, it is improbable that it will occur within the next three months. The board of directors informed you that this knowledge is not to be made public at this time.

You have five full-time employees at the clinic. Because two of these employees are close friends, you feel some conflict about withholding this information from them. You are aware that another clinic in town currently has job openings and that the positions are generally filled quickly.

Assignment: It is important that you staff the clinic for the next three months. When will you notify the staff of the clinic's intent to close? Will you communicate the closing to all staff at the same time? Will you use downward communication? Should the grapevine be used to leak news to employees? When might the grapevine be appropriate to pass on information?

COMMUNICATION MODES

A message's clarity is greatly affected by the mode of communication used. Research by Parker and Coiera (2000) suggests clinical hospital workers tend primarily to use synchronous communication modes such as telephone calls and chance face-to-face meetings with colleagues, even when these channels are not effective. Synchronous communication also contributes to a highly interruptive work environment, increasing the potential for clinical errors.

In general, the more direct the communication, the greater the probability that it will be clear. The more people involved in filtering the communication, the greater the chance of distortion. The manager must evaluate each circumstance individually to determine which mode or combination of modes is optimal for each situation.

The manager uses the following modes of communication most frequently:

- **Written communication.** Written messages (including electronic mail, which will be discussed later in the chapter) allow for documentation. They may, however, be open to various interpretations and generally consume more managerial time. Most managers are required to do a considerable amount of this type of communication and therefore need to be able to write clearly.
- **Face-to-face communication.** Oral communication is rapid but may result in fewer people receiving the information than necessary. Managers communicate verbally upward and downward and formally and informally. They also communicate verbally in formal meetings, with people in peer work groups, and when making formal presentations.
- **Nonverbal communication.** Nonverbal communication includes facial expression, body movements, and gestures and is commonly referred to as body language. Because nonverbal communication indicates the emotional

component of the message, it is generally considered more reliable than verbal communication. There is significant danger, however, in misinterpreting nonverbal messages if they are not assessed in context with the verbal message. Nonverbal communication occurs any time managers are seen (e.g., messages are transmitted to subordinates every time the manager communicates verbally or just walks down a hallway).

- **Telephone communication.** A telephone call is rapid and allows the receiver to clarify the message at the time it is given. It does not, however, allow the receipt of nonverbal messages for either the sender or receiver of the message. Accents may be difficult to understand as well in a multicultural workforce. Because managers today use the telephone so much, it has become an important communication tool, but it does have limits as an effective communication device.

Learning Exercise 19.3

Your Communication Style
Which communication modes do you use most frequently? Which is your preferred mode and why? Which modes are most difficult for you to use and why?

WRITTEN COMMUNICATION WITHIN THE ORGANIZATION

Although communication may take many forms, written communication is used most often in large organizations. Organizational policy, procedures, events, and change may be announced in writing. Job descriptions, performance appraisals, letters of reference, and memos also are forms of written communication.

The written communication issued by the manager reflects greatly on both the manager and the organization. Thus, the manager must be able to write clearly and professionally and to use understandable language. Writing is a learned skill that improves with practice. Because letters constitute much of a manager's writing, HealthCare Education Associates (1988) composed the following suggestions for formal business letters:

- **Know what you want to say before you start writing.** This requires that you think clearly before you can write clearly.
- **Put people into your writing.** When you write about a subject, discuss it in terms of the people affected by it. Avoid words such as administration, authorization, and implementation because they are abstract and impersonal.
- **Use action words.** Action verbs have a stronger impact.
- **Write plainly.** Use familiar, specific, and concrete words. Plain writing is more easily understood and thus is more apt to be read.
- **Use as few words as possible.** Find one good way to make a point, and trust that your reader will understand it.
- **Use simple, direct sentences**. Keep sentences less than 20 words and include only one idea in each. Make positive statements that clearly delineate your position on an issue. Tell the pertinent facts first.

- **Give the reader direction.** Be consistent in the tone of the message to establish a clear point of view.
- **Arrange the material logically.** A logical presentation of facts increases the reliability that the reader attributes to the writer. The material may be organized deductively, inductively, by order of importance, from the familiar to the unfamiliar, in chronological order, by close relationship, or by physical location.
- **Use paragraphs to lead readers.** A paragraph should not exceed eight to ten lines in a memo or five or six lines in a letter.
- **Connect your thoughts.** To do this, you must add enough details, use repetition to tie thoughts together, and select transitional words to tell the reader when you are moving to a new thought.
- **Be clear.** Be certain your pronouns are clearly defined.
- **Express similar thoughts in similar ways.** This will increase the continuity of the message.

Although a business letter's content is very important, its appearance or format also conveys a message. Adequate margins, clear typeface, and the use of appropriate greetings and salutations add to the message's professionalism. **Display 19.2** shows the accepted basic format for any formal business letter.

Display 19.2 | Business Letter Format

Skip four to eight lines, depending on the length of the letter
DATE
Skip four to eight lines
INSIDE ADDRESS—Check the spelling and address for accuracy.
Double space
RE: (pronounced "ray " or "ree," means regarding)—This optional device alerts the reader to the subject of your letter.
Double space
SALUTATION—Write "Dear . . ." Abbreviate titles such as "Mr.," and "Dr."; spell out titles such as "Reverend" and "Senator."
Use a comma (,) for informal letters and a colon (:) for formal letters—if you are on a first-name basis, use a comma; otherwise, use a colon.
If you are uncertain as to the sex of the person to whom you are writing, address by title—"Dear Hospital Administrator" or "Dear Sir or Madam."
Double space
BODY OF LETTER—Single space within the paragraph, and double space between paragraphs. (If you use the indented form, you do not need to double space between paragraphs.)
Double space
COMPLIMENTARY CLOSING—Capitalize the first letter of the first word, and put a comma at the end—"Sincerely,"
Skip four lines if the letter is typed
SIGNATURE (typed)—Place your written signature above your typed name.
Double space
ENCLOSURES—If you are enclosing anything, indicate here, typically with "Enc." or "Encs."

Display 19.2 Business Letter Format

An example of a standard letter format follows.

Healthcare Personnel Associates
Suite 432 Boulevard Building
Somewhere, USA

January 2, 2005

JJ Doe, RN, Director of Nursing
Community Hospital
Somewhere, USA

Re: Project XYZ

Dear Ms. Doe:

We are initiating a new program called Project XYZ to help hospitals and other healthcare agencies in the city meet the increasing need for nurses at competitive costs with a unique pool of experienced professional nurses.

We are launching the project on Wednesday, February 29, from 8 to 9:30 P.M. in the Washington Center on Main Street in Somewhere, USA. We hope you and other interested staff members can attend. Enclosed is the agenda for the meeting.

Please respond to 555-000-5555 or ncn@HPASOC.com by February 26 if you can attend. Light refreshments will be served.

Sincerely,

Nan C. Norse

Nan C. Norse, RN, MBA, President
encl.

Source: Reproduced with permission from Healthcare Education Associates (1998). *Professional writing skills for healthcare managers*, p. 68.

Learning Exercise 19.4

Revising a Formal Business Letter
Read the following formal business letter. Assess the quality of the writing using the criteria listed for writing a business letter. Rewrite the letter so all criteria are met. Be prepared to read your letter to the class.

Mrs. Joan Watkins
October 19, 1991
Brownie Troop 407
Anywhere, USA 00000

Dear Mrs. Watkins:

I am the official Public Relations Coordinator for County Hospital and serve as correspondence officer for requests from public service groups. We have more than 100 requests such as yours every year, so I have a very busy job! You are welcome to come and visit our hospital anytime. My secretary told me you called yesterday and wondered whether we provide tours. There is no charge for our tours. My secretary also told me the average age of your Brownies is 8 years, so it might be most appropriate to have them visit our NICU, PICU, and ER. Please tell the kids about the units in advance so they'll be better prepared for what they will see. The philosophy at our hospital promotes community involvement, so this is one way we attempt to meet this goal. I'll be sure to arrange to have a nursing manager escort the group on your tour. Please call when you have a date and time in mind. I was a Brownie myself when I was 7 years old, so I think this is a terrific idea on your part.

Sincerely,

Ima Verbose, MSN
Personal Relations Coordinator
County Hospital

Communication in a large organization requires tremendous intradepartmental and interdepartmental communication; much of this communication occurs in the form of memos. Memos, unlike letters, are distributed internally within the organization. The primary purpose of most memos is to inform, instruct, recommend, or document. HealthCare Education Associates (1988) suggests the following guidelines for writing effective memos:

- Memos should make the main point at the beginning.
- Only essential information should be given in the memo.
- The memo should be written simply, without inflated or authoritarian language.
- Headings should be used in the memo to direct the reader to specific issues.

Most organizations have an established form for memos. This form is generally in a block format with no indentations from the left-hand margin. **Display 19.3** shows the standard format for an organizational memo.

Display 19.3 Memo Format

Date:
Double space
To: If the memo is to be distributed to more than one person, alphabetical order is the easiest method of listing. You may list by rank if you prefer.
Double space
From:
Double space
Subject: In a few words, state the reason you are writing the memo. This lets the reader know at a glance what you will be talking about.
Triple space
Signature:
Triple space
Copies: You may need to send copies of your memo to different people. You should indicate this here, using the abbreviation "cc:" followed by the names of those receiving copies of the memo.

Source: Reproduced with permission from HealthCare Education Associates (1998). *Professional writing skills for healthcare managers,* p. 68.

The problem with letters and memos is there usually is no feedback mechanism available for the sender to clarify intent. One way to minimize this danger is by having other supervisory personnel read and interpret written communication before distribution.

Learning Exercise 19.5

Writing a Memo
You are a school nurse. In the last two weeks, nine cases of head lice have been reported in four different classrooms. The potential for spread is high, and both the teachers and parents are growing anxious. Compose a memo for distribution to the teachers. Your goals are to inform, reassure, and direct future inquiries. Be sure this memo uses the format shown in Display 19.3 and encompasses the guidelines for memo writing suggested in this chapter.

INTERPERSONAL COMMUNICATION IN A MULTICULTURAL WORKPLACE

Because it is impossible for the individual manager to communicate face to face with each member in the large organization, managers must develop other interpersonal communication skills. These skills include nonverbal communication, verbal communication skills, and listening skills. Perhaps even more importantly, the manager must have the sensitivity and leadership skills to communicate in today's multicultural workplace.

Nonverbal Communication

Ralph Waldo Emerson stated, "What you are speaks so loudly I cannot hear what you say" (Rocchiccioli & Tilbury, 1998, p. 147). Much of our communication occurs through nonverbal channels that must be examined in the context of the verbal content. Generally, if verbal and nonverbal messages are incongruent, the receiver will believe the nonverbal message.

Because nonverbal behavior can be and frequently is misinterpreted, receivers must validate perceptions with senders. The incongruence between verbal and non-verbal leads to many communication problems. The following is a partial list of nonverbal clues that can occur with or without verbal communication:

- **Space.** The space between the sender and receiver influences what is communicated. Although distance implies a lack of trust or warmth, inadequate space, as defined by cultural norms, may make people feel threatened or intimidated. For example, some cultures require greater space between sender and receiver than others. Anglo and African American nurse managers may find themselves backing away from staff members of Hispanic, East Indian, or Middle Eastern origins, who seemingly invade their personal space (Andrews, 1998). Likewise, the manager who sits beside employees during performance appraisals sends a different message than the manager who speaks to the employee from the opposite side of a large and formal desk. In this case, distance increases power and status on the part of the manager; however, the receptivity to distance and the message it implies varies with the culture of the receiver.
- **Environment.** The area where the communication takes place is an important part of the communication process. Communication that takes place in a superior's office is generally taken more seriously than that which occurs in the cafeteria.
- **Appearance.** Much is communicated by our clothing, hairstyles, cosmetics, and attractiveness. The phrase "dressing for success" appropriately defines the impact of dress and appearance on role perception and power; again however, care should be exercised to establish dress policies that incorporate both cultural and gender-related sensitivities (Andrews, 1998).
- **Eye contact.** This nonverbal clue is often associated with sincerity. Eye contact invites interaction. Likewise, breaking eye contact suggests that the interaction is about to cease. Bohannon (2000) states that making eye contact is one of the key components of effective body language. Blinking, staring, or looking away when you begin speaking makes it hard for you to connect with another person emotionally. However, the manager must be aware that, like space, the presence or absence of eye contact is strongly influenced by cultural standards.
- **Posture.** Posture and the way you control the other parts of your body are extremely important. "If you slouch, shuffle, or stoop, you send the message

that you are indifferent. If you wave your arms, clear your throat a lot, or pull on your hair or earlobes frequently, you may come across as insincere and unnatural. If you sit or stand with crossed or folded arms or with your hands stuffed in your pockets, you appear protective, defensive, unwelcoming" (Bohannon, 2000, p. 21). In addition, the weight of a message is increased if the sender faces the receiver, stands or sits appropriately close, and, with head erect, leans toward the receiver.

- **Gestures.** A message accented with appropriate gestures takes on added emphasis. Too much gesturing can, however, be distracting. For example, hand movement can emphasize or distract from the message. Gestures also have a cultural meaning. Nurses from Asian cultures who tend to be less tactile and show affection in a more reserved manner may perceive Anglo or African American nurses to be boisterous, loud, ill mannered, or rude by comparison (Andrews, 1998). Indeed, the use of touch is one gesture that often sends messages that are misinterpreted by receivers from different cultures.
- **Facial expression.** Effective communication requires a facial expression that agrees with your message. Staff perceive managers who present a pleasant and open expression as approachable. Likewise, a nurse's facial expression can greatly affect how and what clients are willing to relate.
- **Timing.** Hesitation often diminishes the effect of your statement or implies untruthfulness.
- **Vocal clues such as tone, volume, and inflection.** All of these clues add to the message being transmitted. Tentative statements sound more like questions than statements, leading listeners to think you are unsure of yourself. Speaking rapidly implies nervousness, and speaking in a monotone voice implies disinterest (Bohannon, 2000). The goal, then, should always be to convey confidence and clarity.

All nurses must be sensitive to nonverbal clues and their importance in communication. This is especially true for nursing leaders. Effective leaders are congruent in their verbal and nonverbal communication, so followers are clear about the messages they receive. Likewise, leaders are sensitive to nonverbal and verbal messages from followers and look for inconsistencies that may indicate unresolved problems or needs. Often organizational difficulties can be prevented because leaders recognize the nonverbal communication of subordinates and take appropriate and timely action.

> Effective leaders are congruent in their verbal and nonverbal communication, so followers are clear about the messages they receive.

Verbal Communication Skills

Highly developed verbal communication skills are critical for the leader–manager. One of the most important verbal communication skills is the art of assertive communication. *Assertive behavior* is a way of communicating that allows people to express themselves in direct, honest, and appropriate ways that do not infringe on another person's rights. A person's position is expressed clearly and firmly using "I" statements. In addition, assertive communication always requires that verbal and nonverbal messages be congruent. To be successful in the directing phase of management, the leader must have well-developed skills in assertive communication.

There are many misconceptions about assertive communication. The first is that all communication is either assertive or passive. Actually, at least four possibilities for communication exist: passive, aggressive, indirectly aggressive or passive-aggressive, or assertive. *Passive* communication occurs when a person suffers in silence, although he or she may feel strongly about the issue. *Aggressive* people express themselves in a direct and often hostile manner that infringes on another person's rights; this behavior is generally oriented toward "winning at all costs" or demonstrating self-excellence. *Passive-aggressive* communication is an aggressive message presented in a passive way. It generally involves limited verbal exchange (with incongruent nonverbal behavior) by a person who feels strongly about a situation. This person feigns withdrawal in an effort to manipulate the situation.

The second misconception is that those who communicate or behave assertively get everything they want. This is untrue because being assertive involves rights and responsibilities. **Display 19.4** lists the rights and responsibilities of the assertive person.

The third misconception about assertiveness is that it is unfeminine. Although the role of women in society in general has undergone tremendous change in the last 100 years, some individuals continue to find great difficulty in accepting that the nurse plays an assertive, active, decision-making role.

Assertive communication is not rude or insensitive behavior; rather, it is having an informed voice that insists on being heard. An assertive communication model helps people unlearn common self-deprecating speech patterns that signal insecurity and a lack of confidence. The nursing profession must be more assertive in its need to be heard. Eventually, a form of peer pressure can emerge that reshapes others and results in an assertive nursing voice.

A fourth misconception is that the terms *assertive* and *aggressive* are synonymous. To be assertive is to not be aggressive, although some cultures find the distinction blurred. Even when faced with someone else's aggression, the assertive

Display 19.4	Rights and Responsibilities of the Assertive Person
Rights	**Responsibilities**
To speak up	To listen
To take	To give
To have problems	To find solutions
To be comforted	To comfort others
To work	To do your best
To make mistakes	To correct your mistakes
To laugh	To make others happy
To have friends	To be a friend
To criticize	To praise
To have your efforts rewarded	To reward others' efforts
To be independent	To be dependable
To cry	To dry tears
To be loved	To love others

(Chenevert, 1988)

communicator does not become aggressive. When under attack by an aggressive person, an assertive person can do several things:

- **Reflect.** Reflect the speaker's message back to him or her. Focus on the affective components of the aggressor's message. This helps the aggressor to evaluate whether the intensity of his or her feelings is appropriate to the specific situation or event. For example, assume an employee enters a manager's office and begins complaining about a newly posted staff schedule. The employee is obviously angry and defensive. The manager might use reflection by stating, "I understand that you are very upset about your schedule. This is an important issue, and we need to talk about it."
- **Repeat the assertive message.** Repeated assertions focus on the message's objective content. They are especially effective when the aggressor overgeneralizes or seems fixated on a repetitive line of thinking. For example, if a manager requests that an angry employee step into his or her office to discuss a problem, and the employee continues his or her tirade in the hallway, the manager might say, "I am willing to discuss this issue with you in my office. The hallway is not the appropriate place for this discussion."
- **Point out the implicit assumptions.** This involves listening closely and letting the aggressor know that you have heard him or her. In these situations, managers might repeat major points or identify key assumptions to show that they are following the employee's line of reasoning.
- **Restate the message by using assertive language.** Rephrasing the aggressor's language will defuse the emotion. Paraphrasing helps the aggressor focus more on the cognitive part of the message. The manager might use restating by changing a "you" message to an "I" message.
- **Question.** When the aggressor uses nonverbal clues to be aggressive, the assertive person can put this behavior in the form of a question as an effective means of helping the other person become aware of an unwarranted reaction. For example, the desperate, angry employee may imply threats about quitting or transferring to another unit. The manager could appropriately confront the employee about his or her implied threat to see if it is real or simply a reflection of the employee's frustration.

As in nonverbal communication, the verbal communication skills of the leader–manager in a multicultural workplace require cultural sensitivity. Even when dealing with staff from the same cultural background, it requires administrative skill to decide whether to speak face to face, send an electronic or paper memo, telephone, or not to communicate about a particular matter at all. This complexity is even greater in the multicultural healthcare setting (Andrews, 1998).

Andrews (1998) suggests the following strategies to promote effective verbal communication in the multicultural workplace:

- Use proper titles of respect. Do not call a person by his or her first name until given permission to do so.
- Be aware of subtle linguistic messages that may convey bias or inequality. For example, referring to a white male as "mister" or "sir" and an African American female by her first name suggests a difference in status.

- Avoid all slang, pejorative, or derogatory terms when referring to persons from a particular ethnicity, race, or religious group.
- Avoid making remarks to staff that they should consider themselves fortunate to be employed by the organization. Do not compare their employment opportunities and conditions to people in their country of origin.
- Avoid using phrases such as "culturally disadvantaged," "socioeconomically disadvantaged," and "culturally deprived" as they suggest inferiority and may be offensive to others. Also avoid use of the term "nonwhite," as it implies that white is the normative standard.
- Do not expect a staff member to know or get along well with all other staff members of the same ethnicity. Although they share the same ethnicity, their uniqueness as individuals creates a diversity of interactions, values, experiences, and beliefs.

Listening Skills

Research has shown that most people hear or actually retain only a small amount of the information given to them. Generally, although the average person spends over half of his or her time listening, only one third of the messages sent are retained. For the leader, the active process of listening is vital for interpersonal communication effectiveness (O'Neil, & Morjikian, 2003). It is important that the leader–manager approach listening as an opportunity to learn appreciation for a cultural perspective of the organization that is different than his or her own (Kerfoot, 1998).

To become better listeners, leaders must first become aware of how their own experiences, values, attitudes, and biases affect how they receive and perceive messages. Second, leaders must overcome the information and communication overload inherent in the middle-management role. It is easy for overwhelmed managers to stop listening actively to the many subordinates who need and demand their time simultaneously.

Finally, the leader must continually work to improve listening skills. The leader who actively listens gives genuine time and attention to the sender, focusing on verbal and nonverbal communication. The leader's primary purpose, then, is to receive the message being sent rather than forming a response before the transmission of the message is complete.

GROUP COMMUNICATION

Managers must communicate with large and small groups, as well as individual employees. Because a group communicates differently than individuals do, it is essential that the manager have an understanding of group dynamics, including the sequence each group must go through before work can be accomplished. Tuckman and Jensen (1977) labeled these stages forming, storming, norming, and performing.

When people are introduced into workgroups, they must go through a process of meeting each other: the *forming stage*. They then progress through a stage where there is much competition and attempts at the establishment of individual identities: the *storming stage*. Next, the group begins to establish rules and design its work: the *norming stage*. Finally, during the *performing stage*, the work actually gets done. **Table 19.1** summarizes each stage.

Some experts suggest there is another phase: *termination* or *closure*. In this phase, the leader guides members to summarize, express feelings, and come to closure. A celebration at the end of committee work is a good way to conclude group effort.

Because a group's work develops over time, the addition of new members to a committee can slow productivity. It takes some time for the group to accept new members. Some developmental stages will be performed again or delayed if several new members join a group. Therefore, it is important when assigning members to a committee to select those who can remain until the work is finished or until their appointment time is over.

> To promote productivity, try to appoint committee members who can serve until the work is finished or until their appointment time is over.

Table 19.1 Stages of Group Process

Group Development Stage	Group Process	Task Process
Forming	Testing occurs to identify boundaries of interpersonal behaviors, establish dependency relationships with leaders and other members, and determine what is acceptable behavior.	Testing occurs to identify the tasks, appropriate rules, and methods suited to the task's performance.
Storming	Resistance to group influence is evident as members polarize into subgroups; conflict ensues and members rebel against demands imposed by the leader.	Resistance to task requirements and the differences surface regarding demands imposed by the task.
Norming	Consensus evolves as group cohesion develops; conflict and resistance are overcome.	Cooperation develops as differences are expressed and resolved.
Performing	Interpersonal structure focuses on task and its completion; roles become flexible and functional; energies are directed to task performance.	Problems are solved as the task performance improves; constructive efforts are undertaken to complete task; more of group energies are available for the task.

Group Dynamics

In addition to forming, storming, and norming, two other functions of groups are necessary for work to be performed. One has to do with the task or the purpose of the group, and the other has to do with the maintenance of the group or support functions. Managers should understand how groups carry out their specific tasks and roles.

Task Roles of Groups

There are 11 tasks that each group performs. A member may perform several tasks, but for the work of the group to be accomplished, all the necessary tasks will be carried out, either by members or by the leader. These roles or tasks follow:

1. **Initiator:** Contributor who proposes or suggests group goals or redefines the problem. There may be more than one initiator during the group's lifetime.
2. **Information seeker:** Searches for a factual basis for the group's work.
3. **Information giver:** Offers an opinion of what the group's view of pertinent values should be.
4. **Opinion seeker:** Seeks opinions that clarify or reflect the value of other members' suggestions.
5. **Elaborator:** Gives examples or extends meanings of suggestions given and how they could work.
6. **Coordinator:** Clarifies and coordinates ideas, suggestions, and activities of the group.
7. **Orienter:** Summarizes decisions and actions; identifies and questions departures from predetermined goals.
8. **Evaluator:** Questions group accomplishments and compares them to a standard.
9. **Energizer:** Stimulates and prods the group to act and raises the level of its actions.
10. **Procedural technician:** Facilitates group action by arranging the environment.
11. **Recorder:** Records the group's activities and accomplishments.

Group-Building and Maintenance Roles

The group task roles contribute to the work to be done; the group-building roles provide for the care and maintenance of the group. Examples of group-building roles include:

- **Encourager:** Accepts and praises all contributions, viewpoints, and ideas with warmth and solidarity.
- **Harmonizer:** Mediates, harmonizes, and resolves conflict.
- **Compromiser:** Yields his or her position in a conflict situation.
- **Gatekeeper:** Promotes open communication and facilitates participation by all members.

- **Standard setter:** Expresses or evaluates standards to evaluate group process.
- **Group commentator:** Records group process and provides feedback to the group.
- **Follower:** Accepts the group's ideas and listens to discussion and decisions.

Organizations need to have a mix of members—enough people to carry out the work tasks but also people who are good at team building. One group may perform more than one function and group-building role.

Individual Roles of Group Members

Group members also carry out roles that serve their own needs. Group leaders must be able to manage member roles so that individuals do not disrupt group productivity. The goal, however, should be management and not suppression. Not every group member has a need that results in the use of one of these roles. The eight individual roles follow:

1. **Aggressor:** Expresses disapproval of others' values or feelings through jokes, verbal attacks, or envy.
2. **Blocker:** Persists in expressing negative points of view and resurrects dead issues.
3. **Recognition seeker:** Works to focus positive attention on himself or herself.
4. **Self-confessor:** Uses the group setting as a forum for personal expression.
5. **Playboy:** Remains uninvolved and demonstrates cynicism, nonchalance, or horseplay.
6. **Dominator:** Attempts to control and manipulate the group.
7. **Help seeker:** Uses expressions of personal insecurity, confusion, or self-deprecation to manipulate sympathy from members.
8. **Special interest pleader:** Cloaks personal prejudices or biases by ostensibly speaking for others.

Managers must be well grounded in group dynamics and group roles because of the need to facilitate group communication and productivity within the organization. However, the leadership role has an even greater impact on group effectiveness. Dynamic leaders inspire followers toward participative management by how they work and communicate in groups. Leaders keep group members on course, draw out the shy, politely cut off the garrulous, and protect the weak.

 Learning Exercise 19.6

Identifying Group Stages and Productivity
Write a list of the various groups with which you are currently involved. Describe the stage of each one. Did it take longer for some of your groups to get to the performing stage than others? If membership in the group changed, describe what happened to the productivity level.

THE IMPACT OF TECHNOLOGY ON ORGANIZATIONAL COMMUNICATION

Richards (2001) argues that a massive communications revolution (paradigm shift) is underway, one that will have profound effects on the art and science of nursing. While nurses as a group have historically been somewhat unsophisticated in informatics potential, new generations of nurses, who have used technology to play, learn, communicate, and form relationships since childhood, will be accustomed to the instantaneous and interactive flow of information and dialogue (Richards, 2001). These nurses will approach and accept technology as an adjunct to their nursing cognizance and not question its presence or use. These "Net nurses" will view technology in the same light as contemporary nurses do their stethoscopes, and will use this resource to continue to provide evidence-based, professional care. Indeed, for these nurses, "collaborative practice will involve a community of electronically connected practitioners providing a richer and more scientific foundation for practice" (Richards, 2001, p. 6).

It is clear that the telecommunication technology growth experienced in the late 20th century will continue to proliferate even more rapidly in the 21st century. This advancing technology may help to balance the constraints being placed on other patient-care resources. Technologies such as electronic mail, faxes, teleconferences, and CD-ROMs are increasing the potential for effective and efficient communication throughout the organization. The use of hospital information system (HIS) configurations such as stand-alone systems, on-line interactive systems, networked systems, and integrative systems has also increased.

McConnell (2000) suggests that technology offers new ways to pull information together and fulfill its potential as a nursing resource. For example, many hospitals now have integrated nurse call systems that simultaneously display patient calls and interface directly with the hospital's information and admission, discharge, and transfer systems. Others use pocket pagers or infrared locators that offer precise, real-time identification and location of caregivers and equipment (McConnell, 2000).

In addition, nurse–managers are increasingly using the *Internet* as both an information source and a communication tool. As a communication tool, the Internet provides access to electronic mail, file transfer protocol, and the World Wide Web. Richards (2001) states that the "Net generation" of nurses will use the Internet as their first point of reference and will demand a fully networked computing environment.

Even the most advanced communication technology, however, cannot replace the human judgment needed by leaders and managers to use that technology appropriately. Examples of the type of communication challenges managers face in such a rapidly evolving technological society include:

- Determining which technological advances can and should be used at each level of the organizational hierarchy to promote efficiency and effectiveness of communication
- Assessing the need for and providing workers with adequate training to appropriately and fully utilize the technological communication tools that may become available to them

- Aligning communication technology with the organizational mission
- Finding a balance between technological communication options and the need for human touch, caring, and one-on-one, face-to-face interaction

Abrahamsen (2003) suggests that organizations face a significant learning curve in applying the new communication technologies available to them. This is because there is such great diversity in user educational needs and motivation to adopt these new technologies. Additionally, Abrahamsen asserts that "technology holds great promise for the healthcare environment while presenting it with countless challenges" (p. 50).

The computer age is not a passing fancy or fad—it has overcome that barrier and is here to stay. Information is indeed power, and as more information becomes available through telecommunications systems, both individuals and organizations will be empowered.

CONFIDENTIALITY

Nurses have a duty to maintain confidential information revealed to them by their patients. This confidentiality can be breached legally only when one provider must share information about a patient so that another provider can assume care. In other words, there must be a legitimate professional need to know.

Indeed, the 1996 Health Insurance Portability and Accountability Act calls for protections and privacy of medical information, including "any information about, whether oral or recorded in any form or medium, that is created or received by a healthcare provider, health plan, public health authority, employer, life insurer, school or university, or health clearing house" (Smith, 2000, p. 294). Enactment of these regulations required putting in place mechanisms and accountabilities to protect patients' privacy.

There is an ethical duty to maintain confidentiality as well. The same level of confidentiality is expected regarding sensitive personal communications between managers and subordinates.

Protecting confidentiality and privacy of personal or patient information has been made even more difficult as a result of increased electronic communication. Indeed, computerization was seen as the most serious threat to medical privacy by 54% of surveyed adults (Smith, 2000). This has occurred because the information available by electronic communication is typically easier to access than traditional information-retrieval methods and because computerized databases are unable to distinguish whether the user has a legitimate right to such information. For example, the federal government has mandated computerized patient records, and many healthcare organizations are moving toward implementation of this mandate. Unfortunately, the discussion and determination of who in the organization should have access to what information are often inadequate before such hardware is put in place, and great potential exists for violations of confidentiality. Clearly, any nurse–manager working with clinical information systems has a responsibility to see that confidentiality is maintained and that any breaches in confidentially are dealt with swiftly and appropriately.

> Any nurse–manager working with clinical information systems has a responsibility to see that confidentiality is maintained.

Learning Exercise 19.7

When Personal and Professional Obligations Conflict

You are a registered nurse employed by an insurance company that provides worker's compensation coverage for large companies. Your job requires that you do routine health screening on new employees to identify personal and job-related behaviors that may place these clients at risk for injury or illness and then to counsel them appropriately regarding risk reduction.

One of the areas you assess during your patient history is high-risk sexual behavior. One of the clients you saw today expressed concern that he might be positive for the AIDS virus because a former girlfriend, with whom he had unprotected sex, recently tested positive for the human immunodeficiency virus (HIV). He tells you that he is afraid to be tested "because I don't want to know if I have it." He seems firm on his refusal to be tested. You go ahead and provide him information about HIV testing and what he can do in the future to prevent transmission of the virus to himself and others.

Later that evening, you are having dinner with your 26-year old sister when she reveals that she has a "new love" in her life. When she tells you his name and where he works, you immediately recognize him as the client you counseled in the office today.

Assignment: What will you do with the information you have about this client's possible HIV exposure? Will you share it with your sister? What are the legal and ethical ramifications inherent in violating this patient's confidentiality? What are the conflicting personal and professional obligations? Would your action be the same if a casual acquaintance revealed to you that this client was her new boyfriend? Be as honest as possible in your analysis.

INTEGRATING LEADERSHIP AND MANAGEMENT IN ORGANIZATIONAL AND INTERPERSONAL COMMUNICATION

Communication is critical to successful leadership and management. A manager has the formal authority and responsibility to communicate with many people in the organization. Cultural diversity and rapidly flourishing communication technologies also add to the complexity of this organizational communication. Because of this complexity, the manager must understand each unique situation well enough to be able to select the most appropriate internal communication network or channel.

After selecting a communication channel, the manager faces an even greater challenge communicating the message clearly, either verbally or in writing, in a language appropriate for the message and the receiver. To select the most appropriate communication mode for a specific message, the manager must determine what should be told, to whom, and when. Because communication is a learned skill, managers can improve their written and verbal communication with repetition.

The interpersonal communication skills are more reflective of the leadership role. Sensitivity to verbal and nonverbal communication; recognition of status, power, and authority as barriers to manager–subordinate communication; and consistent use of assertiveness techniques are all leadership skills. Nurse–leaders who are perceptive and sensitive to the environment and people around them have a keen understanding of how the unit is functioning at any time and are able to intervene appropriately when problems arise. Through consistent verbal and nonverbal communication, the nurse leader is able to be a role model for subordinates.

The integrated leader–manager also uses groups to facilitate communication. Group work is also used to increase productivity. All members of work groups should be assisted with role clarification and productive group dynamics.

Organizational communication requires both management functions and leadership skills. Management functions in communication ensure productivity and continuity through appropriate sharing of information. Leadership skills ensure appraisal and intervention in meeting expressed and tacit human resource needs. Leadership skills in communication also allow the leader–manager to clarify organizational goals and direct subordinates in reaching those goals. Communication within the organization would fail if both leadership skills and management functions were not present.

☀ Key Concepts

- Communication forms the core of management activities and cuts across all phases of the management process.
- Depending on the manager's position in the hierarchy, more than 80% of managerial time may be spent in some type of organizational communication; thus, organizational communication is a management function.
- Because the overwhelming majority of managerial communication time is spent speaking and listening, managers must have excellent interpersonal communication skills.
- Communication in large organizations is particularly difficult due to their complexity and size.
- Managers must understand the structure of the organization and recognize whom their decisions will affect. Both formal and informal communication networks need to be considered.
- The clarity of the message is significantly affected by the mode of communication used. In general, the more direct the communication, the greater the probability of clear communication. The more people involved in filtering the communication, the greater the chance of distortion.
- Written communication is used most often in large organizations.
- A manager's written communication reflects greatly on both the manager and the organization. Thus, managers must be able to write clearly and professionally and use understandable language.
- The incongruence between verbal and nonverbal messages is the most significant barrier to effective interpersonal communication.

- Effective leaders are congruent in their verbal and nonverbal communication, so followers are clear about the messages they receive. Likewise, leaders are sensitive to nonverbal and verbal messages from followers and look for inconsistencies that may indicate unresolved problems or needs.
- To be successful in the directing phase of management, the leader must have well-developed skills in assertive communication.
- Adding new members to an established group disrupts productivity and group development.
- Group members perform certain important tasks that facilitate work.
- Group members also perform roles that assist with group-building activities.
- Some group members will perform roles to meet their own individual needs.
- Most people hear or retain only a small amount of the information given to them.
- Active listening is an interpersonal communication skill that improves with practice.
- Rapidly flourishing communication technologies have great potential to increase the efficiency and effectiveness of organizational communication.

More Learning Exercises and Applications

Learning Exercise 19.8

Identifying and Rephrasing Non-Assertive Responses

Decide if the following responses are an example of assertive, aggressive, passive-aggressive, or passive behavior. Change those that you identify as aggressive, passive, or passive-aggressive into assertive responses.

Situation	Response
1. A coworker withdraws instead of saying what's on his mind. You say:	"I guess you are uncomfortable talking about what's bothering you. It would be better if you talked to me."
2. This is the third time in 2 weeks that your coworker has asked for a ride home because her car is not working. You say:	"You're taking advantage of me and I won't stand for it. It's your responsibility to get your car fixed."
3. An attendant at a gas station neglected to replace your gas cap. You return to inquire about it. You say:	"One of the guys here forgot to put my gas cap back on! I want it found now or you'll buy me a new one."
4. You'd like to have a turn at being in charge on your shift. You say to your head nurse:	"Do you think that, ah, you could see your way clear to letting me be in charge once in a while?"
5. A committee meeting is being established. The proposed time is convenient for other people but not for you. The time makes it impossible for you to attend meetings regularly. When you are asked about the time you say:	"Well, I guess it's OK. I'm not going to be able to attend very much but it fits into everyone else's schedule."
6. In a conversation, a doctor suddenly asks, "What do you women libbers want anyway?" You respond:	"Fairness and equality."
7. An employee makes a lot of mistakes in his work. You say:	"You're a lazy and sloppy worker!"
8. You are the one woman in a meeting with seven men. At the beginning of the meeting, the chair asks you to be the secretary. You respond:	"No. I'm sick and tired of being the secretary just because I'm the only woman in the group."
9. A physician asks to borrow your stethoscope. You say:	"Well, I guess so. One of you doctors walked off with mine last week and this new one cost me $35. Be sure you return it, OK?"
10. You are interpreting the I & O sheet for a physician and he interrupts you. You say:	"You could understand this if you'd stop interrupting me and listen."

Learning Exercise 19.9

Memo to CEO Leads to Miscommunication

Carol White, the coordinator for the multidisciplinary mental health out-patient services of a 150-bed psychiatric hospital, feels frustrated because the hospital is very centralized. She believes this keeps the hospital's therapists and nurse–managers from being as effective as they could if they had more authority. Therefore, she has worked out a plan to decentralize her department, giving the therapists and nurse–managers more control and new titles. She sent her new plan to the CEO, Joe Short, and has just received this memo in return.

Dear Ms. White:

The Board of Directors and I met to review your plan and think it is a good one. In fact, we have been thinking along the same lines for quite some time now. I'm sure you must have heard of our plans. Because we recently contracted with a physician's group to cover our crisis center, we believe this would be a good time to decentralize in other ways. We suggest that your new substance abuse coordinator report directly to the new chief of mental health. In addition, we believe your new director of the suicide prevention center should report directly to the chief of mental health. He then will report to me.

I am pleased that we are both moving in the same direction and have the same goals. We will be setting up meetings in the future to iron out the small details.

Sincerely,

Joe Short, CEO

Assignment: How and why did Carol White's plan go astray? How did her mode of communication affect the outcome? Could the outcome have been prevented? What communication mode would have been most appropriate for Carol White to use in sharing her plan with Joe Short? What should be her plan now? Explain your rationale.

Learning Exercise 19.10

Writing a Letter of Reference

Unit managers are frequently asked to write letters of reference for employees who have been terminated. The information used in writing these letters comes from performance evaluations, personal interviews with staff and patients, evidence of continuing education, and personal observations. Assume that you are a unit manager and that you have collected the following information on Mary Doe, an RN who worked at your facility for three months before abruptly resigning with 48 hour's notice.

Performance Evaluation

Three-month evaluation scant.

- The following criteria were marked "competent": amount of work accomplished, relationships with patients and coworkers, work habits, and basic skills.
- The following criteria were identified as "needing improvement": quality of work, communication skills, and leadership skills.
- No criteria were marked unsatisfactory or outstanding.
- Narrative comments were limited to the following: "has a bit of a chip on her shoulder," "works independently a lot," and "assessment skills improving."

Interviews with Staff

- Coworker RN Judy: "She was OK. She was a little strange—she belonged to some kind of traveling religious cult. In fact, I think that's why she left her job."
- Coworker LVN/LPN Lisa: "Mary was great. She got all her work done. I never had to help her with her meds or AMcare. She took her turn at floating, which is more than I can say for some of the other RNs."
- Coworker RN John: "When I was the charge nurse, I found I needed to seek Mary out to find out what was going on with her patients. It made me real uncomfortable."
- Coworker LVN/LPN Joe: "Mary hated it here—she never felt like she belonged. The charge nurse was always hassling her about little things, and it really seemed unfair."

Patient Comments

- "She helped me with my bath and got all my pills on time. She was a good nurse."
- "I don't remember her."
- "She was so busy—I appreciated how efficient she was at how she did her job."
- "I remember Mary. She told me she really liked older people. I wish she had had more time to sit down and talk to me."

Notes from Personnel File

Twenty-four years old. Graduated from three-year diploma school two years ago. Has worked in three jobs since that time. Divorced and mother of two small children.

Continuing Education
Current CPR card. No other continuing education completed at this facility.
Assignment: Mary Doe's prospective employer has requested a letter of reference to accompany Mary's application to become a hospice nurse/counselor. No form has been provided, so it is important that your response use an appropriate format, such as the one suggested in Display 19.2. Decide which information you should include in your letter and which should be omitted. Will you weigh some information more heavily than other information? Would you make any recommendations about Mary Doe's suitability for the hospice job? Be prepared to read your letter aloud to the class, and justify your rationale for the content you included.

Learning Exercise 19.11

Bringing a Group Together
You are the evening charge nurse of a medical unit. The staff on your unit has voiced displeasure in how requests for days off are handled. Your manager has given you the task of forming a committee and reviewing the present policy regarding requests for days off on the unit. On your committee are four LVNs, three CNAs and five RNs. All shifts are represented. There are three males among the group members and there is a fairly broad range of ethnic and cultural groups.

Tomorrow will be your fourth meeting and you are beginning to get a bit frustrated because the meetings do not seem to be accomplishing much to reach the objectives the group was charged to meet. The objective was to develop a fair method to handle special requested days off that were not part of the normal rotation would be the recommendation of the committee.

On your first meeting you spent time getting to know the members and identified the objective. Various committee members contacted other hospitals and others did a literature search to determine how other institutions handled this matter. During the second meeting, this material was reviewed by all members. On the last meeting the group was very contentious, in fact several raised their voices. Others sat quietly and some seemed to pout. Only the three male members could agree upon anything. One LVN thought that the RNs were too overly represented. One RN thought the policy for day off request should be separated into three different polices, one for each classification. You are not sure how to bring this committee together or what, if any, action you should take.
Assignment: Review the section in this chapter about how groups work. Write a one-page essay on what is happening in the group and answer these questions. Should you add members to the committee? Does your group have too many task members and not enough team-building members? What should be your role in getting the group to perform its task? What could be some strategies you could use that would perhaps bring the group together?

Web Links

Communication Skills Test
http://www.queendom.com/tests/relationships/communication_skills_r_access.html
This 34-question communication skills test takes 15 to 20 minutes to complete and is designed to evaluate your general level of communication skills.

Organizational Communication
http://www.sharedresults.com
Shared Results provides organizational communication assessment and training to develop culture change and entrepreneurial spirit for corporate, non-profit and government organizations.

Stevens, T. G. Harmonious Assertive Communication: Methods to Create Understanding and Intimacy
http://front.csulb.edu/tstevens/c14-lisn.htm
Site index includes assertive conflict resolution, making assertive requests, empathetic listening, and dealing with aggression and manipulation. Also includes Stevens Relationship Questionnaire (SRQ), which explores the relationship between assertive communication skills and relationship happiness.

Improving Listening Skills
http://www.womensmedia.com/seminar-listening.html
Site helps learner develop good listening skills.

References

Abrahamsen, C. (2003). Patient safety: Take the informatics challenge. *Nursing Management, 34*(4), 48–52.

Andrews, M. M. (1998). Transcultural perspectives in nursing administration. *Journal of Nursing Administration, 28*(11), 30–38.

Anthony, M. K., & Preuss, G. (2002). Models of care: The influence of nurse communication of patient safety. *Nursing Economics$, 20*(5), 209–248.

Bohannon, L. F. (2000). Is your body language on your side? *Career World, 29*(3), 21–24.

Brice, A. (Summer, 2000). Access to health service delivery for Hispanics: A communication issue. *Journal of Multicultural Nursing and Health, 6*(2), 7–17.

Chenevert, M. (1988). *Pro-nurse handbook* (3rd ed.). St. Louis: C. V. Mosby.

Chitty, K. K. (2001). *Professional nursing. Concepts and challenges* (3rd ed.). Philadelphia, PA: W. B. Saunders Co.

HealthCare Education Associates. (1988). *Professional writing skills for health care managers: A practical guide.* St. Louis: C. V. Mosby.

Henderson, E. (2003). Communication and managerial effectiveness. *Nursing Management-UK, 9*(9), 30–35.

Jackson, J. M. (1984). The organization and its communication problems. In S. Stone, S. Firisch, S. Vordan (Eds). Management for Nurses. St. Louis: C. V. Mosby.

Kerfoot K. (1998). On leadership : Crating trust *Nursing Economics$, 16*(1), 48–49.

McConnell, E. A. (2000). Get the right information to the right people at the right time. *Nursing Management, 31*(12), 37–38, 40–41.

O'Neil, E. & Morjikian, R. (2003). Nursing leadership: Challenges and opportunities. *Policy, Politics, & Nursing Practice, 4*(3), 173–179.

Parker, J., & Coiera, E. (2000). Improving clinical communication: A view from psychology. *Journal of the American Medical Informatics Association, 7*(5), 453–461.

Ribeiro, V. E., & Blakeley, J. A. (1998). The proactive management of rumor and gossip. In E. C. Hein (Ed.), *Contemporary leadership behavior: Selected readings* (5th ed.). Philadelphia: Lippincott Williams & Wilkins.

Richards, J. A. (2001). Nursing in a digital age. *Nursing Economic$, 19*(1), 6–11.

Rocchiccioli, J. T., & Tilbury, M. S. (1998). *Clinical leadership in nursing.* Philadelphia: W. B. Saunders.

Rudan, V. T., (2003). The best of both worlds: A consideration of gender in team building. *Journal of Nusing Administration, 33*(3), 179–186.

Smith, S. P. (2000). Are you protecting your patients' confidentiality? *Nursing Economic$, 18*(6), 294–297, 319.

Tuckman, B. W., & Jensen, M. A. C. (1977). Stages of small group development revisited. *Group and Organization Studies, 2*(4), 419.

Bibliography

Baker L. H., Reiifsteck, S. W. W., & Mann, W. R. (2003). Perspectives in ambulatory care. Connected: communication for nurses using the electronic medical record. *Nursing Economic$, 21*(2), 85–86.

Blair, P. D. (2003). Make room for patient privacy. *Nursing Management, 34*(6), 28–29.

Calloway, S. D. (2001). Legally speaking. Preventing communication breakdowns. *RN, 64*(1), 71–83.

Fulfer, M. (2001). Nonverbal communication: How to read what's plain as the nose...or eyelid...or chin...on their faces. *Journal of Organizational Excellence, 20*(2), 19–28.

Haggerty, D. (2003). Communication briefs. Unlock the door to clearer communication. *Nursing Management, 34*(1), 52.

Horton, R. L. (2002). Focus on you. Managing difficult conversations: Novice managers face fast learning curve. *AWHONN Lifelines, 6*(3), 250–253.

Lieberman, M. D., & Rosenthal, R. (2001). Why introverts can't always tell who likes them: Multitasking and nonverbal decoding. *Journal of Personality and Social Psychology, 80*(2), 294–311.

McConnell, E. A. (2001)....About communicating clearly. *Nursing, 31*(4), 74–75.

Morand, D. A. (2001). The emotional intelligence of managers: Assessing the construct validity of a nonverbal measure of people skills. *Journal of Business and Psychology, 16*(1), 21–33.

O'Connor, M. (2001). Reframing communication: Conversation in the workplace. *Journal of Nursing Administration, 31*(9), 403–405.

Weiss, R. (2001). Communication strategies. Enhancing relationships with local employers. *Health Progress, 82*(1), 8–9.

What your body language says about you. (2000). *Career World, 29*(3), 2–4.

Woolf, R. (2001). How to talk so people will listen. *Journal of Nursing Administration, 31*(9), 401–402.

Delegation

Delegation is both an art and a science. It includes cognitive, affective, and intuitive dimensions.

—Marjorie Barter

Delegation can be defined simply as getting work done through others or as directing the performance of one or more people to accomplish organizational goals. More complex definitions of delegation, supervision, and assignment, however, have been created by the American Nurses Association (ANA) and the National Council of State Boards of Nursing (NCBSN) in response to the emerging complexity of delegation in today's healthcare arena, where increasing numbers of unlicensed and relatively untrained workers provide direct patient care. Both the ANA and the NCBSN have defined delegation differently (Thomas, Barter, & McLaughlin, 2000). The ANA defines delegation as the transfer of responsibility for the performance of a task from one person to another. The NCBSN defines delegation as transferring to a competent individual the authority to perform a selected nursing task in a selected situation. This second definition suggests that delegation is complex, requiring insight and judgment regarding the environment in which the delegation is to take place and the individuals involved.

Delegation is an essential element of the directing phase of the management process because much of the work accomplished by managers (first-, middle-, and top-level) occurs not only through their own efforts but also through those of their subordinates. For the manager, delegation is not an option but a necessity. Frequently, there is too much work to be accomplished by one person. In these situations, delegation often becomes synonymous with productivity.

There are many good reasons for delegating. Sometimes managers must delegate routine tasks so they are free to handle problems that are more complex or require a higher level of expertise. Managers may delegate work if someone else is better prepared or has greater expertise or knowledge about how to solve a problem. Delegation can also be used to provide learning or "stretching" opportunities for subordinates. Subordinates who are not delegated enough responsibility may become bored, nonproductive, and ineffective. Thus, in delegating, the leader–manager contributes to employees' personal and professional development. The leadership roles and management functions inherent in delegation are shown in **Display 20.1.**

COMMON DELEGATION ERRORS

Delegation is a critical leadership skill that must be learned. Barter (2002) maintains that leaders who delegate effectively are able to synchronize the cognitive, affective, and intuitive dimensions of delegation into a seamless performance. In other words, they are able to think about delegation, to be self-aware regarding their feelings about delegation, and to know certain things about delegation based upon their intuition. Frequent mistakes made by managers in delegating include the following.

Display 20.1 Leadership Roles and Management Functions Associated with Delegation

Leadership Roles

1. Functions as a role model, supporter, and resource person in delegating tasks to subordinates.
2. Encourages followers to use delegation as a time management strategy and team-building tool.
3. Assists followers in identifying situations appropriate for delegation.
4. Communicates clearly and assertively in delegating tasks.
5. Maintains patient safety as a minimum criterion in determining the most appropriate person to carry out a delegated task.
6. Is an informed and active participant in the development of local, state, and national guidelines for UAP scope of practice.
7. Is sensitive to how cultural phenomena affect transcultural delegation.

Management Functions

1. Creates job descriptions and scope of practice statements for all personnel, including UAP, that conform to national, state, and professional recommendations for ensuring safe patient care.
2. Is knowledgeable regarding legal liabilities of subordinate supervision.
3. Accurately assesses subordinates' capabilities and motivation when delegating.
4. Delegates a level of authority necessary to complete delegated tasks.
5. Develops and implements a periodic review process for all delegated tasks.
6. Provides recognition or reward for the completion of delegated tasks.

Underdelegating

Underdelegating frequently stems from the manager's false assumption that delegation may be interpreted as a lack of ability on his or her part to do the job correctly or completely. Delegation need not limit the manager's control, prestige, and power; rather, delegation can extend the manager's influence and capability by increasing what can be accomplished.

Another frequent cause of underdelegating is the manager's desire to complete the whole job personally due to a lack of trust in the subordinates; the manager believes that he or she needs the experience or that he or she can do it better and faster than anyone else. It is important to remember that time spent in training another to do a job can be repaid tenfold in the future. In addition to increased productivity, delegation can also provide the opportunity for subordinates to experience feelings of accomplishment and enrichment.

An additional cause of underdelegation is the fear that subordinates will resent having work delegated to them. Properly delegated work actually increases employee satisfaction and fosters a cooperative working relationship between managers and staff.

> The right to delegate and the ability to provide formal rewards for successful completion of delegated tasks are a reflection of the legitimate authority inherent in the management role.

Display 20.2	**Common Delegating Errors**

Underdelegating
Overdelegating
Improperly delegating

Managers also may underdelegate because they lack experience in the job or in delegation itself. Other managers refuse to delegate because they have an excessive need to control or be perfect. Dye (2000) states, "If leadership is a journey, then respect for its constituents is its fuel and good stewardship is its compass. Respect is the value that multiples each person's desire to deliver better, harder, and consistently excellent performance" (p. 33). The manager who accepts nothing less than perfection limits the opportunities available for subordinate growth and often wastes time redoing delegated tasks.

Some novice managers emerging from the clinical nurse role underdelegate because they find it difficult to assume the manager role. This occurs, in part, because the nurses have been rewarded in the past for their clinical expertise and not their management skills. As managers come to understand and accept the need for the hierarchical responsibilities of delegation, they become more productive and develop more positive staff relationships.

Overdelegating

In contrast to underdelegating, which overburdens the manager, some managers *overdelegate*, burdening their subordinates. Some managers overdelegate because they are poor managers of time, spending most of it just trying to get organized. Others overdelegate because they feel insecure in their ability to perform a task. Managers also must be careful not to overdelegate to exceptionally competent employees, because they may become overworked and tired, which can decrease their productivity.

Improperly Delegating

Improper delegation includes such things as delegating at the wrong time, to the wrong person, or for the wrong reason. It also may include delegating tasks and responsibilities that are beyond the capability of the person to whom they are being delegated or that should be done by the manager. See **Display 20.2** for types of delegating errors.

Delegating decision making without providing adequate information also is an example of improper delegation. If the manager requires a higher quality than "satisficing," this must be made clear at the time of the delegation. Not everything that is delegated needs to be handled in a maximizing mode. In many complex organizations, efforts have been made to delegate decision making to middle-level managers.

EFFECTIVE DELEGATING

Although some balk at the idea of sharing enough information or authority for delegation to be effective, managers can implement a variety of strategies to ensure effective delegation.

Plan Ahead

Plan ahead when identifying tasks to be accomplished. Assess the situation and clearly delineate the desired outcomes.

Identify Necessary Skills and Levels

Identify the skill or educational level necessary to complete the job. Often, legal and licensing statutes determine this. All nurses should be knowledgeable regarding their state's nurse practice act (NPA) and know the following elements of the state's nurse practice act (Barter, 2002):

- The state's NPA definition of delegation
- Items that cannot be delegated
- Items that cannot be routinely delegated
- Guidelines for RNs about tasks that can be delegated
- A description of professional nursing practice
- A description of LVN/LPN nursing practice and unlicensed nursing roles
- The degree of supervision required to complete a task
- The guidelines for lowering delegation risks
- Warnings about inappropriate delegation
- If there is a restricted use of the word "nurse" to licensed staff

The manager should also know the official job description expectations for each worker classification in the organization as it may be more restrictive than the state nurse practice act.

Select Most Capable Personnel

Identify the qualified person best able to complete the job in terms of capability and time to do so. Managers should ask the individuals to whom they are delegating if they are capable of completing the delegated task but should also validate this perception by direct observation. It also is important that the person to whom the task is being delegated considers the task to be important.

Communicate Goal Clearly

Managers should encourage employees to attempt to solve problems themselves; however, employees often need to ask questions about the task or to clarify the desired outcome. When this happens, the manager should clearly communicate what is to be done, including the purpose for doing so, and verify comprehension.

Research by Anthony, Standing, and Hertz (2000a) highlights another concern for the RN in supervising UAP. Their research, which examined the congruence between RN and UAP perceptions of nursing practice, found significant differences in philosophy of patient care and perceived accountability for team and patients between RNs and UAP. In addition, further research by Anthony, et al. (2000a) suggests that while work experience for licensed nurses is associated with positive outcomes for patients, overall experience for UAP was not associated with differences in patient outcomes. Both of these studies suggest that assumptions about the interchangeability of RNs and UAP in the staffing mix must be examined carefully.

It is critical that the RN never lose sight of his or her ultimate responsibility for ensuring that patients receive appropriate, high-quality care. This means that while the UAP may complete non-nursing functions such as bathing, vital signs, and the measurement and recording of intake and output, it is the RN who must analyze that information and then use the nursing process to see that desired patient outcomes are achieved. Only RNs have the formal authority to practice nursing, and activities that rely on the nursing process or require specialized skill, expert knowledge, or professional judgment should never be delegated (Zimmerman, 2001).

The outcomes associated with the increased use of UAP are not yet known. An increasing number of studies suggest a direct link between decreased RN staffing and declines in patient outcomes. Some of these declines in patient outcomes noted in the literature include an increased incidence of patient falls, nosocomial infections, and medication errors (Blegen, Goode, & Reed, 1998; Huston, 1997, 2001; Lichtig, Knauf, & Milholland, 1999).

Cronenwett (1995) developed a strategy assessment guide to assist nurses in determining situations where UAP should be used to assist or substitute for licensed nurses (**Display 20.3**). When scores are low, delegation to UAP can more likely be carried out in a safe manner. As scores rise, delegation to UAP becomes more inappropriate.

Certainly at some point, given the increasing complexity of health care and the increasing acuity of patient illnesses, there is a maximum representation of UAP in the staffing mix that should not be breached. Until those levels are determined, RNs can expect a continued increase in the utilization of UAP. To protect their patients and their professional license, RNs must continue to seek current information regarding national efforts to standardize scope of practice for UAP and professional guidelines regarding what can be safely delegated to UAP.

Barter (2002) states that certain professional responsibilities related to nursing care must never be delegated. These professional responsibilities include patent assessment, nursing diagnosis, care planning, patient teaching, and patient outcome evaluation.

Subordinate Resistance to Delegation

Resistance is a common response by subordinates to delegation. One of the most common causes of subordinate resistance to, or refusal of, delegated tasks is the failure of the delegator to see the subordinate's perspective. Workloads assigned to UAP are generally highly challenging, both physically and mentally. In addition, the UAP frequently must adapt rapidly to changing priorities, often imposed on him or her by more than one delegator. If the subordinate is truly overwhelmed,

Display 20.3	**Strategic Assessment Guide for Nursing's Response to the Use of UAP**

How complex is (are) the task(s) involved?	Very simple			Very complex
	1 2	3	4 5	
What is the potential for harm to clients?	Very low			Very high
	1 2	3	4 5	
How predictable are client responses to the intervention/ tasks?	Very predictable			Very unpredictable
	1 2	3	4 5	
How stable are the conditions of the clients involved?	Very stable			Very unstable
	1 2	3	4 5	
To what extent are problem solving and judgment required during the intervention or task?	Never required			Always required
	1 2	3	4 5	
To what extent are clients monitored by other societal or family agents so that untoward outcomes would be observed?	Continuously			Very sporadically
	1 2	3	4 5	
To what extent would a registered nurse be held liable for an untoward outcome?	Never			Always
	1 2	3	4 5	
How soon could the unlicensed assistive personnel or client be in contact with a professional healthcare provider if needed?	Very soon (min)			Very long time (hrs)
	1 2	3	4 5	
How certain can society be that the unlicensed assistive personnel being considered will have the necessary competencies to perform the tasks or judgments required?	Very certain			Very uncertain
	1 2	3	4 5	
If the patient were your family member, how comfortable would you be with the proposal for unlicensed assistive personnel care?	Very comfortable			Very uncomfortable
	1 2	3	4 5	
How willing are you, as a member of society, to commit fiscal resources to ensure that a registered nurse could be available to cover every person who needed the proposed interventions?	Very unwilling			Very willing
	1 2	3	4 5	

Source: Cronenwett, W. R. (1995). The use of unlicensed assistive personnel: When to support, oppose or be neutral. *Journal of Nursing Administration, 25*(6), 11–12.

additional delegation of tasks is inappropriate and the RN should reexamine the necessity of completing the delegated task personally or finding someone else who is able to complete the task.

Some subordinates resist delegation simply because they believe they are incapable of completing the delegated task. If the employee is capable but lacks self-confidence, the astute leader may be able to use performance coaching to empower the subordinate and build self-confidence levels. If, however, the employee is truly at high risk for failure, the appropriateness of the delegation must be questioned and a task more appropriate to that employee's ability level should be delegated.

Another cause of subordinate resistance to delegation is an inherent resistance to authority. Some subordinates simply need to "test the water" and determine what the consequences are of not completing delegated tasks. In this case, the delegator must be calm but assertive about his or her expectations and provide explicit work guidelines, if necessary, to maintain an appropriate authority power gap. It is an ongoing leadership challenge to instill a team spirit between delegators and their subordinates.

Finally, resistance to delegation may be occurring because tasks are overdelegated in terms of specificity. All subordinates need to believe there is some room for creativity and independent thinking in delegated tasks. Failure to allow for this human need results in disinterested subordinates who fail to internalize responsibility and accountability for the delegated task. The RN should try to mix the UAP more routine, boring tasks with more challenging and rewarding assignments. An additional strategy is to provide the UAP with consistent, constructive feedback, both positive and negative, to foster growth and self-esteem.

When subordinates resist delegation, the delegator may be tempted to avoid confrontation and simply do the delegated task himself or herself. This is seldom appropriate. Instead, the delegator must ascertain why the delegated task was not accomplished and take appropriate action to eliminate these restraining forces.

Learning Exercise 20.3

Dealing with Resistance to Delegation
You are the team leader for 10 patients. An experienced LVN and nurse's aide are also assigned to the team. It is an extremely busy day, and there is a great deal of work to be done. Several times today, you have found the LVN taking long breaks in the lounge or chatting socially at the front desk, despite the unmet needs of many patients. On those occasions, you have clearly delegated work tasks and time lines to her. Several hours later, you follow up on the delegated tasks and find that they were not completed. When you seek out the LVN, you find that she went to lunch without telling you or the aide. You are furious at her apparent disregard of your authority.

Assignment: What are possible causes of the LVN's failure to follow up on delegated tasks? How will you deal with this LVN? What goal serves as the basis for your actions? Justify your choice with rationale.

Delegating to Interdisciplinary Teams

The Joint Commission on Accreditation of Healthcare Organizations (JCAHO) has emphasized the value of interdisciplinary patient care, whereby healthcare professionals from a number of care-giving areas collaborate to meet patients' healthcare needs (Thomassy & McShea, 2001). Although interdisciplinary team members are generally highly trained, self-directed professionals, the team must have a leader to coordinate team members' efforts and to facilitate communication between members. The nurse leader–manager is often called upon as the individual to coordinate such a team. In coordinating the efforts of the interdisciplinary team or in delegating to members of the team, the leader–manager must be sure to recognize the unique expertise of each team member and to delegate accordingly.

Welford (2002) states that transformational leadership requires a greater degree of delegation than other leadership models. Empowerment from appropriate delegation can occur when transformational leaders are clear about boundaries of responsibility and provide adequate information and support. The interdisciplinary team must be managed as a team and not as individual members. There must be respect for employee's ideas and contribution and trust must be placed in the team to carry out assigned roles. Lastly, Welford says there must be recognition of the team's achievements.

Delegating to a Transcultural Work Team

Poole, Davidhizar, and Giger (1995) suggest that six cultural phenomena must be considered when delegating to staff from a culturally diverse background: communication, space, social organization, time, environmental control, and biological variations.

Communication, the first of the cultural phenomena, is greatly affected by cultural diversity in the workforce because dialect, volume, use of touch, context of speech, and kinesics such as gestures, stance, and eye movement all influence how messages are sent and received. For example, delegation delivered in a softer tone may be perceived as less important than delegation received in a loud tone, even if the delegated tasks have equal importance. Similarly, a manager may make an inappropriate assumption about a person's inability to carry out an important delegated task if that person represents a culture that values softer speech and more passive behavior.

Space is another cultural phenomenon influencing delegation. In the United States, the white American middle class prefers an interpersonal space for communication between people of two to three feet, whereas French and African Americans consider this amount of space to be distant and generally unacceptable (Poole et al., 1995). It is important, then, that the delegator recognizes what each staff member's personal space needs are and acts accordingly. If these space needs are not recognized and respected, the likelihood that a delegated task will be heard and followed through on appropriately will be reduced.

Social organization refers to the importance of a group or unit in providing social support in a person's life. For many cultures, the family unit is the single most important social organization. In some cultures, the duty to family always takes precedence over the needs of the organization. In other cultures, this values ranking is less clear, and the employee may experience great intrapersonal conflict in prioritizing delegated work tasks and obligations to the family unit. It is important, then, that the delegator be aware that employees' values differ and be sensitive in delegating critical tasks to employees experiencing stress in the family unit.

Time is also a cultural phenomenon affecting delegation. Cultural groups can be past-, present-, or future-oriented. *Past-oriented* cultures are interested in preserving the past and maintaining tradition. *Present-oriented* cultures focus on maintaining the status quo and on daily operations. *Future-oriented* cultures focus on goals to be achieved and are more visionary in their approach to problems. For example, strategic planning might best be delegated to a person from a future-oriented culture, although the leader–manager should always be alert for opportunities to create new insight and stretching opportunities for subordinates.

Environmental control, the fifth cultural phenomenon, refers to the person's perception of control over his or her environment (internal locus of control). Some cultures believe more strongly in fate, luck, or chance than other cultures, and this may affect how a person approaches and carries out a delegated task. The person who believes he or she has an internal locus of control is more likely to be creative and autonomous in decision making.

The last phenomenon, *biological variations*, refers to the biopsychosocial differences between racial and ethnic groups, such as susceptibility to disease and physiological differences. See **Display 20.4** for a summary of considerations when delegating to a transcultural work team.

All of these cultural phenomena have the potential to affect the relationship between the delegator and his or her subordinates as well as the understanding and implementation of the delegated task. Recognizing that cultural diversity may be a significant factor in delegation is a critical first step. Applying transcultural sensitivity in delegation is, however, what is ultimately needed to create a productive, multicultural work team.

Display 20.4	**Cultural Phenomena to Consider When Delegating to a Transcultural Team**

Communication: especially dialect, volume, use of touch and eye contact
Space: interpersonal space differs between cultures
Social organization: family unit of primary importance in some cultures
Time: cultures tend to be past, present or future oriented
Environmental control: cultures often have either internal or external locus of control
Biological variations: susceptability to diseases (e.g., Tay-Sachs) and physiological differences (e.g., height, color)

Learning Exercise 20.4

Cultural Considerations in Delegation
You are a new charge nurse working on a surgical unit. Today you have one of the recently hired Korean travel nurses working on your unit. This is the end of her second week of orientation on the unit. She also received a month of classroom orientation and enculturation when she was first hired. Today you assign her as one of your team leaders, responsible for a team of LVNs and CNAs. She has been working with another team leader for over a week but this is her first day to have her team totally to herself.

You check with her several times during the morning to see how things are going. She speaks shyly without making eye contact and says "everything is okay." About noon one of the LVNs comes to you and says that the new nurse has not delegated tasks appropriately and is trying to do too much of the work herself. Additionally, some of the other members of the team find her unsmiling behavior and lack of eye contact unsettling.
Assignment: Do you feel that you made an appropriate assignment? Since things do not seem to be going well, what should you do now? In a small group develop a plan of action with the following goals: 1) ensure patient care is accomplished safely, 2) build self-esteem in the Korean nurse, and 3) be a cultural bridge to staff.

INTEGRATING LEADERSHIP ROLES AND MANAGEMENT FUNCTIONS IN DELEGATION

The right to delegate and the ability to provide formal rewards for successful completion of delegated tasks reflect the legitimate authority inherent in the management role. Delegation provides a means of increasing unit productivity. It is also a managerial tool for subordinate accomplishment and enrichment. Delegation, however, is not easy. It requires high-level management skills. Novice managers often make delegation errors such as delegating too late, not delegating enough, delegating to the wrong person or for the wrong reason, and failing to provide appropriate supervision and guidance of delegated tasks. Delegation also requires highly developed leadership skills such as sensitivity to subordinates' capabilities and needs, the ability to communicate clearly and directly, the willingness to support and encourage subordinates in carrying out delegated tasks, and the vision to see how delegation might result in increased personal growth for subordinates as well as increased unit productivity.

With the increased use of UAP in patient care, the need for nurses to have highly developed delegation skills has never been greater. The ability to use delegation skills appropriately will help to reduce the personal liability associated with supervising and delegating to UAP. It will also ensure that clients' needs are met and their safety is not jeopardized.

> The right to delegate and the ability to provide formal rewards for successful completion of delegated tasks reflect the legitimate authority inherent in the management role.

☀ Key Concepts

- Professional nursing organizations and regulatory bodies are actively engaged in clarifying the scope of practice for unlicensed workers and delegation parameters for registered nurses.
- Delegation is not an option for the manager—it is a necessity.
- Delegation should be used for assigning routine tasks and tasks for which the manager does not have time. It also is appropriate as a tool for problem solving, changes in the manager's own job emphasis, and building capability in subordinates.
- In delegation, managers must clearly communicate what they want done, including the purpose for doing so. Limitations or qualifications that have been imposed should be delineated. Although the manager should specify the end product desired, it is important that the subordinate have an appropriate degree of autonomy in deciding how the work is to be accomplished.
- Managers must delegate the *authority* and the *responsibility* necessary to complete the task.
- RNs asked to assume the role of supervisor and delegator need preparation to assume these leadership tasks.
- Assuming the role of delegator and supervisor to UAP increases the scope of liability for the RN.
- Although the Omnibus Budget Reconciliation Act of 1987 established regulations for the education and certification of "nurse's aides" (minimum of 75 hours of theory and practice and successful completion of an examination in both areas), no federal or community standards have been established for training the more broadly defined UAP.
- The RN always bears the ultimate responsibility for ensuring that the nursing care provided by his or her team members meets or exceeds minimum safety standards.
- When subordinates resist delegation, the delegator must ascertain why the delegated task was not accomplished and take appropriate action to remove these restraining forces.
- *Transcultural sensitivity in delegation* is needed to create a productive multicultural work team.

More Learning Exercises and Applications

 Learning Exercise 20.5

Need for Immediate Delegation

You are the charge nurse on the 7 AM to 3 PM shift in an oncology unit. Immediately after report in the morning, you are overwhelmed by the following information:

- The nursing aide reports that Mrs. Jones has become comatose and is moribund. Although this is not unexpected, her family members are not present, and you know they would like to be notified immediately.
- There are three patients who need 0730 parenteral insulin administration. One of these patients had an 0600 blood sugar of 400.
- Mr. Johnson inadvertently pulled out his central line catheter when he was turning over in bed. His wife just notified the ward clerk by the call light system but states she is applying pressure to the site.
- The public toilet is overflowing, and urine and feces are pouring out rapidly.
- Breakfast trays arrived 15 minutes ago, and patients are using their call lights to ask why they do not yet have their breakfast.
- The medical director of the unit has just discovered that one of her patients has not been started on a chemotherapeutic drug she ordered three days ago. She is furious and demands to speak to you immediately.

Assignment: The other RNs are all very busy with their patients, but you do have the following people to whom you may delegate: yourself, a ward clerk, and an IV-certified LVN/LPN. Decide who should do what and in what priority. Justify your decision.

Learning Exercise 20.6

Issues with Delegating Discipline

You are the supervisor of the oncology unit. One of your closest friends and colleagues is Paula, the supervisor of the medical unit. Frequently, you cover for each other in the event of absence or emergency. Today, Paula stops at your office to let you know that she will be gone for seven days to attend a management workshop on the East Coast. She asks that you check on the unit during her absence. She also asks that you pay particularly close attention to Mary Jones, an employee on her unit. She states that Mary, an employee at the hospital for four years, has been counseled repeatedly about her unexcused absences from work and has recently received a written reprimand specifying that she will be terminated if there is another unexcused absence. Paula anticipates that Mary may attempt to break the rules during her absence. She asks that you follow through on this disciplinary plan in the event that Mary again takes an unexcused absence. Her instructions to you are to terminate Mary if she fails to show up for work this week for any reason.

When you arrive at work the next day, you find that Mary called in sick 20 minutes after the shift was to begin. The hospital's policy is that employees are to notify the staffing office of illness no less than two hours before the beginning of their shift. When you attempt to contact Mary by telephone at home, there is no answer.

Later in the day, you finally reach Mary and ask that she come in to your office early the next morning to speak about her inadequate notice of sick time. Mary arrives 45 minutes late the next morning. You are already agitated and angry with her. You inform her that she is to be terminated for any rule broken during Paula's absence and that this action is being taken in accord with the disciplinary contract that had been established earlier.

Mary is furious. She states that you have no right to fire her because you are not her real boss and that Paula should face her herself. She goes on to say, "Paula told me that the disciplinary contract was just a way of formalizing that we had talked and that I shouldn't take it too seriously." Mary also says, "Besides, I didn't get sick until I was getting ready for work. The hospital rules state that I have 12 sick days each year."

Although you feel certain that Paula was very clear about her position in reviewing the disciplinary contract with Mary, you begin to feel uncomfortable with being placed in the position of having to take such serious corrective action without having been involved in prior disciplinary review sessions. You are, however, also aware that this employee has been breaking rules for some time and that this is just one in a succession of absences. You also know that Paula is counting on you to provide consistency of leadership in her absence.

Assignment: Discuss how you will handle the situation. Was it appropriate for Paula to delegate this responsibility to you? Is it appropriate for one manager to carry out another manager's disciplinary plan? Does it matter that a written disciplinary contract had already been established?

Learning Exercise 20.7

How Will You Plan this Busy Morning?
You are a staff nurse who functions as a modular leader on a general medical-surgical unit. The group for which you are responsible is assigned patients in Rooms 401 through 409, with a maximum capacity of 13 patients.

In your unit, a modular type of patient care organization is employed, using a combination of licensed and unlicensed staff. Each module consists of one RN, one LVN/LPN, and one UAP. The LVN/LPN is IV certified and can maintain and start IVs, but cannot hang piggybacks or give IV push medications. The LVN/LPN may give all other medications except IV medications. The RN gives all IV medications. The UAP, with the assistance of his or her modular team members, generally bathes and feeds patients and provides other care that does not require a license.

The RN, as modular leader, divides up the workload at the beginning of the shift between the three modular team members. In addition, he or she acts as a teacher and resource person for the other members of the module.

Today is Wednesday. You have one LVN/LPN and one UAP assigned to work with you—LVN Franklin and UAP Martinez.

LVN Franklin is 26 years old and the mother of four preschool children. Her husband is a city bus driver. UAP Martinez is 53 years old and a grandmother with no children living at home. Her husband died two years ago. She says that work keeps her "happy." The patient roster this morning is as follows:

Room	Patient	Age	Diagnosis	Condition	Acuity level
401	Mrs. Jones	33	Mastectomy for breast CA	2 days postop/fair	II
402	Mrs. Redford	55	Back Pain—Pelvic	Good	I
403	Mrs. Worley	46	Cholecystectomy	2 days postop/ good	III
404-1	Mrs. Smith	83	Parkinson's, CVD hypertension	Fair	II
404-2	Mrs. Dewey	26	PID	Good—home today	I
405-1	Mr. Arthur	71	Metastatic CA	Poor—semi- comatose/ Chemotherapy	IV
405-2	Mr. Vines	34	Possible peptic ulcer	Good—UGI today	III
406-1	Vacant				
406-2	Miss Brown	24	Dilatation and curettage	To OR this a.m.	III

Room	Patient	Age	Diagnosis	Condition	Acuity level
407-1	Mrs. West	41	Myocardial infarction Heparin lock/ telemetry	Fair/from ICU yesterday	III
408-1	Mr. Niles	21	Open reduction femur (MVA)	Fair/3 days postop	III
408-2	Mr. Ford	44	Gastrectomy	Fair/1 day postop	III
409	Mrs. Land	42	Depression	Fair/BA enema today	III

Additional information about patients:
- Mr. Niles is depressed because he believes his football career is over.
- There have been problems with Mr. Ford's IV and his nasogastric tube. Both will need to be replaced today.
- Mrs. Worley requires frequent changes (every two to three hours) of the dressings at the laparoscopy site owing to a high volume of serous drainage.
- Mrs. Jones will need instructions regarding her postoperative activities and has begun to talk about her prognosis.
- Mrs. Land began to talk with you yesterday about her husband's recent death.
- The preparation for the barium enema will result in Mrs. Land's having frequent toileting needs today.
- Mrs. Smith requires assistance with feeding at mealtime.
- Mr. Arthur is no longer able to turn himself in bed.
- Mr. Vines states that being in the same room with a critically ill patient upsets him, and he has asked to move to a new room.

Assignment: How will you make out your assignments this morning? Assign these patients to the LVN/LPN, UAP, and yourself. Be sure to include assessments, procedures, and basic care needs. What will you do if a patient is admitted to your team? Explain the rationale for all your patient assignments. Sample acuity levels are provided to assist in determining patient needs and staffing (see patient roster above).

Learning Exercise 20.8

Evaluating Staffing Safeguards
Interview a middle- or top-level manager of a local healthcare agency. Ascertain the staffing mix at his or her agency. Are there minimum hiring criteria for UAP? Are there written guidelines for determining tasks appropriate for UAP delegation? What educational or training opportunities on delegation are made available to staff who must delegate work assignments on a regular basis?

On the basis of your interview results, write an essay evaluating whether you believe there are adequate safeguards in place at that agency to protect the licensed staff, unlicensed staff, and clients. Would you feel comfortable working in such a facility?

 Learning Exercise 20.9

Deciding Delegation Using the Nurse Practice Act
Which of the following tasks would you be willing to delegate to a UAP? Use your state's Nurse Practice Act as a reference for this case. Discuss your answers in small groups. Did you all agree? If not, what factors were significant in your differences?
1. Uncomplicated wet-to-dry dressing change on patient three days post–hip replacement
2. Every-two-hour checks on patient with soft wrist restraints to assess circulation, movement, and comfort
3. Cooling measures for patient with temperature of 104°F
4. Calculation of IV credits, clearing IV pumps, and completing shift intake/output totals
5. Completing phlebotomy for daily blood draws
6. Holding pressure on insertion site of femoral line that has just been removed
7. Educating a patient about components of a soft diet
8. Testing stool specimens for guaiac blood
9. Performing electrocardiogram testing
10. Feeding a patient with swallowing precautions (high risk of choking post CVA)
11. Oral suctioning
12. Tracheostomy care
13. Ostomy care

Web Links

RN Utilization of Unlicensed Assistive Personnel
http://www.ana.org/readroom/position/uap/uapuse.htm
Position statement of the ANA regarding the utilization of UAP. Effective date December 11, 1992, although ANA work on the UAP issue is ongoing.

Delegation Tips
http://www.liraz.com/tdelegat.htm
Effective delegation will not only give you more time to work on your important opportunities, but you will also help others on your team learn new skills.

The Art of Delegation. By Gerald M. Blair.
http://www.see.ed.ac.uk/~gerard/management/art5.html
Delegation is a skill of which we have all heard—but which few understand.

Project Management Delegation
http://www.see.ed.ac.uk/~gerard/MENG/ME96/Documents/Aspects/delegate.html
Delegation—A key aspect of leadership is delegation.

The Five Rights of Delegation
http://www.state.ma.us/reg/boards/rn/advrul/thefive.htm
The Board of Registration in Nursing (Massachusetts) presents a framework for delegation decision making and accountability based on a model that identifies the five key elements of any delegated act: the right task, the right circumstances, the right person, the right direction/communication, and the right supervision and evaluation.

References

American Nurses Association (ANA). (1992). Progress report on unlicensed assistive personnel: Informal report. Report CNP-CNE-B. Washington DC: ANA.

Anthony, M. K., Standing, T., & Hertz, J. E. (2000a). Factors influencing outcomes after delegation to unlicensed assistive personnel. *Journal of Nursing Administration, 30*(10), 474–481.

Anthony, M. K., Casey, D., Chau, T., & Brennan, P. F. (2000b). Congruence between registered nurses' and unlicensed assistive personnel perception of nursing practice. *Nursing Economic$, 18*(6), 285–293.

Barter, M., McLaughlin, F. E., & Thomas, S. A. (1994). Use of unlicensed assistive personnel by hospitals. *Nursing Economic$, 12*(2), 82–87.

Barter, M (2002). Follow the team leader. *Nursing Management, (33)*10, 55–59.

Blegen, M. A., Goode, C. J., & Reed, L. (1998). Nurse staffing and patient outcomes. *Nursing Research, 47*(1), 43–50.

Cronenwett, L. R. (1995). The use of unlicensed assistive personnel: When to support, oppose, or be neutral. *Journal of Nursing Administration, 25*(6), 11–12.

Dye, C. F. (2000). *Leadership in health care: Values at the top.* Chicago: Health Administration Press.

Fisher, M. (1999). Do your nurses delegate effectively? *Nursing Management, 30*(5), 23–26.

Gordon, S. (1997). What nurses stand for. *The Atlantic Monthly, 279*(2), 80–88.

Hansten, R. I., & Washburn, M. J. (1998). *Clinical delegation skills* (2nd ed.). Gaithersburg, MD: Aspen.

Huston, C. (1996). Unlicensed assistive personnel: A solution to dwindling healthcare resources or the precursor to the apocalypse of registered nursing? *Nursing Outlook, 44*(2), 67–73.

Huston, C. (1997). *The replacement of registered nurses by unlicensed personnel: The impact on three process/outcome indicators of quality.* Unpublished doctoral dissertation, University of Southern California.

Huston, C. (2001). Contemporary staffing mix changes: Impact on postoperative pain management. *Pain Management Nursing, 2*(2), 65–72.

Lichtig, L. K., Knauf, R. A., & Milholland, D. K. (Feb. 1999). Some impacts of nursing on acute care hospital outcomes. *Journal of Nursing Administration, 29*(2), 25–33.

Pew Health Commission Report. (1995). *Critical challenges: Revitalizing the health professions for the twenty-first century.* San Francisco: UCSF Center for the Health Professions.

Poole, V. L., Davidhizar, R. E., & Giger, J. N. (1995). Delegating to a transcultural team. *Nursing Management, 26*(8), 33–34.

Simpkins, R. W. (1997). Using task lists with unlicensed assistive personnel. *Insight, 6*(2), 1–5.

Thomas, S. A., Barter, M., & McLaughlin, F. E. (2000). State and territorial boards of nursing approaches to the use of unlicensed assistive personnel. *JONA's Healthcare Law, Ethics, and Regulation, 2*(1), 13–21.

Thomassy, C. S., & McShea, C. S. (2001). Shifting gears: Jump-start interdisciplinary patient care. *Nursing Management, 32*(5), 40–43.

Welford, C. (2002). Matching theory to practice. *Nursing Management—UK, 9*(4), 7–12.

Zimmerman, P. G. (last updated by Debbie Abraham). (2001). Delegating to unlicensed assistive personnel. Nursing Spectrum Career Fitness [on-line continuing education, self-study module]. Available at: http://nsweb.nursingspectrum.com/ce/ce124.htm Accessed July 13, 2001.

Bibliography

Ahmed, D. S. (June 2000). Practice errors. "It's not my job." *American Journal of Nursing, 100*(6), 25.

Bola, T. V., Driggers, K., Dunlap, C., & Ebersole, M. (2003). Foreign-educated nurses: Strangers in a strange land? *Nursing Management, 34*(7), 39–43.

Cady, R. (2001). Legal issues surrounding the use of unlicensed assistive personnel. *American Journal of Maternal Child Nursing, 26*(1), 49.

Davudhizar, R. (2002). Taking charge by "letting go." *Health Care Manager, 20*(3), 33–38.

Ebright, P. R., Patterson, E. S., Chalko, B. A., & Render, M. L. (2003). Understanding the complexity of registered nurse work I acute care settings. *Nursing Management, 33*(12), 630–638.

Katz, L. W., & Osborne, H. (2002). Simplicity is the best medicine for compliance information: Eight basic steps help improve employee comprehension. *Patient Care Management, 17*(9), 7–9.

Let nurses delegate please . . . A new type of primary care worker is needed. (2000) *Nursing Times, 96*(44), 7.

Nurses urged to delegate duties. (2001). *Nursing Times, 97*(13), 8.

Sadaniantz, B. (2002). To do or to delegate? *Nursing Spectrum, New England, 5*(6), 18.

Sikma, S. K., & Young, H. M. (2001). Balancing freedom with risks: The experience of nursing task delegation in community-based residential care settings. *Nursing Outlook, 49*(4), 193–201.

Spencer, S. A. (2001). Education, training, and use of unlicensed personnel in critical care. *Critical Care Nursing Clinics of North America, 13*(1), 105–118.

Spilsburgy, K., & Meyer, J. (2001). Defining the nursing contribution to patient outcome: Lessons from a review of the literature examining nursing outcomes, skill mix, and changing roles. *Journal of Clinical Nursing, 10*(1), 3–14.

Standing, T., Anthony, M. K., & Hertz, J. E. (2001). Nurses' narratives of outcomes after delegation to unlicensed assistive personnel. *Outcomes Management for Nursing Practice, 5*(1), 18–23.

Wald, A. (2000). Part of management is the art of delegation. *Nursing Spectrum[New York, New Jersey Metro Edition], 12A*(6), 20.

Zimmerman, P. G. (Aug. 2000). The use of unlicensed assistive personnel: An update and skeptical look at a role that may present more problems than solutions. *Journal of Emergency Nursing, 26*(4), 312–317.

Managing Conflict

Peace is not the absence of conflict but the presence of creative alternatives for responding to conflict—alternatives to passive or aggressive responses, alternatives to violence.

—Dorothy Thompson

Conflict is generally defined as the internal or external discord that results from differences in ideas, values, or feelings between two or more people. Because managers have interpersonal relationships with people having a variety of different values, beliefs, backgrounds, and goals, conflict is an expected outcome. Conflict is also created when there are differences in economic and professional values and when there is competition among professionals. Scarce resources, restructuring, and poorly defined role expectations also are frequent sources of conflict in organizations.

Openly acknowledging that conflict is a naturally occurring and expected phenomenon in organizations reflects a tremendous shift from how sociologists viewed conflict a century ago. The current sociological view is that organizational conflict should be neither avoided nor encouraged, but managed. The manager's role is to create a work environment where conflict may be used as a conduit for growth, innovation, and productivity. When organizational conflict becomes dysfunctional, the manager must recognize it in its early stages and actively intervene so that subordinates' motivation and organizational productivity are not adversely affected.

> Conflict is neither good nor bad, and it can produce growth or destruction, depending on how it is managed.

Conflict resolution, or problem solving, appears to be learned less frequently through developmental experiences and instead requires a conscious learning effort. Indeed, recent incidents of violence in schools and among work groups have led corporations and schools to develop programs to teach workers and students how to deal with conflict (Ezarik, 2001; James, 2001). These efforts to reduce conflict violence leads one to believe that the skills necessary to manage conflict effectively can be learned.

This chapter presents an overview of growth-producing versus dysfunctional conflict in organizations. The history of conflict management, categories of conflict, the conflict process itself, and strategies for successful conflict resolution are discussed. Negotiation as a conflict resolution strategy is emphasized. Leadership skills and management functions necessary for conflict resolution at the unit level are outlined in **Display 21.1.**

THE HISTORY OF CONFLICT MANAGEMENT

Early in the 20th century, conflict was considered to be an indication of poor organizational management, was deemed destructive, and was avoided at all costs. When conflict occurred, it was ignored, denied, or dealt with immediately and harshly. The theorists of this era believed that conflict could be avoided if employees were taught the one right way to do things and if expressed employee dissatisfaction was met swiftly with disapproval.

In the mid-20th century, when organizations recognized that worker satisfaction and feedback were important, conflict was accepted passively and perceived as normal and expected. Attention centered on teaching managers how to resolve conflict rather than how to prevent it. Although conflict was considered to be primarily dysfunctional, it was believed that conflict and cooperation could happen simultaneously.

The interactionist theorists of the 1970s, however, recognized conflict as a necessity and actively encouraged organizations to promote conflict as a means of producing growth.

Display 21.1	Leadership Roles and Management Functions Associated with Conflict Resolution

Leadership Roles

1. Is self-aware and conscientiously works to resolve intrapersonal conflict.
2. Addresses conflict as soon as it is perceived and before it becomes felt or manifest.
3. Seeks a win–win solution to conflict whenever feasible.
4. Lessens the perceptual differences that exist between conflicting parties and broadens the parties' understanding about the problems.
5. Assists subordinates in identifying alternative conflict resolutions.
6. Recognizes and accepts the individual differences of staff.
7. Uses assertive communication skills to increase persuasiveness and foster open communication.
8. Role models honest and collaborative negotiation efforts.

Management Functions

1. Creates a work environment that minimizes the antecedent conditions for conflict.
2. Appropriately uses legitimate authority in a competing approach when a quick or unpopular decision needs to be made.
3. When appropriate, formally facilitates conflict resolution involving subordinates.
4. Accepts mutual responsibility for reaching predetermined supraordinate goals.
5. Obtains needed unit resources through effective negotiation strategies.
6. Compromises unit needs only when the need is not critical to unit functioning and when higher management gives up something of equal value.
7. Is adequately prepared to negotiate for unit resources, including the advance determination of a bottom line and possible trade-offs.
8. Addresses the need for closure and follow-up to negotiation.
9. Pursues alternative dispute resolution when conflicts cannot be resolved using traditional conflict management strategies.

Some level of conflict in an organization appears desirable, although the optimum level for a specific person or unit at a given time is difficult to determine. Too little conflict results in organizational stasis, whereas too much conflict reduces the organization's effectiveness and eventually immobilizes its employees (see **Figure 21.1**). With few formal instruments to assess whether the level of conflict in an organization is too high or too low, the responsibility for determining and creating an appropriate level of conflict on the individual unit often falls to the manager.

Conflict also has a qualitative nature. A person may be totally overwhelmed in one conflict situation, yet be able to handle several simultaneous conflicts at a later time. The difference is in the quality or significance of that conflict to the person experiencing it.

Although *quantitative* and *qualitative* conflicts produce distress at the time they occur, they can lead to growth, energy, and creativity by generating new ideas and solutions. If handled inappropriately, quantitative and qualitative conflicts can lead to demoralization, decreased motivation, and lowered productivity.

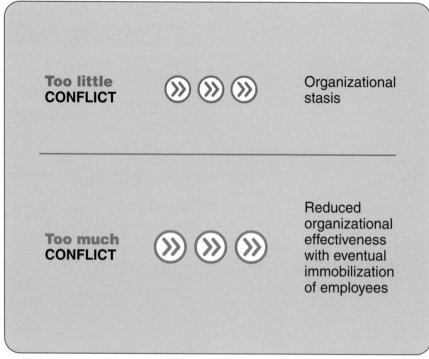

Figure 21.1 The relationship between organizational conflict and effectiveness.

 Learning Exercise 21.1

Thinking and Writing about Conflict
Do you generally view conflict positively or negatively?
Does conflict affect you more cognitively, emotionally, or physically?
How was conflict expressed in the home in which you grew up?
Does the way you handle conflict mirror that of your role models as a child?
Do you believe that you have too much or too little conflict in your life?
Do you feel like you have control over the issues that are now causing
  conflict in your life?
Assignment: Write a one-page essay, answering one of the questions
above.

Nursing managers can no longer afford to respond to conflict traditionally (i.e., to avoid or suppress it) because this is <u>nonproductive.</u> In an era of shrinking healthcare dollars, it has become increasingly important for managers to confront and manage conflict appropriately. The ability to understand and deal with conflict appropriately is a critical leadership skill.

CATEGORIES OF CONFLICT

There are three primary categories of conflict: intergroup, intrapersonal, and interpersonal (see **Figure 21.2**). *Intergroup conflict* occurs between two or more groups of people, departments, or organizations. An example of intergroup conflict might be two political affiliations with widely differing or contradictory beliefs.

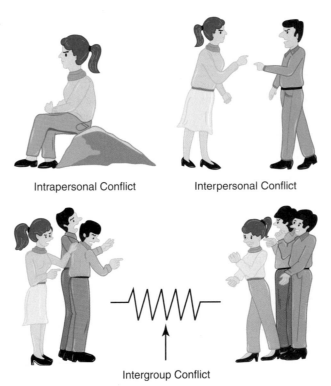

Intrapersonal Conflict

Interpersonal Conflict

Intergroup Conflict

Figure 21.2 Primary categories of conflict.

Intrapersonal conflict occurs within the person. It involves an internal struggle to clarify contradictory values or wants. For managers, intrapersonal conflict may result from the multiple areas of responsibility associated with the management role. Managers' responsibilities to the organization, subordinates, consumers, the profession, and themselves may sometimes conflict, and that conflict may be internalized. Being self-aware and conscientiously working to resolve intrapersonal conflict as soon as it is first felt is essential to the leader's physical and mental health.

Interpersonal conflict, also known as "*horizontal violence*" or "*bullying*," (McKenna, Smith, and Coverdale, 2003) happens between two or more people with differing values, goals, and beliefs. A recent study suggests that interpersonal conflict is a significant issue confronting the nursing profession, especially for new graduates. Because this interpersonal conflict generally is not reported or managed, consequences include absenteeism from work and turnover (McKenna et al., 2003). Similarly, Thomas (2003b) suggests that "horizontal hostility" is rampant in the nursing workforce with nurse colleagues continually criticizing and sniping at each other, with the end result being burnout and stress. "This horizontal violence drains nurses of vitality and undermines institutional attempts to create a satisfied nursing workforce" (p. 91).

Violence and workplace aggression are increasingly being recognized as epidemic in the healthcare workplace. By definition, *workplace aggression* is "any act of physical assault, threatening, or coercive behavior that occurs in a work setting and causes physical or emotional harm" (Del Bel, 2003, p. 31). Del Bel points out that worldwide, nurses are three times more likely than any other service occupational group to experience workplace violence, and U.S. healthcare workers face a 16 times greater risk of violence than other service workers. "Keeping everyone safe is a serious responsibility—one that demands unwavering attention from managers and administrators. While not all workplace aggression is avoidable, research shows that a significant proportion is preventable (p. 31)."

THE CONFLICT PROCESS

Before managers can or should attempt to intervene in conflict, they must be able to assess its five stages accurately. The first stage in the conflict process, *latent conflict*, implies the existence of antecedent conditions, such as short staffing and rapid change. In this stage, conditions are ripe for conflict, although no conflict has actually occurred and none may ever occur. Much unnecessary conflict could be prevented or reduced if managers examined the organization more closely for antecedent conditions. For example, change and budget cuts almost invariably create conflict. Such events, therefore, should be well thought out so interventions can be made before the conflicts created by these events escalate.

If the conflict progresses, it may develop into the second stage: *perceived conflict*. Perceived or substantive conflict is intellectualized and often involves issues and roles. The person recognizes it logically and impersonally as occurring. Sometimes conflict can be resolved at this stage before it is internalized or felt.

The third stage, *felt conflict*, occurs when the conflict is emotionalized. Felt emotions include hostility, fear, mistrust, and anger. It also is referred to as affective conflict. It is possible to perceive conflict and not feel it (i.e., no emotion is attached to the conflict, and the person views it only as a problem to be solved). A person also can feel the conflict but not perceive the problem (i.e., he or she is unable to identify the cause of the felt conflict).

In the fourth stage, *manifest conflict*, also called *overt conflict*, action is taken. The action may be to withdraw, compete, debate, or seek conflict resolution. Catalano (2003) suggests that there are many reasons individuals are uncomfortable with or reluctant to address conflict. These include fear of retaliation, fear of ridicule, fear of alienating others, a feeling that they do not have the right to speak up, and past negative experiences with conflict situations. Indeed, people often learn patterns of dealing with manifest conflict early in their lives, and family background and experiences often directly affect how conflict is dealt with in adulthood.

In addition, gender appears to play a role in how we respond to conflict. Traditionally, men are socialized to respond more aggressively to conflict while women are more apt to try to avoid conflicts or to pacify them. Thomas (2003a) suggests that this is because anger is often a confusing emotion for women as it is often intermingled with hurt and disillusionment despite efforts to objectify conflicts. Thomas goes on to say that despite violations of core values, beliefs, or principles, women are more reluctant than men to confront the conflict for fear of damaging relationships. However, Hunt and Posa (2001) posit that these same gender differences in conflict resolution have resulted in women becoming a vital asset at the peace table, stating "women have been able to bridge the divide even in situations where leaders have deemed conflict resolution futile" (p. 13).

Simmons (2002) suggests, however, a darker side to how women deal with conflict. She describes a world of covert schoolgirl bullying and psychological warfare that she terms *relational aggression*. In such relational aggression, women express conflict nonverbally and indirectly, and yet in an intensely personal manner. Thomas (2003b) appropriately asks whether girlhood is the etiology of the horizontal hostility that is reported to be widespread among nurses.

The final stage in the conflict process is *conflict aftermath*. There is always conflict aftermath, positive or negative. If the conflict is managed well, people involved in the conflict will believe their position was given a fair hearing. If the conflict is managed poorly, the conflict issues frequently remain and may return later to cause more conflict. **Figure 21.3** shows a schematic of this conflict process.

> The aftermath of conflict may be more **significant** than the original conflict if the conflict **has not** been handled constructively.

CONFLICT MANAGEMENT

The optimal goal in resolving conflict is creating a win–win solution for all involved. This outcome is not possible in every situation, and often the manager's goal is to manage the conflict in a manner that lessens the perceptual differences that exist between the involved parties. A leader recognizes which conflict management or resolution strategy is most appropriate for each situation. Common

> The optimal goal in resolving conflict is creating a win–win solution for all **involved.**

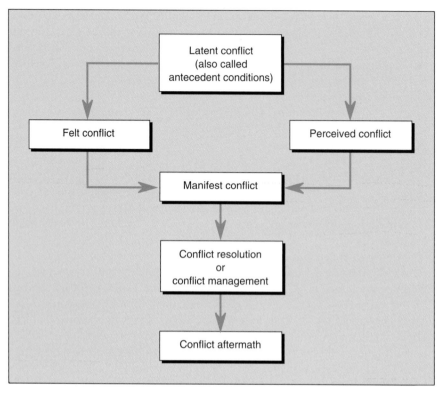

Figure 21.3 The conflict process.

conflict management strategies are identified in **Display 21.2.** The choice of the most appropriate strategy depends on many variables, such as the situation itself, the urgency of the decision, the power and status of the players, the importance of the issue, and the maturity of the people involved in the conflict.

Compromising

In *compromising,* each party gives up something it wants. Although many see compromise as an optimum conflict resolution strategy, antagonistic cooperation may

Display 21.2	**Common Conflict Resolution Strategies**

Compromising
Competing
Cooperating/accommodating
Smoothing
Avoiding
Collaborating

result in a lose–lose situation because either or both parties perceive they have given up more than the other and may, therefore, feel defeated. For compromising not to result in a lose–lose situation, both parties must be willing to give up something of equal value. It is important that parties in conflict not adopt compromise prematurely if collaboration is both possible and feasible.

Competing

The *competing* approach is used when one party pursues what it wants at the expense of the others. Because only one party wins, the competing party seeks to win regardless of the cost to others. Win–lose conflict resolution strategies leave the loser angry, frustrated, and wanting to get even in the future.

Managers may use competing when a quick or unpopular decision needs to be made. It is also appropriately used when one party has more information or knowledge about a situation than the other.

Cooperating

Cooperating is the opposite of competing. In the cooperating approach, one party sacrifices his or her beliefs and allows the other party to win. The actual problem is usually not solved in this win–lose situation. *Accommodating* is another term that may be used for this strategy. The person cooperating or accommodating often collects IOUs from the other party that can be used at a later date. Cooperating and accommodating are appropriate political strategies if the item in conflict is not of high value to the person doing the accommodating. Sullivan (2004) suggests that sometimes it is advisable to lose a battle if the payoff helps you to win the war. The battle is an individual incident and the war is the long-term outcome.

Smoothing

Smoothing is used to manage a conflict situation. One person "smoothes" others involved in the conflict in an effort to reduce the emotional component of the conflict. Managers often use smoothing to get someone to accommodate or cooperate with another party. Smoothing occurs when one party in a conflict attempts to compliment the other party or to focus on agreements rather than differences. Although it may be appropriate for minor disagreements, smoothing rarely results in resolution of the actual conflict.

Avoiding

In the *avoiding* approach, the parties involved are aware of a conflict but choose not to acknowledge it or attempt to resolve it. Avoidance may be indicated in trivial disagreements, when the cost of dealing with the conflict exceeds the benefits of solving it, when the problem should be solved by people other than you, when one party is more powerful than the other, or when the problem will solve itself. The greatest problem in using avoidance is that the conflict remains, often only to reemerge at a later time in an even more exaggerated fashion.

Collaborating

Collaborating is an assertive and cooperative means of conflict resolution that results in a win–win solution. In collaboration, all parties set aside their original goals and work together to establish a supraordinate or priority common goal. In doing so, all parties accept mutual responsibility for reaching the supraordinate goal. Although it is very difficult for people truly to set aside original goals, collaboration cannot occur if this does not happen. For example, a couple experiencing serious conflict over whether to have a baby may first want to identify whether they share the supraordinate goal of keeping the marriage together. A nurse who is unhappy that she did not receive requested days off might meet with her supervisor and jointly establish the supraordinate goal that staffing will be adequate to meet patient safety criteria. If the new goal is truly a jointly set goal, each party will perceive that they have achieved an important goal and that the supraordinate goal is most important. In doing so, the focus remains on problem solving and not on defeating the other party.

Although conflict is a pervasive force in healthcare organizations, only a small percentage of time is spent in true collaboration. Collaboration is rarely used when there is a wide difference in power between the groups or individuals involved. Many think of collaboration as a form of cooperation, but this is not an accurate definition. In collaboration, problem solving is a joint effort with no superior/subordinate, order-giving/order-taking relationships. True collaboration requires mutual respect, open and honest communication, and equitable, shared decision-making powers.

Umiker (1997) suggests that in preparing to collaborate, each person must first analyze the situation by answering these questions:

- What do I want to accomplish, and what is the most I will give up?
- What do I think the other person wants? What covert goals might the other person have?
- What false assumptions or incorrect perceptions might the other person have?
- Which strategy should I use?
- What are my "hot buttons" and what should I do if they are pushed?
- If I plan to use a collaborative approach, what special precautions should be taken?

Krairiksh and Anthony (2001) maintain that collaboration enhances a person's participation in decision making to accomplish mutual goals and therefore is the best method to resolve conflict to achieve long-term benefits. However, because it involves others over whom the manager has no control and because its process is lengthy, it may not be the best approach for all situations. Collaboration remains, however, the best alternative for complex problem solving involving others.

Learning Exercise 21.2

Personal Conflict Solving
It is important for managers to be self-aware regarding how they view and deal with conflict. In your personal life, how do you solve conflict? Is it important for you to win? When was the last time you were able to solve conflict by reaching supraordinate goals with another person? Are you able to see the other person's position in conflict situations? In conflicts with family and friends, are you least likely to compromise values, scarcities, or role expectations?

 Learning Exercise 21.3

Conflicting Personal, Professional, and Organizational Obligations
You are Nurse Jane. You have been working on the oncology unit since your graduation from the state college one year ago. Your supervisor, Mary, has complimented your performance. Lately, she has allowed you to be relief charge nurse on the 3 PM to 11 PM shift when the regular charge nurse is not there.

Occasionally, you have been asked to work on the medical/surgical units when your department has a low census. Although you dislike leaving your own unit, you have cooperated because you felt you could handle the other clinical assignments and wanted to show your flexibility.

Tonight, you have just come to work when the nursing office calls and requests that you help out in the busy delivery room. You protest that you don't know anything about obstetrics and that it is impossible for you to take the assignment. Carol, the supervisor from the nursing office insists that you are the most qualified person; she says, "Just go and do the best you can." Your own unit supervisor is not on duty, and the charge nurse says she does not feel comfortable advising you in this conflict. You feel torn between professional, personal, and organizational obligations.
Assignment: What should you do? Select the most appropriate conflict resolution strategy. Give rationale for your selection and for your rejection of the others. After you have made your choice, read the analysis found in Appendix A.

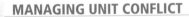 **MANAGING UNIT CONFLICT**

Managing conflict effectively requires an understanding of its origin. Some of the most common sources of organizational conflict are shown in **Display 21.3.** Umiker (1997) suggests that the six most common causes of unit conflict are unclear expectations, poor communication, lack of clear jurisdiction, incompatibilities or disagreements based on differences of temperament or attitudes, individual or group conflicts of interest, and operational or staffing changes.

Display 21.3	**Common Causes of Organizational Conflict**

- Poor communication
- Inadequately defined organizational structure
- Individual behavior (incompatibilities or disagreements based on differences of temperament or attitudes)
- Unclear expectations
- Individual or group conflicts of interest
- Operational or staffing changes
- Diversity in gender, culture, or age

Diversity in gender, culture, and age also has the potential to create conflict in an organization. This occurs as a result of communication difficulties, including language and literacy issues and a growing recognition that some factors are beyond assimilation. In addition, people are currently more willing to celebrate their differences and are not as willing to assimilate into one homogeneous group.

All of these types of unit conflicts can disrupt working relationships and result in lower productivity. It is imperative, then, that the manager is able to identify the origin of unit conflicts and intervene as necessary to promote cooperative, if not collaborative, conflict resolution.

At times, this requires that the manager facilitate conflict resolution between others. The following is a list of strategies a manager may use to deal effectively with organizational or unit conflict:

- **Confrontation.** Many times, subordinates inappropriately expect the manager to solve their interpersonal conflicts. Managers instead should urge subordinates to attempt to handle their own problems. Managers should, however, recommend face-to-face communication for resolving conflicts as e-mails, answering machine messages, and notes are too impersonal for the delicate nature of negative words since "What feels likes a bomb on paper, may feel like a feather in person" (Smith, 2003, para 22).
- **Third-party consultation.** Sometimes managers can be used as a neutral party to help others resolve conflicts constructively. This should be done only if all parties are motivated to solve the problem and if no differences exist in the status or power of the party's involved. If the conflict involves multiple parties and highly charged emotions, the manager may find it helpful to bring in outside experts to facilitate communication and bring issues to the forefront.
- **Behavior change.** This is reserved for serious cases of dysfunctional conflict. Educational modes, training development, or sensitivity training can be used to solve conflict by developing self-awareness and behavior change in the involved parties.
- **Responsibility charting.** When ambiguity results from unclear or new roles, it is often necessary to have the parties come together to delineate the function and responsibility of roles. If areas of joint responsibility exist, the manager must clearly define such areas as ultimate responsibility, approval

mechanisms, support services, and responsibility for informing. This is a useful technique for elementary jurisdictional conflicts. An example of a potential jurisdictional conflict might arise between the house supervisor and unit manager in staffing or between an in-service educator and unit manager in determining and planning unit educational needs or programs.

- **Structure change.** Sometimes managers need to intervene in unit conflict by transferring or discharging people. Other structure changes may be moving a department under another manager, adding an ombudsman, or putting a grievance procedure in place. Often increasing the boundaries of authority for one member of the conflict will act as an effective structure change to resolve unit conflict. Changing titles and creating policies also are effective techniques.
- **Soothing one party.** This is a temporary solution that should be used in a crisis when there is not time to handle the conflict effectively or when the parties are so enraged that immediate conflict resolution is unlikely. Waiting a few days allows most individuals to deal with their intense feelings and to be more objective about the issues (Smith, 2003). Thomas (2003b) suggests eschewing retaliatory hostility by using relaxation techniques or meditation to defuse the immediate anger. Regardless of how the parties are soothed, the manager must address the underlying problem later or this technique will become dysfunctional.

NEGOTIATION

Negotiation in its most creative form is similar to collaboration and in its most poorly managed form may resemble a competing approach. Negotiation frequently resembles compromise when it is used as a conflict resolution strategy. During negotiation, each party gives up something, and the emphasis is on accommodating differences between the parties. People have conflicting needs, wants, and desires that must be constantly compromised. Few people are able to meet all their needs or objectives. Most day-to-day conflict is resolved with negotiation. A nurse who says to another nurse, "I'll answer that call light if you'll count narcotics," is practicing the art of negotiation.

Although negotiation implies winning and losing for both parties, there is no rule that each party must lose and win the same amount. Most negotiators want to win more than they lose, but negotiation becomes destructively competitive when the emphasis is on winning at all costs. A major goal of effective negotiation is to make the other party feel satisfied with the outcome. The focus in negotiation should be to create a *win–win* situation.

Many small negotiations take place every day spontaneously and succeed without any advance preparation. However, not all nurses are expert negotiators. If managers wish to succeed in important negotiations for unit resources, they must (1) be adequately prepared, (2) be able to use appropriate negotiation strategies, and (3) apply appropriate closure and follow-up. To become more successful at negotiating, managers need to do several things before, during, and after the negotiation (see **Display 21.4**).

Display 21.4	Before, During, and After the Negotiation

Before
1. Be prepared mentally by having done your homework.
2. Determine your starting point, trade-offs, and bottom line.
3. Look for hidden agendas, both your own and the parties with whom you are negotiating.

During
1. Maintain composure.
2. Role model good communication skills (speaking and listening), assertiveness, and flexibility.
3. Avoid using destructive negotiation techniques but be prepared to counter them if used against you.

After
1. Restate what has been agreed upon, both verbally and in writing.
2. Recognize and thank all participants for their contributions to a successful negotiation.

Before the Negotiation

For managers to be successful, they must systematically prepare for the negotiation. As the negotiator, the manager begins by gathering as much information as possible regarding the issue to be negotiated. Because knowledge is power, the more informed the negotiator, the greater his or her bargaining power. Adequate preparation prevents others in the negotiation from catching the negotiator off guard or making him or her appear uninformed.

Additionally, individuals must remember that negotiation takes place on two levels. Doland (1998) says the first level is a substance level of who, what, when, where, and how of an issue. This is the area where strategies are prepared. However, Doland cautions that the second level must not be forgotten, which is the human side of every negotiation and interaction. Remember that the "opponents" you face across the bargaining table are individuals like you. The way the other party perceives you as being fair and open to negotiate often plays a role in the decisions that will be reached in the negotiation.

It also is important for managers to decide where to start in the negotiation. Umiker (1997) suggests that managers should initially focus on seeking a bigger pie instead of dividing the pie up. In other words, the negotiators add value to the package rather than seeking concessions from each other.

When this is not possible, the focus must shift to compromise and priority setting. Because managers must be willing to make compromises, they should choose a starting point that is high but not ridiculous. This selected starting point should be at the upper limits of their expectations, realizing that they may need to come down to a more realistic goal. For instance, you would really like four additional full-time RN positions and a full-time clerical position budgeted for your unit. You know that you could make do with three additional full-time

RN positions and a part-time clerical assistant, but you begin by asking for what would be ideal.

It is almost impossible in any type of negotiation to escalate demands; therefore, the manager must start at an extreme but reasonable point. It also must be decided beforehand how much can be compromised. Can the manager accept one full-time RN position or two or three? The very least for which a person will settle is often referred to as the *bottom line*.

The wise manager also has other options in mind when negotiating for important resources. An alternative option is another set of negotiating preferences that can be used so that managers need not use their bottom lines but still meet their overall goal. For instance, you have requested four full-time RN positions and one full-time clerical position. You could get by with three full-time RNs and one part-time clerk. However, you believe strongly that you cannot continue to provide safe patient care unless you are given two RNs and a part-time clerk—your bottom line. However, if the original negotiation is unsuccessful, reopen negotiations by saying that a second option that does not entail increasing the staff would be to float a ward clerk for four hours each day, implement a unit-dose system, require housekeeping to pass out linen, and have dietary pass all the patient meal trays. This way, the overall goal of providing more direct patient care by the nursing staff could still be met without adding nursing personnel.

The manager needs to consider other trade-offs that are possible in these situations. *Trade-offs* are secondary gains, often future-oriented, that may be realized as a result of conflict. For example, while attending college, a parent may feel intrapersonal conflict because he or she is unable to spend as much time as desired with his or her children. The parent is able to compromise by considering the trade-off: eventually, everyone's life will be better because of the present sacrifices. The wise manager will consider trading something today for something tomorrow as a means to reach satisfactory negotiations.

The manager also must look for and acknowledge *hidden agendas*—the covert intention of the negotiation. Usually, every negotiation has a covert and an overt agenda. For example, new managers may set up a meeting with their superior with the established agenda of discussing the lack of supplies on the unit. However, the hidden agenda may be that the manager feels insecure and is really seeking performance feedback during the discussion. Having a hidden agenda is not uncommon and is not wrong by any means. Everyone has them, and it is not necessary or even wise to share these hidden agendas. Managers, however, must be introspective enough to recognize their hidden agendas so they are not paralyzed if the agenda is discovered and used against them during the negotiation. If the manager's hidden agenda is discovered, he or she should admit that it is a consideration but not the heart of the negotiation. For example, although the hidden agenda for increasing unit staff might be to build the manager's esteem in the eyes of the staff, there may exist a legitimate need for additional staff. If, during the negotiations, the fiscal controller accuses the manager of wanting to increase staff just to gain power, the manager might respond by saying, "It is always important for a successful manager to be able to gain resources for the unit, but the real issue here is an inadequate

> The very least **for which** a person will **settle is** often referred **to as the** *bottom line.*

staff." Managers who protest too strongly that they do not have a hidden agenda appear defensive and vulnerable.

During the Negotiation

Negotiation is psychological and verbal. The effective negotiator always looks calm and self-assured. At least part of this self-assurance comes from having adequately prepared for the negotiation. Part of the preparation should have included learning about the people with whom the manager is negotiating. People come in a variety of personality types, and over the course of their careers, managers will come across most, if not all, of these personality types in various negotiations.

Preparation, however, is not enough. In the end, the negotiator must have clarity in his or her communication, assertiveness, good listening skills, the ability to regroup quickly, and flexibility. Strategies commonly used by leaders during negotiation to increase their persuasiveness and foster open communication include the following:

- Use only factual statements that have been gathered in research.
- Listen carefully, and watch nonverbal communication.
- Keep an open mind, because negotiation always provides the potential for learning. It is important not to prejudge. Instead, a cooperative (not competitive) climate should be established.
- Try to understand where the other party is coming from. It is probable that one person's perception is different from another's. The negotiation needs to concentrate on understanding and not just on agreeing.
- Always discuss the conflict. It is important not to personalize the conflict by discussing the parties involved in the negotiation.
- Try not to belabor how the conflict occurred or to fix blame for the conflict. Instead, the focus must be on preventing its recurrence.
- Be honest.
- Start tough so that concessions are possible. It is much harder to escalate demands in the negotiation than to make concessions.
- Delay when confronted with something totally unexpected in negotiation. In such cases, the negotiator should respond, "I'm not prepared to discuss this right now" or "I'm sorry, this was not on our agenda; we can set up another appointment later to discuss that." If asked a question the negotiator does not know, he or she should simply say, "I don't have that information at this time."
- Never tell the other party what you are willing to negotiate totally. You may be giving up the ship too early.
- Know the *bottom line* but try never to use it. If the bottom line is used, the negotiator must be ready to back it up or he or she will lose all credibility. Doland (1998) says that negotiations should always result in both sides improving their positions, but in reality people sometimes have to walk away from the negotiating table if the situation cannot be improved, because not every negotiation can result in terms that are agreeable to each party. If the bottom line is reached, the negotiator should tell the other party that an impasse has been reached and that further negotiation is not possible at this

time. Then the other party should be encouraged to sleep on it and reconsider. The door should always be left open for further negotiation. Another appointment can be made. Both parties should be allowed to save face.

- If either party becomes angry or tired during the negotiation, take a break. Go to the bathroom or make a telephone call. Remember that neither party can effectively negotiate if either is enraged or fatigued.

Destructive Negotiation Tactics

Some negotiators win by using specific intimidating or manipulative tactics. People using these tactics take a competing approach to negotiation rather than a collaborative approach. These tactics might be conscious or unconscious but are used repeatedly because they have been successful for that person. Successful managers do not use these types of tactics, but because others with whom they negotiate may do so, they must be prepared to counter such tactics.

One such tactic is *ridicule*. The goal in using ridicule is to intimidate others involved in the negotiation. If you are negotiating with someone who uses ridicule, maintain a relaxed body posture, steady gaze, and patient smile. Body language must also remain relaxed and nonthreatening.

Another tactic some people use is *ambiguous* or *inappropriate questioning*. For example, in one negotiating situation, the intensive care unit supervisor had requested additional staff to handle open-heart surgery patients. During her bargaining, the CEO suddenly said, "I never did understand the heart; can you tell me about the heart?" The supervisor did not fall into this trap and instead replied that the physiology of the heart was irrelevant to the issue. Because people tend to answer an authority figure, it is necessary to be on guard for this type of diversionary tactic.

Flattery is another technique that makes true collaboration in negotiation very difficult. The person who has been flattered may be more reluctant to disagree with the other party in the negotiation, and thus his or her attention and focus are diverted. One method managers can use to discern flattery from other honest attempts to compliment is to be aware how they feel about the comment. If they feel unduly flattered by a gesture or comment, it is a good indication that they were being flattered. For example, asking for advice or instruction may be a subtle form of flattery, or it may be an honest request. If the request for advice is about an area in which the manager has little expertise, it is undoubtedly flattery. However, exchanging positive opening comments with each other when beginning negotiation is an acceptable and enjoyable practice performed by both parties.

Nurses are also particularly sympathetic to gestures of helplessness. Because nursing is a helping profession, the tendency to nurture is high, and managers must be careful not to lose sight of the original intent of the negotiation—securing adequate resources to optimize unit functioning.

Some people win in negotiation simply by rapidly and *aggressively taking over* and controlling the negotiation before other members realize what is happening. If managers believe this may be happening, they should call a halt to the negotiations before decisions are made. Saying simply, "I need to have time to think this over" is a good method of stopping an aggressive takeover.

The manager needs to be aware of destructive negotiation tactics and develop strategies to overcome them. Destructive negotiation tactics are never a part of collaborative conflict resolution. Leaders use an honest, straightforward approach and develop assertive skills for use in conflict negotiation. Maintaining human dignity and promoting communication require that all conflict interactions be assertive, direct, and open. Conflict must be focused on the issues and resolved through joint compromise.

Closure and Follow-Up to Negotiation

Just as it is important to start the formal negotiation with some pleasantries, it is also good to close on a friendly note. Once a compromise has been reached, restate it so everyone is clear about what has been agreed upon. If managers win more in negotiation than they anticipated, they should try to hide their astonishment. At the end of any negotiation, whether it is a short two-minute conflict negotiation in the hallway with another RN or an hour-long formal salary negotiation, the result should be satisfaction by all parties that each has won something. It is a good idea to follow up formal negotiation in writing by sending a letter or a memo stating what was agreed.

Learning Exercise 21.4

An Exercise in Negotiation Analysis
You are one of a group of staff nurses who believe that part of your job dissatisfaction results from being assigned different patients every day. Your unit uses a system of total patient care, and the head nurse makes assignments. Two staff nurses have gone to the head nurse and requested that she allow each nurse to pick his or her own patients based on the previous day's assignment and the ability of the nurse. The head nurse believes they are being uncooperative because she is responsible for seeing that all the patients get assigned and receive adequate care. She indicates that although she attempts to provide continuity of care, it is often inappropriate because many part-time nurses are used on the unit, and not all the nurses are able to care for every type of patient. At the end of the conference, the two nurses are angry, and the head nurse is irritated. However, the next day, the head nurse says she is willing to meet with the staff nurses. The other nurses believe this is a sign that the head nurse is willing to negotiate a compromise. They plan to get together tonight to plan the strategy for tomorrow's meeting.
Assignment: What are the goals for each party? What could be a possible hidden agenda for each party? What could happen if the conflict escalates? Devise a workable plan that would accomplish the goals of both parties and develop strategies for implementation.

Analysis: A head nurse's goal is to be sure all patients receive safe and adequate care. However, she might have several hidden agendas. One might be that she does not want to relinquish any authority or does not want to devote her energy to the planned change that has been proposed. The staff nurses have goals of job satisfaction and providing more continuity of care; however, their hidden agenda is probably the need for more autonomy and control of the work setting.

If the conflict is allowed to escalate, the staff nurses could begin to disrupt the unit because of their dissatisfaction, and the head nurse could transfer some of the "ringleaders" or punish them in some other way. The head nurse is wise in reconsidering these nurses' request. By demonstrating her willingness to talk and negotiate the conflict, she will be viewed by the staff nurses as cooperative and interested in their job satisfaction.

The staff nurses must realize that they are not going to obtain everything they want in this conflict resolution, nor should they expect that result. To demonstrate their interest, they should develop some sort of workable policy and procedure for patient care assignments, recognizing that the head nurse will want to modify their procedure. Once the plan is developed, the nurses need to plan their strategy for the coming meeting. The following may be their outline:

1. Select as a spokesperson a member of the group who has the best assertive skills but who is not abrasive or aggressive in his or her approach. This keeps the group from appearing overpowering to the head nurse. The other group members will be at the meeting lending their support but will speak only when called on by the group leader. Preferably, the spokesperson also should be someone the head nurse knows well and whose opinion she respects.
2. The designated leader of the group should plan to begin her opening remarks by thanking the head nurse for agreeing to the meeting. In this way, the group acknowledges the authority of the head nurse.
3. There should be a sincere effort by the group to listen to the head nurse and to follow modifications to their plan. They must be willing to give up something also, perhaps some modification in the staffing pattern.
4. As the meeting progresses, the leader of the group should continue to express the goal of the group—to provide greater continuity of patient care—rather than focusing on how unhappy the group is with the present system.
5. At some point, the nurses should show their willingness to compromise and offer to evaluate the new plan periodically.

Ideally, the outcome of the meeting would be some sort of negotiated compromise in patient care assignment, which would result in more autonomy and job satisfaction for the nurses, enough authority for the head nurse to satisfy her responsibilities, and increased continuity of patient care assignment.

ALTERNATIVE DISPUTE RESOLUTION

Sometimes, parties cannot reach agreement through negotiation. In these cases, *alternative dispute resolution* (ADR) may be indicated to keep some privacy in the dispute and to avoid expensive litigation. Types of ADR include mediation, fact-finding, arbitration, and the use of ombudspersons (Epstein, 2003).

Mediation, which uses a neutral third party, is a confidential, legally nonbinding process, designed to help bring the parties together to devise a solution to the conflict. As such, the mediator does not take sides and has no vested interest in the outcome (Epstein, 2003). The mediator's role then becomes one of asking questions to clarify the issues at hand (*fact finding*), listening to both parties, caucusing with parties privately as necessary, making suggestions for areas of improvement, and hopefully, drafting a settlement agreement for both parties to sign (Epstein).

Sometimes, mediators are unable to help conflicted parties come to agreement. When this occurs, formal *arbitration* may be used. Unlike mediation which seeks to help conflicted parties come together to reach a decision themselves, arbitration is a binding conflict resolution process where the facts of the case are heard by an individual who makes a final decision for the parties in conflict.

There are, however, several other types of arbitration. One type is *mediation-arbitration*, in which a third party joins the negotiation process before any serious disputes arise (Ellis & Hartley, 2004). This individual acts only as a mediator unless some deadlock is reached in the negotiation. Then the mediator becomes an official arbitrator.

Another type of arbitration is the *final offer approach* (Ellis & Hartley, 2004). In this approach, the conflicted parties reach agreement on as many issues as possible. A final position for deadlocked issues from each side is then presented to the arbitrator, who is obligated to select only the most reasonable package. Arbitration may be requested from the American Arbitration Association or be available from state, pubic, and private mediation and conciliation services (Ellis & Hartley, 2004).

In addition, individuals experiencing conflict may seek guidance from *ombudspersons*. Ombudspersons generally hold an official title as such within an organization. Their function is to investigate grievances filed by one party against another and to assure that individuals involved in conflicts understand their rights as well as the process that should be used to report and resolve the conflict.

SEEKING CONSENSUS

Consensus is always an appropriate goal in resolving conflicts and in negotiation.

Consensus means that negotiating parties reach an agreement that all parties can support, even it does not represent everyone's first priorities. Consensus decision making does not provide complete satisfaction for everyone involved in the negotiation, as an initially unanimous decision would, but it does indicate willingness by all parties to accept the agreed-upon conditions.

In committees or groups working on shared goals, consensus is often used to resolve conflicts that may occur within the group. To reach consensus often requires the use of an experienced facilitator, and having consensus-building skills is a requirement of good leadership. Building consensus ensures that everyone within the group is heard but that the group will ultimately end up with one agreed-upon course of action. Consensual decisions are best used for decisions that relate to a core problem or need a deep level of group support to implement successfully (Asselin, 2001).

Perhaps the greatest challenge in using consensus as a conflict resolution strategy is that, like collaboration, it is time-consuming. It also requires all the parties involved in the negotiation to have good communication skills and to be open-minded and flexible.

INTEGRATING LEADERSHIP SKILLS AND MANAGEMENT FUNCTIONS IN MANAGING CONFLICT

The manager who creates a stable work environment that minimizes the antecedent conditions for conflict has more time and energy to focus on meeting organizational and human resource needs. When conflict does occur in the unit, managers must be able to discern constructive from destructive conflict. Conflict that is constructive will result in creativity, innovation, and growth for the unit. When conflict is deemed to be destructive, managers must deal appropriately with that conflict or risk an aftermath that may be even more destructive than the original conflict. Consistently using conflict resolution strategies with win–lose or lose–lose outcomes will create disharmony within the unit. Leaders who use optimal conflict resolution strategies with a win–win outcome promote increased employee satisfaction and organizational productivity.

Negotiation also requires both management functions and leadership skills. Well-prepared managers know with whom they will be negotiating and prepare their negotiation accordingly. They are prepared with trade-offs, multiple alternatives, and a clear bottom line to ensure that their unit acquires needed resources. Successful negotiation mandates the use of the leadership components of self-confidence and risk taking. If these attributes are not present, the leader–manager has little power in negotiation and thus compromises the unit's ability to secure desired resources. Other attributes that make leaders effective in negotiation are sensitivity to others and the environment and interpersonal communication skills. The leader's use of assertive communication skills, rather than tactics, results in an acceptable level of satisfaction for all parties at the close of the negotiation.

☀ Key Concepts

- *Conflict* can be defined as the internal discord that results from differences in ideas, values, or feelings of two or more people.
- Because managers have a variety of interpersonal relationships with people with different values, beliefs, backgrounds, and goals, conflict is an expected outcome.
- The most common sources of organizational conflict are communication problems, organizational structure, and individual behavior within the organization.

- Conflict theory has changed dramatically during the last 100 years. Currently, conflict is viewed as neither good nor bad because it can produce growth or be destructive, depending on how it is managed.
- Too little conflict results in organizational stasis, whereas too much conflict reduces the organization's effectiveness and eventually immobilizes its employees.
- The three categories of conflict are *intrapersonal, interpersonal*, and *intergroup*.
- The first stage in the conflict process is called *latent conflict*. Latent conflict implies the existence of antecedent conditions. Latent conflict may proceed to *perceived* or *felt* conflict. *Manifest conflict* also may occur. The last stage in the process is *conflict aftermath*.
- The optimal goal in conflict resolution is creating a *win–win* solution for everyone involved.
- Common conflict resolution strategies include *compromise, competing, accommodating, smoothing, avoiding,* and *collaboration*.
- As a negotiator, it is important to win as much as possible, lose as little as possible, and make the other party feel satisfied with the outcome of the negotiation.
- Because knowledge is power, the more informed a negotiator, the greater his or her bargaining power.
- The leader, while able to recognize and counter negotiation tactics, always strives to achieve an honest, collaborative approach to negotiation.
- The manager must know his or her *bottom line* but try never to use it.
- Closure and follow-up are important parts of the negotiation process.
- *Alternative dispute resolution* usually involves at least one of the elements of *mediation, fact finding, arbitration*, and the use of *ombudspersons*.
- Seeking *consensus*, a concord of opinion, although time-consuming, is an effective conflict resolution and negotiation strategy.

More Learning Exercises and Applications

Learning Exercise 21.5

Choosing the Most Appropriate Resolution Approach

In the following situations, choose the most appropriate conflict resolution strategy (avoiding, smoothing, accommodating, competing, compromising, and collaborating). Support your decision with rationale, and explain why other methods of conflict management were not used.

Situation 1

You are a circulating nurse in the operating room. Usually you are assigned to Room 3 for general surgery, but today you have been assigned to Room 4, the orthopedic room. You are unfamiliar with the orthopedic doctors' routines and attempt to brush up on them quickly before each case today by reading the doctors' preference cards before each case. So far, you have managed to complete two cases without incident. The next case comes in the room, and you realize everyone is especially tense; this patient is the wife of a local physician, and the doctors are performing a bone biopsy for possible malignancy. You prepare the area to be biopsied, and the surgeon, who has a reputation for a quick temper, enters the room. You suddenly realize that you have prepped the area with Betadine, and this surgeon prefers another solution. He sees what you have done and yells, "You are a stupid, stupid nurse."

Situation 2

You are the intensive care unit charge nurse and have just finished an exhausting eight hours on duty. Working with you today were two nurses who work 12-hour shifts. You have each been assigned two patients, all with high acuity levels. You are glad that you are going out of town tonight to attend an important seminar, because you are certainly tired. You also are pleased that you scheduled yourself an eight-hour shift today and that your relief is coming through the door. You will just have time to give report and catch your plane.

It is customary for 12-hour nurses to continue with their previous patients and for assignments not to be changed when 8-hour and 12-hour staff are working together. Therefore, you proceed to give report on your patients to the eight-hour nurse coming on duty. One of your patients is acutely ill with fever of unknown origin and is in the isolation room. It is suspected that he has meningitis. Your other patient is a multiple trauma victim. In the middle of your report, the oncoming nurse says that she has just learned that she is pregnant. She says, "I can't take care of a possible meningitis patient. I'll have to trade with one of the 12-hour nurses." You approach the 12-hour nurses, and they respond angrily, "We took care of all kinds of patients when we were pregnant, and we are not changing patients with just four hours left in our shift."

When you repeat this message to the oncoming nurse, she says, "Either they trade or I go home!" Your phone call to the nursing office reveals that because of a flu epidemic, there are absolutely no personnel to call in, and all the other units are already short-staffed.

Situation 3

You are an RN graduate of a BSN nursing program. Since you graduated six months ago, you have been working at an outpatient emergency clinic and have just recently begun to feel more confident in your new role. However, one of the older diploma educated nurses working with you constantly belittles baccalaureate nursing education. Whenever you request assistance in problem solving or in learning a new skill, she says, "Didn't they teach you anything in nursing school?" The clinic supervisor has given you satisfactory three-month and six-month evaluations, but you are becoming increasingly defensive regarding the comments of the other nurse.

Situation 4

You are the charge nurse on a step down unit. It is your first day back from a two-week vacation. The shift begins in 10 minutes and you sit down to make staffing assignments. The central staffing office has noted that you must float one of your RNs to the oncology unit. When you check the floating roster, you note that Jenny, one of the RNs assigned to work on your unit today, was the last to float. (She floated yesterday.) That leaves you to choose from Mark and Lisa, your other two RNs. According to the float roster, Mark floated 10 days ago and Lisa floated last 11 days ago. You tell Lisa that it is her turn to float.

Lisa states that she floated three times in a row since Mark was on vacation for two weeks last month. Mark says that vacations should not count and that he should not float because it is not his turn. Lisa says that Jenny should float since she floated to oncology yesterday and already knows the patients. Besides, Jenny says that she agreed to come in and work today (on her day off) to help the unit, and she would not have agreed to do this, if she had known she would have to float. Mark says that it is the last day of a six-day stretch and he does not want to float. Jenny says it is not her turn to float and she does not want to float willingly.

 Learning Exercise 21.6

Negotiating the Graduation Ceremony

Often one group is more powerful or has greater status and refuses to relinquish this power position, thus making collaboration impossible. Therefore, negotiating a compromise to a win–win solution, rather than a lose–lose solution, becomes imperative. In the following situation, describe if you could and how you would go about negotiating a win–win solution to conflict.

You are a senior member of a traditional on-campus baccalaureate nursing class. Three years ago, your university implemented an online RN-BSN program. The first students from that program graduated last year and they held a small, private end-of-program ceremony, separate from the on-campus BSN students.

This year, as a result of ongoing state budget cuts, the School of Nursing can no longer subsidize two separate end-of-program ceremonies. This means that the 21 RN-BSN students and the 33 on-campus BSN students must now work together to plan a joint ceremony.

Resistance is high. The two groups of students have not spent any time together and really do not know each other. The on-campus students have been planning their ceremony since they started the nursing program and have collected additional money each semester to fund a formal dinner and dance reception in the evening and breakfast at one of the nicest hotels in town. Money from the School of Nursing would be used to subsidize the cost of a live band and the reception hall. The online students would like to limit the evening reception to cake and punch at the college to reduce the cost since most of them will incur additional travel and lodging costs to attend graduation. They would, however, like to have the School of Nursing use the funds available to host a "picnic in the park" the following day, to which they can bring their families. Both groups perceive that the "other group is trying to control the situation and is not being sensitive to our needs or wants." Both groups have contacted University officials to complain about the situation and a number of students are threatening not to attend the ceremony, if the two groups must be merged.

You have been appointed the unofficial spokesperson for the RN-BSN graduates. Joan is the unofficial spokesperson for the on-campus BSN students. You live only 30 miles from campus so coming to campus to try to resolve the conflict is not a significant hardship.

The faculty member who is the liaison for the end-of-program ceremony has become alarmed at the situation and has contacted both you and Joan. She states that she will cancel the ceremony if the conflict is not resolved. The faculty member agrees to work with you and Joan to mediate the conflict but time is of the essence since the semester ends soon and the on-campus students can get no refund on their reception hall deposit after the end of the current week. She wants the conflict resolved in a win–win situation so that no parties leave angry.

Assignment: Where will you begin? How will you get input from the group you are representing? Would you plan a face-to-face meeting with Joan to attempt to resolve this conflict? What strategies might you use to help both groups win as much as possible and lose as little as possible? Explain your rationale. Remember, you wish to negotiate a compromise, and although you desire a win–win solution, you are limited in time and may not be able to facilitate a true collaboration. How will you deal with conflicted parties who perceive they have lost more than they won? What is your bottom line?

Learning Exercise 21. 7

Behavioral Tactics—Appropriate or Not?
You are a woman who is a unit manager with a master's degree in health administration. You are about to present your proposed budget to the CEO. You have thoroughly researched your budget and have adequate rationale to support your requests for increased funding. Because the CEO is often moody, predicting his response is difficult.

You also are aware that the CEO has some very traditional views about women's role in the workplace, and generally this does not include a major management role. Because he is fairly paternalistic, he is charmed and flattered when asked to assist "his" nurses with their jobs. Your predecessor was fired because she was perceived as brash, bossy, and disrespectful by the CEO. In fact, the former unit manager was one of a series of nursing managers who had been replaced in the last several years because of these characteristics. From what you have been told, the nursing staff did not share these perceptions.

You sit down and begin to plan your strategy for this meeting. You are aware that you are more likely to have your budgetary needs met if you dress conservatively, beseech his assistance and support throughout the presentation, and are fairly passive in your approach. In other words, you will be required to assume a traditionally feminine, helpless role. If you appear capable and articulate, you may not achieve your budgetary goals and may not even keep your job. It would probably not be necessary for you to continue to act this way, except in your interactions with the CEO.
Assignment: Are such behavioral tactics appropriate if the outcome is desirable? Are such tactics simply smart negotiation, or are they destructively manipulative? What would you do in this situation? Outline your strategy for your budget presentation, and present rationale for your choices.

Learning Exercise 21.8

Your First Budget Presentation
You are the head nurse of the new oncology unit. It is time for your first budget presentation to administration. You have already presented your budget to the director of nurses, and although she had a few questions, she was in general agreement. However, it is the policy at Memorial Hospital that each head nurse present her budget to the budget committee, consisting of the fiscal manager, the director of nurses, a member of the board of trustees, and the executive director. You know that money is scarce this year because of the new building, but you really believe you need the increases you have requested in your budget. Basically, you have asked for the following:

- Replace the 22% aides on your unit with 10% LVNs/LPNs and 12% RNs.
- Increase educational time paid by 5% to allow for certification in chemotherapy.
- Provide a new position of clinical nurse specialist in oncology.
- Convert one room into a sitting room and mini-kitchen for patients' families.
- Add shelves and a locked medication box in each room to facilitate primary nursing.
- Provide no new equipment, but replace existing equipment that is broken or outdated.

Assignment: Outline your plan. Include your approach, what is and what is not negotiable, and what arguments you would use. Give rationale for your plan.

Learning Exercise 21.9

Handling Staff–Patient Conflict
You are the supervisor of a rehabilitation unit. Two of your youngest nursing assistants come to your office today to report that a young male quadriplegic patient has been making lewd sexual comments and gestures when they provide basic care. When you question them about their response to the actions of the patient, they maintain that they normally simply look away and try to ignore him, although they are offended by his actions. They are very reluctant to confront the patient directly.

Because it is anticipated that this patient may remain on your unit for at least one month, the nursing assistants have asked you to intervene in this conflict by either talking to the patient or by assigning other nurses responsibility for his care.

Assignment: How will you handle this staff–patient conflict? Is avoidance (assigning different staff to care for the patient) an appropriate conflict resolution strategy in this situation? Will you encourage the nursing assistants to confront the patient directly? What coaching or role playing might you use with them if you choose this approach? Will you confront the patient yourself? What might you say?

Learning Exercise 21.10

Handling Personal Issues in a Professional Manner
You are a male Unit Supervisor of a pediatric trauma unit at Children's
Hospital. Three years ago, you ended a serious romantic relationship with
a nurse named Susan, who was employed at a different hospital in the
same city. The break up was not mutual and Susan was hurt and angry.

Six months ago, Susan accepted a position as a Unit Supervisor at Children's Hospital. This has required you and Susan to interact formally at
department head meetings and informally regarding staffing and personnel issues on a regular basis. Often, these interactions have been marked
by either covert hostility on Susan's part, nonverbal aggression, or sniping
comments. When you attempted to confront Susan about her behavior,
she stated that "she didn't have a problem and that you shouldn't flatter
yourself to think that she does."

The situation is increasingly becoming more difficult to "work around"
and both staff and fellow unit supervisors have become aware of the
ongoing tension. You love your position and do not want to leave Children's Hospital, but it is becoming increasingly apparent that the situation
cannot continue as it is.

Assignment: Answer the following questions:
1. How might gender have influenced the latent conditions, felt/perceived
   conflict, manifest conflict, and conflict aftermath in this situation?
2. What conflict strategies might you use to try to resolve this conflict?
   Avoidance? Smoothing? Accommodation? Competing? Compromise?
   Collaboration?
3. Would the use of a mediator be helpful in this situation?

 Web Links

College Recruiter.com. Suggested Salary Negotiation Guidelines for Recent College
Graduates. Retrieved Nov. 2003 from
http://www.adguide.com/pages/articles/article257.htm
Defines negotiation, explains the process, provides interview and negotiation suggestions

International Council of Nurses (ICN). Retrieved Nov. 8, 2004 from
http://www.icn.ch/sewworkplace.htm
*Includes framework guidelines addressing workplace violence in the health sector as well
as a state of the art paper.*

Teamwork Resolves Conflict (TRC)
http://www.ebl.org/trc.html
*Emphasizes team building as essential to conflict management and includes solved team
building case study (Accessed Nov. 2003).*

The Conflict Processes Section of the American Political Science Association (APSA).
http://www.apsanet.org/~conflict
Conflict processes, datasets, a small working-paper archive, and a newsletter (Accessed Nov. 2003).

References

Asselin, M. (2001). Time to wear a third hat? *Nursing Management, 32*(3), 24–29.

Catalano, J. T. (2003). *Nursing now! Today's issues, tomorrow's trends* (3rd ed.). Philadelphia: F.A. Davis Co.

Del Bel, J. C. (2003). Deescalating workplace aggression. *Nursing Management, 34*(9), 30–34.

Doland, P. (1998). Negotiating price: Improving your bargaining power. *TMA Journal, 18*(3), 58–62.

Ellis, J. R., & Hartley, C. L. (2004). *Nursing in today's world* (8th ed.). Philadelphia: Lippincott, Williams, & Wilkins.

Epstein, D. G. (2003). Mediation, not litigation. *Nursing Management, 34*(10), 40–42.

Ezarik, M. M. (2001). How to be a team player. *Current Health 27*(8), 8–11.

Hunt, S., & Posa, C. (2001). More women to the peace table. *Christian Science Monitor, 93*(121), 13.

James, D. (2001). Constructive conflict. *BRW, 23*(8), 28.

Krairiksh, M., & Anthony, M. K. (2001). Benefits and outcomes of staff nurses' participation in decision making. *Journal of Nursing Administration, 31*(1), 16–23.

McKenna, B. G., Smith, N. A., Poole, S. J., & Coverdale, J. H. (2003). Horizontal violence: Experiences of registered nurses in their first year of practice. *Journal of Advanced Nursing, 42*(1), 90–96.

Simmons, R. (2002). *Odd girl out: The hidden culture of aggression in girls.* New York: Harcourt.

Smith, P. G. (2003). How to handle conflict. *Career World, 32*(3). Available at: http://web7.epnet.com/citation.asp?tb=1&_ug+dbs+0+In+en%2Dus+sid+7E3F9930%2 Accessed November 14, 2003.

Sullivan, E. J. (2004). *Becoming influential: A guide for nurses.* Upper Saddle River, NJ: Pearson/Prentice Hall.

Thomas, S. P. (2003a). Anger: The mismanaged emotion. *MEDSURG Nursing, 12*(2), 103–110.

Thomas, S. P. (2003b). Horizontal hostility. *American Journal of Nursing, 103*(10), 87.

Umiker, W. (1997). Collaborative conflict resolution. *Health Care Supervisor, 15*(3), 70–75.

Bibliography

Alper, S., Tjosvold, A., & Law, K. S. (2000). Conflict management, efficacy, and performance in organizational teams. *Personnel Psychology, 53*(3), 625–643.

Anderson C. (2002). Workplace violence: Are some nurses more vulnerable? *Issues in Mental Health Nursing, 23*(4), 351–366

Andrica, D. C. (2001). Out of a job: Outplacement and severance arrangements. *Nursing Economic$, 19*(1), 35.

Brandt, M. A. (2001). How to make conflict work for you. *Nursing Management, 32*(11), 32–35.

Caffo, B. J. (2003). Never mind who is to blame: Let's deal with our conflicts. *DNA Reporter, 28*(1), 11.

Franklin, E. (2002). A reflective essay: Getting along is highly overrated. *Policy, Politics & Nursing Practice, 3*(2), 93–96.

Hart, K. (2003). Perspectives in leadership. Empowering staff to solve problems. *Nursing Spectrum (Philadelphia TriState), 12*(1), 7.

Homsted, L. (2002). Handling conflict professionally. *Florida Nurse, 50*(4), 12.

Jordan, P. J. (2002). Emotional intelligence and conflict resolution in nursing. *Contemporary Nurse, 13*(1), 94–100.

Kritek, P. (2002). *Negotiating at an uneven table* (2nd ed.). San Francisco: Jossey-Bass.

Lankshear, A. J. (2003). Coping with conflict and confusing agendas in multidisciplinary community mental health teams. *Journal of Psychiatric and Mental Health Nursing, 10*(4), 457.

LeBaron, M. (2002). *Bridging troubled waters.* San Francisco: Jossey-Bass.

Ludwig, G. G. (2003). Manager's corner. Dealing with your enemies. *Emergency Medical Services, 32*(7), 42.

Mamchur, C., & Myrick, F. (2003). Preceptorship and interpersonal conflict: A multidisciplinary study. *Journal of Advanced Nursing, 43*(2), 188–196.

Marco, C. A. (2002). Conflict resolution in emergency medicine. *Annals of Emergency Medicine, 40*(3), 347–349.

Percival, J. (2001). Getting along . . . Getting along with people. *Nursing Standard, 15*(31), 21.

Pettrey, L. (2003, February). Who let the dogs out? Managing conflict with courage and skill. *Critical Care Nurse.* AACN Critical Care Careers 2003, 21–24.

Porter-O'Grady, R. (2003). When push comes to shove: Managers as mediators. *Nursing Management, 34*(10), 34–40.

Roberts, S. J. (2000). Development of a positive professional identity: Liberating oneself from the oppressor within. *Advances in Nursing Science, 22*(4), 71–82.

Sibbald, B. (2001). Conflict-management system need in ERs; jury. *Canadian Medical Association Journal, 165*(1), 74.

Stone, D., Patton, B., & Heen, S. (2000). *Difficult conversations: How to discuss what matters most.* New York, NY: Penguin Putnam.

Valentine, P. E. B. (2001). A gender perspective on *conflict management* strategies of nurses. *Journal of Nursing Scholarship, 33*, 69–74.

Warning: Conflicts may result in more vacancies. (2003). *ED Management, 15*(2), 19–21.

Understanding Collective Bargaining, Unionization, and Employment Laws

Unions don't create the climate in which organizing activity thrives; they simply take advantage of it. The roots of union activity lie in the fertile soil of poor relationships between employees and their leaders.

—H. Forman and G. A. Davis

Factors that have an impact on the directing aspects of management are collective bargaining, unionization, and employment laws. It is possible to maximize these factors, making them positive rather than negative influences on management effectiveness. To accomplish this task, however, managers must first understand the interrelationship of unionization and management, the proliferation of legislation regarding employment practices, and the impact of both on the healthcare industry.

Managers must be able to see collective bargaining and employment legislation from four perspectives: (1) the organization, (2) the worker, (3) general historical/societal, and (4) personal. Managers able to gain this broad perspective will better understand how management and employees can work together cooperatively despite unionization and employment legislation. Many industrialized countries have adopted an attitude of acceptance and tolerance for the difficulties of managing under these influences. However, in the United States, many organizations view these forces with resentment and hostility. This chapter examines the leadership roles and management functions necessary to create a climate in which unionization and legislation are compatible with organizational goals. These leadership roles and management functions inherent in dealing with unions and employment laws are shown in **Display 22.1**.

UNIONS AND COLLECTIVE BARGAINING

Collective bargaining may be defined as activities occurring between organized labor and management that concern employee relations. Such activities include negotiation of formal labor agreements and day-to-day interactions between unions and management. Although first- and middle-level managers usually have little to do with negotiating the labor contract, they are greatly involved with the contract's daily implementation. The middle manager has the greatest impact on the quality of the relationship that develops between labor and management. Terminology associated with unions and collective bargaining is shown in **Display 22.2**.

HISTORICAL PERSPECTIVE OF UNIONIZATION IN AMERICA

Unions have been present in America since the 1790s. Skilled craftsmen formed early unions to protect themselves from wage cuts during the highly competitive era of industrialization. The history of unionization reveals that union membership and activity increases sharply during times of high employment and prosperity and decreases sharply during economic recessions and layoffs.

Union activity also tends to change in response to workforce excesses and shortages. For decades, employment demand for nurses has increased and decreased periodically. High demand for nurses is tied directly to a healthy national economy, and historically this has been correlated with increased union activity. Similarly, when nursing vacancy rates are low, union membership and activity tends to decline.

In addition, nurses' perceptions of the quality of their supervision have always had an impact on unionization rates. The rapid downsizing and restructuring of the

> Management that is perceived to be deaf to the workers' needs provides a fertile ground for union organizers because unions thrive in a climate that perceives the organizational philosophy to be insensitive to the worker.

Display 22.1	Leadership Roles and Management Functions Associated with Unionization and Employment Laws

Leadership Roles

1. Is self-aware regarding personal attitudes and values regarding collective bargaining and employment laws.
2. Recognizes and accepts reasons that people seek unionization.
3. Creates a work environment that eliminates the need for unionization to meet employees' needs.
4. Maintains an accommodating or cooperative approach when dealing with unions and employment legislation.
5. Is a role model for fairness.
6. Is nondiscriminatory in all personal and professional actions.
7. Examines the work environment periodically to ensure that it is supportive for all members regardless of gender, race, age, disability, or sexual orientation.
8. Actively seeks a culturally and ethnically diverse workforce to meet the needs of an increasingly diverse client population.

Management Functions

1. Understands and appropriately implements union contracts.
2. Administers personnel policies fairly and consistently.
3. Works cooperatively with the personnel department and top-level administration when dealing with union activity.
4. Understands and follows labor and employment laws that relate to the manager's sphere of influence.
5. Ensures that the work environment is safe.
6. Is alert for discriminatory employment practices in the workplace.
7. Follows through on investigating any employee reports of discrimination.
8. Ensures that the unit or department meets state licensing regulations.
9. Immediately and fully investigates all complaints regarding violations of the collective bargaining contract and takes appropriate action.

1990s left many nurses feeling that management did not listen to them or care about their needs. Murray (1999) reports that from 1995 to 1998, when hospitals were rapidly downsizing and restructuring, petitions by nurses to unionize increased yearly by 39%, 111%, and over 77%, respectively. This is an unprecedented amount of union activity. However, even with the rise in union membership the past decade, only 20% of nurses belong to collective bargaining units in the United States (Fitzpatrick, 2001).

For many reasons, collective bargaining was slow in coming to the healthcare industry. Until labor laws were amended, unionization of healthcare workers was illegal. Nursing's long history as a service commodity further delayed labor organization in healthcare settings.

Initial collective bargaining in the profession took place in organizations that were deemed government or public. This was made possible by Executive Order

---

Display 22.2 Collective Bargaining Terminology

Agency shop: Also called an *open shop*. Employees are not required to join the union.

Arbitration: Terminal step in the grievance procedure, where a third party reviews the grievance, completes fact finding, and reaches a decision. Always indicates the involvement of a third party. Arbitration may be voluntary on the part of management and labor or imposed by the government in a compulsory arbitration.

Collective bargaining: Relations between employers, acting through their management representatives, and organized labor.

Conciliation and **mediation:** Synonymous terms that refer to the activity of a third party to help disputants reach an agreement. However, unlike an arbitrator, this person has no final power of decision making.

Fact finding: Rarely used in the private sector but used frequently in labor–management disputes that involve government-owned companies. In the private sector, fact finding is usually performed by a board of inquiry.

Free speech: Public Law 101, Section 8 states that "the expressing of any views, argument, or dissemination thereof, whether in written, printed, graphic, or visual form, shall not constitute or be evidence of an unfair labor practice under any provisions of this Act, if such expression contains no threat of reprisal or force or promise of benefit."

Grievance: Perception on the part of a union member that management has failed in some way to meet the terms of the labor agreement.

Lockout: Closing a place of business by management in the course of a labor dispute for the purpose of forcing employees to accept management terms.

National Labor Relations Board: Labor board formed to implement the Wagner Act. Its two manor functions are to (1) determine who should be the official bargaining unit when a new unit is formed and who should be in the unit and (2) adjudicate unfair labor charges.

Professionals: Professionals have the right to be represented by a union but cannot belong to a union that represents nonprofessionals unless a majority of them vote for inclusion in the nonprofessional unit.

Strike: Concerted withholding of labor supply to bring about economic pressure on employers and cause them to grant employee demands.

Union shop: Also called a *closed shop*. All employees are required to join the union and pay dues.

10988, authored in 1962. This order lifted restrictions preventing public employees from organizing. Therefore, collective bargaining by nurses at city, county, and district hospitals and healthcare agencies began in the 1960s.

In 1974, Congress amended the Wagner Act, extending national labor laws to private, nonprofit hospitals; nursing homes; health clinics; health maintenance organizations; and other healthcare institutions. These amendments opened the doors to much union activity for professions and the public employee sector. Indeed, a review of union membership figures readily shows that since 1960, most collective bargaining activity in the United States has occurred in the public and professional sectors of industry, most notably among faculty at institutions of higher education, teachers at primary and secondary levels, and physicians. There has been little growth of unionization in the private and blue-collar sectors since membership peaked in the 1950s.

From 1962 through 1989, there were slow but steady increases in the numbers of nurses represented by collective bargaining agents. In 1989, the National Labor Relations Board (NLRB) ruled that nurses could form their own separate bargaining units, and union activity increased. However, the American Hospital Association immediately sued the American Nurses Association (ANA), and the ruling was halted until 1991 when the Supreme Court upheld the 1989 NLRB decision. **Table 22.1** outlines legislation that led to unionization in health care.

Various unions represent nurses and other healthcare workers. The Service Employees International Union (SEIU) is the largest union in the healthcare industry, representing more than 755,000 healthcare workers, including 110,000 nurses and 20,000 doctors (SEIU, 2003). SEIU is also the largest union of nursing home workers in the United States, representing more than 130,000 employees. Some of the other unions that represent nurses include the ANA; the National Union of Hospital and Health Care Employees of Retail, Wholesale and Department Store Union; American Federation of Labor–Congress of Industrial Organizations (AFL-CIO); the United Steelworkers of America (USWA); the American Federation of Government Employees, AFL-CIO; the American Federation of State, County, and Municipal Employees, AFL-CIO; the International Brotherhood of Teamsters; the American Federation of State, County, and Municipal Employees, which operates mostly in the public sector and the United Auto Workers.

Union representation also varies by state. The states with the most union organizing for all industries, including health care, are New York, California, Pennsylvania, Michigan, and Illinois. The right-to-work states, typically low in union activity, include Arizona, New Mexico, Oklahoma, and Florida (Murray, 2001).

Table 22.1 Labor Legislation

Year	Legislation	Effect
1935	National Labor Act/Wagner Act	Gave unions many rights in organizing; resulted in rapid union growth
1947	Taft-Hartley Amendment	Returned some power to management; resulted in a more equal balance of power between unions and management
1962	Kennedy Executive Order 10988	Amended the 1935 Wagner Act to allow public employees to join unions
1974	Amendments to Wagner Act	Allowed nonprofit organizations to join unions
1989	National Labor Relations Board ruling	Allowed nurses to form their own separate bargaining units

AMERICAN NURSES ASSOCIATION AND COLLECTIVE BARGAINING

One difficult union issue faced by nurse–managers, not typically encountered in other disciplines, stems from the dual role of their professional organization, the ANA. The NLRB recognizes the ANA, at most state levels, as a collective bargaining agent.

The use of state associations as bargaining agents has been a divisive issue among American nurses. Some nurse–managers believe they have been disenfranchised by their professional organization. Other managers recognize the conflicts inherent in attempting to sit on both sides of the bargaining table. For some members of the nursing profession, this issue presents no conflict. Regardless of individual values, there does appear to be some conflict in loyalty. There are no easy solutions to the dilemma created by the dual role held by the ANA. Clarifying these issues begins with the manager examining the motivation of nurses to participate in collective bargaining. The manager must at least try to hear and understand employees' points of view.

Learning Exercise 22.1

The Role of the ANA as Collective Bargaining Agent
How do you feel about the American Nurses Association's (ANA's) certification as a collective bargaining agent? Do you belong to the state student nurses association? Why or why not? Do you plan to join your state ANA? What are the primary driving and restraining forces for your decision? Divide into two groups to debate the pros and cons of having the ANA, rather than other unions, represent nurses.

EMPLOYEE MOTIVATION TO JOIN OR REJECT UNIONS

Knowing that human behavior is goal-directed, it is important to examine what personal goals union membership fulfills. Nurse–managers often tell each other that healthcare institutions differ from other types of industrial organizations. This is really a myth because most nurses work in large and impersonal organizations. The nurse frequently feels powerless and vulnerable as an individual alone in a complex institution.

Six primary motivations for joining a union exist (**Display 22.3**). The first is to increase the power of the individual. Employees know that singly they are much more dispensable. Because a large group of employees is generally less dispensable, nurses greatly increase their bargaining power and reduce their vulnerability by joining a union. This is a particularly strong motivating force for nurses when jobs are scarce and they feel vulnerable. Indeed, during the massive downsizing and restructuring of the 1990s, collective bargaining priorities shifted from wages and benefits to job security.

Display 22.3	**Union Membership: Pros and Cons**

Reasons Nurses Join Unions
1. To increase the power of the individual
2. To increase their input into organizational decision making
3. To eliminate discrimination and favoritism
4. Because of a social need to be accepted
5. Because they are required to do so as part of employment (closed shop)
6. Because they believe it will improve patient outcomes and quality of care

Reasons Nurses Do Not Want to Join Unions
1. A belief that unions promote the welfare state and oppose the American system of free enterprise
2. A need to demonstrate individualism and promote social status
3. A belief that professionals should not unionize
4. An identification with management's viewpoint
5. Fear of employer reprisal
6. Fear of lost income associated with a strike or walkout

When there are nursing shortages, nurses feel less vulnerable, and other reasons to join unions become motivating factors. One motivator driving nurses toward unionization is to communicate their aims, feelings, complaints, and ideas to others. The desire to have input into organizational decision making is often a reason people join unions. A feeling of powerlessness or the perception that administration does not care about employees is a major driving force for unionization.

Because unions emphasize equality and fairness, nurses also join them because they need to eliminate discrimination and favoritism. This might be an especially strong motivator for members of groups that have experienced discrimination, such as women and minorities.

Many social factors also act as motivators to nurses regarding union activity. The fourth motivation for joining a union stems from the social need to be accepted. Sometimes this social need results from family or peer pressure. Because many working-class families have a long history of strong union ties, children are frequently raised in a cultural milieu that promotes unionization.

Another reason nurses sometimes join unions is because the union contract dictates that all nurses belong to the union. This has been a big driving force among blue-collar workers. However, the *closed shop*, or requirement that all employees belong to a union, has never prevailed in the healthcare industry. Most healthcare unions have *open shops*, allowing nurses to choose if they want to join the union.

Finally, some nurses join unions because they believe that patient outcomes are better in unionized organizations due to better staffing and supervised management practices. Research by Seago and Ash (2002) does suggest a positive relationship between patient outcomes and RN unions that goes beyond wages and number of hours. Factors identified by Seago and Ash as potentially leading to this relationship in RN unions are stability in staff, autonomy, collaboration with physicians, and participation in practice decisions.

Just as there are many reasons to join unions, there also are reasons why nurses reject unions (Display 22.3). Perhaps the strongest are societal and cultural factors. Many people distrust unions because they believe unions promote the welfare state and undermine the American system of free enterprise. Other reasons for rejecting unions might be one of six needs. The first is a need to demonstrate that they can get ahead on their own merits.

Professional employees have been slow in forming unions for several reasons that deal with class and education. They argue that unions were appropriate for the blue-collar worker but not for the university professor, physician, or engineer. Nurses rejecting unions on this basis usually are driven by a need to demonstrate their individualism and social status.

Some employees identify with management and thus frequently adopt its viewpoint toward unions. Such nurses, therefore, would reject unions because their values more closely align with management than with workers.

Although employees are protected under the National Labor Relations Act (NLRA), many reject unions because of fears of employer reprisal. Nurses who reject unions on this basis could be said to be motivated most of all by a need to keep their job.

Finally, some nurses reject unions out of the fear of lost income associated with a strike or walkout. Strikes and walkouts are a reality of unionization; however, they are regulated by law. The National Labor Relations Act (NLRA) states in part that "Employees shall have the right to engage in other concerted activities for the purpose of collective bargaining or other mutual aid or protection." The phrase *other concerted activities* refers to "working to rule," "blue flu" epidemics, work slowdowns, filing a barrage of grievances, participating in informational or recognition picketing, contracting government agencies such as the Department of Health or Occupational Safety and Health Administration, and striking (Forman & Powell, 2003). Unions must, however, give employers and the Federal Medication and Conciliation Service (FMCS) 10 days notice of their intent to strike (Forman & Powell).

 Learning Exercise 22.2

Discussing Pros and Cons of Unions
List the reasons you would or would not join a union. Share this with others in your group, and examine the following questions. Would you feel differently about unions if you were a manager? What influences you the most in your desire to join or reject unions? Have you ever felt discriminated against or powerless in the workplace?

Once managers understand the drives and needs behind joining unions, they can begin to address those needs. Organizations with unfair management policies are more likely to become unionized. Fitzpatrick (2001) maintains that the key issues driving current union activity are layoffs and quality of the nurses' work lives.

It is certainly then within managerial power to eliminate some of the needs staff have for joining unions. Managers can encourage feelings of power by allowing subordinates to have input into decisions that will affect their work. Managers also can listen to ideas, complaints, and feelings and take steps to ensure that favoritism and discrimination are not part of their management style. Additionally, the manager can strengthen the drives and needs that make nurses reject unions. By building a team effort, sharing ideas and future plans from upper management with the staff, and encouraging individualism in employees, the manager can facilitate identification of the worker with management.

Steltzer (2001) says that when nurses begin showing signs of job dissatisfaction, when they feel frustrated, stressed or powerless, they are sending a wake-up call to nursing management. Leaders must be alert to employment practices that are unfair or insensitive to employee needs and must intervene appropriately before such issues lead to unionization. However, organizations offering liberal benefit packages and fair management practices may still experience union activity if certain social and cultural factors are present. If union activity does occur, managers must be aware of specific employee and management rights so the NLRA is not violated by either managers or employees.

UNION ORGANIZING STRATEGIES

Murray (2001) suggests that unions have used ten primary organizing strategies to promote union membership since the early 1990s (see **Display 22.4**). The first of these strategies is to "identify new targets," including physicians and home care workers. This increased representation on physicians in collective bargaining has occurred as a result of a 1999 decision by the American Medical Association (AMA) to support the collective bargaining process.

A second strategy has been increased funding. Large unions such as the AFL-CIO have set aside millions of dollars for unions that need financial help in running

---

Display 22.4 Ten Union Organizing Strategies

1. New targets
2. Increased funding
3. Recruitment and training
4. Issue accuracy
5. Corporate campaign
6. Activism
7. Improved contracts
8. Salting
9. Lawsuits
10. Technology

Source: Murray, M. K. (2001). The new economy and new union organizing strategies: Union wins in healthcare. *Journal of Nursing Administration, 31*(7/8), 339–343.

campaigns and increasing organizing funds. A third strategy is recruiting and training new full-time organizers. For example, the AFL-CIO offers the Organizing Institute, Union Summer, and Seminary Summer programs to promote union organizing (Murray, 2001).

Issue identification is a fourth strategy. Issues identified by unions as critical to nurses include the amount of change in the healthcare system, healthcare shortages, reengineering, and managed care. All of these issues have made working nurses question the meaning of loyalty and to ponder whether they have suffered the lion's share on *take-aways* (i.e., lost benefits, weekend plan scheduling changes, staffing shortages, and salary freezes).

The fifth strategy identified by Murray (2001) is corporate campaigns. Unions are refining corporate campaigns with allegations of discrimination, boycotts, rallies, media stories, visits to board members' homes, and one day strikes. Thirteen percent of chief financial officers say that their companies experienced a walkout or a strike during 2000, and 25% say they were threatened with one (On Labor Issues, 2000).

A sixth strategy contributing to labor union wins is activism. Central labor councils, local labor unions, and state labor federations are reaching out to community groups, faith-based organizations, and elected officials in an effort to create unrest and change the environment in which workers organize.

The seventh strategy is focusing contract negotiations on what is deemed most important by workers, e.g., shared decision making and scheduling even more than wages. Unions have increasingly recognized this and shifted their contract negotiations accordingly.

"Salting the bargaining unit" is the eighth strategy identified by Murray (2001) as currently being used by unions to increase membership. *Salting* means that an outsider comes in to organize the union. The United States Supreme Court ruled in 1995 that employees cannot discriminate against paid union organizers who seek jobs to organize nonunion workers. Thus, many unions have "salted" potential union sites with individuals who have union organization as their primary motive.

The ninth strategy is filing lawsuits. Labor unions maintain the goal of breaking employer resolve and demonstrate their ability to protect employees by initiating legal action on behalf of employees against targeted employers (Murray, 2001).

The final strategy is technology. The Internet has made accessing information about how to organize a union very accessible to interested workers. Email has also proven to be an inexpensive and efficient means of mass communication regarding issues critical to the union.

> Although historically unions focused heavily on wage negotiations, the current issues deemed more important by nurses often focus on nonmonetary issues such as guidelines for staffing, float provisions, shared decision making, and scheduling.

MANAGERS' ROLE DURING UNION ORGANIZING

Because of the healthcare industry's movement toward unionization, most nurses will probably be involved with unions in some manner during their careers. Managers who are not employed in a unionized healthcare organization should anticipate that one or more unions will attempt to organize nurses within the next few years. **Display 22.5** shows a list of practices that the organization should have

Display 22.5	**Before the Union Comes**

1. Know and care about your employees.
2. Establish fair and well-communicated personnel policies.
3. Use an effective upward and downward system of communication.
4. Ensure that all managers are well trained and effective.
5. Establish a well-developed formal procedure for handling employee grievances.
6. Have a competitive compensation program of wages and benefits.
7. Have an effective performance appraisal system in place.
8. Use a fair and well-communicated system for promotions and transfers.
9. Use organizational actions to indicate that job security is based on job performance, adherence to rules and regulations, and availability of work.
10. Have an administrative policy on unionization.

in place that will discourage union activity. If the organization waits until the union arrives, it will be too late to perform these functions.

Employees have a right to participate in union organizing under the NLRA, and managers must not interfere with this right. Nurse–managers, as legally defined hospital "supervisors," are legal spokespersons for the hospital. As such, the NLRB closely monitors what they may say and do. Prohibited managerial activities include threatening employees, interrogating employees, promising employees rewards for cessation of union activity, and spying on employees. However, if the astute manager picks up early clues of union activity, the organization may be able to take steps that will discourage unionization of its employees.

The first step in establishing a union is demonstrating an adequate level of desire for unionization by the employees. The NLRB requires that at least 30% of employees sign an interest card before an election for unionization can be held. Most unions, however, will require between 60 and 70% of the employees to sign interest cards before spending the time and money involved in an organizing campaign. Union representatives are generally careful to keep a campaign secret until they are ready to file a petition for election. They do this so they can build momentum without interference from the employer (Forman & Davis, 2002).

After a designated number of cards have been generated, the organization is forced to have an election. At that time, all employees of the same classification, such as registered nurses, would vote on whether they desire unionization. A choice in every such election is *no representation*, which means that the voters do not want a union. During the election, 50% plus 1 of the petitioned unit must vote for unionization, before the union can be recognized.

A process similar to that of certification can also decertify unions. *Decertification* may occur when at least 30% of the eligible employees in the bargaining unit initiate a petition asking to no longer be represented by the union (Forman & Kraus, 2003). Employers, by law, are not allowed to instigate or promote decertification, but may provide employees with information regarding their rights to do so, under the NLRA (Forman and Kraus).

It is important to remember that there are differences between organizing in a healthcare facility and other types of organizations. Generally, the solicitation and distribution of union literature is banned entirely in "immediate patient care areas." Managers should never, however, independently attempt to deal with union-organizing activity. They should always seek assistance and guidance from higher-level management and the personnel department.

The entire list of rights for management and labor during the organizing and establishment phases of unionization is beyond the scope of this book. Throughout the years, Congress has amended various labor acts and laws so that power is balanced between management and labor. At times, the balance of power has shifted to management or labor, but Congress wisely eventually enacts laws that restore the balance. The manager must ensure that the rights of management and employees are protected. The two most sensitive areas of any union contract, once wages have been agreed on, are discipline and the grievance process, which are discussed in Unit 7.

EFFECTIVE LABOR–MANAGEMENT RELATIONS

Before the 1950s, labor–management relations were turbulent. History books are filled with battles, strikes, mass-picketing scenes, and brutal treatment by management and employees. In the last 30 years, employers and unions have substantially improved their relationships. Although evidence is growing that contemporary management has come to accept the reality that unions are here to stay, businesses in the United States are still less comfortable with unions than their counterparts in many other countries. Likewise, unions have come to accept the fact that there are times when organizations are not healthy enough to survive aggressive union demands.

Once management is faced with dealing with a bargaining agent, it has a choice of either accepting or opposing the union. It may actively oppose the union by using various *union-busting techniques*, or it may more subtly oppose the union by attempting to discredit it and win employee trust. Acceptance also may run along a continuum. The company may accept the union with reluctance and suspicion. Although they know the union has legitimate rights, managers often believe they must continually guard against the union encroaching further into traditional management territory.

There also is the type of union acceptance known as *accommodation*. Increasingly common, accommodation is characterized by management's full acceptance of the union, with both union and management showing mutual respect. When these conditions exist, labor and management can establish mutual goals, especially in the areas of safety, cost reduction, efficiency, eliminating waste, and improving working conditions. Porter-O'Grady (2001) believes that this type of relationship has begun to be evidenced between unionized professional nurses and healthcare organizations and refers to this more cooperative interaction as a new model of collective-bargaining relationship. Such cooperation represents the most mature and advanced type of labor–management relations.

The attitudes and the philosophies of the leaders in management and the union determine what type of relationship develops between the two parties in any given organization. When dealing with unions, managers must be flexible. It is critical that they do not ignore issues or try to overwhelm others with power. The rational approach to problem solving must be used.

Unionization of the healthcare industry will undoubtedly expand. It is important to learn how to deal with this potential constraint to effective management. Managers must learn to work with unions and develop the art of using unions to assist the organization in building a team effort to meet organizational goals.

 Learning Exercise 22.3

List and Support Your Reasons For or Against Striking

You are a staff nurse in the intensive care unit in one of your city's two hospitals. You have worked at this hospital for five years, transferring to the intensive care unit two years ago. You love nursing but are sometimes frustrated in your job due to a short supply of nurses, excessive overtime demands, and the stress of working with such critically ill patients.

The hospital has a closed shop, so union dues are deducted from your pay even though you are not actively involved in the union. The present union contract is up for renegotiation, and union and management have not been able to agree on many issues. When management made its last offer, the new contract was rejected by the nurses. Now that the old contract has expired, nurses are free to strike if they vote to do so.

You had voted for accepting the management offer; you have two children to support, and it would be devastating to be without work for a long time. Last night, the nurses voted on whether to return to the bargaining table and try to renegotiate with management or to go out on strike.

Again, you voted for no strike. You have just heard from your friend that the strike vote won. Now you must decide if you are going to support your striking colleagues or cross the picket line and return to work tomorrow. Your friends are pressuring you to support their cause. You know that the union will provide some financial compensation during the strike but believe it won't be adequate for you to support yourself and your children.

You agree with union assertions that the organization has overworked and underpaid you and that it has been generally unresponsive to nursing needs. On the other hand, you believe your first obligation is to your children.

Assignment: List all the reasons for and against striking. Decide what you will do. Use appropriate rationale from outside readings to support your final decision. Share your thoughts with the class. Take a vote in class to determine how many would strike and how many would cross the picket line.

EMPLOYMENT LEGISLATION

Like unionization, the many legal issues involved in hiring and employment have an impact on the directing function. These potential constraints are present regardless of the presence of unions. The American industrial relations system is regarded as one of the most legalistic in the Western world, and it continues to grow. Few aspects of the employment relationship are free from regulation by either state or federal law. Many of these regulations relate to specific aspects of personnel management, such as the laws that deal with collective bargaining or the equal employment laws that regulate hiring. Some personnel regulations are discussed in previous chapters and others are discussed later.

Some observers believe that employment and labor–management laws have become so prescriptive that they preclude experimentation and creativity on the part of management. Others believe that, like collective bargaining, the proliferation of employment laws must be viewed from an historical standpoint to understand their need. Regardless of whether one believes such laws and regulations are necessary, they are a fact of each manager's life.

> The feeling that the employer is fair to all will set the stage for the type of team building so important in effective management.

Being able to handle management's legal requirements effectively requires a comprehension of labor laws and their interpretation. The leader who embraces the intent of laws barring discrimination and providing equal opportunity becomes a role model for fairness.

Employment laws, summarized in **Table 22.2,** fall into one of five categories:

1. **Labor standards:** These laws establish minimum standards for working conditions regardless of the presence or absence of a union contract. Included in this set are minimum wage, health and safety, and equal pay laws.
2. **Labor relations:** These laws relate to the rights and duties of unions and employers in their relationship with each other.
3. **Equal employment:** The laws that deal with employment discrimination are introduced in Chapter 15.

Table 22.2 Employment and Labor Laws

Title of Legislation	Regulation
Fair Labor Standards Act (1938); has been amended many times since 1938	Sets minimum wage and maximum hours that can be worked before overtime is paid
Civil Rights Act of 1964	Sets equal employment practices
Executive Order 11246 (1965) and Executive Order 11375 (1967)	Sets affirmative action guidelines
Age Discrimination Act (1967) and 1978 amendment	Protects against forced retirement
Rehabilitation Act (1973)	Protects the handicapped
Vietnam Veterans Act (1973/1974)	Provides reemployment rights

4. **Civil and criminal laws:** These are statutory and judicial laws that proscribe certain kinds of conduct and establish penalties.
5. **Other legislation:** Nursing managers have some legal responsibilities that do not generally apply to industrial managers. For instance, licensed personnel are required to have a current, valid license from the state in which they practice. Additionally, most states require that employers of nurses report certain types of substance abuse to the state licensing boards. Confidentiality laws also have a significant impact on healthcare organizations.

Labor Standards

Labor standards are regulations dealing with the conditions of the employee's work, including physical conditions, financial aspects, and the amount of hours worked. State and federal employment legislation often overlap; as a general rule, the employer must abide by the stricter of the two regulations.

> State and federal employment legislation often overlap; as a general rule, the employer must abide by the stricter of the two regulations.

Minimum Wages and Maximum Hours

More than 85% of all non-supervisory employees are now covered by the Fair Labor Standards Act (FLSA). This law was enacted by Congress in 1938 and established an hourly minimum wage at that time of 25 cents. Since then, the law has been amended numerous times.

It is often said that in addition to putting a "floor under wages," the FLSA also puts a "ceiling over hours." The latter statement, however, is not quite accurate. The FLSA sets a maximum number of hours in any week beyond which a person may be employed only if he or she is paid an overtime rate. Some states have enacted a law that makes an exception to this weekly rule on overtime. The exception is an 80-hour, 2-week pay period ceiling, after which the employee must receive overtime pay. Overtime pay can be significant, so it is imperative that managers know which standard their organization is using.

"Hours worked" includes all the time the employee is required to be on duty. Therefore, mandatory classes, orientation, conferences, and so on must be recorded as duty time and are subject to the overtime rules. The FLSA does not require time clocks but does require that some record be maintained of hours worked.

The FLSA also regulates the minimum amount of overtime pay, which is at least 1.5 times the basic rate. When state and federal laws differ on when overtime pay begins, the stricter rule usually applies. Some union contracts also have stricter overtime pay agreements than the FLSA.

Federal labor laws exempt certain employees from the minimum wage and overtime pay requirements. Executive employees, administrative employees, and professional employees are the three most notable white-collar exemptions. The functions of the position, rather than the title or the fact that employees are paid a monthly wage, differentiate an exempt employee. Certain students, apprentice learners, and other special circumstances also may qualify an employee for an exemption to FLSA regulations.

In addition, President Bush signed a $328 billion spending bill on January 23, 2004 that, among other things, enacted new regulations that allow companies to pay overtime to fewer white-collar workers, including nurses. Under the new regulations, low-income workers increased their eligibility for overtime compensation while workers earning more than $65,000 a year can now be denied overtime pay if their employers classify them as administrators, professionals, or other exempt employees (Ray, 2004). The personnel department in any large organization is especially helpful to the manager in implementing these labor laws. Managers, however, should have a general understanding of how these laws restrict staffing and scheduling policies.

The *Equal Pay Act of 1963* requires that men and women performing equal work receive equal compensation. Four equal pay tests exist: equal skill, equal effort, equal responsibility, and similar working conditions. This law had a great impact on nursing management when it was enacted. Before 1963, male "orderlies" were routinely paid a higher wage than female "aides" performing identical duties. Although this fact seems incredible today, at the time many managers condoned this widespread practice of blatant wage discrimination. Most healthcare agencies now call these employees "nursing assistants," whether they are male or female, and all are paid the same wage.

Yet data from the 1992 and 1996 National Sample Survey of Registered Nurses suggests that male nurses still earn roughly 12.3% more than female nurses, an amount equal to about $5,361 annually (Kalist, 2002). Approximately 8.6% of this earnings differential can be explained by differences in work productivity and design, but the remaining 91.4% cannot. Kalist suggests that female nurses may have higher quit rates and more career interruptions leading to wage penalties upon reentry into the workforce, but clearly, gender discrimination in pay may still be an issue, despite legislation to prevent it.

Learning Exercise 22.4

Timeclocks
Until the 1950s, most healthcare organizations did not require that employees use a time clock when arriving at or leaving work for meal breaks. Now, time clocks are the norm for hospitals and some other, but not all, healthcare organizations.

Survey several community hospitals, clinics, student health centers, home healthcare facilities, and other organizations that employ nurses. How many of them require nurses to use time clocks? How do you feel about professionals being required to punch or swipe in and out for meal breaks? Discuss this issue in class and with nurses you know.

Labor Relations Laws

In addition to laws regarding collective bargaining, the manager needs to be aware of one section of the Wagner Act (1935) and the Taft-Hartley Amendment (1947), which deal with unfair labor practices by employers and unions.

The original Wagner Act listed and prohibited five *unfair labor practices:*

1. To interfere with, restrain, or coerce employees in a manner that interfered with their rights as outlined under the Act. Examples of these activities are spying on union gatherings, threatening employees with job loss, or threatening to close down a company if the union organizes.
2. To interfere with the formation of any labor organization or to give financial assistance to a labor organization. This provision was included to prohibit "employee representation plans" that were primarily controlled by management.
3. To discriminate with regard to hiring, tenure, and so on to discourage union membership.
4. To discharge or discriminate against an employee who filed charges or testified before the NLRB.
5. To refuse to bargain in good faith.

The original Wagner Act gave so much power to the unions that it was necessary in 1947 to pass additional federal legislation to restore a balance of power to labor–management relations. The Taft-Hartley Amendment retained the provisions under the Wagner Act that guaranteed employees the right to collective bargaining. However, the Taft-Hartley Amendment added the provision that employees have the right to refrain from taking part in unions. In addition to that provision, the Taft-Hartley Amendment added and prohibited the following six unfair labor practices of unions:

1. Requiring a self-employed person or an employer to join a union.
2. Forcing an employer to cease doing business with another person. This placed a ban on secondary boycotts, which were then prevalent in unions.
3. Forcing an employer to bargain with one union when another union has already been certified as the bargaining agent.
4. Forcing the employer to assign certain work to members of one union rather than another.
5. Charging excessive or discriminatory initiation fees.
6. Causing or attempting to cause an employer to pay for unnecessary services. This prohibited *featherbedding*, a term used to describe union practices that prevented the displacement of workers due to advances in technology.

Equal Employment Opportunity Laws

Under the American free enterprise system, employers have historically been able to hire whomever they desired. Today, a transplanted employer of the 1920s might be shocked to see that racial and ethnic minorities, women, the elderly, and the handicapped have acquired substantial rights in the workplace. The first legislation in the area of employment hiring practices resulted from years of discrimination against minorities. More recent legislation has been aimed at eliminating discrimination that occurs because of sex, age, and physical impairment.

Equal employment opportunities have fostered many profound changes in the American workplace. Women, minorities, and the handicapped have had some

Equal employment policies have brought profound changes to the American work force. Many women, minorities, and handicapped individuals have gained employment once denied to them; however, nursing has seen only modest gains in ethnic diversity.

success in gaining jobs previously denied to them. However, only modest gains in achieving ethnic diversity have occurred in nursing. Minority (Black, Asian or Pacific Islander, Hispanic, and American Indian/Alaskan native) representation in the nursing workforce is limited to less than 10% of nurses (246,000 of the 2.65 million registered nurses) despite the fact that almost 28% of the U.S. population represented an ethnic/racial minority as of March 1996 (ANA Press Release, 1999; National Advisory Council on Nurse Education and Practice; 2000).

Giddings and Smith (2001) suggest that discrimination due to sexual orientation also continues to exist in nursing with lesbian nurses reporting both intense scrutiny as well as pressure to keep their lifestyle and identity hidden from others. Indeed, Giddings and Smith refer to this phenomenon as "lesbian invisibility" in nursing, arguing that while we claim to seek diversity in nursing, we fail to respect the differences represented by the lesbian experience.

Civil Rights Act of 1964

The *Civil Rights Act of 1964* laid the foundation for equal employment in the United States. The thrust of Title VII of the Civil Rights Act is twofold: It prohibits discrimination based on factors unrelated to job qualifications, and it promotes employment based on ability and merit. The areas of discrimination specifically mentioned are race, color, religion, sex, and national origin. This act was strengthened by President Lyndon Johnson's Executive Order 11246 in 1965 and Executive Order 11375 in 1967.

President Johnson's executive orders in 1965 and 1967 sought to correct past injustices. Because the government believed that some groups had a long history of being discriminated against, it wanted to build in a mechanism that would assist those groups in "catching up" with the rest of the American work force. Therefore, it created an *affirmative action* component. Affirmative action plans are not specifically required by law but may be required by court order. In most states, affirmative action plans are voluntary unless government contracts are involved. Some states, such as California, have recently voted to eliminate affirmative action in the workplace, arguing that it actually resulted in reverse discrimination. Many organizations, however, have voluntarily put an affirmative action plan in place, if it does not conflict with state regulations.

Affirmative action differs from *equal opportunity*. The EEO legislation is aimed at preventing discrimination. Affirmative action plans are aimed at actively seeking to fill job vacancies with members from groups who are underrepresented, such as women, ethnic minorities, and the handicapped.

The Equal Employment Opportunity Commission (EEOC) is responsible for enforcing Title VII of the Civil Rights Act. The investigatory responsibility of the EEOC is broad. When it finds that a charge of discrimination is justified, the agency attempts to reach an agreement through persuasion and conciliation. When the EEOC is unable to reach an agreement, it has the power to bring civil action against the employer. When discrimination is found, the courts will order restoration of rightful economic status; this means that the employer may be ordered to receive back pay for up to two years. In healthcare organizations, when discrimination was found (such as unequal pay for men and women in nursing assistant jobs), financial awards in class action suits have been extraordinarily high. Managers must be alert for any such discriminatory practices. Some states have fair employment legislation that is stricter than the federal act. Again, the stricter regulations always apply.

Age Discrimination and Employment Act

Enacted by Congress in 1967, the purpose of the *Age Discrimination* and *Employment Act* (ADEA) was to promote employment of older people based on their ability rather than age. In early 1978, the ADEA was amended to increase the protected age to 70. In 1987, Congress voted to remove even this age restriction except in certain job categories. Although some people are alarmed by the removal of mandatory age retirements, trends continue to be toward earlier retirement. However, reversal of this trend may have serious consequences for some organizations. In particular, it could have a significant impact on organizations that are labor-intensive, especially if those labor-intensive organizations also have demanding physical requirements, such as in nursing.

 Learning Exercise 22.5

Addressing Mary's Failing Health

You are the manager of a well-baby newborn nursery. Among your staff is a 73 year-old practical nurse, Mary Jones, who has worked for the hospital for 50 years. No mandatory retirement age exists. This has not been a problem in the past, but Mary's general health is now making this a problem for your unit.

Mary has grown physically fragile. Cataracts have made her vision poor, and she suffers from hypertension. Last month, she began to prepare a little girl for circumcision because she did not read the armband properly.

Your staff has become increasingly upset over Mary's inability to fulfill her job duties. The physicians, however, support Mary and found the circumcision incident humorous. Last week, you requested that Mary have a physical examination, at hospital expense, to determine her physical ability to continue working.

You were not particularly surprised when she returned with medical approval. Her physician spoke very sharply with you, and, although he admitted privately that Mary's health was rapidly failing, he told you that working was her only reason for living. He left you with these words: "Force Mary to retire and she will die within the year."

Assignment: Using your knowledge of age discrimination, patient safety, employee rights, and management responsibilities, decide on an appropriate course of action for this case. Be creative and think beyond the obvious. Be able to support your decisions.

Sexual Harassment

Although job discrimination due to gender became illegal with the Civil Rights Act of 1964, it was not until 1977 that the federal appeals court upheld a claim that a supervisor's verbal and physical advances constituted sexual harassment in the workplace. Since then, sexual harassment has been recognized as a form of sex discrimination that violates Title VII of the Civil Rights Act.

The United States Equal Employment Opportunity Commission (EEOC) (2002) defines *sexual harassment* as unwelcome sexual advances, requests for sexual favors, and other verbal or physical conduct of a sexual nature when submission to or rejection of this conduct explicitly or implicitly affects an individual's employment, unreasonably interferes with an individual's work performance, or creates an intimidating, hostile, or offensive work environment.

The EEOC (2002) states that sexual harassment can occur in a variety of circumstances, including but not limited to the following:

- The victim as well as the harasser may be a woman or a man. The victim does not have to be of the opposite sex.
- The harasser can be the victim's supervisor, an agent of the employer, a supervisor in another area, a coworker, or a nonemployee.
- The victim does not have to be the person harassed but could be anyone affected by the offensive conduct.
- Unlawful sexual harassment may occur without economic injury to or discharge of the victim.
- The harasser's conduct must be unwelcome.

Since the 1977 ruling, allegations of sexual harassment and lawsuits have permeated virtually every type of industry, and the healthcare system is not immune. Nor is sexual harassment in the healthcare workplace confined to the United States: Madison and Minichiello (2001) report that ambiguity about sexual harassment exists in Australia despite fairly aggressive legislation, community scrutiny, medical exposure, and organizational programs aimed at preventing and dealing with sex-based and sexual harassment in the workplace. Madison and Minichiello's research also suggests that sexual harassment in the workplace often involves one harasser who harasses often, rather than the existence of many harassers.

Davidhizar, Erdel, and Dowd (1998) suggest that to deal effectively with sexual harassment, organizations must concentrate on three areas. First, employers must recognize the serious consequences of sexual harassment. Second, both business and health care alike must take preventive strategies to deal with this issue. Third, healthcare supervisors or faculty who are approached with a sexual harassment complaint, whether the accused is a patient, staff member, visitor, or physician, must take complaints seriously and gather data from all involved parties, including any witnesses. A serious, impartial attitude on the part of the supervisor is critical to maintaining staff morale.

In addition, education about sexual harassment should be included in every new employee's orientation and continuing education. "Teams who can recognize sexual harassment when it occurs, evaluate the immediate situation, select an appropriate interpersonal response and then take any further steps necessary decrease the likelihood of harassment occurring" (Davidhizar, Erdel, & Dowd, 1998, p. 43).

Lastly, nurses themselves must take appropriate action when they see such harassment of others or when they themselves are targets of such offenses. When someone makes another uncomfortable in the workplace by the use of sexual innuendoes or jokes or invades another's personal space, the behavior can be clues for recognizing sexual harassment (Madison & Minichiello, 2001).

Learning Exercise 22.6

Confronting Sexual Harassment

You are a new employee at Valley Medical Center's intensive care unit and love your job. Although only 25 years old, you have been a nurse for four years and the last two were spent in a small critical care unit in a rural hospital. You work the 3 P.M. to 11 P.M. shift. Ever since you came to work here, one of the physicians (Dr. Jones) has been especially attentive to you. At first you were flattered, but more recently you have become uncomfortable around him. He sometimes touches you and seems to be flirting with you. You have no romantic interest in him and know he is married. Last night he asked you to meet him for an after-work drink and you refused. He is a very powerful man in the unit and you don't want to alienate him, but you are becoming increasingly troubled by his behavior.

Today you went to your shift charge nurse and told her how you felt and she said, "Oh, he likes to flirt with all the new staff, but he is perfectly harmless." Her comments did not make you feel better. About 7 P.M., Dr. Jones came on the unit and again cornered you in a comatose patient's room and asked you out. You again said no, but you are feeling more anxious by his behavior.

Assignment: Outline an appropriate course of action. What options can you identify? What is your responsibility? What are the driving and restraining forces for action? What support systems for action can you identify? What responsibility does the organization have?

Legislation Affecting Americans with Disabilities

The *Rehabilitation Act of 1973* required all employers with government contracts of more than $25,000 to take affirmative action to recruit, hire, and advance disabled people who are qualified. Similar but less aggressive affirmative action steps were required for other companies doing business with the federal government, with specific requirements depending on the size of the company and the dollar amount of the contract. The Department of Labor was charged with enforcing this act. Although initially there was very slow progress in getting companies to hire those with disabilities, steady progress has been made.

In 1990, Congress passed the *Americans with Disabilities Act* to eliminate discrimination against Americans with physical or mental disabilities in the workplace and in social life. *Disability* is defined as "any physical or mental impairment that limits any major life activity." This includes people with obvious physical disabilities, but also those with cancer, diabetes, human immunodeficiency virus (HIV), or acquired immunodeficiency syndrome (AIDS), and recovering substance users among others.

Veterans Readjustment Assistance Act

The *Veterans Readjustment Act* provides employment rights and privileges for veterans with regard to positions they held before they entered the armed forces. This act was used by some nurses following the Vietnam War and during the nursing surplus following the Persian Gulf War to gain reemployment after military service.

The Occupational Health and Safety Act

The manager needs to be especially cognizant of legislation imposed by the *Occupational Health and Safety Act* (OSHA) and state health licensing boards. OSHA speaks to the employer's requirements to provide a place of employment that is free from recognized hazards that may cause physical harm. The Department of Labor enforces this act. Because it is impossible for the Department of Labor to inspect physically all facilities, most inspections are brought about by employee complaint or employer request. The act allows fines to be levied if employers continue with unsafe conditions.

Since OSHA's inception, many companies have vehemently criticized the act, specifically its administration. Companies also have charged that the cost of meeting OSHA standards has excessively burdened American business.

On the other hand, unions have asserted that the federal government has never staffed or funded OSHA adequately. They have charged that OSHA has been negligent in setting standards for toxic substances, carcinogens, and other disease-producing agents.

Because the risk of discovery and the fine if found guilty are both low, employers often choose to ignore unsafe working conditions. Nurse–managers are in a unique position to call attention to hazardous conditions in the workplace and should communicate such concerns to higher authority. Ongoing controversies regarding safety issues include the cost and effectiveness of universal precautions and immunizations for bioterrorism threats.

Most states also have occupational and safety regulations. Again, the employer must comply with the more stringent regulations. Many of the state licensing boards have additional health regulations that differ from the federal regulations.

STATE HEALTH FACILITIES LICENSING BOARDS

In addition to health and safety requirements, many state boards have regulations regarding staffing requirements. It is the ultimate responsibility of top-level management to maintain the state license to operate. However, all managers are responsible for knowing and meeting the regulations that apply to their unit or department.

For example, if the manager of an intensive care unit has a state staffing level that mandates 12 hours of nursing care per patient per day and requires that the ratio of registered nurses to other staff be 2:1, then the supervisor is obligated to staff at that level or greater. If, during times of short staffing, supervisors are unable to meet this level of staffing, they must apprise upper-level management so that there can be joint resolution.

The variation in state licensing requirements makes a lengthy discussion of them inappropriate for this book. However, managers must be knowledgeable about state licensing regulations that pertain to their level of supervision.

INTEGRATING LEADERSHIP ROLES AND MANAGEMENT FUNCTIONS IN WORKING WITH UNIONS AND EMPLOYMENT LAWS

Unionization and legal constraints will seem less burdensome if managers remember that both primarily protect the rights of patients and employees. If managers perform their jobs well and work for organizations that desire to "do the right thing" by accepting their social responsibility, they need not fear unionization and legal constraints.

If the organization is not unionized, the manager must use the leadership roles of communication, fairness, and shared decision making to ensure that employees do not feel unionization is necessary. Perhaps Forman and Davis (2002) state it best when they say that "unions don't create the climate in which organizing activity thrives; they simply take advantage of it. The roots of union activity lie in the fertile soil of poor relationships between employees and their leaders" (p. 444). The integrated leader–manager is a role model for fairness, knows unit employees well, and sincerely seeks to meet their needs.

When making decisions that deal with unions and employment legislation, the effective leader–manager always seeks to do what is just. Additionally, he or she seeks appropriate assistance before finalizing decisions that involve sensitive legal or contract issues. By incorporating the leadership role, the manager becomes fairer in personnel management. There is increased self-awareness and an understanding of an individual's need to seek unionization and of the necessity for employment legislation.

The effective manager maintains required staffing and ensures a safe working environment. Rights of the organization and the employee are protected as the manager uses personnel policies in a nondiscriminatory and consistent manner. The emphasis is on flexibility and accommodation of employment legislation and union contracts.

☀ Key Concepts

- Historically, union activity is greater during times of labor shortages and economic upswings.
- The ANA acts as both a *professional association* for registered nurses and a *collective bargaining agent*. This dual purpose poses a conflict in loyalty to some nurses.

- People are motivated to join or reject unions as a result of many needs and values.
- Although all managers play an important role in establishing and maintaining effective management–labor relationships, the middle-level manager has the greatest influence on preventing unionization in a nonunion organization.
- It is possible to create a climate in which labor and management can work together to accomplish mutual goals.
- *Labor relations laws* relate to the rights and duties of unions and employers in their relationship with each other.
- *Labor standards* are regulations dealing with the conditions of the employee's work, including physical conditions, financial aspects, and the number of hours worked.
- State and federal employment legislation often overlap; as a general rule, the employer must abide by the stricter of the two regulations.
- Much of the human rights legislation concerning employment practices resulted because of documented discrimination in the workplace.
- Although some legislation makes the job of managing people more difficult for managers, it has resulted in increased job fairness and opportunities for women, minorities, the elderly, and the disabled.

More Learning Exercises and Applications

 Learning Exercise 22.7

Writing About Employment Laws
Many employment laws generate emotion. Usually people feel strongly about at least one of these issues. Select one of the following employment laws, and write a 250-word essay on why you support or disapprove of the law. Choose from the Equal Pay Act of 1963, equal opportunity laws, affirmative action, sexual harassment, or age discrimination.

Learning Exercise 22.8

Dilemma Involving an Expired Nursing License
At your long-term care facility, it is a policy that licensed employees have a current valid license. This is in keeping with the state licensing code. It is always difficult to get people to bring their license in to verify its currency.

You have just come from a meeting with the director. He reminded you that you must not have people performing duties that require a license if the license has expired. You decide to issue a memo stating that you will suspend all employees who have not verified their licenses with you.

Following this, all the LVNs/LPNs brought their licenses in for verification. However, one of the LVNs/LPNs has an expired date on her license. When she is questioned, she admits that she did not mail her payment for relicensure until after she had read your memo. She was hoping to delay showing her license. She was in a financial crisis and that is why she had delayed payment. You call the licensing board, and they state that it will be six weeks before the employee will receive her license. They will not verify her active license status over the telephone.

You consider the following facts. It is illegal to perform duties requiring a license without one. The LVN/LPN had prior knowledge of the licensing laws and hospital policy. The LVN/LPN has been a good employee with no record of prior disciplinary action.
Assignment: Decide what you should do. What alternatives do you have? Provide rationale for your decision.

Learning Exercise 22.9

How Would You Handle This Petition?
Betty Smith, a unit clerk, has come to see you, the nurse–manager of the medical unit, to complain of flagrant discriminatory practices against female employees of University General Hospital. She alleges that women are denied promotional and training opportunities comparable to those made available to men.

She shows you a petition with 35 signatures supporting her allegations. Ms. Smith has threatened to forward this petition to the administrator of the hospital, the press, and the Department of Labor unless corrective action is taken at once. Being a woman yourself, you have some sympathy for Ms. Smith's complaint. However, you believe overall that employees at University General are treated fairly regardless of their sex.

Ms. Smith, a fairly good employee, has worked on your unit for four years. However, she has been creating problems lately. She has been reprimanded for taking too much time for coffee breaks. Personnel evaluations that recommend pay raises and promotions are due next week.
Assignment: How should you handle this problem? Is the personnel evaluation an appropriate time to address the petition? Outline your plan, and give your rationale.

Web Links

American Nurses Association
http://nursingworld.org/uan/
Website of the United American Nurses, a collective bargaining agent, representing 100,000 nurses nationwide—and a full-fledged affiliate of both the American Nurses Association and the AFL-CIO. Site has membership information and news releases.

The U.S. Equal Employment Opportunity Commission (2002). Retrieved Nov. 2004 from
http://www.eeoc.gov/facts/fs-sex.html
Provides facts about sexual harassment.

Employment Workplace Rights
http://www.nolo.com/ChunkEMP/emp.index.html
Covers sexual harassment, fair pay, and privacy rights on the job.

Equal Rights Advocates
http://www.equalrights.org/
A nonprofit law center that advocates for the economic and political equality of women. Online advice and topics such as affirmative action.

Equal Opportunity Publications
http://www.eop.com/
Includes employment issues and statistics concerning ethnic minorities, women, and people with disabilities.

References

American Nurses Association (1999, April 16). *Press release. Population diversity requires more minority registered nurse*s. Available at: http://www.uannurse.com/pressrel/1999/-pr0416.htm. Accessed December 30, 2003.

Davidhizar, R., Erdel, S., & Dowd, S. (1998). Sexual harassment: Where to draw the line. *Nursing Management, 29*(2), 40–43.

Fitzpatrick, M. (2001). Collective bargaining: A vulnerability assessment. *Nursing Management, 32*(2), 40–42.

Forman, H., & Davis, G. A. (2002). The anatomy of a union campaign. *Journal of Nursing Administration, 32*(9), 444–447.

Forman, H., & Kraus, H. R. (2003). Decertification. Management's role when employees rethink unionization. *Journal of Nursing Administration, 33*(6), 313–316.

Forman, H., & Powell, T. A. (2003). Managing during an employee walkout. *Journal of Nursing Administration, 33*(9), 430–433.

Giddings, L. S., & Smith, M. C. (2001). Stories of lesbian invisibility in nursing. *Nursing Outlook, 49*(1), 14–19.

Kalist, D. E. (2002). The gender earnings gap in the RN labor market. *Nursing Economic$, 20*(4), 155–162.

Madison, J., & Minichiello, V. (2001). Sexual harassment in health care. *Journal of Nursing Administration, 31*(11), 534–543.

Meier, E. (2000). Is unionization the answer for nurses and nursing? *Nursing Economic$, 18*(1), 36–38.

Murray, M. K. (1999). Is healthcare reengineering resulting in union organizing of registered nurses? *Journal of Nursing Administration, 29*(10), 4–7.

Murray, M. K. (2001). The new economy and new union organizing strategies: Union wins in healthcare. *Journal of Nursing Administration, 31*(7/8), 339–343.

National Advisory Council on Nurse Education and Practice. (2000). *National agenda for nursing workforce racial/ethnic diversity.* U.S. Department of Health and Human Services. Rockville, MD.

On labor issues. Labor gets louder. (2000). *Institutional Investor, 34*(6), 36.

Porter-O'Grady, T. (2001). Collective bargaining: The union as partner, Part 3. *Nursing Management, 32*(6), 30–32.

Ray, R. (2004, February 9). New overtime legislation may exempt some nurses. *NurseWeek (California),* 2.

Seago, J. A., & Ash, M. (2002). Registered nurse unions and patient outcomes. *Journal of Nursing Administration, 32*(3), 143–151.

Service Employees International Union. (2003). SEIU: America's largest and fastest growing union. Available at: http://www.seiu.org/who/facts.cfm. Accessed December 30, 2003.

Steltzer, T. M. (2001). Part 2, Collective bargaining: A wake-up call. *Nursing Management, 32*(4), 35–37, 48.

United States Equal Employment Opportunity Commission. (2002). Facts about sexual harassment. Available at: http://www.eeoc.gov/facts/fs-sex.html. Accessed December 30, 2003.

Bibliography

Age discrimination: Negative comments on exit-interview form rule out nurse's lawsuit. (2002). *Legal Eye Newsletter for the Nursing Profession, 10*(9), 8.

Bich-Quyen, N. (2001). You're not one of us. *American Journal of Nursing, 101*(1), 77.

Bronner, G. J. (2003). Sexual harassment of nurses and nursing students. *Journal of Advanced Nursing, 42*(6), 637–644.

Cartmail, G. (June 2003). Your rights at work. Capturing ideas and enthusiasm. *Journal of Community Practice, 76*(6), 227

Demoro, R. A. (2003). "It's like representation without representation." *California Nurse, 99*(4), 4–5, 8.

Dowd, S. (April-June 2003). Sexuality, sexual harassment, and sexual humor: Guidelines for the workplace in health care. *Health Care Manager, 22*(2), 144–151.

Fiedler, A., & Hamby, E. (2000). Sexual harassment in the workplace: Nurses' perceptions. *Journal of Nursing Administration, 30*(10), 497–503.

Fitzpatrick, M. (2001). Collective bargaining: A vulnerability assessment. Part 1. *Nursing Management, 32*(2), 40–42.

Forman, H. J., & Powell, T.A. (2003). Management rights. *Journal of Nursing Administration, 33*(1), 7–9.

Gates, D. (2003). Linking practice & research. Dealing with workplace violence—strategies for prevention. *American Association of Occupational Health Nurses (AAOHN) Journal, 51*(6), 243–245.

Johnson, C. L. (2000). Come together. *American Journal of Nursing, 100*(9), 81–82.

Kasoff, J. (2003). Consider this . . . Grievance tracking: Targeting an improvement process. *Journal of Nursing Administration, 33*(7/8), 376.

Murray, M. K. (2001). The new economy and new union organizing strategies: Union wins in healthcare. *Journal of Nursing Administration, 31*(7/8), 339–343.

Labor relations: Charge nurses in nursing home are supervisors, not part of the bargaining unit. (2003). *Legal Eye Newsletter for the Nursing Profession, 11*(7), 8

Letvak, S. (2002). Retaining the older nurse. *Journal of Nursing Administration, 32*(7/8), 387–392.

Martin, S. (2003). Issues update. Solidarity: Union nurses swarm Capitol Hill. *American Journal of Nursing, 103*(8), 65, 67, 69.

Mason, D. J. (2000). The state of the unions. *American Journal of Nursing, 100*(9), 7.

Monarch, K. (2000). Protect yourself from sexual harassment. *American Journal of Nursing, 100*(5), 75.

Our new contract—how we got there and the lesson learned in the process. (2003). *California Nurse, 99*(6), 6, 15

Parish, C. (2003). Unions win right to query pay review body's advice. *Nursing Standard, 17*(43), 4.

Smith, S. P. (2000). Are you protecting your patients' confidentiality?. *Nursing Economic$, 18*(6), 294–297, 319.

You can help win better workers compensation: Your union has been lobbying for injured workers to receive the income they would normally take home when they receive workers' compensation. (2003, Autumn). *Enrolled Nurse, 17.*

Zolot, J. S., & Sofer, D. (2001). To supervise or unionize? That is the question. *American Journal of Nursing, 101*(8), 21.

Zook, R. (2000). Sexual harassment in the workplace. *American Journal of Nursing, 100*(12), 24DDD–26DDD.

CHAPTER

23

Quality Control

Public accountability looms large at U.S. institutions today, forcing a re-evaluation within many organizations of how, and how well, they are accomplishing their goals.

—R. J. Bulger

During the controlling phase of the management process, performance is measured against predetermined standards and action is taken to correct discrepancies between these standards and actual performance. Employees who feel they can influence the quality of outcomes in their work environment experience higher levels of motivation and job satisfaction. Organizations also need some control over productivity, innovation, and quality outcomes. Controlling, then, should not be viewed as a means of determining success or failure but as a way to learn and grow, both personally and professionally.

This unit explores controlling as the fifth and final step in the management process. Because the management process, like the nursing process, is cyclic, controlling is not an end in itself; it is implemented throughout all phases of management. Examples of management controlling functions include the periodic evaluation of unit philosophy, mission, goals, and objectives; the measurement of individual and group performance against preestablished standards; the monitoring of expenses and use of supplies; and the auditing of patient goals and outcomes.

Quality control, a specific type of controlling, refers to activities that are used to evaluate, monitor, or regulate services rendered to consumers. In nursing, the goal of quality care would be to ensure *quality* while meeting intended goals.

For any quality control program to be effective, certain components need to be in place (see **Display 23.1**). First, the program needs to be supported by top-level administration; a quality control program cannot merely be an exercise to satisfy various federal and state regulations. A sincere commitment by the institution, as evidenced by fiscal and human resource support, will be a deciding factor in determining and improving quality of services. In addition, although the organization must be realistic about the economics of rendering services, if nursing is to strive for excellence, then developed quality control criteria should be pushed to optimal levels rather than minimally acceptable levels. Finally, the process of quality control must be ongoing; that is, it must reflect a belief that the search for improvement in quality outcomes is continuous and that care can always be improved.

Although controlling is generally defined as a management function, effective quality control requires the manager to have skill in both leadership and management. Leadership roles and management functions inherent in quality control are delineated in **Display 23.2**.

To understand quality control, the manager must become familiar with the process and the terminology used in quality measurement and improvement activities. This chapter introduces quality control as a specific and systematic process. Audits are presented as tools to measure quality. In addition, the historical impact of

---

Display 23.1 | **Hallmarks of Effective Quality Control Programs**

1. Support from top level administration (fiscal and human resources)
2. Commitment by the organization in terms of fiscal and human resources
3. Quality goals reflect search for excellence rather than minimums
4. Process is ongoing (continuous)

Display 23.2 Leadership Roles and Management Functions Associated with Quality Control

Leadership Roles

1. Encourages followers to be actively involved in the quality control process.
2. Clearly communicates expected standards of care to subordinates.
3. Encourages the setting of high standards to maximize quality, instead of setting minimum safety standards.
4. Promotes quality improvement as an ongoing process.
5. Uses control as a method of determining why goals were not met.
6. Is active in communicating quality control findings and their implications to other health professionals and consumers.
7. Acts as a role model for followers in accepting responsibility and accountability for nursing actions.
8. Distinguishes between clinical standards and resource utilization standards, ensuring that patients receive at least minimally acceptable levels of quality care.
9. Supports/actively participates in research efforts to identify and measure nursing-sensitive patient outcomes.

Management Functions

1. In conjunction with other personnel in the organization, establishes clear-cut, measurable standards of care and determines the most appropriate method for measuring if those standards have been met.
2. Selects and uses process, outcome, and structure audits appropriately as quality control tools.
3. Accesses appropriate sources of information in data gathering for quality control.
4. Determines discrepancies between care provided and unit standards and seeks further information regarding why standards were not met.
5. Uses quality control findings as a measure of employee performance and rewards; coaches, counsels, or disciplines employees accordingly.
6. Keeps abreast of current government, accrediting body, and licensing regulations that affect quality control.
7. Actively participates in state and national benchmarking and "best practices" initiatives.
8. Continually assesses the unit or organizational environment to identify and categorize errors that are occurring, and proactively reworks the processes that led to the errors.

external forces on the development and implementation of quality control programs in healthcare organizations is discussed. Quality control strategies, quality measurement tools, benchmarking, and clinical practice guidelines are introduced.

DEFINING QUALITY HEALTH CARE

Defining and attempting to measure quality of care is not new. In fact, the quality of health care is an idea generally attributed to Ernest Codman, a surgeon who first proposed the "end result idea" in 1869. Codman suggested that hospitals should follow-up on discharged patients to see if treatments were successful and suggested that the surgeon's surgical prowess might make a difference in how well patients recovered. This idea was not well received at the time since it suggested providers had at least some accountability for patient outcomes.

Despite this uneasy start, quality measurement and outcomes accountability have been buzzwords in health care since the 1980s and continue to be at the forefront of almost every healthcare agenda today (Huston, 2003). Defining and measuring quality of care are essential for healthcare providers to demonstrate accountability to insurers, patients, and legislative and regulatory bodies. However, achieving quality care is not only a matter of better training providers or delivering more care. The problem is multi-dimensional and its complexity begins with the very definition of quality care itself (Huston).

The Institute of Medicine (IOM) (1994) defines healthcare quality as "the degree to which health services for individuals and populations increase the likelihood of desired health outcomes and are consistent with current professional knowledge" (p. 3). Huston (2003) suggests that while this definition is widely accepted, parts of it merit further examination. The first is the assertion that quality does not exist unless desired health outcomes are attained. Outcomes are only one indicator of quality. Sometimes, patients receive the best possible care with the information available and poor outcomes occur. At other times, poor care may still result in good outcomes. Thus, while outcomes are an important measure of quality care, it is dangerous to use them as the *only* criteria for quality measurement.

The second implication in the IOM definition that Huston (2003) questions is that for care to be considered high quality, it must be consistent with current *professional* knowledge. Staying current in terms of professional knowledge in today's technological information firestorm is a moving target for even the most dedicated providers. In addition, there continues to be debate about what constitutes professional knowledge. Lee and Estes (2003) report that even with the current emphasis on evidence-based clinical guidelines, some recent studies have suggested that standard preventive and treatment practices do not confer health benefits.

To complicate the issue even further, how quality of care is defined and measured often differs between providers and patients. Bodenheimer (as cited in Lee and Estes, 2003) suggest that physicians often view quality health care as the application of evidence-based medical knowledge to the particular needs and wishes of individual patients but suggest that consumer perceptions about what constitutes quality care may be very different.

Clearly, it is difficult to find a common definition of quality health care that represents the viewpoints of all stakeholders in the healthcare system. What is even more difficult, however, is identifying and elucidating the myriad of factors that play a part in determining whether quality health care exists (Huston, 2003).

> Despite an uneasy start, quality measurement and outcomes accountability have been buzzwords in health care since the 1980s and continue to be at the forefront of almost every healthcare agenda today.

QUALITY CONTROL AS A PROCESS

If defining healthcare quality is problematic, then the measurement of healthcare quality is even more difficult. To make the process more effective and efficient, the collection of both quantitative and qualitative data is used as well as a specific and systematic process. This process, when viewed simplistically, can be broken down into three basic steps:

1. The criterion or standard is determined.
2. Information is collected to determine if the standard has been met.
3. Educational or corrective action is taken if the criterion has not been met.

The first step, as depicted in **Figure 23.1,** is the establishment of control criteria or standards. Measuring performance is impossible if standards have not been clearly established. Not only must standards exist, but leader–managers also must see that all subordinates know and understand the standards. Because standards vary among institutions, employees must know the standard expected of them at their organization. Employees must be aware that their performance will be measured in terms of their ability to meet the established standard. For example, hospital nurses should provide postoperative patient care that meets standards specific to

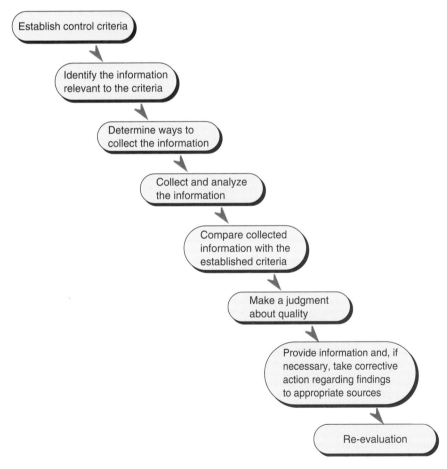

Figure 23.1 Steps in auditing quality control.

their institution. A nurse's performance can be measured only when it can be compared with a preexisting standard.

Many organizations have begun using *benchmarking* as a tool for identifying desired standards of organizational performance. Benchmarking is the process of measuring products, practices, and services against *best-performing organizations*. In doing so, organizations can determine how and why their performance differs from these exemplar organizations and use them as role models for standard development and performance improvement.

Many states have initiated a *best practices* program that invites healthcare institutions to submit a description of a program or protocol relating to improvements in quality of life, quality of care, staff development, or cost-effectiveness practices. Experts review the submissions, examine outcomes, and then designate a "best practice."

The second step in the quality control process includes identifying information relevant to the criteria. What information is needed to measure the criteria? In the example of postoperative patient care, this information might include the frequency of vital signs, dressing checks, and neurological or sensory checks.

The third step is determining ways to collect information. As in all data gathering, the manager must be sure to use all appropriate sources. When assessing quality control of the postoperative patient, the manager could find much of the information in the patient chart. Postoperative flowsheets, the physician orders, and the nursing notes would probably be most helpful. Talking to the patient or nurse also could yield information.

The fourth step in auditing quality control is collecting and analyzing information. For example, if the standards specify that postoperative vital signs are to be checked every 30 minutes for 2 hours and every hour thereafter for 8 hours, it is necessary to look at how often vital signs were taken the first 10 hours after surgery. The frequency of vital signs listed on the postoperative flowsheet is then compared with the standard set by the unit. The resulting discrepancy or congruency gives managers information with which they can make a judgment about the quality or appropriateness of the nursing care. If vital signs were not taken frequently enough to satisfy the standard, the manager would need to obtain further information regarding why the standard was not met and counsel employees as needed. Likewise, the manager should reward employees who provide nursing care that exceeds organizational standards.

In addition to evaluating individual employee performance, quality control provides a tool for evaluating unit goals. If unit goals are consistently unmet, the leader must reexamine those goals and determine if they are inappropriate or unrealistic. There is great danger here that the leader, in a desperate effort to meet unit goals, may lower standards to the point where quality is meaningless. This reinforces the need to determine standards first and then evaluate goals accordingly.

The last step in Figure 23.1 is re-evaluation. If quality control is measured on 20 postoperative charts and a high rate of compliance with established standards is found, the need for short-term re-evaluation is low. If standards are consistently unmet or met only partially, frequent re-evaluation is indicated. Remember that quality control should not be implemented solely as a reaction to a problem.

Effective leaders ensure that quality control is proactive by pushing standards to maximal levels and by eliminating problems in early stages, before productivity or quality is compromised.

THE DEVELOPMENT OF STANDARDS

A *standard* is a predetermined level of excellence that serves as a guide for practice. Standards have distinguishing characteristics; they are predetermined, established by an authority, and communicated to and accepted by the people affected by them. Because standards are used as measurement tools, they must be objective, measurable, and achievable.

Because there is no one set of standards, each organization and profession must set standards and objectives to guide individual practitioners in performing safe and effective care. *Standards for practice* define the scope and dimensions of professional nursing. Since the 1930s, the American Nurses Association (ANA) has played a key role in developing standards for the profession. In 1973, the ANA Congress first established standards for nursing practice, thereby providing a means of determining the quality of nursing that a patient receives, regardless of whether such services are provided by a professional nurse alone or in conjunction with nonprofessional assistants.

Currently, there are more than 20 different ANA Standards for Nursing Practice that reflect different areas of specialty nursing practice (ANA, 2001). *The Standards of Clinical Nursing Practice,* originally published by ANA in 1991 and subsequently revised in both 1998 and 2004, provides a foundation for all registered nurses in clinical practice. These standards consist of Standards of Care and Standards of Professional Performance (see **Display 23.3**). The ANA publication *Scope and Standards for Nurse Administrators* may be of particular interest to nurse–managers. Other developed standards reflect such diverse fields of practice as diabetes nursing, forensic nursing practice, home health nursing practice, gerontological nursing, nursing practice in correctional facilities, parish nursing, oncology nursing, school nursing, psychiatric-mental health nursing practice, nursing informatics, and public health (ANA, 2001). All of these standards exemplify optimal performance expectations for the nursing profession and have provided a basis for the development of organizational and unit standards nationwide.

Organizational standards outline levels of acceptable practice within the institution. For example, each organization develops a policy and procedures manual that outlines its specific standards. These standards may be minimizing or maximizing in terms of the quality of service expected. Such standards of practice allow the organization to measure more objectively unit and individual performance.

One contemporary effort to establish standards for individual nursing practice has been the development of clinical practice guidelines. *Clinical practice guidelines* or *standardized clinical guidelines* provide diagnosis-based, step-by-step interventions for providers to follow in an effort to promote high-quality care while controlling resource utilization and costs. Clinical practice guidelines, such as those developed by the Agency for Health Care Research and Quality (AHRQ), are

| Display 23.3 | **Nursing: Scope and Standards of Practice** |

Standards of Practice

1. ASSESSMENT—The registered nurse collects comprehensive data pertinent to the patient's health or the situation.
2. DIAGNOSIS—The registered nurse analyzes the assessment data to determine the diagnoses or issues.
3. OUTCOMES IDENTIFICATION—The registered nurse identifies expected outcomes for a plan individualized to the patient or the situation.
4. PLANNING—The registered nurse develops a plan that prescribes strategies and alternatives to attain expected outcomes.
5. IMPLEMENTATION—The registered nurse implements the identified plan.
6. EVALUATION—The registered nurse evaluates progress toward attainment of outcomes.

Standards of Professional Performance

7. QUALITY OF PRACTICE—The registered nurse systematically enhances the quality and effectiveness of nursing practice.
8. EDUCATION—The registered nurse attains knowledge and competency that reflects current nursing practice.
9. PROFESSIONAL PRACTICE EVALUATION—The registered nurse evaluates own nursing practice in relation to professional practice standards and guidelines, relevant statutes, rules, and regulations.
10. COLLEGIALITY—The registered nurse interacts with and contributes to the professional development of peers and colleagues.
11. COLLABORATION—The registered nurse collaborates with the patient, family, and others in the conduct of nursing practice.
12. ETHICS—The registered nurse integrates ethical provisions in all areas of practice.
13. RESEARCH—The registered nurse integrates research findings in practice.
14. RESOURCE UTILIZATION—The registered nurse considers factors related to safety, effectiveness, cost, and impact on practice in planning and delivering nursing services.
15. LEADERSHIP—The registered nurse provides leadership in the professional practice setting and the profession.

Source: American Nurses Association (2004). *Nursing: Scope and standards of practice.* Washington, D.C.: Nursebooks.org.

developed following an extensive review of the literature, and suggest what interventions, in what order, will likely lead to the best possible patient outcomes. In other words, clinical practice guidelines reflect *evidence-based practice* (EBP); that is, they should be based on cutting edge research and best practices.

In 1998, the AHRQ and U.S. Department of Health, in partnership with the American Medical Association and American Association of Health Plans–Health Insurance Association of American, launched the *National Guideline Clearinghouse* (NGC). The NGC is a free, updated-weekly, publicly available database of evidence-based clinical practice guidelines and related documents in one easy-to-access location. The website for this clearinghouse and the key features of the NGC are shown in **Display 23.4.**

Display 23.4 | **The National Guideline Clearinghouse: Key Components**

1. Structured, standardized abstracts (summaries) about each guideline and its development.
2. A utility for comparing attributes of two or more guidelines in a side-by-side comparison.
3. Syntheses of guidelines covering similar topics, highlighting areas of similarity and difference.
4. Links to full-text guidelines, where available, and/or ordering information for print copies.
5. Annotated bibliographies on guideline development methodology, structure, implementation, and evaluation.

Source: National Guideline Clearinghouse (11/1/04). About NGC. Retrieved 11/4/04 from
http://www.guideline.gov/about/about.aspx

Some providers eschew clinical practice guidelines, arguing they are "cookbook medicine"; however, the reality is that they likely serve as the best possible guide in caring for specific patient populations that exists today. This does not mean that providers cannot deviate from evidence-based guidelines; they can and do. However, such deviations should be accompanied by the identification of the unique factors of each individual case that call for that deviation. Indeed, studies to date clearly support the relationship between practitioner adherence to guidelines and positive clinical and financial outcomes; however, individual practitioner adherence with core recommendations is inconsistent and highly variable (Dykes, 2003).

AUDITS AS A QUALITY CONTROL TOOL

Whereas standards provide the yardstick for measuring quality care, audits are measurement tools. An *audit* is a systematic and official examination of a record, process, structure, environment, or account to evaluate performance. Auditing in healthcare organizations provides managers with a means of applying the control process to determine the quality of services rendered. Auditing can occur retrospectively, concurrently, or prospectively. *Retrospective audits* are performed after the patient receives the service. *Concurrent audits* are performed while the patient is receiving the service. *Prospective audits* attempt to identify how future performance will be affected by current interventions. The audits most frequently used in quality control include the outcome, process, and structure audits.

Outcome Audit

Outcomes can be defined as the end result of care, or how the patient's health status changed as a result of the intervention. *Outcome audits* determine what results, if any, occurred as a result of specific nursing interventions for patients. These audits assume that the outcome accurately demonstrates the quality of care that was provided. Many experts consider outcome measures to be the most valid indicators of quality care, but until the past decade most evaluations of hospital care have focused on structure and process.

Outcome measurement, however, is not new; Florence Nightingale was advocating the evaluation of patient outcomes when she used mortality and morbidity statistics to publicize the poor quality of care during the Crimean War. In today's era of cost containment, outcome research is needed to determine whether managed care processes, restructuring, and other new clinical practices are producing the desired cost savings without compromising the quality of patient care.

The Joint Commission for Accreditation of Healthcare Organizations (JCAHO) uses outcome criteria established for 24 hours before discharge when reviewing quality of care. Patient records are reviewed after discharge, but the review criteria are stated in terms of expected outcomes that should have occurred 24 hours before discharge. Other postdischarge outcome measures used by JCAHO include the number of sentinel events, overall error rate, number of reports on possible errors or near misses, hospital readmission rates, and rate of hospital acquired infections (Bulger, 2003).

Outcomes are complex, and it is important to recognize that many factors contribute to patient outcomes. There is growing recognition, however, that it is possible to separate the contribution of nursing to the patient's outcome; this recognition of outcomes that are *nursing sensitive* creates accountability for nurses as professionals and is important in developing nursing as a profession. Although outcomes traditionally used to measure quality of hospital care include mortality, morbidity, and length of hospital stay, these outcomes are not highly nursing sensitive. More nursing-sensitive outcome measures for the acute care setting include patient fall rates, nosocomial infection rates, the prevalence of pressure sores, physical restraint use, and patient satisfaction rates.

> The recognition of nursing-sensitive outcomes creates accountability for nurses as professionals and is important in developing nursing as a profession.

One tool that continues to hold promise for linking nursing and patient outcomes is the *Nursing Minimum Data Set* (NMDS) (Huston, 1999). The NMDS was developed by Werley and Lang and represents a decade-long effort to standardize the collection of nursing data. With the NMDS, a minimum set of items of information with uniform definitions and categories is collected to meet the needs of multiple data users. Thus, it creates a shared language that can be used by nurses in any care delivery setting as well as by other health professionals and researchers.

Although the NMDS is gaining recognition across the country, use and implementation have been limited. In 1990, however, the ANA House of Delegates recognized the NMDS as the minimum set of data elements to be included in any electronic patient record system. With it, nursing data can be used to compare nursing effectiveness, costs, and outcomes across clinical settings and nursing interventions.

Another tool that may help to link nursing interventions and patient outcomes is the *Nursing Interventions Classification* (NIC) developed by the Iowa Interventions Project, College of Nursing, Iowa City, Iowa. The NIC is a research-based classification system consisting of independent and collaborative interventions of nurses in all specialty areas and in all settings that provides a common, standardized language for nurses. With 30 diverse classes of care, such as drug management, child-bearing, community health promotion, physical comfort promotion, and perfusion management and multiple domains of interventions, the NIC can be linked with the North American Nursing Diagnosis Association taxonomy, the NMDS, and nursing outcomes to improve patient outcomes. In using NIC, the nurse selects the appropriate class and then chooses from among multiple interventions that promote individualized care (La Duke, 2000).

Process Audit

Process audits are used to measure the process of care or how the care was carried out and assume that a relationship exists between the process used by the nurse and the quality of care provided. Critical pathways and standardized clinical guidelines would be examples of efforts to standardize the process of care. They also provide a tool to measure deviations from accepted best-practice process standards.

Process audits tend to be task-oriented and focus on whether practice standards are being fulfilled. Process standards may be documented in patient care plans, procedure manuals, or nursing protocol statements. For example, a process audit might be used to establish whether fetal heart tones or blood pressures were checked according to an established policy. In a community health agency, a process audit could be used to determine if newborn teaching had been carried out during the first postpartum visit.

 Learning Exercise 23.1

Designing an Audit Tool
You are a public health nurse in a small, nonprofit, visiting nurse clinic. The nursing director has requested that you chair the newly established quality improvement committee because of your experience with developing audit criteria.

Because a review of the patient population indicates that maternal/child visits make up the greatest percentage of visiting nurses' home visits, the committee chose to develop a retrospective process audit tool to monitor the quality of initial postparum visits. The criteria specified that the clients to be included in the audit had been discharged with the infant after less than 12 hours in a birth center or obstetrical unit following uncomplicated vaginal delivery. The home visit would occur no longer than 72 hours after the delivery.
Assignment: Design an audit tool appropriate for this diagnosis that would be convenient to use. Specify percentages of compliance, sources of information, and number of patients to be audited. Limit your process criteria to 20 items. Try solving this yourself before reading the possible solution that follows.
POSSIBLE SOLUTION
When writing audit criteria, define the patient population as clearly as possible first so information can be retrieved quickly. In this case, eliminate complicated births, abnormal newborns, cesarean section births, and home births because these patients will need more assessment and teaching. The performance expectations should be set at 100% compliance, but an allowance should be made for reasonable exceptions. One hundred percent is recommended because if any of these criteria are not recorded in the patient's record, remedial actions should be taken. Select the patient's record as the most objective source of information. It should be assumed that if criteria are not charted, they were not met. Audit 30 charts

to give the agency enough data to make some assumptions, but not too many as to make it economically burdensome to review records. An audit form that could be developed follows:

Nursing Audit Form for Visiting Nurses

Nursing Diagnosis: Initial home visit within 72 hours after uncomplicated vaginal delivery, with normal newborn, occurring in a birth center or obstetrical facility

Source of Information: *Patient's record*

Expected Compliance: *100%, unless specific exceptions are noted*

Number of Records to Be Audited: *30*

After the audit committee reviews the records, a summary should be made of the findings. A summary could look like this:

Summary of Audit Findings

Nursing Diagnosis: Initial home visit, within 72 hours after uncomplicated delivery, with normal newborn, occurring in a birth center or obstetrical facility

Number of Records Audited: 30

Date of Audit: 7/6/05

Summary of Findings: 100% compliance in all areas except mother's temperature (50% compliance) and newborn assessment (70% compliance)

Suggestions for Improving Compliance: Remind nurses to record temperature of mother in record, even if normal. Time might be a factor in newborn assessment because temperature is frequently recorded on subsequent visit. Committee agrees that temperatures should be taken on first home visit and suggests an in-service and staff meeting regarding this area of noncompliance.

Signed, Chair of the Committee

The summaries should be forwarded to the individual responsible for quality improvement, in this case the director of the agency. At no time should individual public health nurses be identified as not having met the criteria. Quality improvement must always be separate from performance appraisal.

Structure Audit

Structure audits assume that a relationship exists between quality care and appropriate structure. A structure audit includes resource inputs such as the environment in which health care is delivered. It also includes all those elements that exist prior to and separate from the interaction between the patient and the healthcare worker. For example, staffing ratios, staffing mix, emergency department wait times, and the availability of fire extinguishers in patient care areas would all be structure measures of quality of care.

Structural standards, which are often set by licensing and accrediting bodies, ensure a safe and effective environment but do not address the actual care provided. An example of a structural audit might include checking to see if patient call lights are in place or if patients can reach their water pitchers. It also might examine staffing patterns to ensure that adequate resources are available to meet changing patient needs.

Learning Exercise 23.2

Identifying Structure, Process, and Outcome Measures
You are a charge nurse on a postsurgical unit. Retrospective survey data reveals that many patients report high levels of postoperative pain in the first 72 hours after surgery. You decide to make a list of possible structure, process, and outcome variables that may be impacting the situation. For example, one of the structure measures you identify is that the narcotic medication carts are located some distance from the patient rooms and that may be contributing to a delay in pain medication administration. One of the process measures you identify is that licensed staff are inconsistent in terms of how soon they make their initial pain assessments on postoperative patients as well as the tools they use to assess pain levels. An outcome measure might be the average wait time from the time a patient requests pain medication until it is administered.
Assignment: Identify at least three additional structure, process, and outcome measures that you might collect data for in an effort to resolve this problem. Select at least one of these measures and specifically identify how you would collect the data. Then describe how you would use your findings to increase the likelihood that future practice on the unit will be evidence based.

TOTAL QUALITY MANAGEMENT/TOYOTA PRODUCTION SYSTEM

Over the past several decades, the American healthcare system has moved from a *quality assurance* (QA) model to one focused on *quality improvement* (QI). The difference between the two concepts is that QA models seek to assure that quality currently exists whereas QI models assume that the process is ongoing and that quality can always be improved. Two models that emphasize the ongoing nature of QI include Total Quality Management and the Toyota Production System.

Total quality management (TQM), also referred to as *continuous quality improvement* (CQI), is a philosophy developed by Dr. W. Edward Deming. Considered the hallmark of highly successful Japanese management systems, TQM is based on the premises that the individual is the focal element on which production and service depend (i.e., it must be a customer-responsive environment) and that the quest for quality in an ongoing process. Thus, identifying and doing the right things, the right way, the first time, and problem-prevention planning—not inspection and reactive problem solving—lead to quality outcomes.

Because TQM is a never-ending process, everything and everyone in the organization are subject to continuous improvement efforts. No matter how good the product or service is, the TQM philosophy says there is always room for improvement. Customer needs and experiences with the product are constantly evaluated. Workers do this data collection, not by a central QA/QI department, thus providing a feedback loop between administration, workers, and consumers. Any problems encountered are approached in a preventive or proactive mode so crisis management becomes unnecessary.

Another critical component of TQM is the empowerment of employees by providing positive feedback and reinforcing attitudes and behaviors that support quality and productivity. Based on the premise that employees have an in-depth understanding of their jobs, believe they are valued, and feel encouraged to improve product or service quality through risk taking and creativity, TQM trusts the employees to be knowledgeable, accountable, and responsible and provides education and training for employees at all levels.

Although the philosophy of TQM emphasizes that quality is placed before profit, the resultant increase in quality of a well-implemented TQM program attracts more customers, resulting in increased profit margins and a financially healthier organization. The 14 quality management principles of TQM as outlined by Deming (1986) are summarized in **Display 23.5.**

 Learning Exercise 23.3

Deming's 14 TQM Principles
Think back to the organization for which you have worked the longest. How many of Deming's 14 principles for total quality management are used in that organization? Do you believe some of the 14 principles are more important than others? Why or why not? Could an organization have a successful quality management program if only some of the principles are used?

Display 23.5	**Total Quality Management Principles**

1. Create a constancy of purpose for the improvement of products and service.
2. Adopt a philosophy of continual improvement.
3. Focus on improving processes, not on inspection of product.
4. End the practice of awarding business on price alone; instead, minimize total cost by working with a single supplier.
5. Improve constantly every process for planning, production, and service.
6. Institute job training and retraining.
7. Develop the leadership in the organization.
8. Drive out fear by encouraging employees to participate actively in the process.
9. Foster interdepartmental cooperation and break down barriers between departments.
10. Eliminate slogans, exhortations, and targets for the workforce.
11. Focus on quality and not just quantity; eliminate quota systems if they are in place.
12. Promote teamwork rather than individual accomplishments. Eliminate the annual rating or merit system.
13. Educate/train employees to maximize personal development.
14. Charge all employees with carrying out the total quality management package.

Source: Deming, W. E. (1986). *Out of the crisis.* Cambridge, MA: MIT Press.

Another more contemporary, customer-focused quality improvement model is the *Toyota Production System* (TPS). This system is a "method of managing people engaged in work that emphasizes frequent rapid problem solving and work redesign that has become the global archetype for productivity and performance" (Thompson, Wolf, & Spear, 2003, p. 585). With TPS, when a patient has an unmet need, the caregiver closest to the problem has the responsibility, resources, teaching, and managerial support to correct it, by determining the root cause and redesigning work to eliminate its recurrence (Thompson, et al.). TPS argues that solving individual problems this way, one at a time where, when, and with whom they occur, prevents larger problems.

Implementing TPS, however, is not easy. It generally requires a change in organizational culture, values, and roles. Because every problem, big or small, must be addressed and immediately so, first-, middle-, and top-level managers must deal with far more requests for problem solving and involvement than in organizations where at least small problems are encouraged to be solved more independently (Thompson, et. al.). In addition, eliminating problems at their root is far different from solving an immediate problem at hand.

Thus, adopting TPS in an organization requires a substantial commitment of leadership time and resources. It also requires a tremendous amount of staff preparation and involvement. However, Thompson, et al. argue that these efforts are offset by "greater quality of care, improved patient safety, lower costs, and increased job satisfaction" (p. 592).

WHO SHOULD BE INVOLVED IN QUALITY CONTROL?

Ideally, everyone in the organization should participate in quality control because each individual is a recipient of the benefits. Quality control gives employees feedback about their current quality of care and how the care they provide can be improved.

Although it is impractical to expect full staff involvement throughout the quality control process, staff should be involved in determining criteria or standards, reviewing standards, collecting data, or reporting. Quality control requires evaluating the performance of all members of the multidisciplinary team. Professionals such as physicians, respiratory therapists, dietitians, and physical therapists contribute to patient outcomes and therefore must be considered in the audit process.

Patients should also be actively involved in the determination of an organization's quality of care. It is important to remember, however, that quality care does not always equate with patient satisfaction. Indeed, patient satisfaction often has nothing to do with whether a patient's health improved during their hospital stay. For example, the quality of food, provision of privacy, satisfaction with a roommate, or noisiness of the nursing station may determine patient satisfaction with a hospital admission. In addition, patient satisfaction may be adversely affected by long waits for call lights to be answered and for transport to ancillary services, such as x-ray. Although these factors are an important component of patient comfort and therefore quality of care, quality is more encompassing and must always include an examination of whether the patient received the most appropriate treatment from the most appropriate provider in a timely fashion.

Quality Measurement as an Organizational Mandate

Organizational accountability for the internal monitoring of cost containment and quality has increased during the last 30 years. Clearly, "nurses today are attempting to do more with less while grappling with faulty error-prone systems that do not focus on patients at the point of care" (Thompson, Wolf, & Spear, 2003 p. 585).

Most healthcare organizations today have complete quality improvement programs and are actively involved in cost containment. Changing government regulations regarding quality control, however, continue to influence management decisions strongly. Managers must be cognizant of changing government and licensing regulations that affect their unit's quality control and standard setting. This awareness allows the manager to implement proactive rather than reactive quality control.

Other factors that are likely to impact quality management in healthcare institutions currently are demographics, technology, financing, and care management (Kirkman-Liff, 2002). Each of these factors impacts how quality is measured, how quality improvement programs are developed, and the government or large employer's roles in regulating quality. For example, given the rapid and dramatic increases in the elderly U.S. population, more attention needs to be given to defining desired outcomes that may be different from a younger population, and more attention needs to be paid to regulating and improving nursing home, home health, and hospice care (Kirkman-Liff).

Similarly, technology with its associated informatics, telemedicine, and E-health gives clinicians a wide variety of screening tools for both more rapid and precise collection of quality data, but "quality assurance will need to assess the appropriateness of decisions concerning the use of this armory" (Kirkman-Liff, 2002, p. 263).

Finance also promises to continue to be a factor affecting health care institutions. Unfortunately, quality assurance and improvement must adjust to the increased financial pressures on healthcare institutions, and resources to expand QA and QI may become limited at a time when consumers are demanding more information and accountability from their providers (Kirkman-Liff, 2002).

Finally, changes in care management will likely require QA and QI projects to span traditional institutional walls, and patients are more likely than ever to be directly involved in the process. The processes of disease management and case management will themselves increasingly incorporate QA and QI (Kirkman-Liff, 2002). An analysis of these four health system changes on quality management is shown in **Display 23.6.**

Factors that impact quality management in healthcare institutions are likely to include demographics, technology, financing, and care management. Each impacts how quality is measured, and how quality improvement programs are developed and regulated.

| Display 23.6 | **Analysis of the Impact of Health System Changes on Quality Management** |

	Measurement of Quality	Quality Assurance and Improvement	Government and Large Employer Regulation of Quality
Demographics Population Demographics	More sensitive measures of quality; recognition that death may not be an adverse outcome; need to measure multicultural sensitivity.	More focus on quality assurance and improvements in the care of elderly.	More focus on nursing home, home health, and hospice quality.
Nursing Demographics	Need to measure multicultural sensitivity.	QA & QI will be able to draw on the maturity and life experiences of older nurses.	
Technology Human Genome Project	Need to measure the appropriate use of new screening tools.	Greater emphasis on decision making concerning use of the most appropriate screening tools, pharmaceuticals, and technology.	Decisions by purchasers on benefit coverage of advanced technologies will affect quality of care.
Pharmaceuticals	Optimal drug prescribing as well as accuracy; patient choice may affect outcomes.		
Medical Technology	Patient choice may affect outcomes.		

(display continues on page 598)

Display 23.6	Analysis of the Impact of Health System Changes on Quality Management		
	Measurement of Quality	**Quality Assurance and Improvement**	**Government and Large Employer Regulation of Quality**
Technology Informatics, Telemedicing, E-health	Greater collection of detailed information allowing more precise quality metrics; rapid access to "real-time" quality measures.	Faster collection of quality data allows almost real-time quality assurance; rich databases for quality-improvement efforts.	Purchasers and regulators will have far more precise and current information on quality; will respond quicker to quality variations.
Financing	Increased patient cost sharing may discourage patient utilization of quality enhancing services; measures must adjust for patient decisions.	Institutions will have problems finding financial resources for quality improvement.	Purchasers may demand greater "value": higher quality at same or lower cost.
Care Management	Quality measurements will include the extent of patient involvement; metrics for case management, disease management, and pain assessment and control will be needed.	Quality assurance and improvement will involve patients and projects that span institutional walls; disease management and case management programs will incorporate QA/QI.	Strength of disease management, case management, and pain assessment and control programs will affect contracting decisions.

Source: Kirkman-Liff, B. (2002). Keeping an eye on a moving target. *Nursing Economics$, (20)*6, 262. Reprinted with permission of the publisher, Jannetti Publications, Inc., East Holly Avenue, Box 56, Pitman, NJ 08071-0056.

EXTERNAL IMPACTS ON QUALITY CONTROL

Although few organizations would argue the significant benefits of well-developed and implemented quality control programs, quality control in healthcare organizations has evolved primarily from external impacts and not as a voluntary monitoring effort. When Medicare and Medicaid (government reimbursement for the elderly, disabled, and financially indigent) were implemented in the early 1960s, healthcare organizations had little need to justify costs or prove that the services provided met patients' needs. Reimbursement was based on the costs incurred in providing the service, and no real ceilings were placed on the amount that could be charged for services. Only when the cost of these programs skyrocketed did the government establish regulations requiring organizations to justify the need for services and to monitor the quality of services.

Professional Standards Review Organizations

Professional Standards Review Board legislation (PL 92-603), established in 1972, was among the first of the federal government's efforts to examine cost and quality. Professional standards review organizations (PSROs) mandated a certification of need for the patient's admission and continued review of care; an evaluation of medical care; and an analysis of the patient profile, the hospital, and the practitioners.

This new "big brother" surveillance and the existence of external controls had a huge effect on the industry. Healthcare organizations began to question basic values and were forced to establish new methods for collecting data, keeping records, providing services, and accounting in general. Because government programs such as Medicare and Medicaid represent such a large group of today's patients, organizations that were unwilling or unable to meet these changing needs did not survive financially.

The Prospective Payment System

The advent of *diagnosis-related groups* (DRGs) in the early 1980s added to the ever-increasing need for organizations to monitor cost containment yet guarantee a minimum level of quality (see Chapter 10). As a result of DRGs, hospitals became part of the prospective payment system (PPS), whereby providers are paid a fixed amount per patient admission regardless of the actual cost to provide the care. Critics of the PPS argue that although DRGS may have helped to contain rising healthcare costs, the associated rapid declines in length of hospital stay and services provided have resulted in a great decline in quality of care.

Clearly, DRGs have resulted in increased acuity levels of hospitalized patients, a decrease in the length of patient stay, and a perception by many healthcare providers that patients are being discharged prematurely. All these factors have contributed to growing levels of dissatisfaction by nurses regarding the quality of care they provide.

Learning Exercise 23.4

Quality of Patient Care
Is the quality of your patient care always as high as you would like it to be? What factors affect this quality? Which ones can you control? In your clinical experiences, have DRGs affected the quality of care provided? How?

The Joint Commission for Accreditation of Healthcare Organizations

The Joint Commission for Accreditation of Health Care Organizations (JCAHO) is an accrediting body for hospitals, long-term care facilities, psychiatric facilities, ambulatory care programs, and home health operations. JCAHO historically has had a tremendous impact on planning for quality control in acute care hospitals. JCAHO was the first to mandate that all hospitals have a QA program in place by 1981. These QA programs were to include a review of the care provided by all clinical departments, disciplines, and practitioners; the coordination and integration of the findings of quality control activities; and the development of specific plans for known or suspected patient problems. Again, in 1982, JCAHO began to require quarterly evaluations of standards for nursing care as measured against written criteria. These new guidelines emphasized the need for continuous review and evaluation of the quality of care provided by professionals (Huston, 1999).

In the late 1990s, JCAHO instituted its *Agenda for Change*, a multiphase, multidimensional set of initiatives directed at modernizing the accreditation process by shifting the focus of accreditation from organizational structure to organizational performance or outcomes. This required the development of clinical indicators to measure the quality of care provided. To further this goal, JCAHO approved a milestone initiative, known as *ORYX*, in February 1997. This initiative integrates outcomes and other performance measures into the accreditation process.

Under ORYX, all organizations accredited by JCAHO were required to select at least one of 60 acceptable performance measurement systems by March 1998 and to enroll in that system by June 30, 1998 (Huston, 1999). Data collection of two clinical measures was to begin by third quarter 1998. Two additional clinical measures were added for implementation in first quarter 1999. Finally, two additional clinical measures (total of six) were to be added by the end of first quarter 2000. Organizations could also volunteer for *ORYX Plus*, an effort by the JCAHO to create a national standardized database of 32 performance measures.

Centers for Medicare and Medicaid Services (CMS)

The *Centers for Medicare* and *Medicaid Services* (CMS), formerly the Health Care Financing Administration (HCFA), play an active role in both setting standards for and measuring quality in health care. With the introduction of the *Medicare Quality Initiative (MQI)*, in November 2001, a new era of public reporting on quality began and health outcomes were targeted as the data source (Harris, 2003).

Harris (2003) describes the four-pronged approach inherent in the Quality Initiative. First, the state survey agencies and CMS conduct regulation and enforcement activities as usual. Second, information is made available to all consumers via a variety of media on the quality of care in target settings. Third, there are ongoing community-based improvement programs for the agencies that report outcomes data for the various quality initiatives. Finally, there is collaboration and partnership among all stakeholders, including quality improvement organizations, state survey organizations, and providers of services. Many believe that this initiative may become the new benchmark in terms of measuring health outcomes and making quality reports readily available to the consumer (Harris, 2003).

National Committee for Quality Assurance

Another external force affecting quality control in healthcare organizations is the *National Committee for Quality Assurance* (NCQA). The NCQA, a private nonprofit organization that accredits managed care organizations, has developed the *Health Plan Employer Data and Information Set* (HEDIS) to compare managed care organizations in the areas of quality of care, access, patient satisfaction, plan membership, service utilization, and financial stability (Huston, 1999). Rather than compare the managed care organizations with each other directly, HEDIS assigns them a grand mean score for the indicators and also provides an analysis of each managed care organization's progress in meeting goals from the U.S. Public Health Service's *Healthy People 2000* (Huston, 1999).

Version 3.0 of HEDIS contains 71 measures that provide numerical and descriptive information about the quality of care, patient outcomes, access and availability of services, utilization, premiums, and the plan's financial stability and operating policies. Future versions are expected to have an even greater number of performance indicators as the growing Medicaid and Medicare segment of the population enrolled in managed care add more specific performance indicators (Huston, 1999). Version 3.0 of HEDIS, with data gathered from nearly 300 health plans, has been compiled into a national database known as *Quality Compass*.

One of the most significant weaknesses of NCQA accreditation is that such accreditation is voluntary and only about half of managed care organizations currently undergo such review (Huston, 1999). Since 1999, however, Medicare and Medicaid have contracted their managed care plans only with health plans that are accredited by the NCQA. More employers are also adopting this policy, with the result that most managed care organizations will need this accreditation in the future to survive fiscally.

Maryland Hospital Association Quality Indicator Project

Another major initiative to measure quality in acute care settings is the *Maryland Hospital Association Quality Indicator Project* (QI Project). The QI Project, a research project that began in 1985 with seven acute care hospitals in Maryland, currently has more than 1,200 hospitals throughout the United States and the United Kingdom participating. It is important to remember that the QI Project is still considered a research project, and as such, the project is not intended to be used to establish performance thresholds or standards of care; however, its benchmark work in indicator identification and measurement is invaluable.

Fourteen quality indicators have been identified in the QI Project for inpatient data collection, five for ambulatory care, eight for psychiatric care, six for long-term care, and four for home care (QI Project website, 2000). Indicators under study are shown in **Displays 23.7, 23.8, 23.9, 23.10,** and **23.11.**

Display 23.7	**Maryland Hospital Association Quality Indicator Project: Inpatient Indicators**

- Device-associated infections in intensive care units
- Device use in intensive care units
- Surgical site infections
- Prophylaxis for surgical procedures
- Inpatient mortality
- Neonatal mortality
- Perioperative mortality
- Management of labor
- Unscheduled readmissions
- Unscheduled admissions following ambulatory procedures
- Unscheduled returns to an intensive care unit
- Unscheduled returns to the operating room
- Isolated coronary artery bypass graft (CABG) peri-operative mortality
- Physical restraint use
- Falls
- Complications following sedation and analgesia in intensive care units, cardiac cath labs, radiology suites, endoscopy suites, and emergency departments

Source: Maryland Quality Indicator Project. Available at: http://www.qiproject.org/Brochure/IndAcute.pdf. Accessed February 14, 2004.

Display 23.8	**Maryland Hospital Association Quality Indicator Project: Acute Care Ambulatory Indicators**

- Unscheduled returns to the emergency department (ED)
- Length of stay in the ED
- ED x-ray discrepancies and patient management
- Patients leaving the ED before treatment is complete
- Cancellation of ambulatory procedures

Source: Maryland Quality Indicator Project. Available at: http://www.qiproject.org/Brochure/IndAcute.pdf. Accessed February 14, 2004.

Display 23.9 Maryland Hospital Association Quality Indicator Project: Psychiatric Care Indicators

- Injurious behaviors (adult and adolescent units)
- Unplanned departures resulting in discharges (adult and adolescent units)
- Transfers/discharges to inpatient acute care (adult units)
- Readmissions to inpatient psychiatric care (adult and adolescent units)
- Use of involuntary restraint (adult and adolescent units)
- Use of seclusion (adult and adolescent units)
- Partial hospitalization (adult units)
- Adult documented falls (adult units)

Source: Maryland Quality Indicator Project. Available at: http://www.qiproject.org/Brochure/IndAcute.pdf. Accessed February 14, 2004.

Display 23.10 Maryland Hospital Association Quality Indicator Project: Long-Term Care Indicators

- Unplanned weight change
- Pressure ulcer prevalence
- Falls
- Unscheduled transfers/discharges to inpatient care
- Nosocomial infection incidence
- Use of physical restraint
- Presence of advance directives
- Psychological well-being

Source: Maryland Quality Indicator Project. Available at: http://www.qiproject.org/Brochure/IndAcute.pdf. Accessed February 14, 2004.

Display 23.11 Maryland Hospital Association Quality Indicator Project: Home Care Indicators

- Unscheduled transfers to inpatient acute care
- Use of emergent care services
- Discharges to nursing home care
- Acquired infections

Source: Maryland Quality Indicator Project. Available at: http://www.qiproject.org/Brochure/IndAcute.pdf. Accessed February 14, 2004.

Participants collect data on any or all of the measures in an indicator set and submit these data to the Project on a quarterly basis. The Project, in turn, provides quarterly comparative feedback to participants in the form of quarterly reports and data analysis (QI Project website, 2000). In addition, participants have access to a wide range of educational and analytical tools and services that are designed to improve their ability to put the data to work. All data submitted to the project are confidential, and participants must agree to maintain the confidentiality of the aggregate rates and related statistical data.

Learning Exercise 23.5

Classifying QI Project Indicators
Look at the inpatient, ambulatory care, psychiatric, and long-term care indicators in use with the QI project. Which ones would be classified as process indicators? Outcome indicators? Structure indicators? Which indicators do you believe would be most difficult to measure?

Multistate Nursing Home Case Mix and Quality Demonstration

There has also been a major move to develop quality indicators in long-term care settings. One of the most significant efforts has been the *Multistate Nursing Home Case Mix* and *Quality demonstration*, funded by the former Health Care Financing Administration (HCFA) (now the Centers for Medicare and Medicaid). This demonstration seeks to develop and implement both a case mix classification system to serve as the basis for Medicare and Medicaid payment, and a quality monitoring system to assess the impact of case mix payment on quality and to provide better information to the nursing home survey process.

Report Cards

In response to the demand for objective measures of quality, a number of health plans, healthcare providers, employer purchasing groups, consumer information organizations, and state governments have begun to formulate healthcare quality report cards. In the early 1990s, California mandated the development of report cards for all hospitals licensed in the state; Ohio and Pennsylvania have similar laws that mandate the dissemination to the public of healthcare institutions' quality performance data. Most states have laws requiring providers to report some type of data. AHRQ has also been exploring the development of a report card for the nation's healthcare delivery system.

It is important to remember, however, that currently most report cards do not contain information about the quality of care rendered by specific clinics, group practices, or physicians in a health plan's network (Huston, 1999). In addition, some critics of healthcare report cards point out that health plans may receive conflicting ratings on different report cards. This is a result of using different performance measures and how each report card chooses to pool and evaluate individual factors. Report cards may also not be readily accessible or may be difficult for the average consumer to understand.

Medical Errors, Appropriateness of Care, and Nursing Dissatisfaction: Ongoing Threats to Quality of Care

One of the largest and most well-known recent studies on quality of health care was a report issued by the Institute of Medicine (IOM), called *To Err is Human* (Kohn, Corrigan, & Donaldson, 2000). This report found that:

- At least 44,000 Americans die each year as a result of medical errors and the number may be as high as 98,000,
- Even when using the lower estimate, deaths due to medical errors become the eighth leading cause of death in this country, and
- More people die in a given year as a result of medical errors than from motor vehicle accidents, breast cancer, or AIDS.

Perhaps the most significant contribution of the IOM report, however, was the conclusions that most of these errors did not occur from individual recklessness. Instead, they occurred because of basic flaws in the way the health delivery system is organized and delivered (Kohn et al., 2000).

The IOM study also looked at the type of errors that were happening. Medication errors stood out as a particularly high risk. Medication errors alone, occurring either in or out of the hospital, were estimated to account for over 7,000 deaths annually, with pediatric patients experiencing harmful medication errors three times more often than adults (Kaushal et al., 2001) and ICU patients suffering more life-threatening medication errors than any other patient population.

And finally, a Commonwealth Fund study in (2002) found that 1.5 million American families (8.1 million households) had experienced a serious drug error—33% of them during a hospitalization.

Other notable studies have looked at quality of health care, but not in terms of errors. Instead, they have attempted to see whether the care given was appropriate in quantity as well as scope. A follow up study by the IOM in (2001), called *Crossing the Quality Chasm*, found large gaps between the preventive, acute, and chronic care people should get and what they actually received. They estimated, for example, that only half the population receives recommended preventive care, only 70% recommended acute care, and only 60% received recommended chronic care. Furthermore, 30% of the acute care and 20% of the chronic care patients actually received care that was contraindicated.

Providers also report quality concerns in the work setting. A (2001) study of 7,299 nurses by the American Nurses Association showed that over half of the nurses (56%) believed that the time available for direct patient care had decreased in the last two years and 76% reported an increased patient care load. Seventy-five percent of the nurses indicated that quality of nursing care had declined in their work setting and cited examples including inadequate staffing, delay in providing basic care, and the discharge of patients without adequate information to continue their care. Even more alarming was the finding that 40% of the nurses surveyed would not feel comfortable having a family member or someone close to them cared for in the facility where they work (ANA).

Another large study of over 80,000 staff nurses in 2001 reported that 20% of the nurses classified the quality of care on their units as fair or poor (Sochalski, 2001). Forty-one percent were moderately or very dissatisfied with their job, with emotional exhaustion a leading cause of their dissatisfaction. And finally, the study reported that the frequency of adverse incidents increased proportionately with their dissatisfaction and emotional exhaustion.

> McGlynn and Brook call for a "war on poor quality" that has the same level of public commitment as the war on cancer or the campaign to put a man on the moon.

McGlynn and Brook (as cited in Lee, & Estes, 2003) call for a "war on poor quality" that has the same level of public commitment as the war on cancer or the campaign to put a man on the moon. This will require sustained public interest to create the momentum to systematically change the healthcare system in a way that improves quality. Increasing consumer knowledge and participation in health care will be imperative in this effort (Huston, 2003).

Another problem that makes addressing medical errors difficult is that a disconnect still exists between consumers' perceptions of the quality of their own health care and the actual quality provided. McGlynn and Brook (as cited in Lee, & Estes, 2003) suggest reports on medical errors have come closest in recent times to breaking through this cognitive dissonance. Although concern about errors has prompted a dialogue, a way must be found to turn this dialogue into a shared understanding of the quality problem without fundamentally undermining trust in the medical care system.

At the institution level, there must be more mandatory reporting of medical errors as well as voluntary efforts. *The Patient Safety and Quality Improvement Act* was introduced in the Senate on June 6, 2002. This bill protects medical-error information voluntarily submitted to new private organizations from being subpoenaed or used in legal discovery and would generally require that the information be treated as confidential (Duff, 2002).

Healthcare organizations also need to a better job of identifying what errors are occurring, categorizing those errors, and examining and reworking the processes that led to the errors (Chaiken, 2001). Ignoring the problem, denying their existence, or blaming the individuals involved in the processes does nothing to eliminate the preventable morbidity, mortality, and waste of resources that poor processes generate each day (Chaiken). Organizational cultures need to change for employees and patients to be comfortable in reporting hazards that can affect patient safety without fear of personal risk.

In addition, the standards and expectations of oversight groups, insurers, and professional groups must be raised. One such effort is the *Leapfrog* group, a conglomeration of nonhealthcare Fortune 500 company leaders who are committed to modernizing the current healthcare system (Milstein, Galvin, Delbanco, Salber, & Buck, 2000). Based upon current research, the Leapfrog group identified three evidence-based standards they believe will provide the greatest impact on reducing medical errors: computerized physician order entry (CPOE), evidence-based hospital referral (EHR), and intensive care unit physician staffing (IPS) (Hudon, 2003). "An understanding of these medically based standards provides nursing an opportunity to consider the potential and actual concerns that span multiple disciplines in their implementation and motivation for future nursing research related to their effect" (Hudon, p. 234).

Finally, if quality health care is to be achieved, the medical liability system and our litigious society must be recognized as potential barriers to systematic efforts to uncover and learn from mistakes that are made in health care (Huston, 2003).

INTEGRATING LEADERSHIP ROLES AND MANAGEMENT FUNCTIONS IN QUALITY CONTROL

Quality control provides managers with the opportunity to evaluate organizational performance from a systematic, scientific, and objective viewpoint. To do so, managers must determine what standards will be used to measure quality care on their units and then develop and implement quality control programs that measure results against those standards. All managers are responsible for monitoring the quality of the product that their units produce; in healthcare organizations, that product is patient care. Managers also must assess and promote patient satisfaction whenever possible.

The manager, however, cannot operate in a vacuum in determining what quality is and how it should be measured. Demands for hard data on quality have increased as regulatory bodies, patients, payers, and hospital managers have required justification of services provided. Managers must be cognizant of rapidly changing quality control regulations and proactively adjust unit standards to meet these changing needs. Limited attention to quality measurement in health care occurred, however, until the past two decades. As we enter the twenty-first century, however, there is an ever-increasing focus on the quality of care and the standardization of quality data collection, and an increased accountability for outcomes from the system level to the individual provider.

Inspiring subordinates to establish and achieve high standards of care is a leadership skill. Leaders role model high standards in their own nursing care and encourage subordinates to seek maximum rather than minimum standards. One way this can be accomplished is by involving subordinates in the quality control process. By studying direct cause–effect relationships, subordinates learn to modify individual and group performance to improve the quality of care provided.

Vision is another leadership skill inherent in quality control. The visionary leader looks at what is and determines what should be. This future focus allows leaders to shape unit goals proactively and improve the quality of care.

And, finally, the integrated leader–manager in quality control must be willing to be a risk taker and to be accountable. In an era of limited resources and cost containment, there is great pressure to sacrifice quality in an effort to contain costs. The self-aware leader–manager recognizes this risk and seeks to achieve a balance between quality and cost containment that does not violate professional obligations to patients and subordinates.

☀ Key Concepts

- Controlling is implemented throughout all phases of management.
- *Quality control* refers to activities that are used to evaluate, monitor, or regulate services rendered to consumers.
- A *standard* is a predetermined baseline condition or level of excellence that constitutes a model to be followed and practiced.
- Because there is no one set of standards, each organization and profession must set standards and objectives to guide individual practitioners in performing safe and effective care.
- *Clinical practice guidelines* provide diagnosis-based, step-by-step interventions for nurses to follow in an effort to promote evidence-based, high-quality care and yet control resource utilization and costs.
- *Benchmarking* is the process of measuring products, practices, and services against those of *best-performing organizations*.
- *Outcome audits* determine what results, if any, followed from specific nursing interventions for patients.
- *Process audits* are used to measure the process of care or how the care was carried out.
- *Structure audits* monitor the structure or setting in which patient care occurs (such as the finances, nursing service structure, medical records, and environmental structure).
- There is growing recognition of the importance of identifying and measuring *nursing-sensitive outcomes* to create accountability for nurses as professionals and in developing nursing as a profession.
- Quality control in healthcare organizations has evolved primarily from external forces and not as a voluntary effort to monitor the quality of services provided.
- Ideally, everyone in an organization should participate in quality control because each person benefits from it.
- As direct caregivers, staff nurses are in an excellent position to monitor nursing practice by identifying problems and implementing corrective actions that have the greatest impact on patient care.

More Learning Exercises and Applications

 Learning Exercise 23.6

Identifying Nursing-Sensitive Outcome Criteria
Some ill patients get better despite nursing care, not as a result of it. However, the quality of nursing care affects patient outcomes tremendously. Do you believe that quality nursing care makes a difference in patients' lives? Identify five criteria you would use to define "quality nursing care." These criteria should reflect what you believe nurses do (nursing sensitive) that makes the difference in patient outcomes. Are the criteria you listed measurable? How?

Learning Exercise 23.7

Working Short Staffed—Again

You are a staff nurse at Mercy Hospital. The hospital's patient census and acuity have been very high for the last six months. Many of the nursing staff have resigned; a coordinated recruitment effort to refill these positions has been largely unsuccessful. The nursing staff is demoralized, and staff frequently call in sick or fail to show up for work. Today, you arrive at work and find that you are again being asked to work short-handed. You will be the only RN on a unit with 30 patients. Although you have two LVNs and two CNAs assigned to work with you, you are concerned that patient safety could be compromised. A check with the central nursing office ascertains that no additional help can be obtained.

   You feel that you have reached the end of your rope. The administration at Mercy Hospital has been receptive to employee feedback about the acute staffing shortage, and you believe they have made some efforts to try to alleviate the problem. You also believe, however, that the efforts have not been at the level they should have been, and that the hospital will continue to expect nurses to work short-handed until some major force changes things. Although you have thought about quitting, you really enjoy the work you do and feel morally obligated to your coworkers, the patients, and even your superiors. Today, it occurs to you that you could anonymously phone the state licensing bureau and turn in Mercy Hospital for consistent understaffing of nursing personnel, leading to unsafe patient care. You believe this could be the impetus needed to improve the quality of care. You also are aware of the action's political risks.

Assignment: Discuss whether you would take this action. What is your responsibility to the organization, to yourself, and to patients? How do you make decisions such as this one, which have conflicting moral obligations?

Learning Exercise 23.8

Examining Mortality Rates

You have been the nursing coordinator of cardiac services at a medium-size urban hospital for the last six months. Among the hospital's cardiac services are open-heart surgery, invasive and noninvasive diagnostic testing, and a comprehensive rehabilitation program. The open-heart surgery program was implemented a little over one year ago. During the last three months you have begun to feel uneasy about the mortality rate of postoperative cardiac patients at your facility. An audit of medical records shows a unit mortality rate that is approximately 30% above national norms.

You approach the unit medical director with your findings. He becomes very defensive and states that there have been a few freakish situations to skew the results but that the open-heart program is one of the best in the state. When you question him about examining the statistics further, he becomes very angry and turns to leave the room. At the door, he stops and says, "Remember that these patients are leaving the operating room alive. They are dying on your unit. If you stir up trouble, you are going to be sorry."

Assignment: Outline your plan. Identify areas in your data gathering that may have been misleading or that may have skewed your findings. If you believe action is still warranted, what are the personal and professional risks involved? How well developed is your power base to undertake these risks? To whom do you have the greatest responsibility?

Learning Exercise 23.9

Weighing Conflicting Obligations

You are the director of a baccalaureate nursing program. In the mid-1990s your school averaged approximately 200 applicants for the 50 student openings each semester. This resulted in the school being very selective about which students would enter the program. Because entering students traditionally had high grade-point averages and had completed almost all non-nursing requirements, the attrition and dropout rate was fairly low, and academic failure was rare.

Currently, because of a severe national nursing shortage coupled with a marked decrease in the number of students seeking nursing as a career, barely enough students apply to fill each entering class. As a result, students meeting only minimal grade-point average requirements and many who haven't met general studies course requirements are accepted into the program. You have seen the attrition and dropout rate quadruple in the last three years, with much of this attrition attributable to academic failure.

Recently, the faculty members have begun discussing changing the academic failure policy in an effort to increase student retention. The current policy results in automatic dismissal from the program if students fail two courses in the major.

Faculty members are concerned that teaching positions will be cut as a result of the decreased enrollment and high attrition. You are aware that the university administration believes that nursing is an expensive major, that this situation is not going to improve in the near future, and that budget cuts may indeed soon be mandated.

You, however, have grave concerns about eliminating or altering the academic failure policy because you believe you are in effect lowering program standards and thus the quality of its end product. You do not believe that students failing two courses in the major would be safe practitioners. You also believe that students in academic difficulty are taking a disproportionate amount of faculty time and energy at the expense of better students.

Assignment: What options are available to you? What obligations do you have to your faculty, to the students, to the public as consumers of health care, and to the university administration? How do you determine an appropriate course of action when these duties conflict?

Web Links

Agency for Healthcare Research and Quality (AHRQ)
http://www.ahcpr.gov

Practical healthcare information, research findings, and data to help consumers, health providers, health insurers, researchers, and policymakers make informed decisions about health care.

Health Grades
http://www.healthgrades.com/public
Report card quality ratings on hospitals, physicians, nursing homes, home health agencies, hospices, and fertility clinics.

National Committee for Quality Assurance (NCQA)
http://www.ncqa.org
Independent, nonprofit organization that assesses and reports on the quality of care delivered by managed care organizations.

References

American Nurses Association (1998). Standards of clinical nursing practice (2nd ed.). Washington, D.C.: American Nurses Association.

American Nurses Association. (2001). *ANA nursing standards.* Available at: http://nursingworld.org/ anp/pdescr.cfm?CNum = 15. Accessed October 2001.

American Nurses Association. (2001). *Analysis of American Nurses Association staffing survey,* Press Release. Available at: http://nursingworld.org/pressrel/2001/pr026.htm. Accessed February 6, 2001.

Bulger, R. J. (2003). *The quest for therapeutic institutions.* Washington, D.C.: Association of Academic Health Centers.

Chaiken, B. P. (2001). Patient safety: Is it really a problem? *Nursing Economic$, 19*(4), 176–177.

Commonwealth Fund. (April 2002). *News release: New study estimates eight million American families experienced a serious medical or drug error.* Available at: http://www.cmwf.org/media/releases/davis534_release04152002.asp. Accessed April 15, 2002.

Crossing the quality chasm: A new health system for the 21st century (2001). Committee on Quality of Health Care in America. Institute of Medicine. Available at http://books.nap.edu/books/0309072808/html/index.html. Accessed November 4, 2004.

Deming, W. E. (1986). *Out of the crisis.* Cambridge, MA: MIT Press.

Duff, S. (2002). Medical-errors reporting system proposed. *Modern Healthcare's Daily Dose.* Available at: http://www.bridgemedical.com/patient_psqia.shtml. Accessed June 5, 2002.

Dykes, P. C. (2003). Practice guidelines and measurement: State of the science. *Nursing Outlook, 51*(2), 65–69.

Harris, M. J. (2003). Medicare quality initiative. *Policy, Politics & Nursing Practice, 4*(4), 263–265.

Hudon, P. S. (2003). Leapfrog standards: Implications for nursing practice. *Nursing Economic$, 21*(5), 233–236.

Huston, C. (1999). Outcomes measurement in health care: Imperatives for professional nursing practice. *Nursing Case Management Journal, 4*(4), 188–195.

Huston, C. (2003). Quality health care in an era of diminished resources: Challenges and opportunities. *Journal of Nursing Care Quality, 18* (4), 295–301.

Institute of Medicine. (1994). *America's health in transition: Protecting and improving quality.* Washington, D.C.: National Academy Press.

Kaushal R., Bates D. W., Landrigan C., McKenna K. J., Clapp M. D., Federico F., & Goldmann, D. A. (2001). Medication errors and adverse drug events in pediatric inpatients. *JAMA, 285*(16), 2114–2120.

Kirkman-Liff, B. (2002). Keeping an eye on a moving target: Quality changes and challenges for nurses. *Nursing Economic$, 20*(6), 258–265, 290.

Kohn, L.T., Corrigan, J. M., & Donaldson, M. S. (Eds.). (2000). *To err is human: Building a safer health system.* Institute of Medicine, Committee on Quality of Health Care in America. Executive Summary, 1–14.

La Duke, S. (2000). NIC puts nursing into words. *Nursing Management, 31*(2), 43–44.

Lee, P. R. & Estes, C. L. (2003). *The nation's health* (7th ed.). Boston: Jones and Bartlett Publishers.

Maryland Quality Indicator Project. Available at: http://www.qiproject.org. Accessed February 14, 2004.

Milstein, A., Galvin, R., Delbanco, S., Salber, P., & Buck, C. (2000). Improving the safety of health care: The Leapfrog initiative. *Effective Clinical Practice, 3*(6) 313–316. Available at:http://www.acponline.org/journals/ecp/novdec00/milstein.pdf. Retrieved January 30, 2004.

Sochalski, J. (2001). Quality of care, nurse staffing, and patient outcomes. *Journal of Policy and Politics. 2*(1): 9–18.

Thompson, D. N., Wolf, G. A., & Spear, S. J. (2003). Driving improvements in patient care: Lessons from Toyota. *Journal of Nursing Administration, 33*(11), 585–595.

Bibliography

Benner, P., Sheets, V., Uris, P., Malloch, K., Schwed, K. & Jamison, D. (2002). Individual, practice, and system causes of errors in nursing. *Journal of Nursing Administration, 32*(10), 509–523.

Black, B. (2000). Can nursing education prepare anyone for today's managed care? *Revolution: The Journal for RNs and Patient Advocacy, 1*(4), 26–28.

Born, P. H., & Simon, C. J. (March/Apr. 2001). Patients and profits: The relationship between HMO financial performance and quality of care. *Health Affairs, 20*(2), 167–174.

Buppert, C. (2000). HEDIS for the primary care provider: Getting an "A" on the managed care report card. *The Nurse Practitioner, 24*(1), 84–99.

Buppert, C. (2000). Measuring outcomes in primary care practice. *The Nurse Practitioner, 25*(1), 88–98.

Burge, P., Cronin, S. N. Kramer, J., & Ober, J. (November 2003). Prepare to draw magnet recognition. *Nursing Management, 34*(11), 32–35.

Campbell, S. M., Roland, M. O., & Buetow, S. A. (2000). Defining quality of care. *Social Science and Medicine, 51*(11), 1611–1625.

Casey, M., & Klingner, J. (2000). HMOs serving rural areas: Experiences with HMO accreditation and HEDIS reporting. *Managed Care Quarterly, 8*(2), 48–59.

Chang, B. L., Lee, J. L., Pearson, M. L., Kahn, M. L., Elliott, M. N., & Rubenstein, L. L. (2002). Evaluating quality of nursing care: The gap between theory and practice. *Journal of Nursing Administration, 32*(7/8), 405–418.

DeLise, D. C., & Leasure, A. R. (2001). Benchmarking: Measuring the outcomes of evidence-based practice. *Outcomes Management for Nursing Practice, 5*(2), 70–74.

Eisenberg, J. M., & Power, E. J. (2000). Transforming insurance coverage into quality health care. *Journal of the American Medical Association, 284*(16), 2100–2109.

Ellis, J. (2001). Introducing a method of benchmarking nursing practice. *Professional Nurse, 16*(7), 1202–1203.

Ellis, J. (2001). Guest editorial. Benchmarking: A way of universalizing the best? *NT-Research, 6*(2), 566–567.

Evans, R. (March 15–21, 2001). Benchmarking is a boon for neglected areas . . . Benchmark will strike at poor care. *Nursing Times, 97*(11), 20.

Future of benchmarking: More data, more sharing, and better patient care: Evidence-based medicine should continue growth. *Healthcare Benchmarks, 8*(5), 49–52.

Landon, B. E., Zaslavsky, A. M., Beaulieu, N. D., Shaul, J. A., & Cleary, P. D. (2001). Health plan characteristics and consumers' assessments of quality. *Health Affairs, 20*(2), 274–286.

Malloch, K., Davenport, S., & Hatler, C. (2003). Nursing workforce management. Using benchmarking for planning and outcomes monitoring. *Journal of Nursing Administration, 33*(10), 538–543.

Marsa, L. (2001, May 7). Demanding overhaul of U.S. health care: A new report by a think tank pushes for standardized guidelines, saying today's patients are at the mercy of a medical industry prone to errors. *Los Angeles Times*, Health, S3.

Marsa, L. (2001, May 14). Health care industry riddled with mistakes, survey shows. *Los Angeles Times*, Health, S3.

Oermann, M., & Wilson, F. L. (2000). Quality of care information for consumers on the Internet. *Journal of Nursing Care Quality, 14*(4), 45–54.

Pantall, J. (2001). Benchmarking in healthcare. *NT-Research, 6*(2), 568–580.

Sochalski, J. (2001). Quality of care, nurse staffing, and patient outcomes. *Journal of Policy and Politics, 2*(1), 9–18.

Steinberg, E. P. (March 2000). The impact of the new HEDIS guidelines: Practical considerations. *American Journal of Managed Care, 6*(4): Suppl: S190–196, S232–234.

Valanis, B. (2000). Professional nursing practice in an HMO: The future is now. *Journal of Nursing Education, 39*(1), 13–20.

Warfield, A. (2001). Outcomes focus thinking: Getting results without the boxing gloves. *Journal of Nursing Administration, 31*(7/8), 337–338.

White, K. M. (2000). HEDIS 2000 update. *Policy, Politics, & Nursing Practice, 1*(2), 104–106.

Performance Appraisal

An effective appraisal process rewards productive employees and assists the professional growth and development of inexperienced and unproductive individuals.

—Mable H. Smith

An additional managerial controlling responsibility is determining how well employees carry out the duties of their assigned jobs. This is done through performance appraisals. In performance appraisals, actual performance, not intent, is evaluated. Performance appraisals let employees know the level of their job performance as well as any expectations the organization may have of them. Performance appraisals also generate information for salary adjustments, promotions, transfers, disciplinary actions, and terminations.

None of the manager's actions is as personal as appraising the work performance of others. Because work is an important part of one's identity, people are very sensitive to opinions about how they perform. For this reason, performance appraisal becomes one of the greatest tools an organization has to develop and motivate staff. When used correctly, performance appraisal can motivate staff and increase retention and productivity; in the hands of an inept or inexperienced manager, however, the appraisal process may discourage and demotivate staff.

A manager's opinions and judgments must be determined in an objective, systematic, and formalized manner because they are used for far-reaching decisions regarding the employee's work life Using a formal system of performance review also reduces the appraisal's subjectivity.

The more professional a group of employees is, the more complex and sensitive the evaluation process becomes. The skilled leader–manager who uses a formalized system appropriately builds a team approach to patient care.

This chapter focuses on the relationship between performance appraisal and motivation and discusses how performance appraisals can be used to determine developmental needs of staff. Emphasis is given to appropriate data gathering, proper implementation of management by objectives (MBO), and peer review. The performance appraisal interview also is explored. Performance management is introduced as a new alternative to the traditional annual performance appraisal. The leadership roles and management functions inherent in performance appraisal are shown in **Display 24.1.**

USING THE PERFORMANCE APPRAISAL TO MOTIVATE EMPLOYEES

Although systematic employee appraisals have been used in management since the 1920s, using the appraisal as a tool to promote employee growth did not begin until the 1950s. Most formal appraisals focus on the professional worker rather than the hourly paid worker, who is often guaranteed automatic pay raises if work meets minimum acceptable criteria.

The evolution of performance appraisals is reflected in its changing terminology. At one time, the appraisal was called a *merit rating* and was tied fairly closely to salary increases. More recently, it was termed *performance evaluation*, but because the term *evaluation* implies that personal values are being placed on the performance review, that term is used infrequently. Some organizations continue to use both of these terms or others, such as competency assessment, effectiveness report, or service rating. Most healthcare organizations, however, use the term *performance*

Display 24.1 Leadership Roles and Management Functions Associated with Performance Appraisal

Leadership Roles

1. Uses the appraisal process to motivate employees and promote growth.
2. Uses appropriate techniques to reduce the anxiety inherent in the appraisal process.
3. Involves employees in all aspects of performance appraisal.
4. Is self-aware of own biases and prejudices.
5. Develops employee trust by being honest and fair when evaluating performance.
6. Encourages the peer review process among professional staff.
7. Uses appraisal interviews to facilitate two-way communication.
8. Provides ongoing support to employees attempting to correct performance deficiencies.
9. Uses coaching techniques that promote employee growth in work performance.
10. Individualizes performance goals and the appraisal interview as needed to meet the unique needs of a culturally diverse staff.

Management Functions

1. Uses a formalized system of performance appraisal.
2. Gathers data for performance appraisals that are fair and objective.
3. Uses the appraisal process to determine staff education and training needs.
4. Bases performance appraisal on documented standards.
5. Is as objective as possible in performance appraisal.
6. Maintains appropriate documentation of the appraisal process.
7. Follows up on identified performance deficiencies.
8. Conducts the appraisal interview in a manner that promotes a positive outcome.
9. Provides frequent informal feedback on work performance.

appraisal because this term implies an appraisal of how well employees perform the duties of their job as delineated by the job description.

An important point to consider if the appraisal is to have a positive outcome is how the employee views the appraisal. If employees believe the appraisal is based on their job description rather than on whether the manager approves of them, they are more likely to view the appraisal as relevant. Management research has shown that the following factors influence whether the appraisal ultimately results in increased motivation and productivity:

- The employee must believe that the appraisal is based on a standard to which other employees in the same classification are held accountable. This standard must be communicated clearly to employees at the time they are hired and may be a job description or an individual goal set by staff for the purpose of performance appraisal.
- The employee should have some input into developing the standards or goals on which his or her performance is judged. This is imperative for the professional employee.
- The employee must know in advance what happens if the expected performance standards are not met.

- The employee needs to know how information will be obtained to determine performance. The appraisal tends to be more accurate if various sources and types of information are solicited. Sources could include peers, coworkers, nursing care plans, patients, and personal observation. Employees should be told which sources will be used and how such information will be weighted.

- The appraiser should be one of the employee's direct supervisors. For example, the charge nurse who works directly with the staff nurse should be involved in the appraisal process and interview. It is appropriate and advisable in most instances for the head nurse and supervisor also to be involved. However, employees must believe that the person doing the major portion of the review has actually observed their work.

- The performance appraisal is more likely to have a positive outcome if the appraiser is viewed with trust and professional respect. This increases the chance that the employee will view the appraisal as a fair and accurate assessment of work performance. Welford (2002) maintains that building trust is a hallmark of transformational leadership and necessary for staff empowerment. A summary of the factors influencing effectiveness of appraisals can be seen in **Display 24.2.**

 Learning Exercise 24.1

Writing About Performance Appraisals
During your lifetime, you probably have had many performance appraisals. These may have been evaluations of your clinical performance during nursing school or as a paid employee. Reflect on these appraisals. How many of them encompassed the six recommendations listed in the chapter? How did the inclusion or exclusion of these recommendations influence your acceptance of the results?
Assignment: Select one of the above six recommendations about which you feel strongly. Write a three-paragraph essay on your personal experience involving this recommendation.

Display 24.2	**Factors Influencing Effective Performance Appraisal**

Appraisal should be based on a standard.
Employee should have input into development of the standard.
Employee must know standard in advance.
Employee must know sources of data gathered for the appraisal.
Appraiser should be someone who has observed employee's work.
Appraiser should be someone the employee trusts and respects.

STRATEGIES TO ENSURE ACCURACY AND FAIRNESS IN THE PERFORMANCE APPRAISAL

A performance appraisal wastes time if it is merely an excuse to satisfy regulations and the goal is not employee growth. If the employee views the appraisal as valuable and valid, it can have many positive effects. Information obtained during the performance appraisal can be used to develop the employee's potential, to assist the employee in overcoming difficulties he or she has in fulfilling the job's role, to point out strengths of which the employee may not be aware, and to aid the employee in setting goals. Because inaccurate and unfair appraisals are negative and demotivating, it is critical that the manager use strategies that increase the likelihood of a fair and accurate appraisal. Although some subjectivity is inescapable, the following will assist the manager in arriving at a fairer and more accurate assessment.

The appraiser should develop an awareness of his or her own biases and prejudices. This helps guard against subjective attitudes and values influencing the appraisal. The appraiser's gender also may influence the accuracy of the performance appraisal. Rudan (2003) states that women leaders view liking, trusting, and helping others as more significant in the workplace than men do. Therefore, female managers are more apt to give a favorable evaluation during performance appraisal than male managers are in an effort to meet affiliation needs. On the other hand, male managers tend to have lower affiliation needs and higher achievement needs; thus, they may be more willing to give constructive criticism even if they expect the employee to be defensive (McMurray, 1993).

Consultation should be sought frequently. Another manager should be consulted when a question about personal bias exists and in many other situations. For example, it is very important that new managers solicit assistance and consultation when they complete their first performance appraisals. Even experienced managers may need to consult with others when an employee is having great difficulty fulfilling the duties of the job. Consultation also must be used when employees work several shifts so information can be obtained from all the shift supervisors.

Data should be gathered appropriately. Not only should many different sources be used in gathering data about employee performance, but the data gathered also need to reflect the entire time period of the appraisal. Frequently, managers gather data and observe an employee just before completing the appraisal, which gives an inaccurate picture of performance. Because all employees have periods when they are less productive and motivated, data should be gathered systematically and regularly. Indeed, Fandray (2001) suggests that annual performance appraisals are falling out of favor with human resource professionals. Instead, companies are turning to a process of ongoing assessment and feedback that emphasizes teamwork and shared leadership.

Accurate record keeping is another critical part of ensuring accuracy and fairness in the performance appraisal. Information about subordinate performance (both positive and negative) should be written down and not trusted to memory. The manager should make a habit of keeping notes about observations, others' comments, and his or her periodic review of charts and nursing care plans. When ongoing anecdotal notes are not maintained throughout the evaluation period, the appraiser is more apt to experience the *recency effect*, in which the importance of recent issues outweighs past performance (Smith, 2003).

Nothing delights employees more than discovering their immediate supervisor is aware of their growth and accomplishments and can cite specific instances in which good clinical judgment was used.

Collected assessments should contain positive examples of growth and achievement and areas where development is needed. Nothing delights employees more than discovering their immediate supervisor is aware of their growth and accomplishments and can cite specific instances in which good clinical judgment was used. Too frequently, collected data concentrate on negative aspects of performance.

Some effort must be made to include the employee's own appraisal of his or her work. Self-appraisal may be performed in several appropriate ways. Employees can be instructed to come to the appraisal interview with some informal thoughts about their performance, or they can work with their managers in completing a joint assessment. One advantage of *management by objectives* (MBO)—the use of personalized goals to measure individual performance—is the manner in which it involves the employee in assessing his or her work performance and in goal setting.

Lastly, the appraiser needs to guard against the three common pitfalls of assessment: the halo effect, the horns effect, and central tendency. The *halo effect* occurs when the appraiser lets one or two positive aspects of the assessment or behavior of the employee unduly influence all other aspects of the employee's performance. The *horns effect* occurs when the appraiser allows some negative aspects of the employee's performance to influence the assessment to such an extent that other levels of job performance are not accurately recorded. The manager who falls into the *central tendency* trap is hesitant to risk true assessment and therefore rates all employees as average. These appraiser behaviors lead employees to discount the

Learning Exercise 24.2

Planning an Employee's First Performance Appraisal
Mrs. Jones is a new LVN/LPN and has been working 3 P.M. to 11 P.M. on the long-term care unit where you are the PM charge nurse. It is time for her three-month performance appraisal. In your facility, each employee's job description is used as the standard of measure for performance appraisal.

Essentially, you believe Mrs. Jones is performing her job well but are somewhat concerned because she still relies on the RNs for even minor patient care decisions. Although you are glad that she does not act completely on her own, you would like to see her become more independent. The patients have commented favorably to you on Mrs. Jones' compassion and on her follow-through on all their requests and needs.

Mrs. Jones gets along well with the other LVNs/LPNs, and you sometimes believe they take advantage of her hard-working and pleasant nature. On a few occasions, you believe they inappropriately delegated some of their work to her.

When preparing for Mrs. Jones' upcoming evaluation, what can you do to make the appraisal as objective as possible? You want Mrs. Jones' first evaluation to be growth producing.

Assignment: Plan how you will proceed. What positive forces are already present in this scenario? What negative forces will you have to overcome? Support your plan with readings from the bibliography at the end of this chapter.

Display 24.3	**Strategies to Ensure Performance Appraisal Accuracy**

Develop self-awareness regarding own biases and prejudices.
Use appropriate consultation.
Gather data adequately over period of time.
Keep accurate anecdotal records for length of appraisal period.
Collect positive data and areas where improvement is needed.
Include employee's own appraisal of their performance.
Guard against halo effect, horns effect, and central tendency trap.

entire assessment of their work. See **Display 24.3** for a summary of performance appraisal strategies.

PERFORMANCE APPRAISAL TOOLS

Since the 1920s, many appraisal tools have been developed. Certain types of tools or review techniques have been popular at different times. Since the early 1990s, the Joint Commission on Accreditation of Healthcare Organizations (JCAHO) has been advocating the use of an employee's job description as the standard for performance appraisal. Currently, JCAHO mandates that acute care hospitals assess, measure, prove, track, and trend the age-specific competency of staff members with specific job titles (Krozek & Scoggins, 2001). In other words, employers must be able to demonstrate that employees know how to plan, implement, and evaluate care specific to the ages of the patients they care for. This continual refinement of critical competencies for professional nursing practice has a tremendous impact on the tools used in the appraisal process.

However, JCAHO makes it very clear that *competence assessments* are not the same as performance evaluations. A competence assessment evaluates whether an individual has the knowledge, education, skills, experience, and proficiency to perform assigned responsibilities; a performance evaluation assesses how well an individual actually performs (Herringer, 2002).

The effectiveness of a performance appraisal system is only as good as the tools used to create those assessments. An effective competence assessment tool should allow the manager to focus on priority measures of performance. The following is an overview of some of the appraisal tools commonly used in healthcare organizations.

Trait Rating Scales

A *rating scale* is a method of rating a person against a set standard, which may be the job description, desired behaviors, or personal traits. The rating scale is probably the most widely used of the many available appraisal methods.

Rating personal traits and behaviors is the oldest type of rating scale. Many experts argue, however, that the quality or quantity of the work performed is a more

Display 24.4	Sample Trait Rating Scale			
Job Knowledge				
Serious gaps in essential knowledge	Satisfactory knowledge of routine	Adequately informed on most phases	Good knowledge of all phases of job	Excellent understanding of the job
1	2	3	4	5
Judgment				
Decisions are often wrong on issues	Makes some decision errors	Good decisions	Sound and logical thinker	Makes good, complex decisions
1	2	3	4	5
Attitude				
Resents suggestions, no enthusiasm	Apathetic but cooperative and accepting	Generally cooperative of new ideas	Openly cooperates and accepts new ideas	Consistently helpful and enthusiastic
1	2	3	4	5

accurate performance appraisal method than the employee's personal traits and that trait evaluation invites subjectivity. Rating scales also are subject to central tendency and halo- and horns-effect errors and thus are not used as often today as they were in the past. Instead, many organizations use two other rating methods, namely the job dimension scale and the behaviorally anchored rating scale (BARS). **Display 24.4** shows a portion of a trait rating scale with examples of traits that might be expected in a registered nurse.

Job Dimension Scales

This technique requires that a rating scale be constructed for each job classification. The rating factors are taken from the context of the written job description. Although job dimension scales share some of the same weaknesses as trait scales, they do focus on job requirements rather than on ambiguous terms such as "quantity of work." **Display 24.5** shows an example of a job dimension scale for an industrial nurse.

Behaviorally Anchored Rating Scales

BARS, sometimes called *behavioral expectation scales,* overcome some of the weaknesses inherent in other rating systems. As in the job dimension method, the BARS technique requires that a separate rating form be developed for each job classification. Then, as in the job dimension rating scales, employees in specific positions work with management to delineate key areas of responsibility. However, in BARS, many specific examples are defined for each area of responsibility; these examples are given various degrees of importance by ranking them from 1 to 9. If

Display 24.5	Sample Job Dimension Rating Scale for an Industrial Nurse					

Job Dimension	5	4	3	2	1
Renders first aid and treats job-related injuries and illnesses					
Holds fitness classes for workers					
Teaches health and nutrition classes					
Performs yearly physicals on workers					
Keeps equipment in good working order and maintains inventory					
Keeps appropriate records					
Dispenses medication and treatment for minor injuries					

(5 = Excellent; 4 = Good; 3 = Satisfactory; 2 = Fair; 1 = Poor)

the highest-ranked example of a job dimension is being met, it is less important than a lower-ranked example that is not.

Appraisal tools firmly grounded in desired behaviors can be used to improve performance and keep employees focused on the vision and mission of the organization. However, because separate BARS are needed for each job, the greatest disadvantage in using this tool with large numbers of employees is the time and expense. BARS also are primarily applicable to physically observable skills rather than to conceptual skills. However, this is an effective tool because it focuses on specific behaviors, allows employees to know exactly what is expected of them, and reduces rating errors.

Although all rating scales are prone to weaknesses and interpersonal bias, they do have some advantages. Many may be purchased, and although they must be individualized to the organization, there is little need for expensive worker hours to develop them. Rating scales also force the rater to look at more than one dimension of work performance, which eliminates some bias.

Checklists

There are several types of *checklist* appraisal tools. The *weighted scale,* the most frequently used checklist, is composed of many behavioral statements that represent desirable job behaviors. Each of these behavior statements has a weighted score attached to it. Employees receive an overall performance appraisal score based on behaviors or attributes. Often merit raises are tied to the total point score (i.e., the employee needs to reach a certain score to receive an increase in pay).

Another type of checklist, the *forced checklist,* requires that the supervisor select an undesirable and a desirable behavior for each employee. Both desirable and undesirable behaviors have quantitative values, and the employee again ends up with a total score on which certain employment decisions are made.

Another type of checklist is the *simple checklist.* The simple checklist is composed of numerous words or phrases describing various employee behaviors or traits. These descriptors are often clustered to represent different aspects of one dimension of behavior, such as assertiveness or interpersonal skills. The rater is asked to check all those that describe the employee on each checklist.

A major weakness of all checklists is that there are no set performance standards. In addition, specific components of behavior are not addressed. Checklists do, however, focus on a variety of job-related behaviors and avoid some of the bias inherent in the trait-rating scales.

Essays

The *essay* appraisal method is often referred to as the *free-form review*. The appraiser describes in narrative form an employee's strengths and areas where improvement or growth is needed. Although this method can be unstructured, it usually calls for certain items to be addressed. This technique has some strengths because it forces the appraiser to focus on positive aspects of the employee's performance. However, a greater opportunity for personal bias undoubtedly exists.

Many organizations combine various types of appraisals to improve the quality of their review processes. Because the essay method does not require exhaustive development, it can quickly be adapted as an adjunct to any type of structured format. This gives the organization the ability to decrease bias and focus on employee strengths.

Self-Appraisals

Employees are increasingly being asked to submit written summaries or *portfolios* of their work-related accomplishments and productivity as part of the self-appraisal process. Portfolios often provide examples of how the employee has implemented clinical guidelines and achieved patient outcomes, as well as including sample patient care documentation (Taylor, 2000). The portfolio also generally includes the employee's goals and an action plan for accomplishing these goals.

There are advantages and disadvantages to using *self-appraisal* as a method of performance review. Although introspection and self-appraisal result in growth when the person is self-aware, even mature people require external feedback and performance validation.

Some employees may look on their annual performance review as an opportunity to receive positive feedback from their supervisor, especially if the employee receives infrequent praise on a day-to-day basis. Asking these employees to perform their own performance appraisal would probably be viewed negatively rather than positively.

In addition, some employees undervalue their accomplishments or may feel uncomfortable giving themselves high marks in many areas. In an effort to avoid this potential influence on their rating, managers may wish to complete the performance appraisal tool before reading the employee's self-analysis, or they should view the self-appraisal as only one of a number of sources of data that should be collected when evaluating worker performance. When self-appraisal is not congruent with other data available, the manager may wish to pursue the reasons for this discrepancy during the appraisal conference. Such an exchange may provide valuable insight regarding the worker's self-awareness and ability to view himself or herself objectively.

Management by Objectives (MBO)

MBO is an excellent tool for determining an individual employee's progress because it incorporates the assessments of the employee and the organization. The focus in this chapter, however, is on how these concepts are used as an effective performance appraisal method, rather than on their use as a planning technique.

Although it is not used frequently in health care, MBO is an excellent method to appraise the performance of the registered nurse in a manner that promotes individual growth and excellence in nursing. The following steps delineate how MBO can be used effectively in performance appraisal:

> ➤ In management by objectives, the focus is on the controllable present and future rather than the uncontrollable past.

1. The employee and supervisor meet and agree on the principal duties and responsibilities of the employee's job. (The job description serves as a guide only.) This is done as soon as possible after beginning employment.
2. The employee sets short-term goals and target dates in cooperation with the supervisor or manager. The manager guides the process so it relates to the position's duties. In addition, the subordinate's goals must not be in conflict with the goals of the organization. In setting goals, it is important that the manager remember that one's values and beliefs simply reflect a single set of options among many; this is especially true in working with a multicultural staff (Taylor, 1998). Professional expectations and values can vary greatly among cultures, and the manager must be careful to resist judgmental reactions and allow for cultural differences in goal setting.
3. Both parties agree on the criteria that will be used for measuring and evaluating the accomplishment of goals. In addition, a time frame is set for completing the objectives, which depends on the nature of the work being planned. Common time frames used in healthcare organizations vary from one month to one year.
4. Regularly, but more than once a year, the employee and supervisor meet to discuss progress. At these meetings, some modifications can be made to the original goals if both parties agree. Major obstacles that block completion of objectives within the time frame are identified. In addition, the resources and support needed from others are identified.
5. The manager's role is supportive, assisting the employee to reach goals by coaching and counseling.
6. During the appraisal process, the manager determines whether the employee has met the goals.
7. The entire process focuses on outcomes and results and not on personal traits.

One of the many advantages of MBO is that the method creates a vested interest in the employee to accomplish goals because employees are able to set their own goals. Additionally, defensive feelings are minimized, and a spirit of teamwork prevails.

MBO as a performance appraisal method has its disadvantages. Highly directive and authoritarian managers find it difficult to lead employees in this manner. Also, the marginal employee frequently attempts to set easily attainable goals. However, research has shown that MBO, when used correctly, is a very effective method of performance appraisal.

Learning Exercise 24.3

Reviewing MBOs as a Part of Performance Appraisal

It is time for Nancy Irwin's annual performance appraisal. She is an RN on a postsurgical unit, dealing with complex trauma patients requiring high-level nursing intensity. You are the evening charge nurse and have worked with Ms. Irwin for the two years since she has graduated from nursing school. Last year, in addition to the regular 1 to 5 rating scale for job expectations, all the charge nurses added an MBO component to the performance appraisal form. In collaboration with his or her charge nurse, each employee developed five goals that were supposed to have been carried out over a one-year period.

In reviewing Ms. Irwin's performance, you use several sources, including your written notes and her charting, and your conclusion is that with her strengths and weaknesses, overall she is a better-than-average nurse. However, you believe she has not grown much as an employee over the past six months. This observation is confirmed by a review of the following:

Objective	Result
1. Conduct a mini-inservice or patient care conference twice monthly for the next 12 months.	Met goal first two months. Last 10 months conducted only six conferences.
2. Will attend five educational classes related to work area; at least one of these will be given by an outside agency.	Attended one surgical nursing wound conference in the city and one in-house conference on TPN.
3. Will become an active member of a nursing committee at the hospital.	Has become an active member of the Policies and Procedures Committee and regularly attends meetings.
4. Reduce the number of late arrivals at work by 50% (from 24 per year to 12).	First three months: not late. Second three months: three late arrivals. Third three months: six late arrivals. Last three months: six late arrivals.
5. Ensure that all patients discharged have discharge instructions documented in their charts.	Anecdotal notes show that Ms. Irwin still frequently forgets to document these nursing actions.

Assignment: As Ms. Irwin's charge nurse, what can you do to ensure that the current appraisal results in greater growth for her? What went wrong with last year's MBO plan? Devise a plan for the performance appraisal.

Analysis: This case could have several different approaches, depending on whether motivation or change theory or another rationale was being implemented to support the decisions. In reality, a manager may employ several different theories in order to increase productivity. However, this case will be solved using only performance appraisal techniques in order to demonstrate that they can also serve as an effective method to control productivity.

There are several aspects that seem to stand out in the information presented in this case. First, it appears that Ms. Irwin is a person who needs to be reminded. She functions well in objective #3 because she received monthly reminders of the meetings, and because she worked with a group of people she was able to make a real contribution to this committee. The similarities among the other four objectives are that (1) they all required Ms. Irwin to work alone to accomplish them and (2) there were no built-in reminders.

Rather than viewing this performance appraisal critically, the charge nurse should expend her energy in developing a plan to help Ms. Irwin succeed in the coming months. Nothing is as depressing or demotivating to an employee as failure. The following plan concentrates only on the MBO portion of Ms. Irwin's performance appraisal and does not center on the rating scale of job performance.

Prior to the Interview	*Rationale*
1. Ask Ms. Irwin to review her objectives from last year and to come prepared to discuss them.	1. Gives the employee opportunity for individual problem solving and personal introspection.
2. Set a convenient time for you and Ms. Irwin and allow adequate time and privacy.	2. Shows interest in and respect for the employee.

At the Interview	*Rationale*
1. Begin by complimenting Ms. Irwin on meeting objective #3. Ask her about her work on the committee, what procedures she is working on, and so forth.	1. Shows interest in and support of employee.
2. Review each of the other four objectives and ask for Ms. Irwin's input. Withhold any evidence or criticism at this point.	2. Allows the employee to make her own judgments about her performance.
3. Ask Ms. Irwin if she sees a pattern.	3. Guide the employee into problem solving on her own.
4. Tell Ms. Irwin that MBO often works better if objectives are reviewed on a more timely basis and ask how she feels about this.	4. This is an offer to assist the employee in achieving improved performance and is not a punitive measure. It allows employee to have input.
5. Suggest that she keep her unmet four objectives and add one new one.	5. Employees should be encouraged to meet objectives unless they were stated poorly or were unrealistic.

6. Work with Ms. Irwin in developing a reminder or check point system that will assist her in meeting her objectives.
7. Do not sympathize or excuse her for not meeting objectives.
8. End on a note of encouragement and support: "I know that you are capable of meeting these objectives."

6. Again, this is helping the employee to succeed. Do not simply tell employees that they should do better; help them identify how.
7. The focus should remain on growth and not on the status quo.
8. Employees often live up to their manager's expectations of them, and if those expectations are for growth, then the chances are greater that it will occur.

Peer Review

> Peer review, when implemented properly, provides the employee with valuable feedback that can promote growth.

When peers rather than supervisors carry out monitoring and assessing work performance, it is referred to as *peer review*. Most likely, the manager's review of the employee is not complete unless some type of peer review data is gathered. Peer review provides feedback that can promote growth. It also can provide learning opportunities for the peer reviewers. Taylor (2000) suggests that peers who work together have a level of insight into each other's clinical practice, and that peer review provides employees with an opportunity to receive better feedback about self-improvement.

The concept of collegial evaluation of nursing practice is closely related to maintaining professional standards. Peer review has the potential for increased professionalism, performance, and professional accountability among practicing staff and is gaining popularity in the United States and internationally (Vuorinen, Tarkka, & Meretoja, 2000). Although the prevailing practice in most organizations is to have managers evaluate employee performance, there is much to be said for collegial review.

Peer review is widely used in medicine and by faculty in universities; however, healthcare organizations have been slow to adopt peer review for the following five reasons:

1. Staff are poorly oriented to the peer review method. Peer review is viewed as very threatening when inadequate time is spent orienting employees to the process and when necessary support is not provided throughout the process.
2. Peers feel uncomfortable sharing feedback with people with whom they work closely, so they omit needed suggestions for improving the employee's performance. Thus, the review becomes more advocacy than evaluation.
3. Peer review is viewed by many as more time-consuming than traditional superior–subordinate performance appraisals.
4. Because much socialization takes place in the workplace, friendships often result in inflated evaluations, or interpersonal conflict may result in unfair appraisals.
5. Because peer review shifts the authority away from management, the insecure manager may feel threatened.

Peer review has its shortcomings, as evidenced by some university teachers receiving unjustified tenure or the failure of physicians to maintain adequate quality control among some individuals in their profession. Additionally, peer review involves much risk taking, is time-consuming, and requires a great deal of energy. However, nursing as a profession should be responsible for setting the standards and then monitoring its own performance. Because performance appraisal may be viewed as a type of quality control, it seems reasonable to expect that nurses should have some input into the performance evaluation process of their profession's members.

Peer review can be carried out in several ways. The process may require the reviewers to share the results only with the person being reviewed, or the results may be shared with the employee's supervisor and the employee. The review would never be shared only with the employee's supervisor.

The results may or may not be used for personnel decisions. The number of observations, number of reviewers, qualification and classification of the peer reviewer, and procedure need to be developed for each organization. If peer review is to succeed, the organization must overcome its inherent difficulties by doing the following before implementing a peer review program:

- Peer review appraisal tools must reflect standards to be measured, such as the job description.
- Staff must receive a thorough orientation to the process before its implementation. The role of the manager should be clearly defined.
- Ongoing support, resources, and information must be made available to the staff during the process.
- Data for peer review need to be obtained from predetermined sources, such as observations, charts, and patient care plans.
- A decision must be made about whether anonymous feedback will be allowed. This is controversial and needs to be addressed in the procedure.
- Decisions must be reached on whether the peer review will affect personnel decisions and, if so, in what manner.

Peer review has the potential to increase the accuracy of performance appraisal. It also can provide many opportunities for increased professionalism and learning. The use of peer review in nursing should continue to expand as nursing increases its autonomy and professional status. See **Display 24.6** for a summary of types of performance appraisal tools.

Display 24.6 Summary of Performance Appraisal Tools

Trait rating scales: Rates an individual against some standard.

Job dimension scales: Rates the performance on job requirements.

Behaviorally anchored rating scales (BARS): Rates desired job expectations on a scale of importance to the position.

Checklists: Rates the performance against a set list of desirable job behaviors.

Essays: A narrative appraisal of job performance.

Self-appraisals: An appraisal of performance by the employee.

Management by objectives: Employee and management agree upon goals of performance to be reached.

Peer review: Assessment of work performance carried out by peers.

Learning Exercise 24.4

Addressing Mary's Change in Behavior

Even in organizations that have no formal peer review process, professionals must take some responsibility for colleagues' work performance, even if informally. The following scenario illustrates the need for peer involvement.

Since your graduation from nursing school, you have worked at Memorial Hospital. Your school room mate, Mary, also has worked at Memorial since her graduation. For the first year, you and Mary were assigned to different units, but you both were transferred to the oncology unit six months ago.

You both work 3 P.M. to 11 P.M., and it is the policy for the charge nurse duties to alternate among three RNs assigned to the unit on a full-time basis. Both you and Mary are among the nurses assigned to rotate to the charge position. You have noticed lately that when Mary is in charge, her personality seems to change; she barks orders and seems tense and anxious.

She is an excellent clinical nurse, and many of the staff seek her out in consultation about patient care problems. You have, however, heard several of the staff grumbling about Mary's behavior when she is in charge. As Mary's good friend, you do not want to hurt her feelings, but as her colleague you feel a need to be honest and open with her.

Assignment: A very difficult situation occurs when personal and working relationships are combined. Describe what, if anything, you would do. Use the readings from the Bibliography to assist you in making a plan.

PLANNING THE APPRAISAL INTERVIEW

> The most accurate and thorough appraisal will fail to produce growth in employees if the information gathered is not used appropriately.

The most accurate and thorough appraisal will fail to produce growth in employees if the information gathered is not used appropriately. Many appraisal interviews have negative outcomes because the manager views them as a time to instruct employees only on what they are doing wrong, rather than looking at strengths as well.

Managers often dislike the appraisal interview more than the actual data gathering. One of the reasons managers dislike the appraisal interview is because of their own negative experiences when they have been judged unfairly or criticized personally. Both parties in the appraisal process tend to be anxious before the interview; thus, the appraisal interview remains an emotionally charged event. For many employees, past appraisals have been traumatizing. Although little can be done to eliminate the often-negative emotions created by past experiences, the leader–manager can manage the interview in such a manner that people will not be traumatized further.

OVERCOMING APPRAISAL INTERVIEW DIFFICULTIES

Feedback, perhaps the greatest tool a manager has for changing behavior, must be given in an appropriate manner. There is a greater chance that the performance appraisal will have a positive outcome if certain conditions are present before, during, and after the interview.

Before the Interview

- Make sure that the conditions mentioned previously have been met (e.g., the employee knows the standard by which his or her work will be evaluated), and he or she has a copy of the appraisal form.
- Select an appropriate time for the appraisal conference. Do not choose a time when the employee has just had a traumatic personal event or is too busy at work to take the time needed for a meaningful conference.
- Give the employee a two- to three-day advance notice of the scheduled appraisal conference so he or she can be prepared mentally and emotionally for the interview.
- Be personally prepared mentally and emotionally for the conference. If something should happen to interfere with your readiness for the interview, it should be canceled and rescheduled.
- Schedule uninterrupted interview time. Hold the interview in a private, quiet, and comfortable place. Forward your telephone calls to another line and ask another manager to answer any pages you may have during the performance appraisal.
- Plan a seating arrangement that reflects collegiality rather than power. Having the person seated across a large desk from the appraiser denotes a power–status position; placing the chairs side by side denotes collegiality.

During the Interview

- Greet the employee warmly, showing that the manager and the organization have a sincere interest in his or her growth.
- Begin the conference on a pleasant, informal note.
- Ask the employee to comment on his or her progress since the last performance appraisal.
- Avoid surprises in the appraisal conference. The effective leader coaches and communicates informally with staff on a continual basis, so there should be little new information at an appraisal conference. Cohen (2000) goes so far as to assert that if the employee first hears about a performance concern during the appraisal, the manager has not been doing his or her job.
- Use coaching techniques throughout the conference.
- When dealing with an employee who has several problems—either new or long-standing—don't overwhelm him or her at the conference. If there are too many problems to be addressed, select the major ones.
- Conduct the conference in a nondirective and participatory manner. Input from the employee should be solicited throughout the interview; however, the manager must recognize that employees from some cultures may be hesitant to provide this type of input. In this situation, the manager must continually reassure the employee that such input is not only acceptable but desired.

- Focus on the employee's performance and not on his or her personal characteristics.
- Avoid vague generalities, either positive or negative, such as "your skills need a little work" or "your performance is fine." Be prepared with explicit performance examples. Be liberal in the positive examples of employee performance; use examples of poor performance sparingly. Use several examples only if the employee has difficulty with self-awareness and requests specific instances of a problem area.
- When delivering performance feedback, be straightforward and state concerns directly. Indirectness and ambiguity are more likely to inhibit communication than enhance it, and the employee is left unsure about the significance of the message.
- Never threaten, intimidate, or use status in any manner. The appraiser must make sure that the person's self-esteem is not threatened, because this will prevent the nurturing of a meaningful and constructive relationship between the manager and employee.
- Let the employee know that the organization and the manager are aware of his or her uniqueness, special interests, and valuable contributions to the unit. Remember that all employees make some special contribution to the workplace.
- Make every effort to ensure that there are no interruptions during the conference.
- Use terms and language that are clearly understood and carry the same meaning for both parties. Avoid words that have a negative connotation. Do not talk down to employees or use language that is inappropriate for their level of education.
- Mutually set goals for further growth or improvement in the employee's performance. Decide how goals will be accomplished and evaluated and what support is needed.
- Plan on being available for employees to return retrospectively to discuss the appraisal review further. There is frequently a need for the employee to return for elaboration if the conference did not go well or if the employee was given unexpected new information. This is especially true for the new employee.

After the Interview

- Both the manager and employee need to sign the appraisal form to document that the conference was held and that the employee received the appraisal information. This does not mean that the employee is agreeing to the information in the appraisal; it merely means the employee has read the appraisal. An example of such a form is shown in **Display 24.7.** There should be a place for comments by both the manager and the employee.
- End the interview on a pleasant note.
- Document the goals for further development that have been agreed on by both parties. The documentation should include target dates for accomplishment,

Display 24.7 Performance Appraisal Documentation Form

Performance appraisal for:

Name: _____

Unit: _____

Prepared by: _____

Reason: _____

(Merit, terminal, end of probation, general reviews)

Date of evaluation conference: _____

Comments by employee:

Employee's signature: _____

(Signature of employee denotes that the evaluation has been read. It *does not* signify acceptance or agreement. Space is provided for any comments employee wishes to make.)

Comments by evaluator:

(These comments are to be written at the time of the evaluation conference and in the presence of the employee.)

_____   _____
Employee's signature (Date)   Evaluator's signature (Date)

support needed, and when goals are to be reviewed. This documentation is often part of the appraisal form.

- If the interview reveals specific long-term coaching needs, the manager should develop a method of follow-up to ensure such coaching takes place.

PERFORMANCE MANAGEMENT

Some experts in human resource management have suggested that annual performance appraisals should be replaced by ongoing *performance management* (Coens, Jenkins, & Block, 2000; Fandray, 2001). In performance management, appraisals are eliminated. Instead, the manager places his or her efforts into ongoing coaching, mutual goal setting, and the leadership training of subordinates. This focus requires the manager to spend more regularly scheduled face-to-face time with subordinates. "Thus, it is people who are managed, rather than paper flow" (Fandray, 2001, p. 40).

In contrast to the annual performance review, which is usually associated with an employee's hire date, the performance management calendar is generally linked to the organization's business calendar (Weizmann, as cited in Fandray, 2001). This way, performance planning is coordinated throughout the entire organization. In this manner, strategic goals for the year can be identified and subordinates' roles to achieve those goals can be openly discussed and planned.

Weizmann also suggests that performance-managed organizations articulate a set of role-based competencies and let every employee know the five or six qualities that define success for every member of the organization, regardless of job description. Then employees can determine how these qualities translate into performance in specific jobs. Expectations, then, are not disputable; they are part of the agreed-upon roles assumed by subordinates (Fandray, 2001).

COACHING: A MECHANISM FOR INFORMAL PERFORMANCE APPRAISAL

Effective managers and astute leaders are aware that day-to-day feedback regarding performance is one of the best methods for improving work performance and building a team approach. The word *coaching* has become a contemporary term to convey the spirit of the manager's role in informal day-to-day performance appraisals. Coaching techniques also should be used in the formal appraisal interview but are especially effective for encouraging and correcting daily work performance. Performance coaching can help people through life transitions, can be instrumental in the mature development of an individual's basic values, can produce high performance in work or other aspects of people's lives, can help people develop a vision and purpose for their endeavors, and can help with career and life planning (Detmer, 2002; Robinson-Walker, 2002). Coaching can guide others into increased competence, commitment, and confidence as well as helping them to anticipate options for making vital connections between their present and future plans.

Manthey (2001) uses the terms *reflective practice* and *clinical coaching* to describe a management strategy that fuses both performance coaching and performance management. In clinical coaching, the manager or mentor meets with an employee regularly to discuss aspects of his or her work. Both individuals determine the agenda jointly with the goal of an environment of learning that can span the personal and professional aspects of the employee's experience. During clinical coaching, employees can discuss things that have made them feel angry or discouraged. They can also get new ideas and information about how to deal with situations from someone who often has experienced the same problems and issues. This shared connection between the manager and employee makes the employee feel validated and part of a larger team. When coaching is combined with informal performance appraisal, the outcome is usually a positive modification of behavior. For this to occur, however, the leader must establish a climate in which there is a free exchange of ideas.

Robinson-Walker (2002) suggests that certain managerial skills are necessary for coaching to succeed and improve work performance. The following tactics will assist managers in becoming effective coaches:

- Be specific, not general, in describing behavior that needs improvement.
- Be descriptive, not evaluative, when describing what was wrong with the work performance.

- Be certain that the feedback is not self-serving but meets the needs of the employee.
- Direct the feedback toward behavior that can be changed.
- Use sensitivity in timing the feedback.
- Make sure the employee has clearly understood the feedback and that the employee's communication also has been clearly heard.

When employees believe that their manager is interested in their performance and personal growth, they will have less fear of the work performance appraisal. When that anxiety is reduced, the formal performance interview process can be used to set mutual performance goals.

INTEGRATING LEADERSHIP ROLES AND MANAGEMENT FUNCTIONS IN CONDUCTING PERFORMANCE APPRAISALS

Performance appraisal is a major responsibility in the controlling function of management. The ability to conduct meaningful, effective performance appraisals requires an investment of time, effort, and practice on the part of the manager. Although performance appraisal is never easy, if used appropriately it produces growth in the employee and increases productivity in the organization.

To increase the likelihood of successful performance appraisal, managers should use a formalized system of appraisal and gather data about employee performance in a systematic manner, using many sources. The manager also should attempt to be as objective as possible, using established standards for the appraisal. The result of the appraisal process should provide the manager with information for meeting training and educational needs of employees. By following up conscientiously on identified performance deficiencies, employees' work problems can be corrected before they become habits.

Integrating leadership into this part of the controlling phase of the management process provides an opportunity for sharing, communicating, and growing. The integrated leader–manager is self-aware regarding his or her own biases and prejudices. This self-awareness leads to fairness and honesty in evaluating performance. This, in turn, increases trust in the manager and promotes a team spirit among employees.

The leader also uses day-to-day coaching techniques to improve work performance and reduce the anxiety of performance appraisal. When anxiety is reduced during the appraisal interview, the leader–manager is able to establish a relationship of mutual goal setting, which has a greater potential to result in increased motivation and corrected deficiencies. The result of the integration of leadership and management is a performance appraisal that facilitates employee growth and increases organizational productivity.

❋ Key Concepts

- The employee *performance appraisal* is a sensitive and important part of the management process, requiring much skill.
- When accurate and appropriate appraisal assessments are performed, the outcomes can be very positive.

- Performance appraisals are used to determine how well employees are performing their job, using the job description as a standard of measurement.
- There are many different types of *appraisal tools,* and selection of the most appropriate tool varies with the type of appraisal to be done and the criteria to be measured.
- The employee must be involved in the appraisal process and must view the appraisal as accurate and fair.
- *Management by objectives* (MBO) has proven to increase productivity and commitment in employees.
- *Peer review* has great potential for developing professional accountability.
- Unless the appraisal interview is carried out in an appropriate and effective manner, the performance appraisal data will be useless.
- Due to past experiences, performance appraisal interviews are highly charged, emotional events for most employees.
- Showing a genuine interest in the employee's growth and seeking his or her input at the interview will increase the likelihood of a positive outcome from the appraisal process.
- Performance appraisals should be signed to show that feedback was given to the employee.
- Informal work performance appraisals are an important management function.
- Leaders should routinely use appropriate coaching techniques to improve work performance on an informal basis.
- In *performance management*, appraisals are eliminated. Instead, the manager places his or her efforts into ongoing coaching, mutual goal setting, and the leadership training of subordinates.

More Learning Exercises and Applications

 Learning Exercise 24.5

Requesting Feedback from Employees
You are the director of a home health agency. You have just returned from a management course and have been inspired by the idea of requesting input from your subordinates about your performance as a manager.

You realize that there are some risks involved but believe the potential benefits from the feedback outweigh the risks. However, you want to provide some structure for the evaluation, so you spend some time designing your appraisal tool and developing your plan.

Assignment: What type of tool will you use? What is your overall goal? Will you share the results of the appraisal with anyone else? How will you use the information obtained? Would you have the appraisal forms signed or anonymous? Who would you include in the group evaluating you? Be able to support your ideas with appropriate rationale.

Learning Exercise 24.6

Making Appraisal Interviews Less Traumatic

You are the new night-shift charge nurse in a large intensive care unit composed of an all-RN staff. When you were appointed to the position, your supervisor told you there had been some complaints regarding the manner in which the previous charge nurse had handled evaluation sessions.

Not wanting to repeat the mistakes, you draw up a list of things you could do to make the evaluation interviews less traumatic. Because the evaluation tool appears adequate, you believe the problems must lie with the interview itself. You put at the top of your list that you will make sure each employee has advance notice of the evaluation.

Assignment: How much advance notice should you give? What additional criteria would you add to the list to help eliminate much of the trauma that frequently accompanies performance appraisal (even when the appraisal is very good)?

Add six to nine items to the list. Explain why you think each of these would assist in alleviating some of the anxiety associated with performance appraisals. Do not just repeat the guidelines listed in this chapter. You may make the guidelines more specific or use the Bibliography for assistance in developing your own list.

 Learning Exercise 24.7

Helping a Seasoned Employee to Grow

Patty Brown is an LVN/LPN who has been employed on your unit for 10 years. She is an older woman and is very sensitive to criticism. Her work is generally of high quality, but in reviewing her past performance appraisals, you notice that during the last 10 years, at least seven times she has been rated unsatisfactory for not being on duty promptly and eight times for not attending staff development programs. Because you are the new charge nurse, you would like to help Patty grow in these two areas.

You have given Patty a copy of the evaluation tool and her job description and have scheduled her appraisal conference for a time when the unit will be quiet. You can conduct the appraisal in the conference room.

Assignment: How would you conduct this performance appraisal? Outline your plan. Include how you would begin. What innovative or creative way would you attempt to provide direction or improvement in the areas mentioned? How would you terminate the session? Be able to give rationale for your decisions.

Learning Exercise 24.8

Could This Conflict Have Been Prevented?

Mr. Jones, a 49-year-old automobile salesman, was admitted with severe back pain. As his primary care nurse, you have established a rapport with Mr. Jones. He has a type A personality and has been very critical of much of his hospitalization. He also was very upset by the quality and quantity of his pain following his laminectomy.

You agreed to ambulate him on your shift three times (at 4 P.M., 7 P.M., and 10:30 P.M.) so he would need to be ambulated only once during the day shift. He does not care for many of the day staff and feels that you help ambulate him better than anyone else. You noted the ambulating routine on his nursing orders.

Yesterday, Joan Martin, a day nurse, believed his bowel sounds were somewhat diminished. She urged him to ambulate more on the day shift, but he refused to do so. (The doctor had ordered ambulation q.i.d.) When Mr. Jones' physician visited, nurse Martin told him that Mr. Jones ambulated only once on the shift. She did not elaborate further to the doctor. The physician proceeded to talk very sternly with Mr. Jones, telling him to get out of bed three times today. Nurse Martin did not mention this incident to you in report.

By the time you arrived on duty and received report, Mr. Jones was very angry. He threatened to sign himself out against medical advice. You talked with his doctor, got the order changed, and finally managed to calm Mr. Jones down. You then wrote a nursing order that read, "nurse Martin is not to be assigned to Mr. Jones again."

When Joan Martin came on duty this morning, the night shift pointed out your notation. She was very angry and went to see the head nurse.

Assignment: Should you have done anything differently? If so, what? Could the evaluation of clinical performance by you and nurse Martin have been done in a manner that would not have resulted in conflict? If you were nurse Martin, what could you have done to prevent the conflict? Be able to discuss this case in relation to professional trust, peer review, and assertive communication.

Learning Exercise 24.9

Addressing Sally's Errors in Judgment

You are a senior baccalaureate nursing student. This is your sixth week of a medical–surgical advanced practicum. Your instructor assigns two students to work together caring for four to six patients. The students alternate fulfilling leader and follower roles and providing total patient care. This is the second full day you have worked as a team with Sally Brown.

Last week, when you were assigned with Sally, she was the leader and made numerous errors in judgment. She got a patient up who was on strict bed rest. She made an intravenous medication error by giving a medication to the wrong patient. She gave morphine too soon because she forgot to record the time in the medication record, and she frequently did not seem to know what was wrong with her patients.

Today, you have been the leader and have observed her contaminate a dressing and forget to check armbands twice when she was giving medications. When you asked her about checking placement of the nasogastric tube, she did not know how to perform this skill. You have heard some of the other students complain about Sally.

Assignment: What is your obligation to your patients, your fellow students, the clinical agency, and your instructor? Outline what you would do. Give rationale for your decisions.

Web Links

Coaching the Caterpillar to Fly: A program for development
http://www.squarewheels.com/coaching/coachcat.html
Interactive "square wheels" exercise and butterfly metaphor that emphasize coaching as a technique for creating trust and team building in organizations.

Guide to Performance Management:
http://www-hr.ucsd.edu/~staffeducation/guide/
Includes overview of performance management, standards of performance, observation and feedback, the appraisal process, performance appraisal models forms, and a bibliography.

Performance Appraisal
http://www.performance-appraisal.com/intro.htm
Outlines basic purposes, methods, benefits, reward issues, conflict and confrontation, common mistakes, and bias effects associated with performance appraisal.

References

Coens, T., Jenkins, M., & Block, P., (2000). *Abolishing performance appraisals: Why they backfire and what to do instead.* San Francisco, CA: Berrett-Koehler Publishers.

Cohen, S. (2000). Managers' fast track. Prepare for your best employee evaluation yet. *Nursing Management, 31*(10), 8.

Detmer, S. S. (2002). Coaching your unit team for results. *Seminars for Nurse Managers, 10*(3), 189–195.

Fandray, D. (2001). The new thinking in performance appraisals. *Workforce, 80*(5), 36–40.

Herringer, J. (2002). Once isn't enough when measuring staff competence. *Nursing Management, 33*(2), 22.

Krozek, C., & Scoggins, A. (2001). *Age-specific competence ... amended to comply with 2001 JCAHO standards.* Glendale, CA: Cinahl Information Systems.

Manthey, M. (2001). Reflective practice. *Creative Nursing, 7*(2), 3–5.

McMurray, C. (1993). Performance appraisal: A measure of effectiveness. *Nursing management, 24*(11), 94–95.

Robinson-Walker, C. (2002). The role of coaching in creating cultures of engagement. *Seminars for Nurse Managers, 10*(2), 150–156.

Rudan, V. T. (2003). The best of both worlds: A consideration of gender in team building. *Journal of Nursing Administration, 33*(3), 179–186.

Smith, M. H. (2003). Empower staff with praiseworthy appraisals. *Nursing Management, 34*(1), 15–18.

Taylor, K. (2000). Tackling the issue of nurse competency. *Nursing Management, 31*(9), 35–37.

Taylor, R. (1998). Check your cultural competence. *Nursing Management, 29*(8), 30–32.

Vuorinen, R., Tarkka, M.. & Meretoja, R. (2000). Peer evaluation in nurses' professional development: A pilot study to investigate the issues. *Journal of Clinical Nursing, 9*(8), 273–281.

Welford, C. (2002). Matching theory to practice. *Nursing Management-UK, 9*(4), 7–12.

Bibliography

Barber, J. L. (2002). A journey into foreign territory: the coach as tour guide. *Seminars for Nurse Managers, 10*(1), 61–67.

Black, R. (2000). On the job: Performance appraisals. Giving and getting feedback. *Canadian Nurse, 96*(7), 37.

Delgado, C. (2002). Student issues. A peer-reviewed program for senior proficiencies. *Nurse Educator, 27*(5), 212–213.

Dolan, G. (2003). Assessing student nurse clinical competency: Will we ever get it right? *Clinical Nurse, 12*(1), 132–141.

Dutton, G. (2001). Making reviews more efficient and fair. *Workforce, 80*(4), 76–82.

Flynn, G. (2001). Getting performance reviews right. *Workforce, 80*(5), 76–77.

Mathews, D. E. (2000). Developing a perioperative peer performance appraisal system. *AORN Journal, 72*(6), 1039–1042, 1044, 1046.

Metcalf, C. (2001, February). The importance of performance appraisal and staff development: A graduating nurse's perspective. *International Journal of Nursing Practice, 1*, 54–46.

Nelson, B. (2000). Are performance appraisals obsolete? *Compensation & Benefits Review, 32*(3), 39–43.

Pulce, R. (2002). Optimising human capital. Performance management. *Seminar for Nurse Managers, 10*(2), 83.

Rotarius, T., & Liberman, A. (2000). Objective employee assessments—Establishing a balance among supervisory evaluations. *Health Care Manager, 18*(4), 1–6.

Scanlan, J. M., Care, W. D., & Gessler, S. (2001). Dealing with the unsafe student in clinical practice. *Nurse Educator, 26*(1), 23–27.

Vuorinen, R., Tarkka, M., & Meretoja, R. (2000). Peer evaluation in nurses' professional development: A pilot study to investigate the issues. *Journal of Clinical Nursing, 9*(2), 273–281.

Wiles, L. L., & Bishop, J. F. (2001). Educational innovations. Clinical performance appraisal: Renewing graded clinical experiences. *Journal of Nursing Education, 40*(1), 37–39.

Zurlinden, J. (2002). Perspectives in leadership. Preparing for a performance review. *Nursing Spectrum, (Florida), 12*(13), 6.

Problem Employees: Rule Breakers, Marginal Employees, and the Chemically or Mentally Impaired

Self-respect is the fruit of discipline; the sense of dignity grows with the ability to say no to oneself. . . .

—Abraham J. Heschel

Employees' perceptions of what they owe the organization and what they owe themselves vary. At times, organizational and individual needs, wants, and responsibilities are in conflict. The coordination and cooperation needed to meet organizational goals require leader–managers to control individual subordinates' urges that are counterproductive to these goals. Subordinates do this by self-control. Managers meet organizational goals by enforcing established rules, policies, and procedures. Leaders do this by creating a supportive and motivating climate and by coaching.

When employees are unsuccessful in meeting organizational goals, managers must attempt to identify reasons for this failure and counsel these employees accordingly. If employees fail because they are unwilling to follow rules or established policies and procedures, or they are unable to perform their duties adequately despite assistance and encouragement, the manager has an obligation to take disciplinary action. However, progressive discipline is inappropriate for employees who are impaired as a result of disease or degree of ability. These employees have special problems and needs and require active coaching, support, and often professional counseling to maintain productivity. Managers must be able to distinguish between employees needing discipline and those who are impaired so that employees can be managed most appropriately.

Regardless of the cause, however, supervisors should be quick to recognize and address inappropriate conduct and poor work performance. Delay only exacerbates such situations (Rafes & Warren, 2001). Indeed, Baum (2000) argues that most employees are confronted by coworkers' sub-par performance on a daily basis. When someone is not performing well, everyone knows it. And when management refuses to act, employees may perceive that their leaders lack the resolve necessary to make the organization successful.

> Not disciplining an employee who should be disciplined jeopardizes an organization's morale.

This chapter focuses on discipline, coaching, and referral as tools in promoting subordinates' growth and meeting organizational goals. The normal progression of steps taken in disciplinary action and strategies for administering discipline fairly and effectively are delineated. Formal and informal grievances are discussed.

In addition, this chapter focuses on two types of employees with special needs: the marginal employee and the impaired employee. Marginal employees are those employees who disrupt unit functioning because the quantity or quality of their work consistently meets only minimal standards. This chapter identifies the challenges inherent in working with marginal employees and presents managerial strategies for dealing with these problem employees.

Impairment, for purposes of this discussion, refers to employees who are unable to accomplish their work at the expected level, as a result of chemical or psychological disease. While the emphasis in this chapter is on chemical impairment (impairment due to drug or alcohol addiction), psychological impairment is increasingly being recognized as a significant problem for employees and the strategies used to deal with both types of impairment often overlap. This chapter profiles chemical addiction among nurses as well as behaviors common to chemically impaired nurses. Steps in the recovery process and the reentry of the recovering chemically impaired nurse into the workforce are also discussed. Leadership roles and management functions appropriate for use with problem employees are shown in **Display 25.1.**

Display 25.1	**Leadership Roles and Management Functions in Creating a Growth-Producing Work Environment Through Discipline and Coaching**

Leadership Roles

1. Recognizes and reinforces the intrinsic self-worth of each employee and the role of successful work performance in maintaining a positive self-image.
2. Encourages employees to be self-disciplined in conforming to established rules and regulations.
3. Assists employees to identify with organizational goals, thus increasing the likelihood that the standards of conduct deemed acceptable by the organization will be accepted by its employees.
4. Is self-aware regarding the power and responsibility inherent in having formal authority to set rules and discipline employees.
5. Serves in the role of coach in performance deficiency coaching.
6. Is self-aware regarding values, biases, and beliefs about chemical abuse.
7. Uses active listening as a support tool in working with chemically and psychologically impaired subordinates, but recognizes own limitations in counseling and refers impaired employees to outside experts for appropriate counseling.
8. Examines the work environment for stressors that contribute to substance abuse and eliminates those stressors whenever possible.

Management Functions

1. Clearly identifies performance expectations for all employees and confronts employees when those expectations are not met.
2. Assigns employees to work roles and situations that successfully challenge or intermittently "stretch" the employee. Does not allow employees to fail repeatedly.
3. Seeks out and completes extensive education about chemical abuse in the work setting. Provides these same opportunities to staff.
4. Acts as a resource to chemically or psychologically impaired employees regarding professional services or agencies that provide counseling and support services.
5. Collects and records adequate objective data when suspicious of employee chemical impairment.
6. Focuses employee confrontations on performance deficits and not on the cause of the underlying problem or addiction.
7. Works with the rule breaker, chemically impaired, and/or marginal employee to develop a remedial plan for action. Ensures that the employee understands the performance expectations of the organization and the consequences of not meeting these expectations.

CONSTRUCTIVE VERSUS DESTRUCTIVE DISCIPLINE

Discipline can be defined as a training or molding of the mind or character to bring about desired behaviors. It is not the same thing as punishment. *Punishment* is defined as an undesirable event that follows an instance of unacceptable behavior and is intended to decrease the frequency of that behavior (Guffey & Helms, 2001). However, discipline has an educational component as well as a corrective one.

Scientific management theory viewed discipline as a necessary means for controlling an unmotivated and self-centered workforce. Because of this traditional philosophy, managers primarily used threats and fear to control behavior. This "big stick" approach to management focused on eliminating all behaviors that could be considered to conflict with organizational goals. Although this approach may succeed on a short-term basis, it is usually demotivating and reduces long-term productivity, because people will achieve only at the level they believe is necessary to avoid punishment. This approach also is destructive because discipline is often arbitrarily administered and is unfair either in the application of rules or in the resulting punishment. Kerfoot and Wantz (2003) concur, arguing that *compliance leadership*, a 17th century leadership model that focuses on compliance and manages by hierarchy and bureaucratic controls, simply doesn't work. Kerfoot and Wantz argue that instead of compliance models, leaders should seek to establish *commitment models* of leadership.

Constructive discipline uses discipline as a means of helping the employee grow, not as a punitive measure. Punishment is frequently included when defining discipline, but it also can be defined as training, educating, or molding. In fact, the word discipline comes from the Latin term *disciplina*, which means teaching, learning, and growing. In constructive discipline, punishment may be applied for improper behavior, but it is carried out in a supportive, corrective manner. Employees are reassured that the punishment given is because of their actions and not because of who they are.

Learning Exercise 25.1

Thinking About Growth-Producing Versus Destructive Discipline
Think back to when someone in authority, such as a parent, teacher, or boss, set limits or enforced rules in such a way that you became a better child, student, or employee. What made this disciplinary action growth-producing instead of destructive? What was the most destructive disciplinary action you ever experienced? Did it modify your behavior in any way?

SELF-DISCIPLINE AND GROUP NORMS

The highest level and most effective form of discipline is *self-discipline*. When employees feel secure, validated, and affirmed in their essential worth, identity, and integrity, self-discipline is encouraged. Ideally, all employees would have adequate self-control and be self-directed in their pursuit of organizational goals. Unfortunately, this is not the case. Instead, group norms often influence individual behavior and make self-discipline difficult. Group norms are group-established standards of expected behavior that are enforced by social pressure. The leader, who understands group norms, is able to work within those norms to mold group behavior. This modification of group norms, in turn, affects individual behavior and thus self-discipline.

Although self-discipline is internalized, the leader plays an active role in developing an environment that promotes self-discipline in employees. Self-discipline is possible only if subordinates know the rules and accept them as valid. It is impossible for employees to have self-control if they do not understand the acceptable boundaries for their behavior, nor can they be self-directed if they do not understand what is expected of them. Therefore, managers must discuss clearly all written rules and policies with subordinates, explain the rationale for the existence of the rules and policies, and encourage questions.

Self-discipline also requires an atmosphere of mutual trust. Managers must believe that employees are capable of and actively seeking self-discipline. Likewise, employees must respect their managers and perceive them as honest and trustworthy. Employees lack the security to have self-discipline if they do not trust their managers' motives. Finally, for self-discipline to develop, formal authority must be used judiciously. If formal discipline is quickly and widely used, subordinates do not have the opportunity to use self-discipline.

FAIR AND EFFECTIVE RULES

Several guidelines must be followed if discipline is to be perceived by subordinates as growth-producing. This does not imply that subordinates enjoy being disciplined or that discipline should be a regular means of promoting employee growth. However, discipline, if implemented correctly, should not permanently alienate or demoralize subordinates.

McGregor (1967) developed four rules to make discipline as fair and growth-producing as possible (see **Display 25.2**). These rules are called "hot stove" rules because they can be applied to someone touching a hot stove.

Unfortunately, most rule breaking is not enforced by using McGregor's rules. For example, many people exceed the speed limit when driving. Generally, people are aware of speed limit regulations, and signs are posted along the roadway as reminders of the rules; thus, there is *forewarning*. There is not, however, *immediacy*, *consistency*, or *impartiality*. Many people exceed the speed limit for long periods before they are stopped and disciplined, or they may never be disciplined at all. Likewise, a person may be stopped and disciplined one day and not the next even though the same rule is broken. Finally, the punishment is inconsistent because some people are punished for their rule breaking, but others are not. Even the penalty varies among people.

Imagine that automobiles had been developed that required drivers to place a built-in electronic sensor on the end of their fingers before the automobile would operate. The purpose of this sensor would be to deliver a low-charge but painful electrical shock every time the car exceeded the posted speed limit. The driver would be forewarned of the consequences of breaking the speed limit rule. If each time the rule was broken, the driver immediately received an electrical

Display 25.2 McGregor's Hot Stove Rules for Fair and Effective Discipline

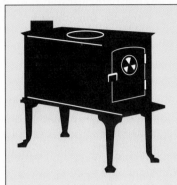

Four elements must be present to make discipline as fair and growth producing as possible:

1. Forewarning
2. Immediate consequences
3. Consistency
4. Impartiality

1. All employees must be *forewarned* that if they touch the hot stove (break a rule), they will be burned (punished or disciplined). They must know the rule beforehand and be aware of the punishment.
2. If the person touches the stove (breaks a rule), there will be *immediate consequences* (getting burned). All discipline should be administered immediately after rules are broken.
3. If the person touches the stove again, he or she will again be burned. Therefore, there is *consistency;* each time the rule is broken, there are immediate and consistent consequences.
4. If any other person touches the hot stove, he or she also will get burned. Discipline must be *impartial*, and everyone must be treated in the same manner when the rule is broken.

shock, and if all automobiles included this feature, speeding would probably be eliminated.

If a rule or regulation is worth having, it should be enforced. When rule breaking is allowed to go unpunished, other people tend to replicate the behavior of the rule breaker. Likewise, the average worker's natural inclination to obey rules can be dissipated by lax or inept enforcement policies because employees develop contempt for managers who allow rules to be disregarded. The enforcement of rules using McGregor's hot stove rules keeps morale from breaking down and allows structure within the organization.

An organization should, however, have as few rules and regulations as possible. A leadership role involves regularly reviewing all rules, regulations, and policies to see if they should be deleted or modified in some way. If managers find themselves spending much of their time enforcing one particular rule, it would be wise to reexamine the rule and consider whether there is something wrong with the rule or how it is communicated.

Learning Exercise 25.2

Rule Breakers and Outdated Rules
Part 1: Think back to "rule breakers" you have known. Were they a majority or minority in the group? How great was their impact on group behavior? What characteristics did they have in common? Did the group modify the rule breaker's behavior, or did the rule breaker modify group behavior?
Part 2: Rules quickly become outdated and need to be deleted or changed in some way. Think of a policy or rule that needs to be updated. Why is the rule no longer appropriate? What could you do to update this rule? Does the rule need to be replaced with a new one?

DISCIPLINE AS A PROGRESSIVE PROCESS

Further action must be taken when employees continue undesirable conduct, either in breaking rules or in not performing their job duties adequately. Managers have the formal authority and responsibility to take progressively stronger forms of discipline when employees fail to meet expected standards of achievement. However, inappropriate discipline (too much or too little) can undermine the morale of the whole team. Determining appropriate disciplinary action, then, is often difficult, and many factors must be considered. Thus, discipline is generally administered using a progressive model.

The *progressive discipline* model was developed in the 1930s in response to the National Labor Relations Act (NLRA) of 1935 (Guffey & Helms, 2001). The NLRA required that discipline and discharge be based on *just cause*. This model follows four progressive steps to address identical offenses committed by an employee.

Generally, the first step of the disciplinary process is an *informal reprimand* or *verbal admonishment*. This reprimand includes an informal meeting between the employee and manager to discuss the broken rule or performance deficiency. The manager suggests ways in which the employee's behavior might be altered to keep the rule from being broken again. Often, an informal reprimand is all that is needed for behavior modification.

The second step is a *formal reprimand* or *written admonishment*. If rule breaking recurs after verbal admonishment, the manager again meets with the employee and issues a written warning about the behaviors that must be corrected. This written warning is very specific about what rules or policies have been violated, the potential consequences if behavior is not altered to meet organizational expectations, and the plan of action the employee is expected to take to achieve expected change. Both the employee and the manager should sign the warning to signify that the problem or incident was discussed. The employee's signature does not imply that the employee agrees with everything on the report, only that it has been discussed. The employee must be allowed to respond in writing to the reprimand, either on the form itself or by attaching comments to the disciplinary report; this allows the employee to air any differences in perception between the manager and the employee. One copy of the written admonishment is then given to the employee, and another copy is retained in the employee's personnel file. **Display 25.3** presents a sample reprimand form.

Display 25.3 **Sample Written Reprimand Form**

Employee name

_____

Position _____ Date of hire _____
Person completing report _____
Position _____ Date report completed _____
Date of incident(s) _____ Time _____
Description of incident:

Prior attempts to counsel employee regarding this behavior (cite date and results of disciplinary conferences):

Disciplinary contract (plan for correction) and time lines:

Consequences of future repetition:

Employee comments: (Additional documentation or rebuttal may be attached)

_____   _____
Signature of individual making the report   Employee signature

Date _____   Date _____

Date and time of follow-up appointment to review disciplinary contract:

Learning Exercise 25.3

Deciding Upon Disciplinary Action

You are a supervisor in a neurological care unit. One morning, you receive a report from the night-shift RNs, nurse Caldwell and nurse Jones. Neither of the nurses reports anything out of the ordinary, except that a young head-injury patient has been particularly belligerent and offensive in his language. This young man was especially annoying because he appeared rational and then would suddenly become abusive. His language was particularly vulgar. You recognize that this is fairly normal behavior in a head-injury patient, but yesterday morning his behavior was so offensive to his neurosurgeons that one of them threatened to wash his mouth out with soap.

After both night nurses leave the unit, you receive a phone call from the house night supervisor. She relates the following information: When the supervisor made her usual rounds to the neuro unit, nurse Caldwell was on a coffee break and nurse Jones was in the unit with two LVNs/LPNs. Nurse Jones reported that nurse Caldwell became very upset with the head-injury patient because of his abusive and vulgar language and had taped his mouth shut with a four-inch piece of adhesive tape. Nurse Jones had observed the behavior and had gone to the patient's bedside and removed the piece of tape and suggested that nurse Caldwell go get a cup of coffee.

The supervisor observed the unit several times following this, and nothing else appeared to be remiss. She stated that nurse Jones said no harm had come to the patient and that she was reluctant to report the incident but believed perhaps one of the supervisors should counsel nurse Caldwell. You thank the night supervisor and consider the following facts in this case:

- Nurse Caldwell has been an excellent nurse but is occasionally judgmental.
- Nurse Caldwell is a very religious young woman and has led a rather sheltered life.
- Taping a patient's mouth with a four-inch piece of adhesive tape is very dangerous, especially for someone with questionable chest and abdominal injuries and neurological injuries.
- Nurse Caldwell has never been reprimanded before.

You call the physician and explain what happened. He says that he believes there was no harm done. He agrees with you that it is up to you whether to discipline the employee and to what degree. However, he believes most of the medical staff would want the nurse fired.

You phone the nurse and arrange for a conference with her. She tearfully admits what she did. She states that she lost control. She asks you not to fire her, although she agrees this is a dischargeable offense. You consult with the administration, and everyone agrees that you should be the one to decide the disciplinary action in this case.

Assignment: Decide what you would do. You have a duty to your patients, the hospital, and your staff. List at least four possible courses of action. Select from among these choices, and justify your decision.

The third step in progressive discipline is usually a *suspension from work* without pay. If the employee continues the undesired behavior despite verbal and written warnings, the manager should remove the employee from his or her job for a brief time, generally a few days to several weeks. Such a suspension gives employees the opportunity to reflect on their behavior and plan how they might modify their behavior in the future.

The last step in progressive discipline is *involuntary termination* or dismissal. In reality, many people terminate their employment voluntarily before reaching this step, but the manager cannot count on this happening. Termination should always be the last resort when dealing with poor performance. However, if the manager has given repeated warnings and rule breaking or policy violations continue, then the employee should be dismissed. Although this is difficult and traumatic for the employee, the manager, and the unit, the cost in terms of managerial and employee time and unit morale of keeping such an employee is enormous.

When using progressive discipline, the steps are followed progressively only for repeated infractions of the same rule. For example, although an employee has previously received a formal reprimand for unexcused absences, discipline for a first-time offense of tardiness should begin at the first step of the process. Also remember that although discipline is generally administered progressively, some rule breaking is so serious that the employee may be suspended or dismissed with the first infraction. When using progressive discipline in all but the most serious infractions, the slate should be wiped clean at the conclusion of a predesignated period. Little justification exists for holding infractions against employees in perpetuity if the employee has modified his or her behavior. **Table 25.1** presents a progressive discipline guide for managers.

DISCIPLINARY STRATEGIES FOR THE NURSE–MANAGER

It is vital that managers recognize their power in evaluating and correcting employees' behavior. Because a person's job is very important to him or her—often as a part of self-esteem and as a means of livelihood—disciplining or taking away a person's job is a very serious action and should not be undertaken lightly. The manager can implement several strategies to increase the likelihood that discipline will be fair and produce growth.

The first strategy the manager must use is to investigate thoroughly the situation that has prompted the employee discipline. A supervisor must investigate all allegations of misconduct even if they initially appear to have no basis or are anonymously reported (Rafes & Warren, 2001).

Questions the manager might ask include: Was the rule clear? Did this employee know he or she was breaking a rule? Is cultural diversity a factor in this rule breaking? Has this employee been involved in a situation like this before? Was he or she disciplined for this behavior? What was his or her response to the corrective action? How serious or potentially serious is the current problem or infraction? Who else was involved in the situation? Does this employee have a history of other types of disciplinary problems? What is the quality of this employee's performance in the

Table 25.1 Guide to Progressive Discipline

Offense	First Infraction	Second Infraction	Third Infraction	Fourth Infraction
Gross mistreatment of a patient	Dismissal			
Discourtesy to a patient	Verbal admonishment	Written admonishment	Suspension	Dismissal
Insubordination	Written admonishment	Suspension	Dismissal	
Intoxication while on duty (this offense is difficult to prove)	Verbal admonishment	Written admonishment	Dismissal	
Use of intoxicants while on duty	Dismissal			
Neglect of duty	Verbal admonishment	Written admonishment	Suspension	Dismissal
Theft or willful damage of property	Written admonishment	Dismissal		
Falsehood	Verbal admonishment	Written admonishment	Dismissal	
Unauthorized absence	Verbal admonishment	Written admonishment	Dismissal	
Abuse of leave	Verbal admonishment	Written admonishment	Suspension	Dismissal
Deliberate violation of instruction	Verbal admonishment	Written admonishment	Suspension	Dismissal
Violation of safety rules	Verbal admonishment	Written admonishment	Dismissal	
Fighting	Verbal admonishment	Written admonishment	Suspension	Dismissal
Inability to maintain work standards	Verbal admonishment	Written admonishment	Suspension	Dismissal
Excessive unexcused tardiness*	Verbal admonishment	Written admonishment	Dismissal	

*The first, second, and third infractions do not mean the first, second, and third time an employee is late, but the first, second, and third time that unexcused tardiness becomes excessive as determined by the manager.

work setting? Have other employees in the organization also experienced the problem? How were they disciplined? Could there be a problem with the rule or policy? Were there any special circumstances that could have contributed to the problem in this situation? What disciplinary action is suggested by organizational policies for this type of offense? Has precedent been established? Will this type of disciplinary action keep the infraction from recurring? The wise manager will ask all these questions so a fair decision can be reached about an appropriate course of action.

Another strategy the manager should use is always to consult with either a superior or the personnel department before dismissing an employee. Most organizations have very clear policies about which actions constitute grounds for dismissal and how that dismissal should be handled. To protect themselves from charges of willful or discriminatory termination, managers should carefully document the behavior that occurred and any attempts to counsel the employee. Managers also must be careful not to discuss with one employee the reasons for discharging another employee or to make negative comments about past employees, which may discourage other employees or reduce their trust in the manager.

Performance Deficiency Coaching

Performance deficiency coaching is another strategy the manager can use to create a disciplined work environment. This type of coaching may be ongoing or problem centered. *Problem-centered coaching* is less spontaneous and requires more managerial planning than *ongoing coaching*. In performance deficiency coaching, the manager

 Learning Exercise 25.4

Writing a Performance Deficiency Coaching Plan
You are the professional staff coordinator of a small emergency care clinic. Historically, the clinic is busiest on weekend evenings, when the majority of drunk-driving injuries, stabbings, and gunshot wounds occur. In addition, many use the clinic on weekends to take care of non-emergency medical needs that were not addressed during regular physician office hours. Jane has been an RN at the clinic since it opened two years ago. She is well liked by all the employees and provides a sense of humor and lightheartedness in what is usually a highly stressful environment.

Jane has a reputation for being a "party animal." She is known to begin partying after work on Friday night and close down the bars Saturday morning. During the last three months, Jane has called in sick five of the seven Saturday evenings she was scheduled to work. The other employees have worked understaffed on what is generally the busiest night of the week, and they are becoming angry. They have asked you to talk to Jane or to staff an additional employee on the Saturday evenings Jane is assigned to work.

Assignment: You have decided to begin performance deficiency coaching with Jane. Write a possible coaching scenario that includes the following:

- The problem stated in behavioral terms
- An explanation to the employee of how the problem is related to organizational functioning
- A clear statement of possible consequences of the unwanted behavior
- A request for input from the employee
- Employee participation in the problem solving
- A plan for follow-up on the problem

Display 25.4	Performance Deficiency Coaching Scenario

Coach: I am concerned that you have been regularly coming into report late. This interrupts the other employees who are trying to hear report and creates overtime because the night shifts must stay and repeat report on the patients you missed. It also makes it difficult for your modular team members to prioritize their plan of care for the day if the entire team is not there and ready to begin at 0700. Why is this problem occurring?

Employee: I've been having problems lately with an unreliable babysitter and my car not starting. It seems like it's always one thing or another, and I'm upset about not getting to work on time, too. I hate starting my day off behind the eight ball.

Coach: This hospital has a longstanding policy on attendance, and it is one of the criteria used to judge work performance on your performance appraisal.

Employee: Yes, I know. I'm just not sure what I can do about it right now.

Coach: What approaches have you tried in solving these problems?

Employee: Well, I'm buying a new car, so that should take care of my transportation problems. I'm not sure about my babysitter, though. She's young and not very responsible, so she'll call me at the last minute and tell me she's not coming. I keep her, though, because she's willing to work the flexible hours and days that this job requires, and she doesn't charge as much as a formal day-care center would.

Coach: Do you have family in the area or close friends you can count on to help with childcare on short notice?

Employee: Yes, my mother lives a few blocks away and is always glad to help, but I couldn't count on her on a regular basis.

Coach: There are employment registry lists at the local college for students interested in providing childcare. Have you thought about trying this option? Often, students can work flexible hours and charge less than formal day-care centers.

Employee: That's a good idea. In fact, I just heard about a childcare referral service that also could give me a few ideas. I'll stop there after work. I realize that my behavior has affected unit functioning, and I promise to try to work this out as soon as possible.

Coach: I'm sure these problems can be corrected. Let's have a follow-up visit in two weeks to see how things are going.

actively brings areas of unacceptable behavior or performance to the attention of the employee and works with him or her to establish a plan to correct deficiencies. Because the role of coach is less threatening than that of enforcer, the manager becomes a supporter, and helper. Performance-deficiency coaching helps employees, over time, to improve their performance to the highest level of which they are capable. As such, the development, use, and mastery of performance deficiency coaching should result in improved performance for all. The scenario depicted in **Display 25.4** is an example of performance deficiency coaching.

The Disciplinary Conference

When coaching is unsuccessful in modifying behavior, the manager must take more aggressive steps and use more formal measures, such as a *disciplinary conference*. After thoroughly investigating an employee's offenses, managers must confront the employee with their findings. This occurs in the form of a disciplinary conference. The following steps are generally part of the disciplinary conference.

Reason for Disciplinary Action

Begin by clearly specifying why the employee is being disciplined. The manager must not be hesitant or apologetic. Novice managers often feel uncomfortable with the disciplinary process and may provide unclear or mixed messages to the employee regarding the nature or seriousness of a disciplinary problem. Managers must assume the authority given to them by their role. A major responsibility in this role is evaluating employee performance and suggesting appropriate action for improved or acceptable performance.

Employee's Response to Action

Give the employee the opportunity to explain why the rule was not followed. Allowing employees feedback in the disciplinary process ensures them recognition as human beings and reassures them that your ultimate goal is to be fair and promote their growth.

Rationale for Disciplinary Action

Explain the disciplinary action you are going to take and why you are going to take it. Although the manager must keep an open mind to new information that may be gathered in the second step, preliminary assessments regarding the appropriate disciplinary action should already have been made. This discipline should be communicated to the employee. The employee who has been counseled at previous disciplinary conferences should not be surprised at the punishment, because it should have been discussed at the last conference.

Clarification of Expectations for Change

Describe the expected behavioral change and list the steps needed to achieve this change. Explain the consequences of failure to change. Again, do not be apologetic or hesitant, or the employee will be confused about the seriousness of the issue. Because they may lack self-control, employees who have repeatedly broken rules need firm direction. It must be very clear to the employee that timely follow-up will occur.

Agreement and Acceptance of Action Plan

Get agreement and acceptance of the plan. Give support, and let the employee know that you are interested in him or her as a person. Remember too that the leader–manager administers discipline to promote employee growth rather than to impose punishment. Although the expected standards must be very clear, the leader imparts a sense of genuine concern for and desire to help the employee grow. This approach helps the employee recognize that the discipline is directed at the offensive behavior and not at the individual. The leader must be cautious, however, not to relinquish the management role in an effort to nurture and counsel. The leadership role is to provide a supportive environment and structure so the employee can make the necessary changes.

> Disciplinary **problems, if** unrecognized or **ignored,** generally do **not go** away; they get **worse.**

All discipline, even informal admonishments, should be conducted in private.

In addition to understanding what should be covered in the disciplinary conference, the leader must be sensitive to the environment in which discipline is given. Although the employee must receive feedback about his or her rule breaking or inappropriate behavior as soon as possible after it has occurred, the manager should never discipline in front of patients or peers. If more than an informal admonishment is required, the manager should inform the employee of the unacceptable action and then schedule a formal disciplinary conference later.

All formal disciplinary conferences should be scheduled in advance at a time agreeable to both the employee and manager. Both will want time to reflect on the situation that has occurred. Allowing time for reflection should reduce the situation's emotionalism and promote employee self-discipline, because employees often identify their own plan for keeping the behavior from recurring.

In addition to privacy and advance scheduling, the length of the disciplinary conference is important; it should not be so long that it degenerates into a debate, nor so short that both the employee and manager cannot provide input. If the employee seems overly emotional or if great discrepancies exist between the manager's and employee's perceptions, an additional conference should be scheduled. Employees often need time to absorb what they have been told and to develop a plan that is not defensive.

The Termination Conference

At times, the disciplinary conference must be a termination conference. Although many of the principles are the same, the termination conference differs from a disciplinary conference in that planning for future improvement is eliminated. The following steps should be followed in the termination conference:

1. Calmly state the reasons for dismissal. The manager must not appear angry or defensive. Although managers may express regret that the outcome is termination of employment, they must not dwell on this or give the employee reason to think the decision is not final. The manager should be prepared to give examples of the behavior in question.
2. Explain the employment termination process. State the date on which employment is terminated as well as the employee's and organization's role in the process.
3. Ask for employee input. Termination conferences are always tense, and raw, spontaneous emotional reactions are common. Listen to the employee, but do not allow yourself to be drawn emotionally into his or her anger or sorrow. Always stay focused on the facts of the case and attempt to respond without reacting.
4. End the meeting on a positive note if possible. The manager should also inform the employee what, if any, references will be supplied to prospective employers. Finally, it is usually best to allow the employee who has been dismissed to leave the organization immediately. If the employee continues to work on the unit after dismissal has been discussed, it can be demoralizing for all the employees who work on that unit.

GRIEVANCE PROCEDURES

Growth can occur only when employees perceive that feedback and discipline are fair and just. When employees and managers perceive "fair" and "just" differently, the discrepancy can usually be resolved by a more formal means called a *grievance procedure*. The grievance procedure is essentially a statement of wrongdoing or a procedure to follow when one believes a wrong has been committed. This procedure is not limited to resolving discipline discrepancies; employees can use it any time they believe they have not been treated fairly by management. This chapter, however, focuses specifically on grievances that result from the disciplinary process.

Most grievances or conflicts between employees and management can be resolved informally through communication, negotiation, compromise, and collaboration. Generally though, even informal resolution has well-defined steps that should be followed.

If the employee and management are unable to resolve their differences informally, a formal grievance process begins. The steps of the formal grievance process are generally outlined in all union contracts or administrative policy and procedure manuals. Generally these steps include the progressive lodging of formal complaints up the chain of command. If resolution does not occur at any of these levels, a formal hearing is usually held. Several people or a small group is impaneled, much in the same way as a jury, to make a determination of what should be done. Such groups are often at risk of favoring the individual employee over the all-powerful institution. This tendency reinforces the need for the manager to have clear, objective, and comprehensive written records regarding the problem employee's behavior and attempts to counsel.

If the differences cannot be settled through a formal grievance process, the matter may finally be resolved in a process known as arbitration. In *arbitration*, both sides agree on the selection of a professional mediator who will review the grievance, complete fact-finding, and interview witnesses before coming to a decision.

Although grievance procedures extract a great deal of time and energy from both employees and managers, they serve several valuable purposes. Grievance procedures can settle some problems before they escalate into even larger ones. The procedures also are a source of data to focus attention on ambiguous contract language for labor–management negotiation at a later date. Perhaps the most important outcome of a grievance is the legitimate opportunity it provides for employees to resolve conflicts with their superiors. Employees who are not given an outlet for resolving work conflicts become demoralized, angry, and dissatisfied. These emotions affect unit functioning and productivity. Even if the outcome is not in the favor of the person filing the grievance, the employee will know that the opportunity was given to present the case to an objective third party, and the chances of constructive conflict resolution are greatly increased. In addition, managers tend to be fairer and more consistent when they know that employees have a method of redress for arbitrary managerial action.

Rights and Responsibilities in Grievance Resolution

Employees and managers have some separate and distinct rights and responsibilities in grievance resolution, but many rights and responsibilities overlap. Although it is easy to be drawn into the emotionalism of a grievance that focuses on one's perceived rights, the manager and employee must remember that they both have rights and that these rights have concomitant responsibilities. For example, although both parties have the right to be heard, both parties are equally responsible to listen without interrupting. The employee has the right to a positive work environment but has the responsibility to communicate needs and discontent to the manager. The manager has the right to expect a certain level of productivity from the employee but has the responsibility to provide a work environment that makes this possible. The manager has the right to expect employees to follow rules but has the responsibility to see that these rules are clearly communicated and fairly enforced.

Both the manager and the employee must show good will in resolving grievances. This means that both parties must be open to discussing, negotiating, and compromising and must attempt to resolve grievances as soon as possible. The ultimate goal of the grievance should not be to win, but to seek a resolution that satisfies both the person and the organization.

In many cases, the manager can eliminate or reduce his or her risk of being involved in a grievance by fostering a work environment that emphasizes clear communication and fair, constructive discipline. Employees also can eliminate or reduce their risk of being involved in a grievance by being well informed about the labor contract, policies and procedures, and organizational rules. If both employee and employer recognize their rights and responsibilities, the incidence of grievances in the workplace should decrease. When mutual problem solving, negotiation, and compromise are ineffective at resolving conflicts, the grievance process can provide a positive and growth-producing resolution to disciplinary conflict.

DISCIPLINING THE UNIONIZED EMPLOYEE

It is essential that all managers be fair and consistent in disciplining employees regardless of whether a union is present. The presence of a union does, however, usually entail more procedural, legalistic safeguards in administering discipline, and a well-defined grievance process for employees who believe they have been disciplined unfairly. For example, the manager of non-unionized employees has greater latitude in selecting which disciplinary measure is appropriate for a specific infraction. Although this gives the manager greater flexibility and latitude, discipline between employees may be inconsistent.

On the other hand, unionized employees generally must be disciplined according to specific, preestablished steps and penalties within an established time frame. For example, the union contract may be very clear that excessive unexcused absences from work must be disciplined first by a written reprimand, then a three-day work suspension, and then termination. This type of discipline structure is generally fairer to the employee but allows the manager less flexibility in evaluating each case's extenuating circumstances.

Another aspect of discipline that may differ between unionized and non-unionized employees is following due process in disciplining union employees. *Due process* means that management must provide union employees with a written statement outlining disciplinary charges, the resulting penalty, and the reasons for the penalty. Employees then have the right to defend themselves against such charges and to settle any disagreement through formal grievance hearings.

Another difference between unionized and non-unionized employee discipline lies in the burden of proof. In disciplinary situations with non-unionized employees, the burden of proof typically falls on the employee. With union employees, the burden of proof for the wrongdoing and need for subsequent discipline falls on management. This means that managers disciplining union employees must keep detailed records regarding misconduct and counseling attempts.

Finally, another common difference between unionized and non-unionized employees is that most non-union employees are classified as *at will*, meaning that they are subject to dismissal "at the will" of the employer. The *at-will doctrine,* which is applicable in many states, permits an employer to terminate employment for any or no reason and at the discretion of the supervisor. In states that do not subscribe to the employment-at-will doctrine, or in organizations that have union representation for employees, employers must have good and legal cause to dismiss an employee. Managers who have "at-will" employees are generally advised not to provide any specific reason for dismissal other than that the employee did not meet the employer's expectations (Rafes & Warren, 2001). It must be noted, however, that even when the employment-at-will doctrine is applicable, there are numerous exceptions, and an employer must be knowledgeable about each exception. Such exceptions where at-will dismissal would not apply might include when employment is being terminated based on membership in a protected legal group such as race, sex, pregnancy, national origin, religion, disability, age, or military status (Rafes & Warren, 2001).

The contract language used by unions regarding discipline may be very specific or very general. Most contracts recognize the right of management to discipline, suspend, or dismiss employees for just cause. Just cause can be defined as having appropriate rationale for the actions taken. For just cause to exist, the manager must be able to prove that the employee violated established rules, that corrective action or penalty was warranted, and that the penalty was appropriate for the offense. These contracts also generally recognize the right of the employee to submit grievances when he or she believes these actions have been taken unfairly or are discriminatory in some way.

Managers are responsible for knowing all union contract provisions that affect how discipline is administered on their units. Managers also should work closely with others employed in human resources or personnel positions in the organization. These professionals generally prove to be invaluable resources in dealings with union employees.

THE MARGINAL EMPLOYEE

Marginal employees are another type of problem employee; however, traditional discipline is generally not constructive in modifying their behavior. This is because marginal employees often make tremendous efforts to meet competencies, yet usually manage to meet only minimal standards at best. Marginal employees usually do not warrant dismissal, but they contribute very little to overall organizational efficiency. All organizations have at least a few such employees. Managing such employees then is often a frustrating and tiring task for managers.

Managers typically try multiple strategies to deal with marginal employees. One common strategy is simply to transfer the employee to another department, section, or unit. While clearly some marginal employees may be more successful on one unit than another, the more common end result of this solution is that the problem is simply transferred from one unit to another and the marginal employee experiences yet another failure.

Other managers choose to dismiss marginal employees or attempt to talk them into early retirement or resignation. Again, this does little to help the marginal employee succeed. Other managers simply choose to ignore the problem and attempt to "work around" the employee. This is not always possible, however, and the end result is frequently resentment from coworkers who have to carry the burden of finishing work the marginal employee was unable to accomplish.

The most time-intensive option in dealing with marginal employees is coaching. With this strategy, the manager attempts to improve the marginal employee's performance through active coaching and counseling. While this strategy holds the greatest promise for personal growth in the marginal employee, there is no guarantee that the employee's performance will improve or that the end results will justify the time and energy costs to the manager.

The strategy chosen for dealing with the marginal employee often varies with the level of the manager. Ignoring the problem is a passive response and is more frequently used by lower-level managers. Higher-level managers tend to employ the more active measures of coaching, transferring, and dismissal.

In addition, the nature of the organization plays a role in determining what strategy is used to deal with the marginal employee. Government-controlled organizations are more apt to use passive measures, whereas managers in organizations with other sponsors are more apt to use active measures. The size of the organization also influences how managers deal with the marginally productive employee. Baum (2000) recommends that companies with fewer than 100 employees dismiss employees who are not performing well, because an organization that relies on subpar performers is missing out on opportunities to be successful.

However, in larger organizations the trend has been toward passive managerial coping strategies with marginal employees. It is important for the manager to remember that each person and situation is different and that the most appropriate strategy depends on many variables. Looking at past performance will help determine if the employee is merely burnt out, needs educational or training opportunities, is unmotivated, or just has very little energy and only marginal skills for the job. If the latter is true, then the employee may never become more than a marginal employee, no matter what management functions and leadership skills are brought into play. Learning Exercise 25.5, which has been solved for the reader (see the Appendix), depicts alternatives managers may consider in dealing with the marginal employee.

Learning Exercise 25.5

The Marginal Employee

You are the oncology supervisor in a 400-bed hospital. There are 35 beds on your unit, which is generally full. It is an extremely busy unit, and your nursing staff needs high-level assessment and communication skills in providing patient care. Because the nursing care needs on this floor are unique and because you use primary nursing, it has been very difficult in the past to float staff from other units when additional staffing was required. Although you have been able to keep the unit adequately staffed on a day-to-day basis, there are two open positions for registered nurses on your unit that have been unfilled for almost three months.

Historically, your staff members have been excellent employees. They enjoy their work and are highly productive. Unit morale has been exceptionally good. However, in the last three months, the staff has begun complaining about Judy, a full-time employee who has been on the unit for about four months.

Judy has been a registered nurse for about 15 years and has worked in oncology units at other facilities. References from former employers identified Judy's work as competent, although little other information was given. At Judy's six-week and three-month performance appraisals, you coached her regarding her barely adequate work habits, assessment and communication skills, and decision making. Judy responded that she would attempt to work on improving her performance in these areas, because working on this unit was one of her highest career goals.

Although Judy has been receptive to your coaching and has verbalized to you her efforts to improve her performance, there has been little observable difference in her behavior. You have slowly concluded that Judy is probably currently working at the highest level of which she is capable and that she is a marginal employee at best. The other nurses believe Judy is not carrying her share of the workload and have asked that you remove her from the unit.

Try to solve this exercise on your own before reading the solution in the Appendix. The traditional problem-solving process is used as a decision-making tool in the solution.

THE CHEMICALLY IMPAIRED EMPLOYEE

Nursing administrators may face no management problem more costly or emotionally draining than that of nurses whose practice is impaired by substance abuse or psychological dysfunction. Substance misuse is defined by Lillibridge, Cox, and Cross (2002) as maladaptive patterns of psychoactive substance abuse indicated by continued use even when faced with recurrent occupational, social, psychological or physical problems as well as/or use in dangerous situations. Effective management demands that the organization take an active role in assuring patient safety by immediately removing these employees from the work setting. However, managers also have a responsibility to help these employees deal with their disease so that they can return to the workforce in the future as productive employees.

Modlin and Montes (1964) first documented chemical dependency in the health professions in studies in the late 1940s although there is little doubt that chemical dependency has been around as long as alcohol and drugs have been. The exact magnitude of chemical impairment within nursing is not known, and estimates vary widely, but a review of the literature suggests that somewhere between 6% and 14% of all nurses are chemically impaired. In addition, the chemical impairment rate of health professionals is generally acknowledged as being greater than that of the general public.

One difference, however, between chemically impaired health professionals and other addicts, is that chemically impaired nurses and physicians tend to obtain their drugs of choice through legal channels, such as legitimate prescriptions that were written for them, or diversionary measures on the job, rather than purchasing them illegally on the street (Danis, 2003). Indeed, in spite of narcotic-dispensing machines, such as the Pyxis and Baxter, introduced to reduce the diversion of these drugs, workplace theft has been identified as the most frequent source of illegally obtained narcotics (Danis, 2003). In fact, the majority of disciplinary actions by licensing boards are related to misconduct resulting from chemical impairment, including the misappropriation of drugs for personal use and the sale of drugs and drug paraphernalia to support the nurse's addiction (Cherry & Jacob, 2002).

Although alcohol is the most frequently abused substance, meperidine (Demerol) is a drug of choice while oxycodone (Oxycontin), and clonazepam (Klonopin) are increasing in popularity (National Institute on Drug Abuse, n.d.). Other frequently abused chemicals include such benzodiazepines as diazepam (Valium), and narcotic drugs such as morphine and pentazocine (Talwin). Barbiturates may replace alcohol in the workplace so that the employee may feel a similar effect without having alcohol detectable on the breath.

The type of work setting also seems to be a predictor of chemical impairment for nurses. Research suggests that nurses who experience higher levels of workplace stress, such as critical care or the emergency department, as well as those with greater or more frequent access to controlled substances, have a greater incidence of abuse (Storr, Trinkoff, & Anthony, 1999; Bell, McDonough, Ellison, & Fitzhugh, 1999). Indeed, participants in a qualitative, phenomenological study by Lillibridge et al. (2002) defended their use of substances in order to deal with the stress of their work.

Recognizing the Chemically Impaired Employee

Although most nurses have finely tuned assessment skills for identifying patient problems, they generally are less sensitive to behaviors and actions that could signify chemical impairment of an employee or colleague. Sensitivity to others and to the environment is a leadership skill.

The profile of the impaired nurse may vary greatly, although several behavior patterns and changes are noted frequently. These behavior changes can be grouped into three primary areas: personality/behavior changes, job performance changes, and time and attendance changes. **Displays 25.5, 25.6, and 25.7** show characteristics of each of these categories.

Display 25.5 **Common Personality/Behavior Changes of the Chemically Impaired Employee**

- Increased irritability with patients and colleagues, often followed by extreme calm
- Social isolation; eats alone, avoids unit social functions
- Extreme and rapid mood strings
- Euphoric recall of events or elaborate excuses for behaviors
- Unusually strong interest in narcotics or the narcotic cabinet
- Sudden dramatic change in personal grooming or any other area
- Forgetfulness ranging from simple short-term memory loss to blackouts
- Change in physical appearance, which may include weight loss, flushed face, red or bleary eyes, unsteady gait, slurred speech, tremors, restlessness, diaphoresis, bruises and cigarette burns, jaundice, and ascites
- Extreme defensiveness regarding medication errors

Display 25.6 **Common Job Performance Changes of the Chemically Impaired Employee**

- Difficulty meeting schedules and deadlines
- Illogical or sloppy charting
- High frequency of medication errors or errors in judgement affecting patient care
- Frequently volunteers to be medication nurse
- Has a high number of assigned patients who complain that their pain medication is ineffective in relieving their pain
- Consistently meeting work performance requirements at minimal levels or doing the minimum amount of work necessary
- Judgment errors
- Sleeping or dozing on duty
- Complaints from other staff members about the quality and quantity of the employee's work

Display 25.7 **Common Time and Attendance Changes of the Chemically Impaired Employee**

- Increasingly absent from work without adequate explanation or notification; most frequent absence on a Monday or Friday
- Long lunch hours
- Excessive use of sick leave or requests for sick leave after days off
- Frequent calling in to request compensatory time
- Arriving at work early or staying late for no apparent reason
- Consistent lateness
- Frequent disappearances from the unit without explanation

As the employee progresses into a deeper stage of chemical dependency, managers can more easily recognize these behaviors. Typically, in the earliest stages of chemical dependency, the employee uses the addictive substance primarily for pleasure, and although the alcohol or drug use is excessive, it is primarily recreational and social. Thus, substance use generally does not occur during work hours, although some secondary effects of its use may be apparent.

As chemical dependency deepens, the employee develops tolerance to the chemical and must use the substance in greater quantities and more frequently to achieve the same effect. At this point, the person has made a conscious lifestyle decision to use chemicals. There is a high use of defense mechanisms, such as justifying, denying, and bargaining about the drug. Often, the employee in this stage begins to use the chemical substance both at and away from work. By this stage of chemical dependency, work performance generally declines in the areas of attendance, judgment, quality, and interpersonal relationships, and an appreciable decline in unit morale, as the result of an unreliable and unproductive worker, begins to be apparent.

In the final stages of chemical dependency, the employee must continually use the chemical substance, even though he or she no longer gains pleasure or gratification. The employee, physically and psychologically addicted, generally harbors a total disregard for self and others. Because the need for the substance is so great in this stage, the employee's personal and professional lives are focused on the need for drugs, and the employee becomes unpredictable and undependable in the work area. Assignments are incomplete or not done at all; charting may be sloppy or illegible; frequent judgment errors occur. Because the employee in this stage must use drugs frequently, there are often signs of drug use during work hours. Narcotic vials are missing. The employee may be absent from the unit for brief periods of time with no plausible excuse. Mood swings are excessive, and the employee often looks physically ill.

The bottom line is that chemically impaired employees should be removed from the work setting long before they reach this stage. The reality, however, is that the identification of chemical impairment is often very difficult. Even when chemical impairment is suspected, managers may not be aware of nurses who are at risk nor may they know how to proceed (Ponech, 2000). Nursing school courses generally focus on the physiological effects of alcohol and other drugs, dealing little with the psychological process of addiction and even less with chemical dependency in nurses. Because of this limited knowledge about chemical impairment, many nurses are ill prepared to deal with chemical impairment.

Confronting the Chemically Impaired Employee

Unlike most alcoholics or intravenous narcotic users, healthcare professionals do not achieve clandestine peer approval for their addictive behavior. Indeed, research by Lillibridge et al. (2002) found that the fear of discovery, and the subsequent loss of livelihood and identity associated with being a nurse, was central to the lived experience of substance impaired nurses. Thus, physicians and nurses are much less likely to admit, even to colleagues, that they are using, much less that they are

In contrast to non-nurse addicts, nurses usually use their drugs in private, rather than with friends, to protect their professional identity.

addicted to, a controlled substance. Frequently, they deny their chemical impairment even to themselves.

This self-denial is perpetuated because nurses and managers traditionally have been slow to recognize and reluctant to help these colleagues. Substance impaired nurses in the Lillibridge et al. (2002) study reported that "they felt let down because other nurses and the profession failed to recognize and confront their substance abuse problem" (p. 224). This is changing. Many state boards of nursing now have treatment programs for nurses, (discussed later in this chapter), and as managers gain more information about chemical impairment, how to recognize it, and how to intervene, more employees are being confronted with their impairment.

The first step in dealing with the chemically impaired employee actually occurs before the confrontation process. In the data- or evidence-gathering phase, the manager collects as much hard evidence as possible to document suspicions of chemical impairment in the employee. All behavior, work performance, and time and attendance changes presented in the displays in this chapter should be noted objectively and recorded in writing. If possible, a second person should be asked to validate the manager's observations. In suspected drug addiction, the manager also may examine unit narcotic records for inconsistencies and check to see that the amount of narcotic the nurse signed out for each patient is congruent with the amount ordered for that patient.

Proving alcohol impairment is more difficult because an employee can generally hide alcoholism more easily than drug addiction. Because few nurses drink while on duty, the manager will have to observe for more subtle clues, such as the smell of alcohol on the employee's breath. If the organization's policy allows for it, the manager may wish to require an employee suspected of alcohol impairment while on duty to have a serum alcohol analysis. If the employee refuses to cooperate, the organization's policy for documenting and reporting this incident should be followed.

If at any time the manager suspects that an employee is chemically influenced and thus presents a potential hazard to patient safety, the employee must be immediately removed from the work environment and privately confronted with the manager's perceptions. The manager should decisively and unemotionally tell the employee that he or she will not be allowed to return to the work area because of the manager's perception that the employee is chemically impaired. The manager should arrange for the employee to be taken home so that he or she is not allowed to drive while impaired. A formal meeting to discuss this incident should be scheduled within the next 24 hours.

This type of direct confrontation between the manager and the employee is the second phase in dealing with the employee suspected of chemical impairment. Although some employees admit their problem when directly confronted, most use defense mechanisms (including denial) because they may not have admitted the problem to themselves. Denial and anger should be expected in the confrontation. If the employee denies having a problem, documented evidence demonstrating a decline in work performance should be shared. The manager must be careful to keep the confrontation focused on the employee's performance deficits and not allow the discussion to be directed to the cause of the underlying problem or addiction. These are issues and concerns that the manager is unable to address. The manager also must be careful not to preach, moralize, scold, or blame.

Confrontation should always occur before the problem escalates too far. However, in some situations, the manager may have only limited direct evidence but still may believe that the employee should be confronted because of rapidly declining employee performance or unit morale. There is, however, a greater risk that confrontation at this point may be unsuccessful in terms of helping the employee. If direct confrontation is unsuccessful, it may have been too early; the employee may not have been desperate enough or may still be in denial. In these situations, job performance will probably continue to be marginal or unsatisfactory, and progressive discipline may be necessary. If the employee continues to deny chemical impairment and work performance continues to be unsatisfactory despite repeated constructive confrontation, dismissal may be necessary.

 Learning Exercise 25.6

The Chemically Impaired Colleague
Write a two-page essay which speaks to the following:
Has your personal or professional life been affected by a chemically impaired person? In what ways have you been affected? Has it colored the way you view chemical abuse and chemical impairment? Do you believe you will be able to separate your personal feelings about chemical abuse from the actions you must take as a manager in working with chemically impaired employees? Have you ever suspected a work colleague of chemical abuse? What, if anything, did you do about it? If you did suspect a colleague, would you approach him or her with your suspicions before talking to the unit manager? Describe the risks involved in this situation.

The last phase of the confrontation process is outlining the organization's plan or expectations for the employee in overcoming the chemical impairment. This plan is similar to the disciplinary contract in that it is usually written and outlines clearly the rehabilitative measures that should be undertaken by the employee and consequences if remedial action is not sought. Although the employee is generally referred informally by the manager to outside sources to help deal with the impairment, the employee is responsible for correcting his or her work deficiencies. Time lines are included in the plan, and the manager and employee must agree on and sign a copy of the contract.

The Manager's Role in Assisting the Chemically Impaired Employee

Clearly, the incidence of chemical impairment in health professionals is substantial. On a personal level, a person suffers from an illness that may go undetected and untreated for many years. On a professional level, the chemically impaired employee affects the entire healthcare system. Nurses with impaired skills and judgment jeopardize patient care. The chemically impaired nurse also compromises teamwork and continuity as colleagues attempt to pick up the slack for their impaired team member. The personal and professional cost of chemical impairment demands that nursing leaders and managers recognize the chemically impaired employee as early as possible and provide intervention.

Because of the general nature of nursing, many managers find themselves wanting to nurture the impaired employee, much as they would any other person who is sick. However, this nurturing can quickly become enabling. In addition, the employee who already has a greatly diminished sense of self-esteem and a perceived loss of self-control may ask the manager to participate actively in his or her recovery. This is one of the most difficult aspects of working with the impaired employee. Others who have greater expertise and objectivity should assume this role.

The manager also must be careful not to feel the need to diagnose the cause of the chemical addiction or to justify its existence. Protecting patients must be the top priority, taking precedence over any tendency to protect or excuse subordinates. The manager's role is to identify clearly performance expectations for the employee and to confront the employee when those expectations are not met. This is not to say that the manager should not be humanistic in recognizing the problem as a disease and not a disciplinary problem, or that he or she should be unwilling to refer the employee for needed help. Although the manager may suggest appropriate help or refer the impaired employee to someone, a manager's primary responsibility is to see that the employee becomes functional again and can meet organizational expectations before returning to the unit.

In addition, the manager can play a vital role in creating an environment that decreases the chances of chemical impairment in the work setting. This may be done by controlling or reducing work-related stressors whenever possible and by providing

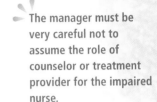

The manager must be very careful not to assume the role of counselor or treatment provider for the impaired nurse.

Learning Exercise 25.7

Working Under the Influence
There have been rumors for some time that Mrs. Clark, one of the night nurses on the unit you supervise, has been coming to work under the influence of alcohol. Fellow staff have reported the odor of alcohol on her breath, and one staff member stated that her speech is often slurred. The night supervisor states that she believes "this is not my problem," and your night charge nurse has never been on duty when Mrs. Clark has shown this behavior. This morning, one of the patients whispered to you that he thought Mrs. Clark had been drinking when she came to work last night. When you question the patient further, he states, "Mrs. Clark seemed to perform her nursing duties okay, but she made me nervous." You have decided you must talk with Mrs. Clark. You call her at her home and ask her to come to your office at 3 P.M.
Assignment: Determine how you are going to approach Mrs. Clark. Outline your plan, and give rationale for your choices. What flexibility have you built into your plan? How much of your documentation will be shared with Mrs. Clark?

mechanisms for employee stress management. The manager also should control drug accessibility by implementing, enforcing, and monitoring policies and procedures related to medication distribution. Finally, the manager should provide opportunities for the staff to learn about substance abuse, its detection, and available resources. "Educating nurses to recognize the signs of substance misuse assists in early intervention and is critical for long-term recovery" (Lillibridge et al., 2002, p. 227).

The Recovery Process

Although most authors disagree on the name or number of steps in the recovery process, they do agree that certain phases or progressive observable behaviors suggest that the person is recovering from the chemical impairment. In the first phase, the impaired employee continues to deny the significance or severity of the chemical impairment but does reduce or suspend chemical use to appease family, peers, or managers. These employees hope to reestablish their substance abuse in the future.

In the second phase, as denial subsides, the impaired employee begins to see that the chemical addiction is having a negative impact on his or her life and begins to want to change. Frequently, people in this phase are buoyant with hope and commitment but lack maturity about the struggles they will face. This phase generally lasts about three months.

During the third phase, the person examines his or her values and coping skills and works to develop more effective coping skills. Frequently, this is done by aligning himself or herself with support groups that reinforce a chemical-free lifestyle. In this stage, the person realizes how sick he or she was in the active stage of the disease and is often fraught with feelings of humiliation and shame.

In the last phase, people gain self-awareness regarding why they became chemically addicted, and they develop coping skills that will help them deal more effectively with stressors. As a result of this, self-awareness, self-esteem, and self-respect increase. When this happens, the person is able to decide consciously whether he or she wishes to and should return to the workplace.

State Board of Nursing Treatment Programs

Although chemical dependency can impair nurses' physical, psychological, social, and professional functioning, the problem was largely ignored until the late 1970s when the American Nurses Association (ANA) began efforts to secure assistance for chemically and mentally impaired nurses (Haack & Yocom, 2002). This assistance occurred primarily in the form of *diversion programs* (also called *intervention* or *peer assistance programs*). A diversion program is a voluntary, confidential program for registered nurses whose practice may be impaired due to chemical dependency or mental illness.

The goal of a diversion program is to protect the public by early identification of impaired registered nurses and by providing these nurses access to appropriate intervention programs and treatment services. Public safety is protected by immediate suspension of practice, when needed, and by ongoing careful monitoring of the nurse (California Board of Registered Nursing, n.d, para 2.) In addition to rehabilitating nurses with chemical dependence, most diversion programs also serve nurses impaired by certain mental illnesses such as anxiety, depression, bipolar disorder, and schizophrenia (Sloan & Vernarec, 2001). Some programs cover nurses with physical disabilities as well. Rasmussen (2001) reports that at least 30 states now have such treatment programs in place.

Sloan and Vernarec (2001) identified several factors that have led state boards to adopt diversion programs. First, a punitive system creates barriers to reporting and keeps impaired nurses from getting help. Nurse colleagues or practitioners who are treating an impaired nurse may well hesitate to report something that could cost a nurse his or her job and license. From an employer's standpoint, the fear of litigation often makes it easier to dismiss a nurse without charges of misconduct. But this practice leaves the nurse, who is at risk of harming patients and him or herself, free to seek work elsewhere. Even if a nurse is reported to the state board, a purely disciplinary approach to impairment not only shows a lack of compassion, it does not adequately protect the public. A board investigation can take months, even up to two years, during which time the nurse in question can continue working without restraint. If the nurse is licensed in another state, he or she can simply move away to avoid disciplinary action altogether (Sloan & Vernarec, 2001).

Finally, an alternative program is cheaper to administer than an investigation. In the diversion program set up by the California Board of Registered Nursing, the cost of participation in a four-year program for chemical dependence is about a third the cost of pursuing traditional discipline for a single violation (California Board of Nursing, 2001).

Diversion programs are voluntary and confidential. In addition to helping the nurse with recovery, the programs offer assistance to the employers and staff in coping with employee substance abuse. Impaired nurses who refuse participation in diversion programs are subject to disciplinary review by their state board of nursing and possible license revocation.

 Learning Exercise 25.8

Researching Your State Board of Nursing's Recovery Program
Determine if your state board of nursing offers some type of recovery program for chemically impaired nurses and for mentally ill nurses. You may either call the board or use the Internet. Research the following questions:
- Is the program voluntary and confidential?
- What is the rate of recidivism?
- What types of monitoring mechanisms are in place?
- What is the length of the program?
- Are nurses allowed to continue practicing while completing the treatment program?
- Are there practice restrictions?

Assignment: Write a one-page report of your findings.

Diversion programs have a good success rate. The California program reports that over 800 registered nurses have successfully completed the Board of Registered Nurses' Diversion Program since it began in 1985 (California Board of Registered Nursing, n.d.). To successfully complete the program, a nurse must demonstrate a change in lifestyle that supports recovery and have a minimum of 24 consecutive months of clean, random body-fluid test results. A nurse with a history of mental illness must demonstrate the ability to identify the symptoms or triggers of the disease and be able to take immediate action to prevent an escalation of the disease (California Board of Registered Nursing, n.d). Generally speaking, diversion programs employ a zero tolerance policy and RNs who violate the conditions set forth for completing the diversion program are subject to immediate disciplinary action (Sloan & Vernarec, 2001).

Reentry of the Chemically Impaired Employee into the Workplace

Because chemically impaired nurses recover at varying rates, predicting how long this process will take is difficult. Many experts believe impaired employees must devote at least one year to their recovery without the stresses of drug availability, overtime, and shift rotation. Success in reentering the work force depends on factors such as the extent of their recovery process and individual circumstances. Again, although managers must show a genuine personal interest in their employee's rehabilitation, their primary role is to be sure that the employee understands that the organization has the right to insist on unimpaired performance in the workplace. The following are generally accepted reentry guidelines for the recovering nurse:

- No psychoactive drug use will be tolerated.
- The employee should be assigned to day shift for the first year.
- The employee should be paired with a successful recovering nurse whenever possible.
- The employee should be willing to consent to random urine screening with toxicology or alcohol screens.
- The employee must give evidence of continuing involvement with support groups, such as Alcoholics Anonymous or Narcotics Anonymous. Employees should be encouraged to attend meetings several times each week.
- The employee should be encouraged to participate in a structured aftercare program.
- The employee should be encouraged to seek individual counseling or therapy as needed.

These guidelines should be a part of the employee's return to work contract. Mandatory drug testing, however, invokes questions about privacy rights and generally should not be implemented without advice from human resources personnel or legal counsel.

Humanistic leaders recognize the intrinsic self-worth of each individual employee and strive to understand the unique needs these workers have. If the leader genuinely cares about and shows interest in each employee, employees learn to trust, and the helping relationship has a chance to begin.

Managers have the responsibility to be proactive in identifying and confronting chemically impaired employees. Prompt and appropriate intervention by managers is essential for positive outcomes. Organizations have an ethical responsibility to actively assist these employees to return as productive members of the workforce.

INTEGRATING LEADERSHIP ROLES AND MANAGEMENT FUNCTIONS THROUGH DISCIPLINE

The leader recognizes that all employees have intrinsic worth and assists them in reaching their maximal potential. Because individual abilities, achievement drives, and situations vary, the leader recognizes each employee as an individual with unique needs and intervenes according to those specific needs. In some situations, such as frequent rule breaking, discipline may be the most effective tool for ensuring that employees succeed. In the case of the chemically impaired, psychologically impaired, or marginal employee, coaching and assisting the employee to get the treatment they need is the primary management responsibility.

Both roles require leadership and management skills. In administering discipline, the leader actively shapes group norms and promotes self-discipline. The leader also is a supporter, motivator, enabler, and coach and the humanistic attributes of the leadership role make employees want to follow the rules of the leader and thus the organization. In dealing with the employee with special needs (marginal employee, psychologically or chemically impaired), the leader serves more as a coach and resource person, than as a counselor, disciplinarian, or authority figure.

The manager, however, must enforce established rules, policies, and procedures and although good managerial practice greatly reduces the need for discipline, some employees still need external direction and discipline to accomplish organizational goals. Discipline allows employees to understand clearly the expectations of the organization and the penalty for failing to meet those expectations. Clearly, the manager's primary obligation is to see that patient safety is assured and that productivity is adequate to meet unit goals. The manager uses the authority inherent in his or her position to provide positive and negative sanctions for employee behavior in an effort to meet these goals.

The integrated leader–manager blends these unit productivity needs and human resource needs, however, selecting and implementing appropriate strategies to meet both goals is difficult. The leader–manager, however, believes that each employee has the potential to be a successful and valuable member of the unit and intervenes accordingly to meet each one's special needs.

☀ Key Concepts

- It is essential that managers be able to distinguish between employees needing *progressive discipline* and those who are chemically impaired, psychologically impaired, or marginal employees so that the employee can be managed in the most appropriate manner.
- *Discipline* is a necessary and positive tool in promoting subordinate growth.

- The optimal goal in *constructive discipline* is assisting employees to behave in a manner that allows them to be self-directed in meeting organizational goals.
- To ensure fairness, rules should include McGregor's "hot stove" components of forewarning, immediate application, consistency, and impartiality.
- If a *rule* or *regulation* is worth having, it should be enforced. When rule breaking is allowed to go unpunished, groups generally adjust to and replicate the low-level performance of the rule breaker.
- As few rules and regulations as possible should exist in the organization. All rules, regulations, and policies should be regularly reviewed to see if they should be deleted or modified in some way.
- Except for the most serious infractions, discipline should be administered in progressive steps, which include *verbal admonishment, written admonishment, suspension,* and *dismissal.*
- In *performance deficiency coaching,* the manager actively brings areas of unacceptable behavior or performance to the attention of the employee and works with him or her to establish a short-term plan to correct deficiencies.
- The *grievance procedure* is essentially a statement of wrongdoing or a procedure to follow when one believes that a wrong has been committed. All employees should have the right to file grievances about disciplinary action that they believe has been arbitrary or unfair in some way.
- The presence of a union generally entails more procedural, legalistic safeguards for administering discipline and a well-defined grievance process for employees who believe they have been disciplined unfairly.
- Because *chemical and psychological impairment* are diseases, traditional progressive discipline is inappropriate because it cannot result in employee growth.
- The profile of the impaired nurse may vary greatly, although typically behavior changes are seen in three areas: personality/behavior changes, job performance changes, and time and attendance changes.
- Nurses and managers traditionally have been slow to recognize and respond to chemically impaired colleagues.
- Confronting an employee suspected of chemical impairment should always occur before the problem escalates and before patient safety is jeopardized.
- The manager should not assume the role of counselor or treatment provider or feel the need to diagnose the cause of the chemical addiction. The manager's role is to identify clearly performance expectations for the employee and to confront the employee when those expectations are not met.
- Strategies for dealing with *marginal employees* vary with management level, the nature of the healthcare organization, and the current prevailing attitude toward passive or active intervention.

More Learning Exercises and Applications

 Learning Exercise 25.9

Determining an Appropriate Action When Proof Is Unavailable

You are the supervisor of a pediatric acute care unit. One of your patients, Joey, is a five-year-old boy who sustained 30% third-degree burns, which have been grafted and are now healing. He has been a patient in the unit for approximately two months. His mother stays with him nearly all the waking hours and generally is supportive of both him and the staff.

In the last few weeks, Joey has begun expressing increasing frustration with basic nursing tasks, has frequently been uncooperative, and has, in your staff's opinion, become very manipulative. His mother is frustrated with Joey's behavior but believes that it is understandable given the trauma he has experienced. She has begun working with the staff on a mutually acceptable behavior modification program.

Although you have attempted to assign the same nurses to care for Joey as often as possible, it is not possible today. This lack of continuity is especially frustrating today because the night shift has reported frequent tantrums and uncooperative behavior. The nurse you have assigned to Joey is Monica. Monica is a good nurse but has lacked patience in the past with uncooperative patients. During the morning, you are aware that Joey is continuing to act out. Although Monica begins to look more and more harried, she states that she is handling the situation appropriately.

When you return from lunch, Joey's mother is waiting at your office. She furiously reports that Joey told her that Monica hit him and told him he was "a very bad boy" after his mother had gone to lunch. His mother believes physical punishment was totally inappropriate, and she wants this nurse to be fired. She also states that she has contacted Joey's physician and that he is on his way over.

You call Monica to your office, where she emphatically denies all the allegations. Monica states that, during the lunch hour, Joey refused to allow her to check his dressings and that she followed the behavior modification plan and discontinued his television privileges. She believes his accusations further reflect his manipulative behavior. You then approach Joey, who tearfully and emphatically repeats the story he told to his mother. He is consistent about the details and swears to his mother that he is telling the truth. None of your staff was within hearing range of Joey's room at the time of the alleged incident. When Joey's doctor arrives, he demands that Monica be fired.

Assignment: Determine your action. You do not have proof to substantiate either Monica's or Joey's story. You believe that Monica is capable of the charges but are reluctant to implement any type of discipline without proof. What factors contribute the most to your decision?

Learning Exercise 25.10

What Type of Discipline is Appropriate?
Susie has been an RN on your medical-surgical unit for 18 months. During that time, she has been a competent nurse in terms of her assessment and organizational skills and her skills mastery. Her work habits, however, need improvement. She frequently arrives 5 to 10 minutes late for work and disrupts report when she arrives. She also frequently extends her lunch break 10 minutes beyond the allotted 30 minutes. Her absence rate is twice that of most of your other employees.

You have informally counseled Susie about her work habits on numerous past occasions. Last month, you issued a written reprimand about these work deficiencies and placed it in Susie's personnel file. Susie acknowledged at that time that she needed to work on these areas but that her responsibilities as a single parent were overwhelming at times and that she felt demotivated at work. Every day this week, Susie has arrived 15 minutes late. The staff are complaining about Susie's poor attitude and have asked that you take action.

You contemplate what additional action you might take. The next step in progressive discipline would be a suspension without pay. You believe this action could be supported given the previous attempts to counsel the employee without improvement. You also realize that many of your staff are closely watching your actions to see how you will handle this situation. You also recognize that suspending Susie would leave her with no other means of financial support and that this penalty is somewhat uncommon for the offenses described. In addition, you are unsure if this penalty will make any difference in modifying Susie's behavior.
Assignment: Decide what type of discipline, if any, is appropriate for Susie. Support your decision with appropriate rationale. Discuss your actions in terms of the effects on you, Susie, and the department.

Learning Exercise 25.11

Discipline and Insubordination

You are the coordinator of a small, specialized respiratory rehabilitation unit. Two other nurses work with you. Because all of the staff are professionals, you have used a very democratic approach to management and leadership. This approach has worked well, and productivity has always been high. The nurses work out schedules so there are always two nurses on duty during the week, and they take turns covering the weekends, at which time there is only one RN on duty. With this arrangement, it is possible for three nurses to be on duty one day during the week, if there is no holiday or other time off scheduled by either of the other two RNs.

Several months ago, you told the other RNs that the state licensing board was arriving on Wednesday, October 16, to review the unit. It would, therefore, be necessary for both of them to be on duty because you would be staying with the inspectors all day. You have reminded them several times since that time.

Today is Monday, October 14, and you are staying late preparing files for the impending inspection. Suddenly, you notice that only one of the RNs is scheduled to work on Wednesday. Alarmed, you phone Mike, the RN who is scheduled to be off. You remind him about the inspection and state that it will be necessary for him to come to work. He says that he is sorry that he forgot about the inspection but that he has scheduled a three-day cruise and has paid a large, nonrefundable deposit. After a long talk, it becomes obvious to you that Mike is unwilling to change his plans. You say to him, "Mike, I feel this borders on insubordination. I really need you on the 16th, and I am requesting that you come in. If you do not come to work, I will need to take appropriate action." Mike replies, "I'm sorry to let you down. Do what you have to do. I need to take this trip, and I will not cancel my plans."

Assignment: What action could you take? What action should you take? Outline some alternatives. Assume it is not possible to float in additional staff because of the specialty expertise required to work in this department. Decide what you should do. Give rationale for your decision. Did ego play a part in your decision?

 Web Links

Addiction Recovery Resources for the Professional
http://www.lapage.com/arr/
Identifies resources for chemically impaired healthcare professionals.

Employee Relations: Positive Discipline
http://www.bizmove.com/personnel/m4i4.htm
Defines positive discipline and proposes guidelines for establishing a climate of positive discipline outlines strategies.

Employee Discipline and Termination Checklist
http://www.workplaceissues.com/freereports.htm
This checklist provides questions designed to be a guide for use in the proper discipline or dismissal of an employee.

Monitoring, Reentry and Relapse. Prevention for Chemically Dependent Healthcare Professionals
http://www.nursingceu.com/NCEU/courses/monitoring/index.htm
One unit CEU course on chemical dependency and health care professionals.

References

Baum, G. (2000). Ready, aim, fire. *Forbes, 165*(8), 174–175.

Bell, D.M., McDonough, J.P., Ellison, J.S., & Fitzhugh, E.C. (1999). Controlled drug misuse by certified registered nurse anesthetists. *American Association Nurse Anesthetists Journal, 67*(2), 133–140.

California Board of Registered Nursing. (2001). What is the diversion program? Available at: http://www.rn.ca.gov/div/whatisdiv.htm. Accessed December 16, 2003.

Cherry, B., & Jacob, S. R. (2002). *Contemporary nursing. Issues, trends, and management* (2nd ed.). St. Louis: Mosby.

Danis, S. J. (2003). The impaired nurse. Education/CE. Self Study Module. *Nursing Spectrum.* Available at: http://nsweb.nursingspectrum.com/ce/ce153.htm. Retrieved December 16, 2003.

Guffey, C. J., & Helms, M. M. (2001). Effective employee discipline: A case of the Internal Revenue Service. *Public Personnel Management, 30*(1), 111–128.

Haack, M. R., & Yocom, C. J. (2002). State policies and nurses with substance abuse disorders. *Journal of Nursing Scholarship, 34*(1), 89–94.

Kerfoot, K., & Wantz, S. L. (2003). Compliance leadership: The 17th century model that doesn't work. *Nursing Economics, 21*(1), 42–44.

Lillibridge, J., Cox, M., & Cross, W. (2002). Uncovering the secret: Giving voice to the experiences of nurses who misuse substances. *Journal of Advanced Nursing, 39*(3), 219–229.

McGregor, D. (1967). *The professional manager.* New York: McGraw-Hill.

Modlin, H. C., & Montes, A. (1964). Narcotics addiction in physicians. *American Journal of Psychiatry,* 121, 358–363.

National Institute on Drug Abuse (NIDA). (n.d.). Pain medications and other prescription drugs. Available at: http://www.drugabuse.gov/infofax/painmed.html. Retrieved December 16, 2003.

Ponech, S. (2000). Telltale signs. *Nursing Management, 31*(5), 32–38.

Rafes, R., & Warren, E. (April 2001). Hiring and firing in community colleges: Caveats and considerations for protecting institutions and employees. *Community College Journal of Research & Practice, 25*(4), 283–297.

Rasmussen, E. (March 19, 2001). Clean and Sober. *Nurseweek.* Retrieved 11/4/04 from http://www.nurseweek.com/news/features/01-03/sober.asp

Sloan, A., & Vernarec, E. (2001). Impaired nurses: Reclaiming careers. *RN Web Archive.* Available at: http://www.rnweb.com/be_core/ADS?filename=/be_core/content/journals/r/data/2001/0201/impaired2.html&title=Impaired+nurses%3A+Reclaiming+careers&navtype=r&site=r&query=chemical+addiction. Accessed December 16, 2003.

Storr, C.L., Trinkoff, A.M., & Anthony, J.C. (1999). Job strain and non-medical drug use. *Drug Alcohol Dependency, 55*(1–2), 45–51.

Trinkoff, A.M., Zhou, Q., Storr, C.L.,& Soeken, K.L. (1999). Workplace access, negative prescriptions, job strain, and substance abuse in registered nurses. *Nursing Research, 49*(2), 83–90.

West, M. M. (2002). Early risk indicators of substance abuse among nurses. *Journal of Nursing Scholarship, 34*(2), 187–193.

Bibliography

Bain, V. (2000). How to diagnose and treat poor performance. *Journal for Quality & Participation, 23*(5), 38–42.

Castledine, G. (2003). Professional misconduct case studies. Case 97: Physical abuse. Senior staff nurse who physically abused clients in a home. *British Journal of Nursing, 12*(14), 837.

Collins, S. E. (2003). Legally speaking. The trouble with bending the rules. *RN, 66*(7), 69–70, 72, 78.

Domrose, C. (2001, February 9). New beginnings. *Nurse Week (California),* 30–32.

Fedor, P. F. (2000). 30-day limit on reprimands. *Nursing, 30*(10), 12.

Feskanich, D. et al. (2002). Stress and suicide in the Nurses' Health Study. *J Epidemiol Community Health, 56*(2), 95–98.

Forman, H., & Merrick, F. (2003). Discipline. Learning the rules of the management high road. *Journal of Nursing Administration, 33*(2), 65–67.

Holman, T. L. (2001). Reconcilable differences. *Emergency Medical Services, 2*(1): Suppl: 4, 7.

Kany, K. (2000). Workplace rights. Patient vs. employment abandonment. *American Journal of Nursing, 100*(6), 73.

Kasoff, J. (2003). Grievance tracking. Targeting an improvement process. *Journal of Nursing Administration, 33*(7/8), 376.

Lachman, V. D. (2000). Coaching techniques. *Nursing Management, 31*(1), 15–19.

LaDuke, S. (2000). The effects of professional discipline on nurses. *American Journal of Nursing, 100*(6), 26–34.

LaDuke, S. (2001). Professional misconduct: Issues related to hiring and firing. *Journal of Nursing Administration, 31*(9), 408–413.

Liden, R. C., Wayne, S. J., & Kraimer, M. L. (2001). Managing individual performance in work groups. *Human Resource Management, 40*(1), 63–72.

Morrison, C. (2000). Fear of addiction. *American Journal of Nursing, 100*(70), 81.

Murphy, V. (2000). HR toolbox. Read my lips: perfect your verbal counseling skills: The first step in disciplining problem employees. *EMS Manager and Supervisor, 2*(2), 2–3.

Murphy, V. (2000). HR toolbox. Problem employees part II: create meaningful written reprimands: The second step in disciplining problem employees. *EMS Manager and Supervisor, 2*(3), 2–3.

Murphy, V. (2000). HR toolbox. Trial before fire: pre-disciplinary hearings are your third step in progressive discipline. *EMS Manager and Supervisor, 2*(4), 2–3.

Murray, B. (2003). Recruitment & retention report. Positive discipline reaps retention. *Nursing Management, 34*(6), 19–20, 22.

Raphael, T. (2001). Dealing with disgruntled employees. *Workforce, 80*(1), 12–15.

Samet, J. H., Friedmann, P. D., & Saitz, R. (2001). Benefits of linking primary medical care and substance abuse services. *Archives of Internal Medicine, 161,* 85–91.

Trossman, S. (2003). Issues update. Nurses' addictions: Finding alternatives to discipline. *American Journal of Nursing, 103*(9), 27–28.

What is Peer Assistance Services and how did this agency materialize? An interview with Elizabeth M. Pace, MSM, RN, CEAP. (2001). *Journal of Addictions Nursing, 13*(1), 49–51.

Learning Exercise 9.5

A Busy Day at the Public Health Agency
Here is how one nurse handled interruptions and still had time for lunch.

Time	Task	Rationale
8:00 A.M.	Assign lunch breaks: 11:30–12:30—receptionist 12:30–1:30—clerical worker 12:00–1:00—you	Because you have a lunch engagement at noon, make sure other employees know when their lunch times must be.
	Finish reports	Because reports are due tonight, this would be the immediate task to be accomplished. Plan to finish these by 9 A.M.
8:30 A.M.	Supervisor's request	Ask her when she needs the information. Tell her an estimate using primary diagnoses is now available but that an accurate figure that includes secondary diagnoses must wait until you have time to go through your 150 family case files, which will be next week.
9:00 A.M.	Client with pregnant daughter/ chest clinic drop-ins	The pregnancy takes priority over the chest clinic drop-ins. Ask the receptionist to start the paperwork on drop-ins while you spend 30 minutes with the mother.
9:30 A.M.	Phone call	Delegate this to the receptionist.
9:30 A.M.	Dental clinic referral	Delegate this duty to the clerical worker.
10:00 A.M.	Client call	Because this person is confused and you don't have available information, ask that he come in at 10 A.M. tomorrow with his bills.
10:45 A.M.	Families with food vouchers	Ask receptionist to finish paperwork and interviews on the families. Then quickly review information and sign vouchers. These families should not have had such a long wait. Make a note to find out what happened, and later counsel office staff about the delay.
11:45 A.M.	Drug call	Talk with client. Make a referral to a local drug clinic, and make an appointment for a part-time psychiatrist at the clinic. Do not get too involved on the phone with the client because it is better to make the appropriate referrals.

Learning Exercise 12.3

Cultures and Hierarchies
Below is an analysis of how one might approach a problem involving a non-nursing department but affecting the nurses' work and the nursing staff.

Analysis: Data Assessment
1. A copy of the organization chart was given to you when you were hired. The formal structure is a line-and-staff organization. The housekeeping department head is below the nursing director and the nursing section supervisor but at the same level as the immediate clinic supervisor. The housekeeping department head reports directly to the maintenance and engineering department head.
2. The county administrator has stated she has an open-door policy. You do not know if this means that bypassing department heads is acceptable or merely that the administrator is interested in the employees. An important reason for not skipping intermediate supervisors when communicating is that they must know what is going on in their departments. A manager's position, value, and status are strengthened if he or she serves as a vital and essential link in the vertical chain of command.
3. You have twice attempted to talk with your immediate supervisor; however, whether you followed up regarding your supervisor's action on the complaint is unclear.
4. You are a new employee and therefore probably do not know how the formal or informal structure works. This newness might render the complaints less credible.
5. Possible risks include creating trouble for the housekeeping staff or their immediate supervisor, being labeled a troublemaker by others in the organization, and alienating your immediate supervisor.
6. Before proceeding, you need to assess your own values and determine what is motivating you to pursue this issue.

Alternatives for Action
There are many choices available to you.
1. You can do nothing. This is often a wise choice and should always be an alternative for any problem. Some problems solve themselves if left alone. Sometimes the time is not right to solve the problem.
2. You can talk with the county health administrator. Although this involves some risk, the possibility exists that the administrator will be able to take action. At the very least, you will have unburdened your problem on someone.
3. You can talk directly with the individual housekeepers by using "I" messages, such as, "I get angry when the housekeeping staff take naps, and the bathrooms are dirty." Perhaps if feelings and frustrations were shared, you would learn more about the problem. Maybe there is a reason for their behavior; maybe they only socialize during their breaks. This alternative involves some risk: The housekeepers might look on you as a troublemaker.

4. Have all the evening staff sign a petition, and give it to the immediate supervisor. Forming a coalition often produces results. However, the supervisor could view this action as overreacting or meddlesome and might feel threatened.

5. Go to the housekeeping staff's department head and report them. In this way, you are saving some time and going right to the person who is in charge. However, this might be unfair to the housekeepers and certainly will create some enemies for you.

6. Follow up with the immediate supervisor. You could request permission to take action yourself and ask how best to proceed. This would involve your immediate supervisor and keep her informed. However, it also shows that you are willing to take risks and devote some personal time and energy to solving the problem.

Selecting an Alternative

This problem has no right answer. Under certain conditions, various solutions could be used. Under most circumstances, it is more fair to others and efficient for you to select the third alternative listed. However, because you are new and have little knowledge of the formal and informal organizational structure, your wisest choice would be alternative 6. New employees need to seek guidance from their immediate supervisors.

For this follow-up session with the supervisor to be successful, you need to do the following:

1. Talk with the supervisor during a quiet time.

2. Admit to personally "owning" the problem without involving colleagues.

3. Acknowledge that legitimate reasons for the housekeepers' actions may exist.

4. Request permission to talk directly with the housekeepers. Role-play an appropriate approach with the supervisor.

You must accept the consequences of your actions. However, your attempt to correct the problem may motivate your supervisor to pursue the problem directly with the housekeeping staff's supervisor. If this is the action your supervisor takes, you should ask to speak with the housekeeping staff directly first. If, after talking with the housekeeping staff, you decide a problem still exists and you elect to address that problem, then you should return to your immediate supervisor before proceeding.

Analysis of the Problem Solving

Would you have solved this problem differently? What are some other alternatives that could have been generated? Have you ever gone outside the chain of command and had a positive experience as a result?

Learning Exercise 13.5

Turning Lemons into Lemonade

This is the strategy that Sally Jones used to solve the conflict between her and Bob Black.

In analyzing this case, one must forego feelings of resentment regarding Bob's obvious play for control and power. In reality, what real danger does his empire building pose for the director of nursing? Isn't Sally really just ridding herself and her staff of clerical duties and interruptions?

A certain amount of power is inherent in the ability to hire. Employees develop a loyalty for the person who actually hires them. Because Sally Jones or her designee will still actually make the final selection, Bob's proposal should result in little loss of loyalty or power.

Let's look at what the real Sally Jones did to solve this conflict. When she was able to see that Bob was not stripping her of any power, Sally was capable of using some very proactive strategies. Here was a chance for her to appear compromising, thereby increasing her esteem in the CEO's eyes and gaining political clout in the organization.

When she met with Jane Smith and Bob, Sally began by complimenting Bob on his ideas. Then she suggested that because nurses were in the habit of coming to the nursing department to apply for positions and because human resources offices were rather cold and formal places, stationing the new personnel clerk in the nursing office would be more convenient and inviting. Sally knew that the human resources department lacked adequate space and that the nursing office had some extra room. She went on to say that because some of her unit clerks were very knowledgeable about the hospital organization, Bob might want to interview several of them for the new position. Although an experienced unit clerk would be difficult to replace, Sally said she was willing to make this sacrifice for the new plan to succeed.

The CEO, very impressed with Sally's generous offer, turned to Bob and said, "I think Sally has an excellent idea. Why don't you hire one of her clerks and station her in the nursing office?" Jane then said to Sally, "Now, do we understand that the clerk will be Bob's employee and will work under him?"

Sally agreed with this because she felt she had just pulled off a great power play. Let's examine what Sally won in this political maneuver.

1. She gained by not competing with Bob, therefore not making him her enemy.
2. She gained by impressing the CEO with her flexibility and initiative.
3. She gained a new employee.

Although the new employee would be working for Bob with the salary charged to his cost center, the clerk would be Sally's former employee. Because the clerk would be working in the nursing office, she would have some allegiance to Sally. In addition, the clerk would be doing all the work that Sally and her assistants had been doing and at no cost to the nursing department.

When Sally first received Bob's memo, she was angry; her initial reaction was to talk to the CEO privately and complain about Bob. Fortunately, she did not do this. It is nearly always a political mistake for one manager to talk about another behind his or her back and without his or her knowledge. This generally reflects unfavorably on the employee, with a loss of respect from the supervisor.

Another option Sally had was to compete with Bob and be uncooperative. Although this might have delayed centralizing the personnel department, in the end Bob undoubtedly would have accomplished his goal, and Sally would not have been able to reap such a great political victory.

The later effects of this political maneuver were even more rewarding. The personnel clerk remained loyal to Sally. Bob became less adversarial and more cooperative with Sally on other issues. The CEO gave her a sly grin later in the week and said, "Great move with Bob Black." This case might be concluded by saying that this is an example of someone being given a lemon and then making lemonade.

Learning Exercise 18.3

Crossword Puzzle—A Review of Motivational Theory
Solution

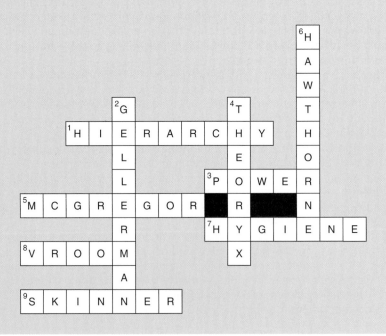

Learning Exercise 21.3

Conflicting Personal, Professional, and Organizational Obligations
The following is conflict resolution strategy used by you when the nursing office supervisor (Carol), who considers you to be competent and responsible, asked you to help cover the workload in the delivery room. Although this supervisor believes you can do the job, you think that you do not know enough about labor and delivery nursing to be effective. Here are some strategies you can use to resolve the conflict.

Analysis
You need to examine your goal, the supervisor's goal, and a goal on which you can both agree. Your goal might be protection of your license and doing nothing that would bring harm to a patient. Carol's goal might be to provide assistance to an understaffed unit. A possible supraordinate goal would be for neither you nor Carol to do anything that would bring risk or harm to the organization.

The following conflict resolution strategies were among your choices:

Accommodating
Accommodating is the most obvious wrong choice. If you really believe you are unqualified to work in the delivery room, this strategy could be harmful to patients and your career. Such a decision would not meet with your goal or the supraordinate goal.

Smoothing or Avoiding
Because you have little power and no one is available to intervene on your behalf, you are unable to choose either of these solutions. The problem cannot be avoided, nor will you be able to smooth the conflict away.

Compromising
In similar situations, you might be able to negotiate a compromise. For instance, you might say, "I cannot go to the delivery room, but I will float to another medical–surgical area if there is someone on another medical–surgical unit who has OB experience." Alternatively, you could compromise by stating, "I feel comfortable working postpartum and will work in that area if you have a qualified nurse from postpartum that can be sent to the delivery room." It is possible that either solution could end the conflict, depending on the availability of other personnel and how comfortable you would feel in the postpartum area. Often, someone attempting to problem solve, such as the supervisor in this case, becomes so overburdened and stressed that other alternatives are not apparent.

Collaborating

If time allows and the other party is willing to adopt a common goal, this is the preferred method of dealing with conflict. However, the power holder must view the other as having something important to contribute if this method of conflict management is to be successful. Perhaps you could convince Carol that the hospital and she could be at risk if an unqualified RN was assigned to an area requiring special skills. Once the supraordinate goal is adopted, you and Carol would be able to find alternative solutions to the problem. There are always many more ways to solve a problem than any one person can generate.

Competing

Normally, competing is not an attractive alternative for resolving conflict, but sometimes it is the only recourse. Before using competition as a method to manage this conflict, you need to examine your motives. Are you truly unqualified for work in the delivery room, or are you using your lack of experience as an excuse not to float to an unfamiliar area that would cause you anxiety? If you are truly convinced that you are unqualified, then you possess information that the supervisor does not have (a criterion necessary for the use of competing as a method of conflict resolution). Therefore, if other methods for solving the conflict are not effective, you must use competition to solve the conflict. You must win at the expense of the supervisor's losing. You risk much when using this type of resolution. The supervisor might fire you for insubordination or, at best, she may view you as uncooperative. The most appropriate method for using competition in this situation is an assertive approach. An example would be repeating firmly but nonaggressively, "I cannot go to the delivery room to work because I would be putting patients at risk. I am unqualified to work in that area." This approach is usually effective. You must not work in an area where patient safety would be at risk. It would be morally, ethically, and legally wrong for you to do so. (*Note*: The legal implications of this case are discussed in Chapter 5.)

Learning Exercise 25.5

The Marginal Employee
As the nursing supervisor of a 35-bed oncology unit in a 400-bed hospital, this is how you may solve the problems posed by a marginal employee (Judy) on your staff.
1. Identify the problem: The marginal performance of one employee is affecting unit morale.
2. Gather data to analyze the causes and consequences of the problem. The following information should be gathered and considered:
   • Judy has been a registered nurse for 15 years and probably has always been a marginal employee.
   • Judy states she is highly motivated to be an oncology nurse.
   • Judy has been coached on several occasions regarding how she might improve her performance and no improvement is evident.
   • It is difficult to recruit and retain staff nurses for this unit.
   • The unit is already short two full-time RN positions.
   • Judy's performance is not unsatisfactory; it is only marginal.
   • The other nurses on the floor considered Judy's performance to be disruptive enough to ask you to remove her from the floor.
3. Identify alternative solutions.
   Alternative 1—Terminate Judy's employment.
   Alternative 2—Transfer Judy to another floor.
   Alternative 3—Continue coaching Judy, and help her identify specific and realistic goals about her performance.
   Alternative 4—Do nothing and hope the problem resolves itself.
   Alternative 5—Work with the other staff nurses to create a work environment that will make Judy want to be transferred from the unit.
4. Evaluate the alternatives.
   Alternative 1—Although this would provide a rapid solution to the problem, there are many negative aspects to this alternative. Judy, although performing at a marginal level, has not done anything that warrants discipline or termination. Although some staff have requested her removal from the unit, this action could be viewed as arbitrary and grossly unfair by a silent minority. Thus, employees' sense of security and unit morale could decrease even more. In addition, it would be difficult to fill Judy's position.
   Alternative 2—This alternative would immediately remove the problem from the supervisor and would probably please the staff. This alternative merely transfers the problem to a different unit, which is counterproductive to organizational goals. This might be an appropriate alternative if the supervisor could show that Judy could be expected to perform at a higher level on another unit. It is difficult to predict how Judy would feel about this alternative. Judy is probably aware of the other staff's frustration with her, and a transfer would provide at least temporary shelter from her colleagues' hostility. In addition, although Judy would

be pleased that she was not dismissed, she would appropriately view the transfer as her failure. This recognition is demoralizing, and the opportunity for her to fulfill a long-term career goal would be denied.

Alternative 3—This alternative requires a long-term and time-consuming commitment on the part of the manager. There is inadequate information in the case to determine whether the supervisor can make this type of commitment. In addition, there is no guarantee that setting short-term, specific, and realistic goals will improve Judy's work performance. It should, however, increase Judy's self-esteem and reinforce her supervisor's interest in her as a person. It also retains a registered nurse who is difficult to replace. This alternative does not address the staff's dissatisfaction.

Alternative 4—There are few positive aspects to this alternative other than that the supervisor would not have to expend energy at this point. The problem, however, will probably snowball, and unit morale will get worse.

Alternative 5—Although most would agree that this alternative is morally corrupt, there are some advantages. Judy would voluntarily leave the unit, and the supervisor and staff would not have to deal with the problem. The disadvantages are similar to those cited in Alternative 1.

5. Select the Appropriate Solution

   As in most decisions with an ethical component, there is no one right answer, and all the alternatives have desirable facets. Alternative 3 probably presents the least number of undesirable attributes. The cost to the supervisor is in time and effort. There is really little to lose in attempting this plan to increase employee productivity, because there are no replacements to fill the position anyway. Losing Judy by dismissal or transfer merely increases the workload on the other employees due to short staffing. It also cannot help the employee.

6. Implement the Solution

   In implementing Alternative 3, the supervisor should be very clear with Judy about her motives. She also must be sure that the goals they set are specific and realistic. Although the staff may continue to verbalize their unhappiness with Judy's performance, the supervisor should be careful not to discuss confidential information about Judy's coaching plan with them. The manager should, however, reassure the staff that she is aware of their concerns and that she will follow the situation closely.

7. Evaluate the Results

   The supervisor elected to review her problem solving six months after the plan was implemented. She found that although Judy was satisfied with her performance and appreciative of her supervisor's efforts, her performance had not improved appreciably. Judy continued to be a marginal employee but was meeting minimal competency levels. The supervisor did find, however, that the staff seemed more accepting of Judy's level of ability and rarely verbalized their dissatisfaction with her anymore. In general, unit morale increased again.

Glossary

accountability — internalized responsibility whereby an individual agrees to be morally responsible for the consequences of his actions. (12)*

ad hoc structure — loose bureaucratic structure, usually temporary. (12)

administrative agencies — organizations given authority to act by the state legislative body and create rules and regulations that enforce statutory laws. (5)

administrative cases — legal situations in which an individual is sued by a state or federal governmental agency assigned the responsibility of implementing governmental programs. (5)

administrative man — decision maker who has only fragmented knowledge and has difficulty predicting consequences; chooses from only a few alternatives; therefore final choice is "satisficing" rather than maximizing. (1)

Administrative Simplification plan — portion of HIPAA aimed at restructuring the coding of health information to simplify the digital exchange of information among healthcare providers and to improve the efficiency of healthcare delivery. (5)

advanced directives — written instructions regarding end-of-life care completed by competent individuals, to be implemented should they become incapacitated in the future. (5)

advocacy — helping others to grow and self-actualize by informing others of their rights and ascertaining that they have sufficient information on which to base their decisions. (6)

affirming the consequences — type of illogical thinking in which one decides that if *B* is good, and one is doing *A*, then *A* must not be good. (1)

androgogy — adult learning. (16)

applied ethics — application of normative ethical theory to everyday problems. (4)

arguing from analogy — type of inaccurate thinking that occurs when a component is present in two separate concepts, and one assumes that since *A* is present in *B*, then *A* and *B* are alike in all respects. (1)

assault — conduct that makes a person fearful and produces a reasonable apprehension of harm. (5)

authoritarian — leadership style characterized by strong control over the work group, coercion, commands, downward communication, a single decision maker, emphasis on status, and punitive criticism. (3)

authority — the official power to act. (12)

*Numbers in parentheses following the definition indicate the chapter in which the term is discussed.

authority–power gap — the gap that sometimes exists between a position of authority and subordinate response. (13)

autonomy — ethical principle which suggests that each individual should have freedom of choice and be able to accept the responsibility for that choice. (4)

battery — intentional and wrongful physical contact with a person that entails an injury or offensive touching. (5)

beneficence — ethical principle which suggests that the actions one takes should be done in an effort to promote good. (4)

breach of duty — violation of the standard of care. (5)

capital expenditure budget — expenses to cover major purchases (e.g., real estate) and acquisitions (e.g., MRI equipment); composed of long-term and short-term components. (10)

career development — planning and implementation of career plans; a life process involving the individual and his or her employer(s). (11)

case management — collaborative process that assesses, plans, implements, coordinates, monitors, and evaluates options and services to meet an individual's health needs through communication and available resources. (14)

centralized decision making — decisions that are made by a few managers at the top of the hierarchy. (12)

centralized staffing — form of staffing in which staffing decisions are made by personnel in a central office or staffing center. (17)

certification programs — programs designed to recognize advanced knowledge in a particular specialty, which is demonstrated by passing a written examination and meeting practice requirements. (5)

chain of command — the formal paths of communication and authority. (12)

change agent — a person skilled in the theory and implementation of planned change. (8)

chunking — presenting independent items of information and grouping them together into one unit. (16)

civil cases — legal situation in which one individual sues another monetarily to compensate for a perceived loss. (5)

clinical ethics committees — group formed to assist with problem solving regarding patient health issues such as end-of-life concerns. (4)

closed-unit staffing — occurs when the staff members on a unit make a commitment to cover all absences and needed extra help themselves, in return for not being pulled from the unit in times of low census. (17)

coercive power — power based on fear of punishment. (13)

competence — the ability to meet the requirements of a particular role. (16)

confidentiality — ethical principle which holds that there is an obligation to observe the privacy of another and to hold certain information in strict confidence. (4)

constitution — system of fundamental laws or principles that govern a nation, society, corporation, or another aggregate of individuals, used to establish the basis of a governing system for the future and the present. (5)

controllable expenses — expenses that can be controlled or varied by a manager. (10)

controlling — final phase of the management process; in this phase, performance is measured against predetermined standards and action is taken to correct discrepancies between these standards and actual performance. (2)

copayment — in healthcare circles, the amount of money enrollees pay out of their pocket at the time a service is provided. (10)

court decisions — judicial or decisional laws made by the courts to interpret legal issues that are in dispute. (5)

criminal cases — legal situation in which a person faces charges generally filed by the state or federal attorney general for crimes committed against an individual or society. (5)

critical pathways — also called clinical pathways; predetermined courses of progress that patients should be making after admission for a specific diagnosis or after a specific surgery. (10)

cross-training — providing personnel with varying educational backgrounds and expertise, the skills necessary to take on tasks normally outside their scope of work and to move between work environments and function knowledgeably. (17)

decentralized decision making — diffused decision making; allows problems to be solved by the lowest practical managerial level. (12)

decentralized staffing — form of staffing in which the unit manager is often responsible for covering all scheduled staff absences, reducing staff during periods of decreased patient census or acuity, adding staff during periods of high patient census or acuity, preparing monthly unit schedules, and preparing holiday and vacation schedules. (17)

decision making — complex, cognitive process employed to choose a particular course of action; implies that there was doubt about several courses of action and that a choice was made to eliminate the uncertainty. (1)

defamation — communicating to a third party false information that injures a person's reputation; causes economic damage; diminishes the esteem, respect, goodwill, or confidence that others have for the person; or causes adverse, derogatory, or unpleasant opinions of him. (5)

defendant — party in a lawsuit that is alleged to have caused injury to the plaintiff. (5)

democratic — leadership style characterized by moderate control, motivation using economic and ego awards, direction via suggestions and guidance, interactive communication, group decision making, and constructive criticism. (3)

deontological theories — beliefs of ethical decision making that arise from the intent of the action that the decision maker takes; includes duty-based, rights-based, and intuitionist ethical reasoning. (4)

diagnosis-related groups (DRGs) — predetermined payment schedules reflecting historical costs for treatment of specific patient conditions. (10)

directing — fourth phase of the management process; also referred to as coordinating or activating; in this "doing" phase of management, managers direct the work of subordinates. (2)

disease management (also called population-based health care and continuous health improvement) — a comprehensive, integrated approach to the care and reimbursement of high-cost, chronic illnesses across treatment settings regardless of reimbursement patterns. (14)

doctrine of charitable immunity — legal concept which holds that a charitable (nonprofit) hospital cannot be sued by a person who has been injured as a result of a hospital employee's negligence. (5)

driving forces — forces that propel a system toward the change. (8)

duty-based reasoning — ethical framework in which decisions are made because an obligation exists to do something or to refrain from doing something. (4)

economic man — decision maker who has complete knowledge of the problem or situation, a complete list of possible alternatives, a rational system of ordering preference of alternatives, and the ability to select the choice that will maximize utility function. (1)

emotional intelligence — process of regulating both feelings and expressions; leaders with emotional intelligence possess the ability to identify emotions in themselves and others, use emotions in their thought processes, manage emotions in themselves and others, and understand and reason with emotions. (3)

empowerment — an interactive process that develops, builds, and increases power through cooperation, sharing, and working together. (13)

entrepreneurial case management — independent case management consultants contract with patients, family members, physicians, or insurance companies to coordinate all aspects of care, in the home and in any level of care needed. (14)

ethical dilemmas — situations in which one must choose between two or more undesirable alternatives. (4)

ethical frameworks — guides used to assist in clarifying personal values and beliefs in order to facilitate the solution of an ethical problem; four of the most commonly used ethical frameworks are utilitarianism, duty-based reasoning, rights-based reasoning, and intuitionism. (4)

ethics — the systematic study of what a person's conduct and actions ought to be with regard to self, other human beings, and the environment. (4)

enculturation — see socialization. (16)

expert power — power gained through knowledge or skill. (13)

express consent — witnessing a written consent; role of nurse in express consent is to be sure that the patient has informed consent and to seek remedy if he or she does not. (5)

expressed policies — policies that are delineated either verbally or in writing. (7)

false imprisonment — unlawful confinement within fixed boundaries, or restraint of movement, produced by physical, emotional, or chemical means. (5)

feminist power (also called *self-power*) — the power a person gains and maintains over his or her own life; personal power that comes from maturity, ego integration, security in relationships, and self-confidence. (13)

fidelity — ethical principle that suggests that individuals should be faithful to their commitments and promises. (4)

fixed expenses — expenses that do not vary (e.g., mortgage payment). (10)

flat organizational designs — an effort to remove hierarchical layers by flattening the scalar chain and decentralizing the organization. (12)

flex time — system that allows employees to select the time schedules that best meet their personal needs while still meeting work responsibilities. (17)

float pool — group of employees who agree to cross-train on multiple units so that they can work additional hours during periods of high census or worker shortages. (17)

foreseeability of harm — having the knowledge or availability of information that not meeting the standard of care can result in harm. (5)

formal organizational structure — highly visible plan that defines roles and functions, managerial authority, responsibility, and accountability; rank and hierarchy are evident. (12)

functional nursing care — care organized by task with specific tasks (e.g., blood pressure measurement, wound care) being performed by different nursing personnel rather than one nurse. (14)

goal — desired result toward which effort is directed; the aim of the philosophy. (7)

Good Samaritan laws — statute intended to protect healthcare providers from potential liability if they volunteer their professional skills away from the workplace in an emergency situation, provided that actions taken are not grossly negligent. (5)

governmental immunity — common law rule stating that governments cannot be held liable for the negligent acts of their employees while carrying out government activities. (5)

group HMO — independent physician group contracted directly by a parent HMO. (10)

Health Insurance Portability and Accountability Act (HIPAA) — Federal act passed in 1996 directed at protecting the privacy of health information and improving the portability and continuity of health insurance coverage. (5)

health maintenance organizations (HMOs) — A prepaid organization that provides healthcare to voluntarily enrolled members in return for a preset amount of money on a per-person, per-month basis. Also includes a licensed health plan that places at least some of the providers at risk for medical expenses as well as health plans that utilize designated (usually primary care) physicians as gatekeepers (although some HMOs do not). Common types of HMOs include staff, independent practice association (IPA), group, and network. (10)

home health case management — service that manages the needs of the chronically ill in the home setting; includes coordinating wound care, infusion therapy services, physical therapy, speech therapy, occupational therapy, durable medical equipment, medication monitoring, and skilled nursing services. (14)

hospice case management — coordination of end-of-life care. (14)

implied consent — used in an emergency situation when it is impossible to gain informed consent; consists of the physician stating in the medical record that the patient is unable to provide signed consent but that treatment is immediately needed and is in the patient's best interest. (5)

implied policies — policies that are neither written nor expressed verbally, but usually have developed over time and follow a precedent. (7)

inactivism — type of conventional planning in which energy is spent preventing change and maintaining conformity. (7)

incident reports — records of unusual or unexpected incidents that occur in the course of a client's treatment; typically considered confidential and cannot be subpoenaed by clients or used as evidence in their lawsuits in most states. (5)

indoctrination — induction, orientation, and socialization of employees. (15)

informal organizational structure — unplanned and hidden structure that is generally social with blurred or shifting lines of authority and accountability. (12)

informational power — power gained by possession of information that others must have to accomplish their goals. (13)

informed consent — signature of a patient on a consent form for surgery or procedure indicating that he or she has received full disclosure of all pertinent information regarding the surgery or procedure, and that he or she understands all potential benefits and risks associated with the procedure. (5)

institutional licensure — shifting the responsibility for professional licensure from regulatory boards, such as a Board of Registered Nursing, to an institution or agency. (5)

insurance case management (**also called** *third-party payor case management)* — case manager resolves disputes between providers, patients, and the insurer regarding needed levels of care and authorizations for reimbursement. (14)

intentional torts — legal wrongs committed against a person or property, independent of a contract, that render the person who commits them liable for damages in a civil action; direct invasion of someone's legal rights. (5)

interactional theory — premise that leadership behavior is generally determined by the relationship between the leader's personality and the specific situation. (3)

internship — an extended orientation program that lasts longer than short-term acclimation to a job or profession. (16)

interview — a verbal interaction between individuals for a particular purpose. (15)

intuitionism — ethical framework which allows the decision maker to review each ethical problem or issue on a case-by-case basis, primarily using intuition to compare the relative weights of goals, duties, and rights. (4)

Independent Practice Association (IPA) — an intermediary that negotiates contracts with individual physicians or groups to provide services for HMOs. (10)

job profile — an analysis of the criteria that defines top performers in a specific job. (15)

joint liability — legal concept in which the healthcare providers and healthcare organization share liability for wrongdoing. (5)

justice — ethical principle stating all equals should be treated equally and unequals should be treated according to their differences. (4)

laissez-faire — leadership style characterized by minimal control, motivation occurring rarely and only when requested by group, little direction, interactive communication, dispersed decision making, group emphasis, and lack of criticism. (3)

leader — a person who influences and guides direction, opinion, and course of action; often requires taking risks, and challenging the status quo. (3)

leadership — process of persuading and influencing others toward a goal, through mostly noncoercive means; typically composed of a wide variety of roles. (3)

legitimate power position — also called authority; power gained by a title or official position within an organization. (13)

license — legal document permitting a person to offer special skills and knowledge to the public in a particular jurisdiction, when such practice would otherwise be unlawful. (5)

line organization — authority and responsibility are clearly defined; typical bureaucratic structure. (12)

long-range plans (**also called** *strategic plans)* — complex organizational plans that involve a long period (usually 3 to 10 years). (7)

malpractice (**also called** *professional negligence)* — failure of a person with professional training to act in a reasonable and prudent manner. (5)

managerial decision-making model — decision-making model which includes the following steps: setting objectives, searching for alternatives, evaluating alternatives, choosing, implementing, and following up or controlling. (Goal setting step eliminates weakness of traditional problem solving process.) (1)

mandatory overtime — employees are forced to work additional shifts, often under threat of patient abandonment. (17)

matrix structure — formal vertical and horizontal chain of command that focuses on function (tasks required to produce the product), and product (end result of the function). (12)

Medicaid — a federal–state cooperative health insurance plan for the financially indigent. (10)

mentoring — a distinctive interactive relationship between two individuals, occurring most commonly in a professional setting with the *mentor* consciously deciding to assist the protégé (or *mentee*) in attaining expert status and in furthering his or her career development. (16)

mission statement — brief statement identifying the reason that an organization exists, the organization's constituency, and the organization's position regarding ethics, principles, and standards of practice; also called a purpose statement. (7)

modular nursing — a mini-team (two or three members) approach to nursing care that allows the professional nurse more time for planning and coordinating team members; the small nursing team requires less communication, allowing members better use of their time for direct patient care activities. (14)

monochronic style — preference for completing one activity or task at a time. (9)

moral distress — conflict that occurs when one knows the right thing to do, but institutional or other constraints make it difficult to pursue the desired course of action. (4)

moral uncertainty — conflict that occurs when one is unsure what moral principles or values apply in an ethical conflict, or even if there is an ethical or moral problem. (4)

multidisciplinary action plan (MAP) — combination of a *critical pathway* and a *nursing care plan*; all healthcare providers follow the care MAP to facilitate expected outcomes. (14)

negligence — the omission to do something that a reasonable person, guided by the considerations that ordinarily regulate human affairs, would do; or doing something that a reasonable and prudent person would not do. (5)

network groups — colleagues who meet to discuss professional issues and pending legislation. (6)

network HMOs — the HMO contracts with multiple independent physician group practices. (10)

networking — forming coalitions and alliances. (13)

new performance budgeting — budgeting for specific outcomes and results. (10)

noncontrollable expenses — expenses that cannot be controlled or varied by a manager. (10)

nonmaleficence — ethical principle which states that if one cannot do good, then one should at least do no harm. (4)

normative–reeducative strategies — a group of change strategies that relies on group process to effect change by socializing and influencing people so change will occur. (8)

nursing process — theoretical system for solving problems and making decisions that includes the following steps: assess, diagnose, plan, implement, and evaluate. (1)

objectives — explicit, measurable, observable or retrievable, and obtainable measures that detail how and when goals are to be accomplished. (7)

operating budget — budgetary expenses that change in response to the volume of service. (10)

organization chart — vehicle that depicts the formal relationships, lines of communication, and authority within an organization. (12)

organizational climate — how employees perceive an organization. (12)

organizational culture — set of symbols and interactions that defines an organization's ways of thinking, behaving, and believing as well as its values, language, tradition, customs, and "sacred cows" that are absolute and not open to discussion or change. (12)

organizational ethics committees — multidisciplinary group formed to assist with problem solving regarding difficult or ambiguous value issues related to patient care or organizational activities. (4)

organizational structure — the way in which a group is formed, its lines of communication, and its means for channeling authority and making decisions. (12)

organizing — second phase of the management process; in this phase, relationships are defined, procedures are outlined, equipment is readied and tasks are assigned; also involves establishing a formal structure that provides the best possible coordination or use of resources to accomplish unit objectives. (2)

overgeneralizing — type of inaccurate thinking that occurs when one believes that because *A* has a particular characteristic, every other *A* also has the same characteristic; stereotypical thinking. (1)

paternalism — ethical principle that suggests that one person assumes the authority to make a decision for another; typically justified only to prevent a person from coming to harm. (4)

patient's bill of rights — statement of patient rights that is legally binding when backed by law or state regulations; not legally binding when issued by healthcare organizations and professional associations but should be considered professionally binding. (6)

Patient Self Determination Act (PSDA) — law enacted in 1991 requiring federally funded healthcare organizations to provide education for staff and patients on issues concerning treatment and end-of-life issues. (5)

per-diem employee — employees who generally have the flexibility to choose if and when they want to work. In exchange for this flexibility, they receive a higher rate of pay, but usually no benefits. (17)

personnel budget — budgeted expenses to cover the cost of personnel; includes actual worked time (also called productive time or salary expense) and time the organization pays the employee for not working (nonproductive or benefit time), such as cost of benefits, new employee orientation, employee turnover, sick and holiday time, and education time. (10)

philosophy — a statement of the values and beliefs that guide an organization; provides the basic foundation for directing all planning to achieve the mission. (7)

plaintiff — injured party in a lawsuit. (5)

planned change — change that results from a well thought-out and deliberate effort to make something happen. (8)

planning — first phase of the management process; a proactive and deliberate process that requires deciding in advance what to do, who is to do it, and how, when, and where it is to be done; involves choice. (2)

point-of-service (POS) plan — health insurance plan whereby a patient has the option, at the time of service, to select a provider outside the parent HMO network, but pays a higher premium as well as a copayment for the flexibility to do so. (10)

policies — plans reduced to statements or instructions that set boundaries for action taking and decision making. (7)

political action committees — groups that attempt to persuade legislators to vote in a particular way. (6)

politics — the art of using legitimate power wisely. (13)

polychronic style — preference for doing two or more activities or tasks simultaneously. (9)

power–coercive strategies — change strategies based on the application of power by legitimate authority, economic sanctions, or political clout of the change agent; these strategies include influencing the enactment of new laws and using group power for strikes or sit-ins. (8)

preactivisim — type of future-oriented planning in which technology is utilized to accelerate change. (7)

preceptor — an experienced person or colleague who provides knowledge and emotional support, as well as a clarification of role expectations on a one-to-one basis. (16)

preferred provider organization (PPO) — health insurance organization that renders services on a fee-for-service basis but provides financial incentives to consumers (they pay less if they seek care within the PPO). (10)

preponderance of evidence — burden of proof required to be found guilty in a civil case in which the judge or jury must believe that it was more likely than not, that the accused individual was responsible for the injuries of the complainant. (5)

*primary nursing (also called *relationship-based nursing)* — patient care delivery that requires a one-to-one relationship between a nurse and a patient; all nursing staff must be RNs, with the primary RN assuming 24-hour responsibility for planning the care of one or more patients from admission or the start of treatment to discharge or treatment end. (14)

privacy rules — portion of HIPPA directed at ensuring strong privacy protections for patient without threatening access to care. (5)

*proactive planning (also called *interactive planning)* — type of planning in which the past, present, and future are considered and attempts are focusing on planning the future rather than reacting to it. (7)

problem solving — systematic process that focuses on analyzing a difficult situation and includes a decision-making step; differs from decision making in that it requires problem identification. (1)

procedures — plans that establish customary or acceptable ways of accomplishing a specific task and delineate a sequence of steps of required action. (7)

procrastination — putting off an activity or decision until a future time, to postpone, or to delay needlessly. (9)

product liability — legal concept in which a provider is held responsible for injury caused by malfunctioning equipment, especially if she or he had prior knowledge of the equipment's defect. (5)

professional code of ethics — set of principles or basic beliefs, established by a profession, to guide the individual practitioner to achieve ethical practice. (4)

professional negligence — see *malpractice.*

queen bee syndrome — activities and behaviors used to keep others from power. (13)

rational–empirical strategies — change strategies that use current research as evidence to support the change; the strategy assumes that resistance to change comes from ignorance or superstition and that change will result from facts documenting the need for change. (8)

reasonable and prudent — the average judgment, foresight, intelligence, and skill that would be expected of a person with similar training and experience. (5)

recruitment — the process of actively seeking out or attracting applicants for existing positions. (15)

referent power — power obtained because of identification with a leader or with what that leader symbolizes. (13)

res judicata — legal doctrine meaning a "thing or matter settled by judgment"; this doctrine applies only when a competent court has decided a legal dispute and when no further appeals are possible. (5)

resocialization — the learning of new values, skills, attitudes, and social rules as a result of changes in roles, environment, workplace, responsibilities, and the like. (16)

respondeat superior **(also called** *vicarious liability)* — legal concept meaning "the master is responsible for the acts of his servants;" indicates that an employer should be held legally liable for the conduct of employees whose actions he or she has a right to direct or control. (5)

responsibility — a duty or an assignment. (12)

responsibility accounting — each category of an organization's revenues—expenses, assets, and liabilities—is someone's responsibility. (10)

restraining forces — forces that divert a system from change. (8)

reward power — ability to grant rewards to others. (13)

rights-based reasoning — ethical framework in which decisions are made based on the belief that some things are a person's just due, basic claim, or entitlement, with which there should be no interference. (4)

role model — someone worthy of imitation. (16)

rules — plans that define acceptable action or nonaction. (7)

sanctions — the bestowing of rewards and punishments. (16)

satisficing — term used to describe decisions that may not be ideal but result in solutions that are "good enough." (1)

scalar chain — the decision-making hierarchy or pyramid. (12)

servant leadership — type of leadership in which individuals lead by placing others, such as employees, customers, and the community, first. (3)

service line organization — similar to the matrix design; can be used in some large institutions to address the shortcomings that are epidemic to traditional large bureaucratic organizations. (12)

shared governance — egalitarian organizational governance shared among board members, committees, and management. (12)

short-term planning — operational planning that focuses on achieving specific tasks usually over a period of one hour to three years. (9)

situational or contingency leadership theory — belief that leaders must adapt their leadership style accordingly to the task to be accomplished, the needs of a given situation, and the maturity of the subordinates. (3)

socialization (**also called** *enculturation*) — process by which a person acquires the technical skills of his or her society, the knowledge of the kinds of behavior that are understood and acceptable in that society, and the attitudes and values that make conformity with social rules personally meaningful. (16)

span of control — number of people directly reporting to any one manager or officer. (12)

staff development — the indoctrination, training, and education of staff members. (16)

staff HMO — physician providers are salaried by the HMO and under direct control of the HMO. (10)

staffing — third phase of the management process; in this phase, the manager recruits, selects, orients, and promotes personnel development to accomplish the goals of the organization. (2)(15)

standard of care — the skills and learning commonly possessed by members of a profession; generally are the minimal requirements that define an acceptable level of care. (5)

stare decisis — legal doctrine meaning "to let the decision stand"; uses precedents as a guide for decision making. (5)

statutes — laws that govern; statutes are officially enacted (voted on and passed) by a legislative body and compiled into codes, collections of statutes, and ordinances. (5)

strategic plans — see *long range plans*. (7)

subordinate advocacy — situation in which managers assist subordinates to resolve problems and live with the solutions at the unit level. (6)

team nursing — ancillary personnel collaborate in providing care to a group of patients under the direction of a professional nurse, who is responsible for knowing the condition and needs of all the patients assigned to the team and for planning individual care. (14)

teleological theories — beliefs of ethical decision making that support decisions that favor the common good (utilitarian). (4)

time management — making optimal use of available time. (9)

torts — legal wrongs committed against a person or property, independent of a contract that renders the person who commits them liable for damages in a civil action. (5)

total patient care — nurses assume total responsibility for meeting all the needs of assigned patients during their time on duty; the oldest mode of organizing patient care. (14)

traditional problem-solving model — widely used, and perhaps best-known, problem-solving model which includes seven steps: identifying the problem, gathering data, exploring alternative solutions, evaluating alternatives, selecting the appropriate solution, implementing the solution, and evaluating the results. (1)

training — an organized method of ensuring that people have knowledge and skills for a specific purpose and that they have acquired the necessary knowledge to perform specific duties and activities. (16)

transactional leader — individual who leads by focusing on the day-to-day operations and management tasks of an organization. (3)

transformational leader — individual who leads by vision and has the ability to empower others with this vision. (3)

utilitarianism — ethical framework in which an individual makes decisions based on what provides the greatest good for the greatest number of people. (4)

utility — ethical principle stating that what is best for the common good outweighs what is best for the individual. (4)

values — beliefs that guide behavior. (7)

variable expenses — expenses that vary with volume (e.g., payroll). (10)

variance tracking — documentation of when and why a patient's care varies from the clinical pathway. (14)

veracity — ethical principle related to the need for truth telling or the acceptability of deception. (4)

vicarious liability — see *respondeat superior*. (5)

vision statement — statement outlining the future aim or function of an organization. (7)

whistleblowers — individuals who speak out about organizational practices they believe may be harmful or inappropriate. (6)

workers' compensation case management — case management directed at preventing worker injuries, when possible, and managing such injuries when they occur. (14)

workload measurement system — system that evaluates work performance as well as necessary resource levels; captures census data, care hours, patient acuity, and patient activities. (17)

workplace advocacy — ensuring that the work environment is both safe and conducive to professional and personal growth for subordinates. (6)

Index

Page numbers followed by letters *d, f,* and *t* indicate displays, figures, and tables, respectively.

NOTES

NOTES

NOTES

NOTES

NOTES

NOTES